second edition

EMBALMING

History, Theory, & Practice

Robert G. Mayer
Licensed Embalmer and Funeral Director
Pittsburgh, Pennsylvania

Adjunct Professor
Pittsburgh Institute of Mortuary Science
Pittsburgh, Pennsylvania

With a foreword by

Gordon S. Bigelow, PhD
Executive Director
American Board of Funeral Service Education

APPLETON & LANGE
Stamford, Connecticut

Copyright © 1996 by Appleton & Lange
A Simon & Schuster Company
Copyright © 1990 by Appleton & Lange

96 97 98 99 00 / 10 9 8 7 6 5 4 3 2 1

Prentice Hall International (UK) Limited, *London*
Prentice Hall of Australia Pty. Limited, *Sydney*
Prentice Hall Canada, Inc., *Toronto*
Prentice Hall Hispanoamericana, S.A., *Mexico*
Prentice Hall of India Private Limited, *New Delhi*
Prentice Hall of Japan, Inc., *Tokyo*
Simon & Schuster Asia Pte. Ltd., *Singapore*
Editora Prentice Hall do Brasil Ltda., *Rio de Janeiro*
Prentice Hall, *Upper Saddle River, New Jersey*

Library of Congress Cataloging-in-Publication Data

Mayer, Robert G.
    Embalming : history, theory, and practice / Robert G. Mayer ; with
a foreword by Gordon S. Bigelow. -- 2nd ed.
        p.   cm.
    Includes bibliographical references and index.
    ISBN 0-8385-1468-5 (case : alk. paper)
    1. Embalming.   I. Title.
    [DNLM: 1. Embalming.   WA 844 M469e 1996]
RA622.M39   1996
6149.6--dc20
DNLM/DLC
for Library of Congress   96–4861
                                                              CIP

Acquisitions Editor: Tracey Roth
Production Editor: Jennifer Sinsavich
Designer: Libby Schmitz
PRINTED IN THE UNITED STATES OF AMERICA

ISBN 0-8385-1468-5
9 780838 514689
90000

Editorial Consultants

George H. Poston, PhD
President
Commonwealth Institute of Funeral Service
Houston, Texas

Dale E. Stroud
Former Associate Professor
Mortuary Science Department
University of Minnesota
Minneapolis, Minnesota

*This book is dedicated
to all who teach and
to all who labor
in the practice of the art and science
of Embalming.*

Contributing Authors

These authors' contributions appear essentially unchanged.

James M. Dorn, MS
Chairman, Embalming Sciences
Cincinnati College of Mortuary Science
Cincinnati, Ohio

Jerome F. Fredrick, PhD
Director of Chemical Research
Dodge Chemical Company
Bronx, New York

Barbara M. Hopkins, PhD
Associate Professor and Chair
Chemistry Department
Xavier University
Cincinnati, Ohio

Edward C. Johnson
Funeral Director—Instructor of Embalming
Chicago, Illinois

Gail R. Johnson
Funeral Director—Instructor of Clinical Embalming
Chicago, Illinois

Robert G. Mayer
Licensed Embalmer and Funeral Director
Pittsburgh, Pennsylvania

Adjunct Professor
Pittsburgh Institute of Mortuary Science
Pittsburgh, Pennsylvania

Leandro Rendon, MS
Director of Research and Educational Programs
The Champion Company
Williamsburg, Virginia

Gordon Rose, PhD
Former Professor and Chairman
Mortuary Science Department
Wayne State University
Detroit, Michigan

Melissa J. Williams
Funeral Director
Chicago, Illinois

Contributors

John Alsobrooks, MS
Associate Professor, Funeral Service Program
Vincennes University Junior College
Vincennes, Indiana

James H. Bedino, BAS, BS
Director of Research
The Champion Company
Springfield, Ohio

R. Stanley Barnes
Funeral Director
Canton, Ohio

Brian A. Broznick
Executive Director
Pittsburgh Transplant Foundation
Pittsburgh, Pennsylvania

Daniel Buchanan, MA
President
Gupton-Jones College of Funeral Service
Decatur, Georgia

William Counce, PhD
Funeral Service Education Department
Jefferson State College
Birmingham, Alabama

Emmet Crahan
Dodge Chemical Company
Jay, New York

Kenneth Curl, PhD
Chairman
Funeral Service Education Department
University of Central Oklahoma
Edmond, Oklahoma

Donald E. Douthit, MS
Supervisor of Clinical Services
Cincinnati College of Mortuary Science
Cincinnati, Ohio

Dan Flory, PhD
President
Cincinnati College of Mortuary Science
Cincinnati, Ohio

Arthur Grabowski
Former Chairman
Mortuary Science Department
State University of New York College of Technology
Canton, New York

Marvin E. Grant, MEd
Former Chairman
Mortuary Science Department
East Mississippi Community College
Scooba, Mississippi

Ralph Klicker, MSEd
Director
Thanos Institute
Buffalo, New York

John Kroshus, PhD
Associate Professor and Chairman
Mortuary Science Department
University of Minnesota
Minneapolis, Minnesota

Daniel Lawlor
Embalmer and Funeral Director
Providence, Rhode Island

Terry McEnany, MA
Dean
Simmons Institute
Syracuse, New York

Stuart E. Moen, MA
Dean
Commonwealth Institute of Funeral Service
Houston, Texas

Frank P. Nagy, PhD
Associate Professor
Department of Anatomy
Wright State University Medical School
Dayton, Ohio

F. Jay Nation
Pittsburgh Institute of Mortuary Science
Pittsburgh, Pennsylvania

N. Thomas Rogness, MA
Former Instructor
Institute of Funeral Service
Houston, Texas

Shelly J. Roy
Funeral Director
York, Alabama

Donald W. Sawyer
Director of Embalming Education
Dodge Chemical Company
Castro Valley, California

Dale E. Stroud
Former Associate Professor
Mortuary Science Department
University of Minnesota
Minneapolis, Minnesota

Brenda L. Tersine, MA
Former Instructor
Mortuary Science Department
Hudson Valley Community College
Troy, New York

John R. Trout
Funeral Service Education Department
Northampton Area Community College
Bethlehem, Pennsylvania

Todd W. VanBeck, MA
Director
Education Programs
The Lorwen Group
Cincinnati, Ohio

Kenneth R. Whittaker
Dean of Students
Dallas Institute of Funeral Service
Dallas, Texas

Contents

Foreword xiii

Acknowledgments xv

Introduction .xvii

Part I. The Theory and Practice of Embalming .1

1. Fundamentals of Embalming: Legal Aspects, Methods, and Order of Embalming .3
2. Professional Performance Standards 27
3. Environment and Personal Health Considerations 37
4. Technical Orientation of Embalming 51
5. Death—Agonal and Preembalming Changes 85
6. Embalming Chemicals 109
7. Use of Embalming Chemicals 127
8. Anatomical Considerations 143
9. Embalming Vessel Sites and Selections 157
10. Embalming Analysis 179
11. Preparation of the Body Prior to Arterial Injection 191
12. Distribution and Diffusion of Arterial Solution 215
13. Injection and Drainage Techniques 235
14. Cavity Embalming 253
15. Preparation of the Body After Arterial Injection 269

16. Age and General Body Considerations . .285
17. Preparation of Autopsied Bodies 303
18. Preparation of Bodies of Organ Donors .319
19. Delayed Embalming 333
20. Discolorations 347
21. Moisture Considerations 369
22. Vascular Considerations 385
23. Effect of Drugs on the Embalming Process 393
24. Selected Conditions 403

Part II. The Origin and History of Embalming and History of Modern Restorative Art 419

Edward C. Johnson, Gail R. Johnson, and Melissa J. Williams

Part III. Glossary 479

Prepared by the Embalming Course Content Committee of the American Board of Funeral Service Education

Part IV. Selected Readings 495

The Mathematics of Embalming Chemistry: Part I. A Critical Evaluation of "One-Bottle" Embalming Chemical Claims 497

Final Report on Literature Search on the Infectious Nature of Dead Bodies for the Embalming Chemical Manufacturers Association, September 1, 1968 499

Multiple Death Disaster Response Handbook .502

Occupational Exposure to Formaldehyde in Mortuaries .507

Formaldehyde Vapor Emission Study in
    Embalming Rooms .... .511
Reported Studies on Effects of Formaldehyde
    Exposure .... .512
Dangers of Infection .... .514
In-Use Evaluation of Glutaraldehyde as a
    Preservative–Disinfectant in
    Embalming .... .516
The Antimicrobial Activity of Embalming
    Chemicals and Topical Disinfectants on the
    Microbial Flora of Human Remains ..... .519

The Microbiologic Evaluation and Enumeration
    of Postmortem Specimens from Human
    Remains .... .522
Recommendations for Prevention of HIV
    Transmission in Health-Care Settings ..... .525
CDCs Universal Precautions in the Context of
    Medical Waste Management .... .532
Can Magnesium Sulfate Be Safely Used to Rid the
    Body of Fluid in the Lower Extremities? ...534

Index .... .537

Foreword

"You must express your grief at the death of a loved one, and then you must go on. The eyes of the dead must be gently closed and the eyes of the living must be gently opened."

Jan Brugler, 1973

This book has come to be viewed as the most up-to-date and complete text/reference work on embalming in existence. Since its 1990 introduction, it has gone through two printings, and thousands of copies have been purchased by libraries, funeral service education academic departments in colleges and universities, and funeral homes as a ready reference guide for preparation room personnel, both in the United States and abroad. Now, after five years of use, the second edition of the book is presented to the reader. This new edition incorporates the best of the first edition and adds material which reflects changes to the field of embalming during the interim period.

The original work was the result of joint efforts of the American Board of Funeral Service Education and the National Funeral Directors Association. Work on the book began in 1984, stimulated by Glenn McMillen, the President of the NFDA, and David Fitzsimmons, then President of the Cincinnati College of Mortuary Science. Through their efforts, funding was identified and Dr. Frank Nagy of Wright State University School of Medicine, was selected as first draft editor. The book eventually incorporated ideas and text from over three dozen funeral service educators, practitioners, and suppliers. The primary author, Robert Mayer, utilized these many inputs during his writing of the final draft. His final work, the first edition, was the result of the review of literally thousands of pages of articles and monographs on embalming. A distinguished funeral service educator at the Pittsburgh Institute of Mortuary Science, Mr. Mayer devoted much of two years of his busy life to bring the first edition of the book to its successful conclusion. He has devoted the same energy and time to ensuring that the second edition is as good as, and in many areas, an improvement over the first edition. Mr. Mayer insists on high quality in all he does and the second edition of this book is an excellent example of this trait. He approaches his professional and personal life with enthusiasm, energy and humor. We are fortunate to have been able to enlist his skills.

The process undertaken for the second edition was extensive. It began in 1994 when the author joined eight other instructors at an embalming teaching course rewriting workshop in Denver, Colorado. Shortly thereafter, Robert Mayer selected a small editorial team consisting of Professor Dale Stroud, then at the University of Minnesota, and Dr. George Poston, President of the Commonwealth Institute of Funeral Service, Houston, Texas. Together they read and discussed each individual page of the first edition, noting areas in which changes were either necessary or desirable. All teaching programs in Funeral Service Education were solicited for their comments. Mr. Mayer took the results of this review and planned the second edition. Several chapters were extensively rewritten, while others remain essentially intact from the former book. Illustrations have been widely updated. The second edition review and rewriting work extended over much of 1995 and produced a completely reviewed, accurate, and timely new work. *Embalming: History, Theory and Practice*, second edition, is the result and is presented with pride by the author and with enthusiastic endorsement by the American Board of Funeral Service Education.

The foreword statement from the first edition is equally true for the Second Edition:

"This book covers embalming as no other book ever has. It is useful as a teaching text and, in that regard, follows the American Board of Funeral Service Education curriculum guide on this subject. It is also useful as an historical or technical reference for the funeral service practitioner or the lay reader."

Gordon S. Bigelow, PhD
Executive Director
American Board of Funeral Service Education
March, 1996

Acknowledgments

In July of 1994 in Denver, Colorado, the American Board of Funeral Service Education held an Embalming Curriculum Review conference. The purpose of the two day meeting was to establish, for the first time, an Embalming Glossary of Terms which would be appended to the basic course content in embalming. The workshop activities were overseen by James Augustine of the Milwaukee Area Technical College serving as the Curriculum Chair. The Embalming Committee was chaired by Dale Stroud from the University of Minnesota and co-chaired by Dr. George Poston, then of Southern Illinois University. Eleven educators formed the committee. Because of the broad scope of a glossary almost every division of the embalming curriculum was discussed. The discussions were often in great depth—this form of open idea exchange brought to light many obsolete areas of the syllabus. In addition, the discussion introduced new concepts that needed to be added to the curriculum. It truly was a rare opportunity for all involved in the teaching of embalming who participated. Not only was a glossary established at these two days of meetings but the foundation was also laid for this second edition of *Embalming: History, Theory, and Practice.* I would like to thank those committee members who were present for these discussions: John Chew, Lynn University; William Counce, Jefferson State University; James Dorn, Cincinnati College; Marcus Gray, American Academy–McAllister Institute; Tim Kowalski, Worsham College; Doug Metz, Cypress College; George Poston, now with Commonwealth College; Byron Stout, Cypress College; Dale Stroud, University of Minnesota; and Ken Whittaker, Dallas Institute.

In January 1995, Dale Stroud, George Poston, and I met in Houston to outline the changes reflected in this edition. George Poston later had the monumental task of editing this edition. Dale Stroud has reviewed the photography and the glossary in this edition.

I am grateful for the services of James H. Bedino, Director of Research for the Champion Chemical Company, who has reviewed the chemistry chapters of this edition. Through the help of Robert W. Ninker of the Illinois Funeral Directors Association and George Fulton an ethical discussion has been introduced into the first chapter. Review of the OSHA and FTC sections of Chapter 1 has been done by NFDA General Counsel Scott Gilligan and NFDA OSHA Counsel Edward Ranier. James Dorn and Barbara Hopkins of Cincinnati have made a contribution in Chapter 23 on the preparation of bodies involved with radioactive isotopes. Linda F. Harris of Sunnyvale, California, has redrawn all of the line illustrations. Finally I am most grateful to Edward C. Johnson, his wife Gail R. Johnson, and daughter Melissa Williams for their new section titled "The History of Modern Restorative Art."

I am grateful to all who have made contributions to this edition and certainly to the first edition of this text. Their names appear in the contributors section. The National Funeral Directors Association and the American Board of Funeral Service Education have given not only time to this text but much needed monies. Dr. Gordon Bigelow of the American Board of Funeral Service Education has faithfully overseen this project from its inception. I am most grateful to him for his patience and guidance.

Robert G. Mayer
Pittsburgh, Pennsylvania
March, 1996

Introduction

The second edition of the text *Embalming: History, Theory, and Practice* is designed as a basic texbook for the student of mortuary science and as a reference text for the practitioner. Incorporated into the text is the *Basic Course Content Curriculum and Glossary* used by all colleges of mortuary science throughout the United States. The basic course content curriculum has been developed, reviewed, and updated by a committee of the American Board of Funeral Service Education. The text seeks to go beyond the basic course curriculum and attempts to approach the subject of embalming from the practical view as well as from the theoretical.

The early chapters of this book give a background of the environment in which the preparation of the body occurs. These chapters also elaborate on the chemicals used to prepare the body, review the anatomical sites used for arterial fluid injection, and explain the various methods of arterial injection and drainage as well as the physical and chemical means by which embalming fluid comes into contact with the body proteins to preserve and sanitize the dead human remains.

The primary thrust of this writing is to design the embalming techniques and treatments based on the conditions which the embalmer can observe—not so much on a particular cause of death or a drug medication that may have been administered during life. The cause of death and drug treatments are generally not known by the embalmer at the time the body is prepared.

In the past 30 years the type and nature of the dead human body have changed. The widespread use of drugs, chemotherapy, and transplantation of organs has allowed persons to live much longer lives. The result is that disease processes continue in the body for weeks, months, and even years longer than they would have done years ago. The embalmer sees more and more bodies with advanced arteriosclerosis, edema, emaciation, jaundice, and secondary infections. The many strains of bacteria and viruses that have become drug resistant has brought about a greater need for the embalmer to take extraordinary precautions in the handling and embalming of dead human bodies.

More and more bodies are being prepared after full or partial autopsy. In addition, the donation of tissue after death has increased and will continue to do so. Two chapters are devoted to the problems created by these postmortem activities.

The later chapters of the text deal with the specific conditions generally found in the dead human body that have the most significant influence on the type of embalming treatment used. The chapter on "Embalming Analysis" helps the embalmer to acquire a clearer picture of the five or six basic treatments in most embalming routines (based upon the conditions present in the body at the time of the preparation).

Every attempt has been made to adhere as closely as possible to the guidelines established in the course content outlines approved in October, 1995 by the American Board of Funeral Service Education. The order of this book is optional for the instructor, and individual instructors are encouraged to teach this subject in the progression they find most suitable for their programs of instruction.

An attempt has been made to make each chapter a complete entity. For this reason, a number of topics are repeated. This saves the student or practitioner the time of having to reference items discussed in various chapters.

As there are, no doubt, more than 100 companies (large and small) that manufacture embalming chemicals, discussion regarding the use of arterial chemicals is very general. It is important to remember that most fluid companies make 10 or more arterial fluids. It is most difficult to be specific when there is such a large variety of arterial embalming chemicals from which to choose.

As this text is being published new formaldehyde- and phenol-free embalming chemicals are being developed. If proved to be successful, we will no doubt see a radical change in the chemicals and their use which we employ in arterial embalming. This change should be as radical as the introduction of formaldehyde as an embalming agent was in 1895! Throughout this text we have recommended the use of restricted cervical injection in the preparation of the unautopsied body. We have through practical experience found that this technique best suits the needs for the most successful preparation of almost all unautopsied bodies. You will find this technique repeated throughout the text.

A new addition to this edition is the "History of Modern Restorative Art." The subjects of embalming and restorative art are quite interdependent. Nowhere else is the history of the subject of restorative art presented in any greater detail than in this essay on the subject presented in this text. Together these two histories trace the development of the art and science of embalming in the United States from its inception to its present status.

Finally, a large selection of detailed studies are presented for an in-depth look into some of the current embalming problems. These articles focus on handling the dead body from both communicable and infectious diseases. Emphasis is also placed on recent environmental studies that will assist the embalmer in recognizing the environmental health hazards that exist in handling embalming chemicals and preservative powders.

Whether the reader of this book is a student or a long-time practitioner, it is agreed that "we can all do a little better work." It is hoped that this writing will help the embalmer to better understand and overcome many of the complex problems that today's practitioner faces.

second edition

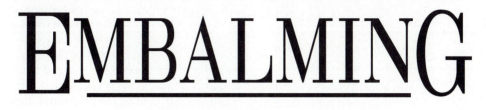

EMBALMING

History, Theory, & Practice

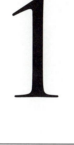

part

The Theory and Practice of Embalming

1

Fundamentals of Embalming: Legal Aspects, Methods, and Order of Embalming

Embalming is governed principally by the legislature of the individual states. Two principal bodies may have control of the care and disposition of dead human remains. These two legislative groups are a Board of Health (or Bureau of Vital Records) and the governing body that controls funeral directing and embalming in many states—a State Board of Embalmers and Funeral Directors. These two groups promulgate and enforce statutory law as well as rules and regulations governing the disposition of dead human bodies.

Permission to embalm should be obtained from those with the right and duty of disposal. Permission may be obtained orally in most states, with the actual consent form signed later during the arrangement conference.

In recent years two federal agencies have come to play a very important role in the activities of the funeral home preparation room. The Federal Trade Commission (FTC) has established regulations that (1) require the funeral director to fully explain, to a party making funeral arrangements, the necessity and purpose of embalming (or allowing them the choice not to have the body embalmed), (2) provide for the proper permission for the embalming to be secured, and (3) require a full disclosure of all costs and charges for goods and services performed in the transportation, handling, and preparation of the body. A second federal agency is the Occupational Safety and Health Administration (OSHA), which has set standards governing the safety of workers in the work areas of the funeral home and safety in working with hazardous chemicals. Also, the standards provide for proper protection for employees working with and disposing of bloodborne pathogenic and other infectious wastes. In addition, many states have agencies related to these federal departments, such as the State Department of Environmental Protection. These agencies promulgate regulations and standards often more demanding than the federal governing bodies. The embalmer must be current on standards required by both of these state and federal governing bodies.

FEDERAL TRADE COMMISSION

In April 1984, the federal government through the FTC promulgated a rule governing the activities of funeral directors and embalmers. The rule, which is commonly referred to as the Funeral Rule, was amended by the FTC in 1994. It is most important that all embalmers be fully aware of the statutes and rules and regulations of the state in which they are practicing. These rules differ from state to state, but the Funeral Rule applies to ALL states. For this reason the following excerpts are reprinted from the *Federal Register:*

3

Misrepresentations

Embalming Provisions—Deceptive Acts or Practices. In selling or offering to sell funeral goods or funeral services to the public, it is a deceptive act or practice for a funeral provider to:

1. Represent that state or local law requires that a deceased person be embalmed when such is not the case
2. Fail to disclose that embalming is not required by law except in certain special cases

Preventive Requirements. To prevent these deceptive acts or practices as well as the unfair or deceptive acts or practices defined in §453.4(b) (1) and §453.5 (2) [of the Funeral Rule], funeral providers must:

1. Not represent that a deceased person is required to be embalmed for:
   A. Direct cremation;
   B. Immediate burial; or
   C. A closed casket funeral without viewing or visitation when refrigeration is available and when state or local law does not require embalming; and
2. Place the following disclosure on the general price list, required by §453.2 (b) (4) in immediate conjunction with the price shown for embalming: "Except in certain special cases, embalming is not required by law. Embalming may be necessary, however, if you select certain funeral arrangements, such as a funeral with viewing. If you do not want embalming, you usually have the right to choose an arrangement that does not require you to pay for it, such as direct cremation or immediate burial." The phrase "except in certain special cases" need not be included in this disclosure if state or local laws in the area(s) where the provider does business do not require embalming under any circumstances.

Services Provided Without Prior Approval

Unfair or Deceptive Acts or Practices. In selling or offering to sell funeral goods or funeral services to the public, it is an unfair or deceptive act or practice for any provider to embalm a deceased body for a fee unless:

1. State or local law or regulation requires embalming in the particular circumstances regardless of any funeral choice which the family might make; or
2. Prior approval for embalming (expressly so described) from a family member or other authorized person; or
3. The funeral provider is unable to contact a family member or other authorized person after exercising due diligence, has no reason to believe the family does not want embalming performed, and obtains subsequent approval for embalming already performed (expressly so described). In seeking approval, the funeral provider must disclose that a fee will be charged if the family selects a funeral which requires embalming, such as a fu-

neral with viewing, and that no fee will be charged if the family selects a service which does not require embalming, such as direct cremation or immediate burial.

Preventive Requirement. To prevent these unfair or deceptive acts or practices, funeral providers must include on the itemized statement of funeral goods and services selected, required by §453.2 (b) (5), the statement: "If you selected a funeral that may require embalming, such as a funeral with viewing, you may have to pay for embalming. You do not have to pay for embalming you did not approve if you selected arrangements such as direct cremation or immediate burial. If we charge for embalming, we will explain why below.*"

OSHA HAZARD COMMUNICATION STANDARD

The Occupational Safety and Health Administration requires employers to communicate to their employees information regarding hazardous chemicals to which they are exposed in the workplace. This Hazard Communication Standard applies to every employer regardless of size as of May 23, 1988. The hazard communication rule requires chemical manufacturers and distributors to supply purchasers of hazardous chemicals with specific information regarding such hazards by labels on containers and material safety data sheets (generally designated by MSDSs) which must accompany the first shipment of a hazardous chemical. The manufacturer is responsible for identifying which chemicals are hazardous and describing such hazards by labels and MSDSs.

Summary of the Standard

Every employer, regardless of size, is required to comply with OSHA's revised rule. In summary, the rule requires employers to institute a hazard communication program, provide affected employees with certain training regarding hazardous chemicals, and establish a file of MSDSs for hazardous chemicals used in the workplace.

The hazard communication program that must be established by employers sets forth the employer's commitment to compliance with the law and identifies the company officer with overall responsibility. A company officer should be assigned for overall compliance with the standard. This is an advisory action rather than a mandate. This individual will have the responsibility for the oversight of the initial and ongoing activities that have to be undertaken to comply with the rule. The program also sets forth information on labeling in-plant containers, MSDSs, and employee training.

---

*Review and update provided by Scott Gilligan, Esq., National Funeral Directors Association General Counsel.

Employee training is required for employees exposed to hazardous chemicals and should include a written checklist of procedures for handling hazardous chemicals under routine situations, procedures for emergencies such as spills, the measures employees are expected to take to protect themselves from exposure to hazards, explanation of labels and MSDSs, and the location and availability of the MSDSs. In addition, a funeral director's training program will necessarily conform to the training requirements of OSHA's recently promulgated standard on formaldehyde.

Material Safety Data Sheets

The keystone of the Hazard Communication Standard is the MSDS provided for each hazardous chemical used in the workplace. Employees who are exposed to hazardous chemicals must know the location of the company MSDS file and such employees must always have immediate access to such file. In emergencies such access may be crucial.

The MSDS sets forth the chemical name of the substance; physical and chemical characteristics such as the flash point; physical hazards including the potential for fire, explosion, and reactivity; and health hazards including symptoms of exposure and medical conditions recognized as being aggravated by exposure. The MSDS sets forth precautions for safe handling and emergency and first aid procedures.

The chemical manufacturer or distributor must send an MSDS with the first shipment of a hazardous chemical; however, funeral directors may have received an MSDS with previous shipments prior to their coverage by the OSHA rule. In the event the director does not receive an MSDS, it is his or her responsibility to contact the supplier to obtain one.

Environmental Protection Agency Regulations

Ninety days after the effective date of coverage by the OSHA Hazard Communication Standard, newly covered employers will be subject to the Environmental Protection Agency (EPA) Community Right-to-Know Rule. Failure to comply with this rule could subject an employer to a $25,000 fine. Under the EPA rule every company that stores 10,000 pounds of a hazardous chemical or 500 pounds of any chemical designated by the EPA as "extremely hazardous" must file an MSDS with its state emergency response commission and local emergency planning committee and local fire department.

(Formaldehyde is a chemical listed on the EPA list of extremely hazardous substances.) By March 1 of the first year after newly covered employers become subject to the EPA rule, any employer who stores 10,000 pounds of any hazardous chemical or 500 pounds of extremely hazardous chemical must file more detailed reports

(called Tier I reports) with the state and local agencies and fire department. Employers who store chemicals in the designated amounts will be required to file such Tier I reports annually thereafter. Two years and three months after an employer becomes covered by the EPA regulations, employers who store smaller amounts of hazardous chemicals will be required to file MSDSs and by March 1 of the third year of coverage, such employers must file Tier I reports with the appropriate agencies. Although the current regulations provide that the employers on those dates will be required to file reports for hazardous chemicals stored in *any* amount, the EPA has indicated that it will study the effect of the regulations and will at some future date set specific final stage threshold amounts for reporting. The actual dates on which the funeral directors who store the designated amounts of hazardous or extremely hazardous chemicals must file MSDSs and Tier I reports cannot be stated definitely at this time since all reporting dates are based on the effective date of the coverage of the OSHA hazard communications rule.

Penalties for Noncompliance with OSHA Rule

Compliance with OSHA regulations is most important, as failure to comply can result in costly penalties and time-consuming hearings and other administrative procedures. Compliance should ensure that employees of funeral homes will be provided with maximum safety in the workplace. Many of the communication and safety procedures are designed to alert employees to health hazards resulting from unsafe work practices. Consequently, the long-range benefits of compliance with the OSHA rules go beyond simple avoidance of legal penalties. Many of the health hazards that are set forth on the MSDS are conditions that could manifest themselves in future years. Failure to comply with the OSHA Hazard Communication Standard could result in an alleged exposure and injury by an employee subjecting a funeral director to a workers' compensation claim. This is because each of the 50 states has a workers' compensation law for claims resulting from on-the-job injuries or illnesses that bars employees from filing a lawsuit against their employer. The only exception to this, in some states, is when there is a *deliberate* intent to injure an employee by the employer. Where this exception exists, it is usually narrowly interpreted against the employee, thereby limiting the employee's remedy to a compensation claim for most employment-related injuries or illnesses.

REQUIREMENTS OF THE STANDARD

As of May 23, 1988, all employers must be in compliance with all provisions of the Hazard Communication

Standard. There are four basic elements within the standard:

1. Acquisition and maintenance of MSDSs
2. Maintenance of proper container labeling
3. Employee information and training
4. A comprehensive written program in which you describe how the objectives listed above will be met

The standard covers all employees exposed to work site chemicals. "Exposure" includes any contact on a routine basis, or the chance for contact in a foreseeable emergency. Employees exposed in isolated, nonroutine instances may not be considered to be covered by the standard; however, an MSDS should be available for any hazardous or toxic chemical in the employee work area, including for "potential" exposure.

The standard covers all chemicals that expose employees to a health or physical hazard. With respect to a mixture, a material is covered if it contains 1% or more of hazardous ingredient (0.1% for carcinogens, teratogens, or mutogens). The Funeral Service Database provides a list of the most commonly found chemicals used in funeral service, and can be helpful in identifying those products for which you must obtain a MSDS. It is included as an integral part of this compliance manual.

As a general rule, however, check the product label. *If there is any type of precautionary statement on the label, request the MSDS.* Materials labeled without a precautionary statement can be assumed to be exempt.

Summary Statement

The Hazard Communication Standard is a requirement of the Federal Department of Labor and OSHA. It took effect May 23, 1988. The following is a summary of how you can fulfill your obligations as an employer:

1. Acquire a three-ring binder. Label it MSDSs or Hazard Communication Standard.
2. Prepare a list of the hazardous and toxic substances found on the job site. Place this in the binder along with the MSDSs.
3. Obtain MSDSs from each supplier whose product you use. A copy of the MSDS has been included in shipments of products containing hazardous substances. Be sure you have all MSDSs for materials used by your employees.
4. Arrange the MSDSs in alphabetical order, by product name, three-hole punch them, and insert them on the left-hand side of your three-ring binder.
5. Conduct your own inspection of the preparation room to ensure that all containers carry the appropriate hazard warnings. Allow no product to remain that is not identified.

6. Determine where the three-ring binder will be located in your funeral home. If you have branch operations, each workplace must have a similar manual.
7. Gather your employees who have any contact with the chemicals for a training session. Explain the Hazard Communication Standard to them. Acknowledge that you and your firm are interested in providing a safe work environment.
8. Tell your employees where the binder, MSDSs, and training program will always be maintained so they can readily find it in the preparation room. Identify a person, you or an employee, who will be responsible for keeping the manual up to date. Be sure your staff knows who is responsible for the manual.
9. Outline for your employees emergency procedures in the event there is a spill or other exposure they sustain to hazardous substances.
10. Follow the training program and communicate to your employees methods of detecting the presence of a hazardous chemical, explain the dangers of those chemicals you use, outline safety precautions to protect employees, and give them details of the hazard communication program including an explanation of the labeling system, the MSDSs, and how employees can obtain the appropriate hazard information.
11. Ask employees for any questions and answer or obtain answers to their inquiries.
12. Be certain to review the Hazard Communication Standard with any employee you hire in the future who has a need to know.
13. Encourage employees and take the initiative to make the work area as safe as you can.

MATERIAL SAFETY DATA SHEETS

It is the supplier's obligation to provide, and the employer's obligation to acquire, an MSDS on each hazardous work site chemical covered by the law. The MSDS provides the health and safety information required to formulate your comprehensive written program and employee training program. The MSDS provides information on manufacturer identity, hazardous ingredients, health and physical hazards, employee protection, spill and leak detection and cleanup, and proper disposal technique. Most are published on OSHA Form 174; however, this is not required as long as all the information is contained within the alternate form.

The employer must keep a collection of MSDSs for the chemicals found within each work area. This collection and accompanying alphabetical index must be kept readily accessible to the employees in the work area.

In addition to the alphabetical index of the MSDSs kept with each collection, a master MSDS list must be included in your written program. The master list may be segregated by work area or comprehensive for the facility. The written program must also include a description of how your facility will meet the requirements to acquire and maintain the MSDSs for all regulated materials on the work site.

SAMPLE MSDS PROGRAM

1. Name of person responsible for acquisition of MSDSs and a brief description of duties.

   Sally Able, purchasing agent, is responsible for requesting MSDSs on all purchases of hazardous materials. Sally requests the MSDS unless she knows, from checking the master list, that the MSDS has been previously required. If any employee finds a particular MSDS is missing for a product, Sally is notified immediately, and she requests the MSDS from the purchaser.

2. Name(s) of person(s) responsible for maintenance of MSDSs in each work area.
   _____Rod Jones_____ supervisor, embalming area
   _____Ruth Jones_____ supervisor, janitorial staff
3. Location and availability of MSDSs for each work area.

   MSDSs are available for inspection during each employee break, before and after each work shift, and at any time in the case of an emergency. The collection of MSDSs is kept in each work area supervisor's work desk.

Container Labeling

All containers of hazardous materials must be marked with the name of the product as it appears on the MSDS and "appropriate" hazard warnings. The purpose of the label is to provide immediate "at-a-glance" information to the user.

As a general rule, end users of chemicals are not required to relabel containers, unless the original label becomes defaced. If you transfer a material into a new container, you must label it. The one exemption to this requirement is for a container intended for immediate employee use. These containers do not require a label. The exemption applies only when the portable container is for the immediate use of the employee who performs the transfer.

Some employers also use alternate labeling programs. If you do use one of these alternate programs, you

need to include a description of the program in your written plan.

The employer may use tags, tickets, or placards if conventional labeling is inappropriate. Labels must be in English, and other languages may be added.

SAMPLE LABEL PROGRAM

1. Label program description
   [] reliance on manufacturers' labels
   [] alternate program (name of program)
   Note: If you use an alternate program, attach a description of it to this work sheet.
2. Name of person responsible for ensuring proper labels on incoming containers and a brief description of duties.
   Joe Able, receiving clerk, checks all incoming shipments for a proper label. Any materials without proper labels are segregated in the receiving area. He notifies Sally Able immediately, who requests a label from the supplier.
3. Name(s) of person(s) responsible for maintenance of proper labeling in each work area.
   _____Rod Jones_____, supervisor embalming area
   _____Ruth Jones_____, supervisor janitorial staff
   Each work area supervisor is responsible for proper container labeling in their work areas.

INTRODUCTION TO THE HAZARD COMMUNICATION STANDARD

Employee Training Program

I. Explain the Standard.
   A. In recent years, many states have enacted right-to-know laws. In brief, these laws simply gave employees or workers the right to know of any potentially hazardous materials that might be in the workplace, precautions to be exercised in handling such materials, permissible exposure limit for those materials, and proper first aid in the event of accidental overexposure.
   B. More recently, OSHA, a division of the U.S. Department of Labor, has issued a Hazard Communication Standard, which preempts all state right-to-know laws. (The reader should be directed to check for additional requirements if the funeral home is located in a state that operates its own OSHA enforcement program.) In summary, the Standard requires that chemical manufacturers evaluate potential hazards in their products and

communicate those hazards to employers, and that the employer must *communicate* those hazards to all employees who might have exposure to those hazards. The last point is the purpose of this training program.

II. All Containers in the Preparation Room Must Be Labeled.

  A. Show and review and familiarize employee(s) with labels bearing hazard warnings.

  B. Instruct employees that there should be no *un*labeled containers in the workplace; that they are not to place or store anything in unlabeled containers; and that they are not to use anything from an unlabeled container, unless the contents have been satisfactorily and adequately identified and any hazard is fully understood.

III. Show and Explain MSDS Form.

  A. Explain that the warning label on a package is only a *warning. Full* disclosure of the hazards, precautions to be taken in handling the material, and first aid treatments will be found on the MSDS for that product. Most warning labels will include the words, "See MSDS."

  B. Review a typical MSDS with the employee(s), line by line, pointing out hazardous components, the nature of the hazard, the permissible exposure limit (PEL), protective equipment recommended, and first aid measures.

  C. Define: carcinogen, corrosive, irritants, highly toxic, toxic, sensitizer, and target organ effects. Be certain employee understands terms used in preparing MSDSs.

IV. Designate Place Where MSDSs Will Be Kept.

  A. Show employee where MSDSs will be kept in the preparation room. (Preferably in a loose leaf binder, so marked as to be easily identified. The designated place should be one that is easily accessible to all workers—and conspicuous. If it is kept in a cabinet or drawer, it should be one that is opened regularly and frequently.)

  B. Instruct employee that the MSDS binder is not to be removed from the premises. Whenever used, it *must* be returned to the designated, permanent location.

  C. While a manufacturer must supply an MSDS on request, it is the employer's responsibility to request an MSDS for any hazardous material in the workplace for which an MSDS is not presently on hand. If an employee has authority to order supplies, she or

he should be instructed to be certain that an MSDS for any hazardous material ordered is on hand or should request one promptly. Further, if any employee should discover that an MSDS for any hazardous substance has not been received, or lost, or for whatever reason is not in the binder, she or he will immediately notify the employer in order that it may be requested (in writing and copy saved) from the supplier of the product.

V. Explain Safe Handling of Hazardous Materials We Use.

  A. When working with a hazardous substance or pouring such material on when there is any risk of spilling or splashing on the hands, rubber gloves will be worn; pouring will be done carefully to avoid splashing.

  B. Whenever injection chemicals are in an embalming machine, whether in use or not, the cover will be kept on the reservoir (tank). All bottle caps will be replaced promptly after use.

  C. *When hazardous materials are being used in the preparation room, the ventilation or exhaust system will be in operation.*

  D. Containers of hazardous substances will not be handled with wet hands or gloves, which could cause the container to slip from one's hands and cause an accidental spill.

VI. Explain National Institute for Occupational Safety and Health (NIOSH)-Approved Respirator and Dust Mask and Fit Masks. Label Mask for Each Person Who Works in Preparation Room.

  A. New masks must be fitted and adjusted to the individual employee when they are received not when they are needed. Masks will have a designated storage space, where the mask will be readily accessible in the event that it is needed, and where the mask will be kept clean and ready for use at all times.

VII. Explain Method of Cleaning Up Spills.

  A. Regardless of how small the spill, it should be cleaned up promptly, and the exhaust system should be turned up to maximum capacity. If it is an ounce or two of arterial or cavity fluid, it may be wiped up with a cloth or other absorbent material. The cloth should then be rinsed under running water or in 2 gallons of water in a sink or pail to dilute the material. Rubber gloves must be worn in doing this cleanup.

  B. If the spill of liquid is of a greater amount, turn exhaust system to maximum, wear gloves, goggles, and a respirator. Cover the spill with absorbent material. If the spill contains formaldehyde, spray it with a small amount of household ammonia to neutralize the formaldehyde. When liquid is absorbed, place it in an open container and remove it to a well-ventilated area, preferably outside, for the liquid to evaporate. Place in a plastic bag and dispose of it in accordance with applicable regulations.

  C. If the spill is a powder, avoid breathing fumes or dust. Eliminate ignition sources. Sweep up and put in disposable container. Cover container. Pick up any remaining film with a wet mop. Dry in a well ventilated area.

  D. *Caution:* If the spill or situation causes you dizziness or discomfort, exit the preparation room to recover before attempting to complete the clean up.

VIII. Ask Employee for Any Questions He or She Might Have.

  A. Ask trainees if they have any questions about any of the several areas covered. Explain that you will get answers from the manufacturers or the appropriate government agency if you don't have them. Again, remind employees where the MSDSs are kept. Assure them that they are there for their reference. Also explain that the company's written Hazard Communication Program is kept in a file in the office and is available for them to read at any time. Finally, assure employees that the company is not only concerned with complying with the law, but also its desire to maintain a safe and comfortable working environment.

IX. Ask Employee to Sign Form Indicating He or She Has Received the Employee Training.

  A. To comply with the OSHA Hazard Communication Standard, it is essential that we be able to prove that we have provided this training to all employees who are exposed to hazardous substances. So, I will ask you to sign this form.

NONROUTINE TASKS TRAINING

The Hazard Communication Standard requires employers to include a description of the method used to train employees about nonroutine hazards in their written plan. This description should include the method by which the training is given, such as classroom instruction, monthly safety meetings, or personalized instruction. A description of the training materials, such as MSDSs and reference documents, should be included.

SAMPLE NONROUTINE HAZARDS TRAINING PROGRAM

1. Name of person responsible for training employees on the hazards of nonroutine tasks. John Able, Owner
2. Description of the training method:
   Nonroutine tasks will be discussed in the monthly employee meeting. If the task must be performed before the next scheduled monthly meeting, John will give personal training to the employee. John will review the following:
   > If an MSDS is available, it will be reviewed for any nonroutine chemical being used.
   > The product label will be reviewed.
   > Personal protective gear will be discussed.
   > The step-by-step directions will be studied.
   > Emergency procedures will be reviewed.

COMPREHENSIVE WRITTEN HAZARD COMMUNICATION PROGRAM

Each employer is required to develop and maintain a comprehensive written program that describes how the requirements of the standard will be met. For most employers, the following criteria must be addressed in the written program:

1. Acquisition and maintenance of MSDSs
2. Proper container labeling
3. Employee information and training
4. A list of MSDSs, either segregated by work area or comprehensive for the facility
5. Employee training about the hazards of nonroutine tasks

The employer is required to maintain one copy of the written program in a central location. The written program must be made readily accessible for employee inspection. If your facility is inspected by a federal OSHA representative, you will be asked to produce this document for review by the inspector.

FUNERAL SERVICE DATABASE

The following three examples represent chemicals commonly used in the preparation room. A complete list of hazardous chemicals may be obtained by contacting the National Funeral Directors Association for its publication, *Hazard Communication Program.** Hazardous chemicals may be obtained from the MSDSs. It is important to understand that the severity of the health effects listed for the chemicals will depend on the amount

---

*National Funeral Directors Association, 11121 West Oklahoma Ave, Milwaukee, WI, 53227.

of material in the product, the frequency and duration of your exposure, and your individual susceptibility.

Examples: Hazardous Chemicals

Acetone (Dimethyl Ketone)
Health Effects:
A narcotic in high concentrations that can cause skin irritation from defatting of tissue. Prolonged inhalation can cause headache, dryness, throat irritation. A dangerous fire risk when exposed to heat, flame, or oxidizers.
Found in:
    accessory embalming chemicals
    external sealing composition
    lip tint
    solvents
    sealants
        OSHA PEL:1000 ppm[†]
        ACGIH TLV: 750 ppm, 1000 ppm STEL

Formaldehyde. When in aqueous solution, the term formalin is often used.
Health Effects
Severe irritant via all routes of entry. A known sensitizer/allergen. Contact with eyes may cause corneal clouding, permanent eye damage. Skin contact can cause a cracked, white, scaly dermatitis. Chronic exposure can cause a hardening and tanning of the skin. Sensitive persons can develop an allergic eczematous dermatitis and hives. Ingestion can yield severe inflammation of nose, eyes, mouth, throat, and stomach, often accompanied by severe stomach pain. It can be fatal.

Inhalation can yield severe eye and throat irritation, difficulty in breathing, also coughing and burning in the throat and eye tearing. Prolonged or repeated exposures can yield respiratory impairment. In higher concentrations, symptoms can include pulmonary edema, pneumonitis, also asthma and bronchitis. Formaldehyde is a potential cancer hazard associated with nasopharyngeal, oropharyngeal, and lung cancers in humans. It is a moderate fire and explosion risk when exposed to heat or flame. It can react violently with strong oxidizers.
Found in:

embalming adhesive gel	preservative cream
feature builder	arterial embalming
embalming spray	chemicals
sanitizing embalming	preservative/disinfectant gel
spray	supplemental embalming gel

accessory embalming   bleaching agent
  chemical   cavity embalming fluid/gel
incision sealer
pre-injectih chemicals
    OSHA PEL: 0.75 ppm TWA 2 ppm/15 min STEL

Phenol
Health Effects:
Highly irritating and corrosive to tissue. The contact site will become white, soft, wrinkled, with a delayed, intense burning sensation followed by local anesthesia and possibly gangrene. Phenol is absorbed readily through the skin, which has resulted in fatal overexposure. Contact with the eye can cause severe damage and blindness. Highly toxic via ingestion. Corrosion and possible perforation of lips, mouth, throat, esophagus and stomach can result. Symptoms include nausea, possibly vomiting, and severe abdominal cramps.

Inhalation of vapor is highly irritating to eyes and respiratory tract. Systemic effects from all routes of exposure include central nervous system depression, weakness, headache, dizziness, tinnitus, weak pulse, dypsnea, cyanosis, shock, frothing from nose and mouth, lung edema, possibly death.

Chronic poisoning can result in *gastrointestinal disturbances, nervous disorders, skin rash,* and *discoloration.* Liver, kidney, spleen, pancreas damage may occur. Chronic dermatitis from phenol contact is common in industry. It is a moderate fire risk when exposed to heat, flame, or oxidizers.
Found in:

embalming cauterant   accessory embalming
embalming chemical   chemical
  disinfectant
cavity embalming fluid/gel
  preservative/disinfected gel

    ACGIH TLV:5 ppm
    OSHA PEL: 5ppm TWA

The following is a sample listing of commonly used chemicals found in the compounding of products used in the preparation room. Each of these toxic chemicals is explained in detail on the MSDS that accompanies the product in which they are contained, similar to the three previously detailed examples:

Acetone	Camphor
Alkyl dimethylbenzyl	Chlorine salts
ammonium chloride	Chloroform
Amaranth	Cresol
Amitrole	Diethanolamine
2-Butoxyethanol	Diethylene glycol

[†]Pel, permissible exposure limit; ACG1H, American Congress of Governmental Industrial Hygienists; TLV, threshold limit value; STEL, short-term exposure limit.

Dimethylformamide
Ethyl acetate
Ethyl alcohol
Ethylene dichloride
Ethylene glycol
Ethylene glycol
   monomethyl ether
Formaldehyde
Formic acid
Glutaraldehyde
Hexylene glycol
Isobutane
Isopropyl alcohol
Methyl alcohol
Methyl ethyl ketone
2,2'-Methylenebis(4-
   chlorophene)
Methylene chloride
Mineral spirits

Molding plaster
Nitrocellulose
Orthodichlorobenzene
Oxalic acid
Paradichlorobenzene
Paraformaldehyde
p-tert-Pentylphenol
Phenol
Propane
Propylene glycol
Quartz
Quaternary ammonium
   compounds
Sodium hypochlorite
Sodium pentachlorophenate
Talc
Toluene
1,1,1-Trichloroethane
Trichloroethylene

Safe Chemical Practices

1. Know the chemical. Always check the label before using a material. Follow label warnings and directions. Obtain an MSDS for more complete product safety information.
2. Use protective gear.
3. Check for lack of ventilation and other physical hazards before using a hazardous chemical.
4. Know the correct emergency and first aid procedures.
5. No eating, drinking, or smoking in areas where hazardous materials are used or stored. Use good personal hygiene to protect against accidental ingestion.
6. Do not mix chemicals unless specifically instructed to do so on the label or the MSDS.
7. Clean up spills promptly.
8. Dispose of hazardous waste properly. Avoid reusing containers.

FEDERAL STANDARDS

1988—OSHA's Formaldehyde Rule

The OSHA Formaldehyde Rule* is a revised standard, not a new one. It reduces the permissible exposure limit (PEL) from 1 part formaldehyde in 1 million parts of air (ppm) to 0.75 ppm as a time-weighted average (TWA) over an 8-hour workday. The short-term exposure limit (STEL) is reduced from 5 ppm for 30 minutes to 2 ppm for 15 minutes. The revision also establishes an "action level" of 0.5 ppm as an 8-hour TWA. The rule also pro-

*Printed by permission of the Dodge Chemical Co., PO Box 193, Cambridge, MA, 02140.

vides for monitoring, medical surveillance, record keeping, annual employee training, medical removal protection, and hazard control plan.

The standard became effective February 2, 1988. OSHA allowed 6 months for completion of initial monitoring, or until August 2nd. The results of the initial monitoring dictate the other steps that must be taken. Let us now, by example, look at what is entailed at various levels of exposure. I start with the "worst case" first.

Example A. Initial monitoring shows a formaldehyde level above the PEL or STEL. This might be 1.1 ppm as a TWA (exceeds PEL) or 2.1 ppm for 15 minutes (exceeds STEL). The work area (preparation room) must then be posted at all entrances as follows:

DANGER—FORMALDEHYDE
IRRITANT AND POTENTIAL CANCER HAZARD
AUTHORIZED PERSONNEL ONLY

The employer must immediately, by engineering controls and work practices, attempt to reduce exposure to or below the PEL or STEL. If this cannot be accomplished, the employer must provide employees with full-face respirators, comply with fitting regulations, allow time away from the work area, as needed, for employees to wash their faces and face pieces, and on and on.

All employees must complete a medical questionnaire under the supervision of a licensed physician at the time of assignment to the work area. Based on that questionnaire, the physician determines whether or not the employee must undergo a physical examination. Exposure monitoring, medical surveillance, respirator fit testing, and employee training must be repeated annually. Exposure monitoring records will be kept for 30 years. Respirator fit testing records will be kept until replaced by a more recent record.

Example B. Initial monitoring reveals formaldehyde exposure within the PEL—under 0.75 ppm—but above the action level as a TWA over an 8-hour workday. Entrances to the work area need not be posted and employees need not wear respirators; however, exposure monitoring must be repeated every 6 months and the previously outlined medical surveillance and record keeping must be carried out.

Example C. Initial monitoring indicates exposure to be below the action level—below 0.5 ppm. The monitoring must be done, obviously, while embalming is in progress, as that is when the employee has exposure to formaldehyde. To qualify for the exemption from periodic monitoring, medical surveillance, and so on, the results from two consecutive monitoring samples, taken at least 7 days apart, must show that the exposure is below action level and the STEL. Employees must be notified of monitoring results in writing within 15 days of receipt of the report. If at a later time a new process or work practice that might increase exposure levels is introduced into the work area, the monitoring would have to be repeated. The principal engineering control for formaldehyde exposure in the preparation room is ventilation. The most important factor in the ventilation system is the location of the exhaust. It should be at the foot of the embalming table and below the level of the tabletop. The air replacement or intake should ideally be high on the opposite wall. Thus, fresh air is being blown toward the embalmer, while chemical fumes (as well as odors from the body and microorganisms) are being drawn down and away from the breathing zone. Formaldehyde gas is heavier than air, so we are merely helping it along when our exhaust pulls it down.

It certainly is advisable to consult a good ventilation engineer when installing or changing an air exchange system. The required number of air changes per hour is determined by the contents of the room, whether or not more than one embalming will be in progress at the same time, the shape of the room, and other factors. As a rough rule of thumb, for a single-table room, the number of air changes ranges from 12 to 20. It is highly desirable to have the exhaust motor on a high–medium–low switch for very obvious reasons. One should consider warming the incoming air in cold climates in winter and cooling it in warm climates in summer to maintain a comfortable working environment.

"Work practice" controls are nothing more than commonsense steps taken to avoid extra formaldehyde fumes into the atmosphere of the work area. Here are a few very obvious ideas:

- Always keep the lid on the embalming machine, except when it must be removed for filling.
- Replace the cap promptly on all bottles after pouring required quantities. This is a minor source of fumes, but "every little bit hurts."
- Do not treat autopsy viscera in an open container. Use a covered pail or closed viscera bag.
- Cover waste or drainage sinks, when in use, with a sheet of clear plastic, such as plexiglass, with holes for the aspirator and table drainage hoses, or, make a disposable cover with such products as Saran Wrap.
- Use a drainage tube with rubber tubing to the table drain to remove drainage from the embalmer's breathing zone.
- Keep post aspirator running on the "floor" of the abdominal cavity to collect return drainage when injecting an autopsied body.
- Cover all waste receptacles at all times. A piece of cotton or gauze used to wipe up a small spill and placed in an open waste receptacle will obviously contribute to the formaldehyde ppm.

- When using a "cavity compress" or external preservative, cover the area with light plastic and perhaps seal it with adhesive tape to contain the fumes.

In addition, there are background contributors:

- The mop standing in a bucket of water in the corner: When there is a spill, the mop is used to pick it up, and then put back in the bucket, where it gives off fumes. Add a bit of ammonia to the water in the bucket to neutralize any formaldehyde that might be picked up by the mop.
- The wood blocks so commonly used to position the arms and legs: Some have never been painted. On others, the paint has worn or chipped off. In either case, the wood has become saturated over time with embalming chemicals. Such blocks should be soaked in a mild solution of ammonia to neutralize the formaldehyde and dried thoroughly in the sun if possible. They should then be painted with a highgloss enamel that will not be penetrated by the embalming solution.
- One of those "I've got to fix that first chance I get" leaks in the embalming machine: The kind that is not very serious, just enough to keep the base of the machine wet. These are usually corrected by tightening a connection.

How can you get an idea of what the level of formaldehyde is in your work area when it is in use? The National Institute for Occupational Safety and Health gives these guidelines. Slight eye irritation occurs when one first enters an area with 0.05 to 0.5 ppm formaldehyde present. At 0.15 to 1ppm, the odor becomes apparent. At 2 to 3 ppm, eye irritation becomes more noticeable and one begins to feel a tingling sensation or irritation in the nostrils and throat.

Once you are satisfied that you have implemented all of the good work practices you can come up with, and have eliminated all possible background sources, you are ready to do that "initial monitoring." A good question to ask yourself at this point is, "Am I as ready as I would want to be if I knew the OSHA inspector would arrive tomorrow morning while I'm embalming?"

If you were able to answer that question with a "yes," there are several possibilities for getting the monitoring done. In urban areas, a quick source of help is the Yellow Pages. Look under *Industrial Hygiene Consultant*. In most states, the Department of Labor or the Department of Health will do the monitoring. In at least some states, it is a free service. Still another possibility would be a university if there is one within reasonable traveling distance of your funeral home. The great majority would have an industrial hygienist on the staff who would do free-lance monitoring.

Because of the relatively small amounts of formaldehyde-containing products used in the preparation room

and because of the manner in which they are used and handled, the only necessary protection against formaldehyde, as I see it, is rubber gloves and waterproof aprons. The purpose of both, of course, is protection against splashes while pouring chemical into the injector and from drainage on the table. If there is *any* possibility that an employee's eyes may be splashed with solutions containing 0.1% or greater formaldehyde, the employer *must* provide suitable eye wash facilities within the imme-
...ency use. There is a specific re-
... of the eyes and skin with liq-
...re formaldehyde be prevented
...tective clothing made of a ma-
...maldehyde and the use of other
...h as goggles and face shields,
...ation.
...that funeral service can live
...grees, because according to fig-
...idard, the overwhelming ma-
...ould have levels of formalde-
...vel" in the preparation. Just a
...EL. With a well-designed ex-
...ork practices, I believe those
...he same time, they will be pro-
...more comfortable work envi-

...a in 1982–1983, 44 randomly
...e monitored for formaldehyde
...ded the new PEL. That is not
...nothing but sit back and wait
...isit. Every funeral home owner
...the air exchange system in the
...rtain that it is adequate. Such
...tate board regulations in most
...k the work practices and back-
...ehyde fumes. Finally, have the
...g completed. If you are below
...have nothing to do, except to
...rtain that the exhaust is being
...d work practices are being ob-

...ppeared in the *Federal Regis-*
...including preamble, the rule,

For a copy of the complete rule, you should write OSHA Office of Publications, U.S. Department of Labor, Room N-3101, 200 Constitution Avenue, NW, Washington, DC 20210. Or, you may telephone 1–202–523–9667. Simply request the final rule on Occupational Exposure to Formaldehyde.

See Selected Readings for additional information.

OSHA's Bloodborne Pathogen Standard to Include Embalmers

In the *Federal Register* for December 6, 1991, OSHA published its Final Standard for the Protection of Health Care Workers Against Bloodborne Pathogens. The rule applies to all persons in occupations in which there is exposure to blood, products made from human blood, body fluids that might contain traces of blood, and other potentially infectious materials.

To prevent exposure the regulation requires an Exposure Control Plan, the use of personal protective equipment, a hepatitis B immunization program, annual employee training, the use of biohazard warning labels, and record keeping. It also requires postexposure evaluation and follow-up in the event of an exposure incident.

The first step to compliance is exposure determination. The employer must identify the tasks and procedures in which occupational exposure may occur. Then the employer must list job descriptions that may be reasonably expected to involve skin, eye, mucous membrane, or parenteral contact with blood or other potentially infectious materials. This list would obviously include embalmers and apprentices. In addition, it might include persons making first calls or removals, persons on ambulance duty if the funeral home offers this service. and persons cleaning the preparation room or laundering reusable gowns and sheets, if other than those previously listed. The occupational exposure of each listed employee must then be documented. Other funeral home personnel who would not be reasonably or routinely expected to have exposure in the normal course of their duties need not be listed.

The employer must prepare a written exposure control plan. The plan is to be designed to minimize or eliminate employee exposure. The plan must include exposure determination and the schedule and method of implementation for each part of the standard, and it must be reviewed and updated when any changes are made in the duties and tasks of the employees.

To understand the pathogen rule, it is important that we understand *universal precautions,* a term originated by the Centers for Disease Control and Prevention (CDC).* In brief, it is a method of infection control in which all human blood and certain human body fluids are treated as if known to be infectious for human immunodeficiency virus (HIV), hepatitis B virus (HBV), and other bloodborne pathogens. The practice makes particularly good sense for embalmers, as embalming is often done before the cause of death is known. Even when the cause of death is known to be something other than bloodborne disease, that is not necessarily positive proof that a bloodborne disease was not also present. If all bodies are treated as though the person had died of a bloodborne infection, there will be no need for second guessing.

The employer must provide and ensure that employees use necessary and appropriate personal protec-

---

*See Selected Readings for the complete CDC Universal Precautions.

tive equipment. This would include such items as gloves, gowns, waterproof aprons, head and foot coverings, and face shields or eye protection. Gloves, gowns, aprons, and face shields would seem to be appropriate and adequate for normal embalming operations; however, if there is potential for splashing of blood or other potentially infectious materials on the head, head covers, surgical caps, or hoods must be worn. Fluidproof shoe covers should be worn if there is potential for shoes to become contaminated and/or soaked with blood or other potentially infectious materials. Personal protective equipment must be readily available in appropriate sizes to all personnel with occupational exposure. Cleaning, laundering, or disposal of personal protective equipment shall be provided at no cost to the employee. Disposable or surgical gloves must be replaced as soon as possible when they are torn or punctured. They should not be washed or disinfected for reuse if the integrity of the glove is not compromised.

Work practice controls must be spelled out and enforced. Such controls would include immediate hand washing after removal of gloves. All protective equipment must be removed immediately on leaving the work area and placed in a designated area or container for storage, washing, decontamination, or disposal. Used needles and other sharps should not be sheared, bent, broken, recapped, or resheathed by hand. Sharps are to be disposed in closable, puncture-resistant, disposable containers that are leakproof on the sides and bottom and that bear proper warning labels or are color coded (red). Eating, drinking, smoking, application of cosmetics, and handling of contact lenses are prohibited in work areas. No food or drink should be stored in refrigerators where blood is stored or in other areas of possible contamination. All procedures involving blood or other potentially infectious body fluids should be performed in such a manner as to minimize splashing, spraying, and aerosolization.

Employers must ensure that the work area is maintained in a clean and sanitary condition, in accord with a written schedule for cleaning and disinfection. This could be on completion of embalming or at the end of the work shift. All instruments, equipment, and environmental and working surfaces must be properly cleaned and disinfected after contact with blood or other potentially infectious materials. All pails, containers, and receptacles intended for reuse that have a potential for becoming contaminated with blood or other potentially infectious materials should be inspected, cleaned, and disinfected on a regularly scheduled basis or as soon as possible on visible contamination.

All infectious waste destined for disposal must be placed in closable, leakproof containers or bags that are color coded or labeled. Disposal of all infectious waste shall be in accordance with applicable federal, state, and local regulations.

Hepatitis B vaccination must be made available to all employees who have occupational exposure. If an employee declines a vaccination, he or she must sign a specifically worded declination. If an employee at first declines HBV vaccination but later decides to accept it, it must be provided. In the event of a needle stick or other accidental exposure, the employer shall make available to the employee a confidential medical evaluation and follow-up.

The record keeping required by the proposed standard must include medical records and training records. The medical record should include the name and social security number of the employee, a copy of the employee's HBV vaccination records, and a copy of the results of physical examinations, medical testing, and follow-up procedures as they relate to the employee's ability to receive vaccination or to postexposure evaluation after an exposure incident; also required are the employer's copy of the physician's written opinion and a copy of the information provided to the physician. These medical records must be kept confidential, except as provided by the standard or as may be required by law. Medical records will be maintained for the duration of employment, plus 30 years. Training records must include the dates of training, a summary of the training, the names of the person or persons conducting the training and the names of all persons receiving the training. Training records must be maintained for 3 years from the date on which the training occurred.

Individual states will also be developing hazardous waste guidelines. It is most important that funeral establishments be familiar with these state regulations which, in most instances, will be more stringent than the OSHA rule.*

EMBALMER ETHICS†

In the United States, where Judeo-Christian tradition has fostered respect for the human dead and considerations of public health require protection of the living against infection or contagion, the preparation of dead human bodies is entrusted to a specialized group: licensed embalmers.

Ethical Practice

Ethics is the science of rectitude and duty. Its subject is morality and its sphere is virtuous conduct. It treats the

---

*These OSHA sections were contributed by Arnold J. Dodge of the Dodge Chemical Company, Cambridge, MA. The OSHA sections were reviewed and updated in 1995 by Edward M. Ranier, Esq., NFDA Occupational Safety and Hazard Counsel.
†Developed by George Fulton and the Illinois Funeral Directors Association, Robert W. Ninker, Executive Director.

various aspects of rights and obligations. In essence, ethics is a set of principles that governs conduct for the purpose of establishing harmony in all human relations. For practical purposes, ethics is fair play.

In the absence of a specific set of rules by which men and women are governed or through which they learn to govern themselves in their relations with others, they are dependent on traditional customs and practices as rules of conduct. This section, therefore, is intended to suggest some desirable uniform rules of conduct by which any embalmer may be guided in the practice of embalming. No code can specify all the duties of the embalmer in every circumstance that confronts him or her. This section is designed to serve as a guide in promoting professional attitudes and ensuring ethical conduct in many of the situations where neither custom nor tradition has provided a standard of practice that serves the best interests of the public and the profession.

Judicious Counsel

Experience qualifies embalmers to be of great value to those whom they serve and it is their professional obligation to give judicious counsel. In accordance with the wishes of the family, the embalmer should advise them concerning their expectations for a visitation, with viewing, when circumstances dictate the need for special attention such as restoration, any necessary invasive procedures, or embalmer's need for available photos of the deceased to aid him or her in embalming and feature setting, taking into account any of the deceased's cosmetic or hairdressing preferences.

Whenever the service is made challenging, because of the circumstances of the death, the embalmer should communicate realistic expectations to the family or through the arranging funeral director. Misrepresentation is unethical and unprofessional. Representations concerning embalming and restoration should be full and factual.

Body Donation, Organ Donation, Autopsy

The embalmer should support the wishes of families who choose to authorize organ and/or tissue donation although the facts about known delays should also be factually presented. Likewise, the embalmer should support the wishes of individuals or families who choose body donations or are asked, by others, to authorize an autopsy.

The embalmer shares with all medical and hospital personnel the professional responsibility of cooperating with all groups and in supporting all measures that promote the health, safety, and welfare of the public. Courtesy, tact, and discretion should characterize all of the embalmer's professional actions.

Embalmers should never aid or abet an unlicensed person, where licensure is required, to represent herself or himself as a licensed embalmer or to engage in practices reserved to the holder of an embalming license.

Confidentiality

The family must be able to rely on confidentiality between themselves, the funeral director, and the embalmer on all matters relating to cause and manner of death.

The embalmer may be privy to other matters shared with him or her by the family. All such confidences must be assured by the embalmer and funeral director.

Defamation of Others

Comments by one embalmer concerning another funeral director or embalmer should always be selected with care. Insinuations, nonfactual statements, or overplay of facts that have the intent or effect of harming another professional should be avoided at all times.

Enticement of Another Embalmer

It is unethical for an embalmer to willfully entice the employees of another firm with the purpose of unduly hampering, injuring, or prejudicing that firm or professional.

Accommodation of the Family

Not every family may wish or be able to pay for a visitation, with viewing, but may express an earnest desire to view the remains in the preparation room. To the extent possible, embalmers should attempt to accommodate the families in this regard and should present the remains with features set and whatever other preparations are feasible. Such accommodation may be considered the family's right to check the embalmer's quality control.

Knowing the value of viewing, for many people, the embalmer, through his or her efforts, may provide a family with an acceptable memory picture, even when circumstances may not allow a public viewing.

Identification

The embalmer has responsibility to ascertain that he or she has a properly identified body and must manage the care and internal identification of the remains that there can be no mistake, especially when viewing is not planned or cremation is the method of final disposition.

Observing Laws, Rules, and Regulations

The embalmer is duty-bound and legally responsible for ensuring that he or she observes all legal and regulatory requirements of federal, state, or local government. The embalmer also has the responsibility for informing the funeral home owner, if he or she is not the owner, of the resources or capital investments required to meet OSHA standards, any applicable EPA requirements, or other measures needed to be in compliance.

Maintaining Competence

The embalmer has a moral and ethical responsibility to ensure that he or she receives whatever continuing education is necessary to maintain skills commensurate with professional practice.

State-of-the-art changes in practices and procedures should be known to and practiced by the embalmer at all times.

Health Protection and Sanitation

The embalmer is ethically responsible for protecting the health of any person who is allowed to enter the preparation room for any reason, and for restricting entry to any person not authorized to be in the preparation room. That responsibility includes appropriate sanitation procedures to maintain a safe working area for any individual. The embalmer is responsible for safe sheltering so that no person has possible access to the human remains.

Proper Care of the Deceased

The embalmer should deliver and document quality care of the deceased body.

The embalming procedures used should be documented for possible future reference. A record of clothing or other personal articles or valuables received by the firm would be appropriate. In addition, any written permission to embalm or a record of the expressed permission should be maintained.

CORONER OR MEDICAL EXAMINER

In addition to state and federal rules pertaining to preparation of the body, the embalmer is also responsible for reporting any suspicious circumstances surrounding the death to the coroner or medical examiner. It is important that the funeral personnel in charge of arrangements ascertain who will sign the certificate of death if the nature of the death is such that the coroner or medical examiner must be notified to investigate. The following list (issued by the Ohio Department of Health) shows the types of deaths about which the coroner or medical examiner must be notified. *This list applies to only one state. It is important that the embalmer be familiar with the requirements of the state in which he or she is practicing.*

I. **Accidental deaths: all forms including death arising from employment**
   A. Anesthetic accident (death on the operating table or prior to recovery from anesthesia)
   B. Blows or other forms of mechanical violence
   C. Burns and scalds
   D. Crushed beneath falling objects
   E. Cutting or stabbing
   F. Drowning (actual or suspected)
   G. Electric shock
   H. Explosion
   I. Exposure
   J. Firearms
   K. Fractures of bones, not pathological (such cases to be reported even when fracture is not primarily responsible for death)
   L. Falls
   M. Carbon monoxide poisoning (resulting from natural gas, automobile exhaust, or other)
   N. Hanging
   O. Heat exhaustion
   P. Insolation (sunstroke)
   Q. Poisoning (food, occupational, narcotic, sedative, and other)
   R. Strangulation
   S. Suffocation (foreign object in bronchi, by bed clothing or other means)
   T. Vehicular accidents (automobile, street car, bus, railroad, motorcycle, bicycle, or other)

II. **Homicidal deaths: including those involving child abuse**

III. **Suicidal deaths**

IV. **Abortions—criminal or self-induced: When the manner of death falls within the above classifications, such death must be reported to the coroner even though the survival period subsequent to onset is 12 months.**

V. **Sudden deaths: When in apparent health or in any suspicious or unusual manner including**
   A. Alcoholism
   B. Sudden death on the street, at home, in a public place, at place of employment
   C. Deaths in unknown circumstances, whenever there are no witnesses or where little or no information can be elicited concerning the deceased person (deaths of this type include those persons whose dead bodies are found in the open, in places of temporary shelter, or in their home under conditions that offer no clues as to the cause of death)
   D. Deaths that follow injuries sustained at place of employment whenever the circumstances surrounding such injury may ultimately be the subject of investigation

1. Industrial infections (anthrax, septicemia following wounds including gas bacillus infections, tetanus, etc.)
2. Silicosis
3. Industrial poisonings (acids, alkalies, aniline, benzene, carbon monoxide, carbon tetrachloride, cyanogen, lead, nitrous fumes, etc.)
4. Contusions, abrasions, fractures, burns (flame, chemical, or electrical) received during employment which in the opinion of the attending physician are of sufficient import, either as the cause or contributing factor to the cause of death, to warrant certifying them on the death certificate

E. All stillborn infants where there is suspicion of illegal interference
F. Death of persons where the attending physician cannot be found, or death of persons who have not been attended by a physician within 2 weeks prior to the date of death
G. All deaths occurring within 24 hours of admission to a hospital unless the patient has been under continuous care of a physician for a natural disease that is responsible for death

EXAMPLE FORMS

The suggested authorization forms in Figures 1–1, 2, and 3 give the funeral home permission to take possession of the body and allow the body to be embalmed. Figure 1–4 is the form used when the family does not request embalming.

Personal Property

Personal property of the deceased, including jewelry and clothing worn at the time of the death, are often brought into the funeral home. Figure 1–5 is a sample record for personal property inventory, which includes the location of the removal and who removed the property.

Jewelry or other personal items placed on the deceased or within the casket during the time of visitation, which are to be returned to the family, should be documented in writing. This note should be placed in a position where it will be seen at the closing of the casket (e.g., on the casket lid, along the seal of the casket, at the location of the casket locking device).

Embalming Documentation

The embalming of the body should always be documented. The preparation of an embalming report (Fig. 1–6) is most important if the body is to be shipped to an-

other funeral home. A copy of this document should accompany the body. Some funeral homes also prepare an autopsy report and return it to the pathology department of the hospital where the autopsy was performed. The autopsy report can be used to express concerns about the autopsy protocol when it directly interferes with the preparation of the body.

Organ Donations

When death occurs at the residence, the funeral director may be called on to secure permission for the donation of specific organs. Many organs such as the whole eyes, corneas, or kidneys may be removed at the funeral home. The funeral director and embalmer should be familiar with the guidelines of their state for the donation of organs. Consult Chapter 18 for more detailed information on the legal requirements for organ donation. A sample donor form is included for reference (Fig. 1–7).

THE EMBALMING PROCESS IN SUMMARY

Embalming can be defined as a process of chemically treating the dead human body to reduce the presence and growth of microorganisms, to retard organic decomposition, and to restore an acceptable physical appearance.

The embalming process acts on the body proteins. It changes the proteins' colloidal nature by establishing many crosslinkages that were not formerly present between adjacent proteins. This forms a latticework of inert, firm material that can no longer serve as food for bacteria. Likewise, this new protein form cannot be broken down by enzymes from body cells or bacteria.

Body proteins have many reactive centers and a great affinity to hold water. Embalming destroys these reactive centers, and the new aprotein-like structure no longer has the ability to retain water. As a result enzymes, which break down or decompose proteins, can no longer act on the new protein structures. Thus, the tissues are temporarily preserved. Likewise, the embalmed tissue becomes drier, for it has lost its ability to hold large amounts of moisture.

Enzymes have the ability to react with body proteins, fats, and carbohydrates and break down (decompose) these body substrates. Embalming preservatives also act on the enzymes, for they are a form of protein. Embalming chemicals destroy the pathogenic bacteria of the body, because they react with the proteins that make up these organisms. The embalming(preservative) solution converts the body proteins to a more stable, longer-lasting substance. In addition, the preservatives destroy the body and bacterial chemicals (enzymes) that break down the body tissues after death. Finally, the microor-

AUTHORIZATION FOR RELEASE AND EMBALMING

The undersigned hereby authorize

_____
Name of Institution or Person

to release the body of _____
Deceased

to _____ and/or
Name of Funeral Home

its agents and authorize said funeral home and/or its agents to care for, embalm and otherwise prepare said body for burial and/or other disposition.

I (we) hereby represent that I am (we are) of the same and nearest degree of relationship to the deceased and/or are legally authorized or charged with the responsibility for such burial and/or other disposition.

_____   _____
Name   Relationship

_____   _____
Name   Relationship

_____   _____
Name   Relationship

Witness _____

Date _____

Figure 1–1. Authorization form for release and embalming a body. *(From Resource Manual, Milwaukee, WI: National Funeral Directors Association; 1979, with permission.)*

ganisms found in the body (pathogenic and nonpathogenic) are destroyed, for their protein "bodies" are also converted to an inactive state. Thus, the body, to a certain extent, is sanitized. The likelihood of it remaining a source of disease-producing microbes, or their products, is reduced.

By conversion or inactivation of the protein of the body, the protein of enzymes, and the protein of bacteria, the body is sanitized and temporarily preserved. The length of preservation varies, depending on many intrinsic body factors, extrinsic environmental factors, and the ability of the embalmer to obtain as much contact be-

AUTHORIZATION TO EMBALM

The undersigned hereby authorize _____
Name of Funeral Home

and/or its agents, to care for, embalm and otherwise prepare for burial and/or other disposition of the body of _____
Deceased

I (we) hereby represent that I am (we are) of the same and nearest degree of relationship to the deceased and/or are legally authorized or charged with the responsibility for such burial and/or other disposition.

_____   _____
Name   Relationship

_____   _____
Name   Relationship

_____   _____
Name   Relationship

Witness _____

Date _____

Figure 1–2. Authorization form to embalm body. *(From Resource Manual, Milwaukee, WI: National Funeral Directors Association; 1979, with permission.)*

NECESSARY INFORMATION

1. Name of Deceased _____ Age _____
   Home address _____ City _____ State & Zip _____
2. Where is deceased _____
3. Is autopsy scheduled: ( ) Yes ( ) No - if yes Time _____ Date _____
   Can the body be embalmed before the autopsy ( ) Yes ( ) No
4. *Who called:* Name _____ Phone No. _____
   Relationship to deceased _____ Other _____
5. Who will be making arrangements: _____
   Address _____ Phone No. _____
   Relationship to deceased _____
6. When will arrangements be made: Date _____ Time _____ AM/PM
7. Other information: _____
   _____
8. When was call received: Date _____ Time _____ AM/PM
9. Signature of person taking call _____

. . . .

AUTHORIZATION TO TAKE POSSESSION OF BODY

( ) _____ , _____ , a family member.
         (name)   *(relationship)*

( ) _____ , _____ , a person acting upon instructions of the family.
         (name)   *(capacity)*

( ) _____ , _____ , a legally authorized local official.
         (name)   *(title)*

Requested that our firm, including our proper agents, take possession of the body of *(deceased)* _____
_____ This request received at *(time)* _____ AM/PM, on *(date)* _____
by the undersigned.

_____   _____
(Firm Name)   *(Signature of person receiving request)*

. . . .

AUTHORIZATION FOR EMBALMING OF BODY

( ) _____ , _____ , a legally authorized family member.
         (name)   *(relationship)*

( ) _____ , _____ , a legally authorized representative of the family.
         (name)   *(capacity)*

( ) _____ , _____ , a legally authorized local official.
         (name)   *(title)*

Read, or was read the following statement and granted the permission therein: "Permission is given for embalming the body of *(deceased)* _____ " This oral permission was granted at *(time)* _____ AM/PM *(date)* _____ and received by _____
(Firm Name) _____   _____
                                              (Signature of person receiving permission)
If person granting permission available sign here _____

. . . .

CONCURRENCE WITH VERBAL AUTHORIZATIONS

The above verbal authorizations were given, to the best of my knowledge, as recorded

_____   _____
(Signature of person authorized to arrange for service)   *(Date)*

Figure 1–3. First Call and Authorization Report. *(From Resource Manual, Milwaukee, WI: National Funeral Directors Association; 1979, with permission.)*

tween a sufficient amount of preservative chemical and the millions and millions of proteins within the body. Under the right conditions bodies may be preserved as long as several hundred years or as temporarily as only a few days. *There is no measure by which the degree or length of preservation can be measured.*

Another purpose of embalming is to restore the deceased to a natural form and color. This is called **restora-**tion. The goal of restoration of the dead human body is not so much to make the deceased look lifelike, but rather to try and remove from the body the devastation caused by many long-term diseases and illnesses. Other purposes include removal of the disfigurement created by the long-term usage of therapeutic drugs and removal of the visible postmortem changes that may have begun to appear.

AUTHORIZATION FOR REMOVAL AND DISPOSITION WITHOUT EMBALMING

The undersigned hereby direct and authorize the _____

name of funeral home

and/or its agents, to remove and take possession of the body of _____

(deceased)

_____ and to provide for the final disposition of said body by ( ) earth burial, ( ) entombment, ( ) cremation, ( ) burial at sea, ( ) other _____
We direct that there be no embalming or other preparation or care of the body. The undersigned also wish hereby to indicate the desire (not to have) (to have) rites/ceremonies with the casketed body present.

The undersigned do further state that they (have) (have not) identified the body of the above named decedent and assume all responsibility and/or liability of anyone whomsoever for mistaken identity.

The undersigned do hereby agree to indemnify and hold harmless the above-named funeral home, its officers, agents and employees from any claims or causes of action, including a reasonable attorney's fee for the defense thereof arising out of their act of identification or failure to identify, or arising out of their decision not to embalm, or arising out of any other decision indicated by this agreement which may result in mental or physical distress or anguish or harm or financial loss to themselves or to others.

_____	_____
Name	Relationship to deceased
Name	Relationship to deceased
Name	Relationship to deceased

Witness _____

Date _____

Figure 1–4. Authorization form for removal and disposition without embalming. *(From Resource Manual, Milwaukee, WI: National Funeral Directors Association; 1979, with permission.)*

Time Body Received at Funeral Home _____   Page No. _____
MEMO OF CLOTHING AND EFFECTS
NAME _____   _____   Date _____
Removed from _____   By _____

☐ BLOUSE	☐ HOUSECOAT	☐ P.Js.	☐ SLIPPERS	☐ UNDERWEAR
☐ BRA	☐ NECKTIE	☐ SHIRT	☐ SLIP	☐ VEST
☐ COAT	☐ NIGHTGOWN	☐ SHOES	☐ SKIRT	☐ OVERNIGHTER
☐ DRESS	☐ NIGHTSHIRT	☐ SOX	☐ SWEATER	☐ SUIT CASE
☐ GIRDLE	☐ PANTS	☐ STOCKINGS	☐ TOPCOAT	☐ CASH $_____
				☐ KEYS

Valuables and Jewelry _____
Medical Devices (i.e., pacemaker) _____
_____
_____

Disposition Authorized by _____   Date _____

member of family

☐ Give to Family at once
☐ We dispose

Date _____   _____
Signature of Funeral Director

Figure 1–5. Example of the form used to inventory personal property of the deceased. *(From Resource Manual, Milwaukee, WI: National Funeral Directors Association: 1979, with permission.)*

```
┌──────────────────────────────────────────────────────────────────────────────────┐
│         CONFIDENTIAL   EMBALMING REPORT   CONFIDENTIAL                              │
│  Date _____ Case No. _____ Funeral Record No. _____ │
│                                                                                    │
│  History and Description                                                           │
│  Name of deceased _____ Address _____ │
│                                                                                 AM │
│  Place of death _____ Date _____ 19____ Time _____ PM │
│  Age _____ Sex _____ Color or Race _____ Height _____ Approximate Weight _____ │
│        Long _____                                                                   │
│  Beard Short _____ Moustache _____ Eyes _____ Teeth _____ Hair _____ │
│  Scars, Birth Marks, Moles, Warts, Tattoo—Describe: _____ │
│  Cause of Death _____ How ascertained _____ │
│  Medical Attendant or Coroner _____ Address _____ │
│                                                                                 AM │
│  Received at funeral home:  Date _____ 19____ Time _____ PM │
│  Permission to embalm received on the ____ day of _____, 19____ from _____. │
│  Body tagged as contagious or infectious yes no   If yes description opposite side │
│  Condition of Body Before Embalming:                                               │
│  Normal _____ clean _____ dirty _____ evidence of disease _____ emaciation _____ evidence of surgery _____ │
│  evidence of external wounds _____ eruptions _____ dropsical _____ postmortem pigmentation _____ skin _____ │
│  slip _____ gas _____ tumors _____ ulcerations _____ mutilations _____ purge (type) _____ rigor mortis _____ │
│  Autopsy (type) _____ Authorized by _____ Performed by _____         │
│  Remarks: _____ │
│  Protective attire worn by embalmer_____ │
│                                                                                    │
│  Embalming performed with or without incident to embalmer_____ if with describe medical treatment on opposite side │
│                                                                                    │
│  Embalming:                                                                        │
│  Elapsed time between death and start of embalming: _____ │
│  Arteries used for injection _____ │
│  Veins used for drainage _____ │
│  Auxiliary drainage methods used _____ │
│  Method of injection: Hand pump _____ Gravity _____ Pressure machine _____ │
│  Fluid used: A _____ B _____ C _____ │
│   (Trade name    preinjection          arterial              cavity                │
│    and index)                                                                      │
│                         D _____                                  │
│                             co-injection                                           │
│  Fluid Dilution  (Ounces to one gallon):                                           │
│  1st _____ 2nd _____ 3rd _____ 4th _____          │
│  Cavity fluids  (ounces injected undiluted): _____ │
│  Other cavity treatment _____ Treatment _____ │
│  Parts receiving poor circulation _____ and treatment _____ │
│  Restorative art treatment _____ Authorized by _____ │
│  Cosmetics used _____ │
│  Length of time required to complete operation _____ │
│  Note: Place additional remarks or sketches on reverse side.                       │
│                                                                                    │
│  Condition of Body After Embalming:                                                │
│  Condition of body at completion of operation _____ │
│  Condition of body at time of funeral _____ │
│  Special postembalming treatment required _____ │
│  _____ │
└──────────────────────────────────────────────────────────────────────────────────┘
```

Figure 1–6. Example of a form used to document the embalming process. (From Resource Manual, Milwaukee, WI: National Funeral Directors Association; 1979, with permission.)

Embalming the body allows for its transport to a distant point without the remains arriving in a decomposed and unsanitary state. It allows for the body to be viewed by relatives and friends (if that is their custom) even though the death may have occurred thousands of miles from the location where the funeral ceremonies are held. Preserving the body also allows more time for the arrangement and planning of the funeral. It gives relatives and friends in distant locations the opportunity to be present and allows the body to be

---

CONSENT BY NEXT-OF-KIN FOR THE DONATION OF ORGANS AND TISSUES

I/WE _____ as next-

(name of next-of-kin)

of-kin and* _____ of _____

(relationship)   (name of donor)

for humanitarian reasons hereby give consent for the donation of his/her

_____ for the purposes

(specify donated organs or tissues)

of transplantation or research, if medically suitable, after the time of his/her death has been determined by the attending physician.

I/WE understand that these gifts are made to the Pittsburgh Transplant Foundation and that the recovery, distribution and determination of use of these gifts will be coordinated by the Foundation in accordance with medical and ethical standards. The Foundation will be responsible for the costs related to the organ and tissue recovery.

I/WE understand that death has been determined and its time recorded based on the fulfillment of brain death criteria. I/WE understand that artificial support of heartbeat and respiration will be continued during the recovery of vital organs and discontinued upon completion of the procedure. I/WE give consent for the recovery of the organs and tissues specified above under the circumstances described. I/WE also authorize the Pittsburgh Transplant Foundation to obtain complete medical history, autopsy findings (if performed), and tissue specimens for immunology studies necessary to insure the safety of the organs and tissues for transplantation.

_____ (date)   _____ (date)
(signature of next-of-kin)   (signature of next-of-kin)

_____ (date)   _____ (date
(signature of witness)   (signature of witness)

_____
(Organ Procurement Coordinator)

*The Uniform Anatomical Gift Act establishes the following order of priority: (1) spouse; (2) adult son or daughter; (3) either parent; (4) adult brother or sister; (5) guardian of the person of the decedent; (6) any other person authorized or under obligation to dispose of the body.

Figure 1–7. Sample donor form. *(From Resource Manual, Milwaukee, WI: National Funeral Directors Association; 1979, with permission.)*

viewed without the adverse effects of decomposition being evidenced.*

Embalming consists basically of two processes: arterial embalming and cavity embalming. In *arterial embalming*, the preservation solution (generally 3 or 4 gallons) is injected into a large artery of the body. Blood is removed simultaneously from a large vein of the body to make room for this preservative solution. The preservative solution flows through the arterial and venous routes in the same course followed by blood in the living body. The basic difference is that the heart is no longer the central starting point for the fluid flow. Embalming solution is distributed from the arch of the aorta and does not flow through the chambers of the heart as blood does in the living. A portion of the embalming solution passes through the capillaries of the body and enters the tissue spaces. Here, it makes contact with the body cells and brings about the conversion of body proteins.

Cavity embalming is the treatment of the organs in the abdominal and thoracic cavities. Many of these organs are hollow and their contents are not reached by the embalming solution. The contents of these hollow organs and any liquids or gases that may have accumulated in the body cavities are removed. To do this, the embalmer inserts a long needle into the abdominal wall. This process is called *aspiration*. As it is impossible to see if the tissues of the organs are receiving arterial solution, a very strong preservative solution is injected through the same abdominal opening. This process is called *cavity fluid injection*.

Supplemental Methods of Embalming

In addition to arterial and cavity embalming there are several supplemental methods of embalming. These methods are generally used to preserve and sanitize local areas of the body that have not received arterial fluid or to treat areas that have received insufficient amounts of preservative chemicals. These supplemental methods include hypodermic and surface embalming. Hypodermic and surface embalming may be used as the primary meth-

---

*Many studies have shown that confrontation with the dead human body by relatives and friends helps to enforce the fact that the death has occurred. This contact can help release emotions that can often be the beginning of the emotional healing process after death.

ods for embalming for the preservation of an infant, fetus, visceral tissue, or a severed or mutilated portion of the body.

Hypodermic embalming is the sanitation and preservation of a local body area by subcuticular injection of a suitable chemical. The chemical injected may be a solution of arterial fluid, cavity fluid, or a supplemental preservative chemical. The solution may be injected by hypodermic needle, syringe, or an infant trocar attached by tubing to the pressurized embalming machine.

Surface embalming (penetration–absorption) is the sanitizing and preservation of a local area by application of a suitable chemical to the surface of the body. The chemical may be an arterial fluid, a cavity chemical, an accessory embalming chemical, or an autopsy gel. Compresses of cotton or gauze can be used to apply the chemical. The autopsy gel may be viscous enough to be brushed on the surface of the skin. External compresses should always be covered with plastic to limit undesirable fumes. Surface embalming can be applied to external skin surfaces or to internal surfaces as in the application of compresses under the eyelids, within the mouth, or in the autopsied body from within the body cavities.

Embalming Sequence

The following embalming chronologies provide an overview of the entire embalming procedure from start to finish. The first suggested chronology gives the step-by-step procedure for embalming the adult *unautopsied* body; the second chronology gives the sequence of treatments for preparation of the *autopsied* adult body.

Suggested Chronology for Embalming the Unautopsied Adult Body

The steps that follow are the general order for embalming the unautopsied adult body. Note that the steps need not be taken in this recommended order. For example, features can be set before, during, or even after arterial embalming; many embalmers prefer to suture incisions after cavity embalming, as the aspiration of the organs relieves the pressure on the vascular system and reduces the chance of incision leakage. The embalmer should be appropriately attired and gloved when handling the dead human body. The embalming report should be prepared throughout the embalming of the body.

After the body has been placed on the embalming table the following steps are suggested:

1. Remove all clothing from the body. Be certain to examine for any valuables. If rings or jewelry are present, make a list. Some embalmers prefer to tape rings to fingers or affix them with a string. Jewelry such as necklaces, religious articles, and watches should be removed and carefully stored.

    A. Soiled clothing should either be destroyed or cleaned.
    B. All contaminated bedding (such as sheets and hospital gowns) should be destroyed or properly laundered.

2. Disinfect the body with a droplet spray or with a disinfectant solution that is sponged onto the body. Allow the disinfectant time to work. Disinfect all body orifices and swab these orifices with cotton. Remove all material from the mouth and throat. A nasal tube aspirator can also be used to remove material from the mouth, throat, and nasal passages.

3. Position the body. Rigor mortis should be relieved at this time. Limbs can be flexed and exercised and hands extended and manipulated. The head should be elevated above the chest and the chest elevated above the abdomen. Slightly tilt the head to the right. The hands can remain at the sides or even down over the table at this point. This allows the blood to gravitate into the hands and help expand the vessels. Once arterial injection has begun and the hands show signs of fluid distribution, they can be placed in the correct position. Special blocking is necessary for arthritic conditions or where limbs have atrophied. Attempt to straighten the limbs by wrapping them with cloth strips. It is not recommended that any tissue be cut to extend limbs.

4. Wash the body surface with a germicidal warm-water soapy solution. Give particular attention to face and hands. The hair should be washed. At this time the fingernails can be cleaned. It is much easier to get any dirt out from under the nails at this time than after arterial embalming. Clean using a brush; an instrument may tear the skin under the nail and a discoloration will result. Use solvents to remove any surface stains. Thoroughly dry the body.

5. Shave the facial hair. Any facial hair remaining may interfere with the later cosmetic application. Be certain to check if a mustache or beard is to be removed or merely trimmed. If there is any doubt, the beard or mustache can be shaved after embalming once the family has been consulted. Removal of facial hair is much simpler than reconstruction of a mustache or beard. Facial hair should be removed from all bodies, including women and children.

6. Close the mouth using an appropriate method such as the needle injector method or suturing. If dentures are available, they should be properly cleaned and disinfected. If dentures or teeth are absent a replacement of cotton or a "mouth former" can be substituted. The eyes should be cleaned and closed using cotton or an "eyecap." If fever blisters are present on the lips or if there is crusted material along the eyelashes, using a soft rag or gauze moistened with

warm water will easily remove these items. A solvent such as trichloroethylene or the "dry hair washes" also serves as a good cleaner. Care should be taken at this point to straighten the nostrils with cotton and to carefully clip any nostril hairs that may be visible. Some embalmers prefer at this time to place a light coating of massage cream over the face, hands, and neck. This cream should not be placed over discolored areas where opaque cosmetics will later be applied. Surface compresses of bleach (phenol or formaldehyde) can be placed on blood or pathological discolorations at this time.

7. Select the artery that will be used for injection and the vein that will be used for drainage. This choice is based on the embalming analysis.

8. Select the arterial fluid and prepare the embalming solution.

9. Inject the embalming solution. The pressure and the rate of flow of the injection are determined by the embalming analysis. Look for signs of arterial solution distribution. Where fluid is lacking, manipulate the injection methods to encourage even distribution of the fluid throughout the body. Four questions need to be asked at this stage of embalming: (i) How much solution is needed? (ii) What should the strength of the solution be? (iii) Which areas of the body *are* and which *are not* receiving solution? (iv) When has the body or body areas received sufficient arterial solution?

10. After arterial injection, make an analysis of the body to determine if all areas have been perfused with sufficient arterial solution. If areas are lacking fluid, secondary points of injection can be injected. In addition, areas that cannot be reached by arterial injection can be embalmed using hypodermic injection and surface preservative techniques at this time.

11. Remove arterial tubes and drainage devices and dry and tightly suture incisions.

12. You can now aspirate the body. Some embalmers prefer to delay this process for several hours. Condition of the body helps to dictate whether cavity embalming should be done immediately after arterial injection or several hours later.

13. After aspiration, inject the cavities via the trocar with an undiluted cavity fluid. Size and condition of the body determine the amount of fluid to inject. For the average body, 32 to 48 ounces is generally satisfactory. After cavity fluid injection, close the openings(s) in the abdominal wall with a trocar button or by suture.

14. Remove any surgical drains and close the openings by suture. Remove all intravenous lines or products of other invasive procedures into the vascular system and seal any punctures. Remove a pacemaker if the body is to be cremated. Disinfect colostomy openings with a phenol solution and close by suture. Open, drain, disinfect, and suture any unhealed surgical incisions.

15. Rewash the hair and the body. Dry the body thoroughly, being certain to roll the body to one side so the back, shoulders, and buttocks areas can be dried. After washing and drying, apply surface glue to all sutured areas. At this time, check the mouth to be certain it is dry and free from any purge material. If there has been purge or blood in the oral cavity, this cotton should be replaced with dry cotton. Now, the mouth and the eyes can be glued. The anal orifice can be packed with cotton saturated with cavity fluid or autopsy gel. By delaying this treatment until this time, fecal matter will have had time to exit during the cavity embalming process.

16. If reaspiration of the cavities is to be performed it is usually done several hours after completion of the embalming.

17. Clean and fill the embalming machine with clean water. By filling the machine now, gases such as chlorine have time to escape prior to the next use of the machine. Instruments can be cleaned and all waste properly disposed.

18. Dress the body in plastic garments (pants, coveralls, stockings or a unionall) and place some embalming powder within the garment. If necessary, plastic stockings can also be used.

19. Cosmetic treatment will now follow.

Suggested Chronology for Embalming the Autopsied Adult Body

Employing Universal Precautions, the embalmer should be properly attired prior to any handling of the deceased. The embalming process needs to be documented using an embalming report. Notation in the report should be made of the type of autopsy performed; organs and tissues removed; and organs, tissues, and personal effects that are returned with the body.

1. Place the autopsied body on the center of the preparation table. Spray with a droplet surface disinfectant. Wash the body with a good liquid soap using warm water. Take care to remove blood stains from the autopsy. Pay particular attention to the hands and cleaning of the fingernails. The hair can be rinsed; however; because of the cranial autopsy, the hair will need rewashing after embalming.

2. Open the autopsy temporary sutures and aspirate any liquids that have accumulated within the cavities. Spray the inside walls of the cavities with a droplet disinfectant spray.

3. Examine the extent of the autopsy. If a partial autopsy has been performed the extent should

be evaluated. If the eyes have been removed the procedure for treatment can begin at this time. Rigor mortis can be relieved by flexing, bending, and massaging the limbs. This allows for a temporary positioning of the body.

4. Shave the facial hair.
5. Clean the oral cavity and replace dentures or, if they are not available, replace missing teeth or dentures with cotton or a "mouth former." The mouth can be held closed by needle injector wires or sutures. If the tongue has been removed, the oral cavity can be swabbed with a phenol cautery agent on cotton. The area can also be painted with autopsy gel.
6. Clean areas around the eyes. The eyes can be closed using cotton or an "eyecap."
7. Prepare the arterial solution. Strength and quantity depend on conditions of the body.
8. Raise the arteries that will be used to inject the legs. Place the arterial tubes into the arteries. Drainage will be taken by letting the drainage collect in the body cavities. Control over drainage may be obtained by using a hemostat clamped to the vein.
9. Inject the legs. Give attention to the distribution of the fluid. Increase pressure or rate of flow to establish uniform distribution. Areas not reached can be treated by hypodermic injection later.
10. Prepare the arteries that will be used to inject the arms—the subclavian arteries or the right and left axillary arteries. Drainage can be controlled by the use of a hemostat applied to the accompanying veins.
11. Inject the arms. Be certain good distribution is achieved through all the fingers. If distribution is not complete the radial or ulnar arteries can be raised and injected at this time.
12. Isolate and place arterial tubes into the right and left common carotid arteries. Inject the left side of the head *first*, then inject the right side of the face. Leakage from the internal carotid arteries in the base of the skull can be controlled with hemostats.
13. Prepare a strong solution. Diluted cavity fluid or a strong arterial solution can be used. With a small trocar inject the buttocks, trunk walls, shoulders, and back of the neck (any trunk areas where arterial fluid is absent or insufficient). All this can be done from within the cavities.
14. Aspirate and dry the cranial, abdominal, thoracic, and pelvic cavities. Coat the inside walls of the cavities with an autopsy gel. This gel should also be placed on the reflected scalp.

15. Fill the cavities with an absorbent sheeting that can also be soaked with cavity fluid. The neck areas can be filled with cotton or kapoc to achieve a natural look. If the viscera is being returned to the cavities the neck will have to be filled out with cotton or kapoc. Likewise, the pelvic cavity should be filled with cotton or kapoc. Place the bag containing the viscera into the cavities. A minimum of two bottles of concentrated cavity fluid should be poured into the bag over the viscera.*
16. Suture the abdominal and thoracic cavities closed. Use a strong linen thread. The baseball suture provides an airtight suture.
17. Anchor the calvarium into position. Suture the scalp closed beginning on the right side of the head and ending on the left. A worm suture helps to stretch the scalp tissue.
18. Wash the body and hair. The body and hair should be thoroughly dried and the body should be turned and dried underneath.
19. Apply a surface sealer to the autopsy sutures of the thorax and abdomen.
20. Glue the mouth and eyes.
21. Place the body in plastic garments. Place some embalming powder into the garments.
22. The body is now ready for cosmetic application and dressing.

KEY TERMS AND CONCEPTS FOR STUDY AND DISCUSSION

1. Define the following terms:
   Arterial embalming
   Cavity embalming
   Disinfection
   Embalming
   Hypodermic embalming
   Preservation
   Restoration
   Surface embalming
   Universal Precautions
2. Explain the OSHA formaldehyde standard.
3. With reference to your state laws and the FTC, explain how permission must be obtained for the embalming of the body.
4. Briefly outline the OSHA Hazard Communication Standard.
5. In your community what deaths must be reported to the coroner or medical examiner.
6. Outline the embalming of an unautopsied body.
7. Outline the embalming of an autopsied body.

*There are several types of visceral treatments.

8. What are the objectives of embalming?
9. Explain what the embalming process actually does to the body protein.

BIBLIOGRAPHY

Dhonau CO. *Manual of Case Analysis*. Cincinnati, OH: 1924.

Dodge AJ. *OSHA's Formaldehyde Rule*. Director, May, 1988.

Dodge AJ. OSHA's proposed bloodborne pathogen standard to include embalmers. *Dodge Mag.* 1989;81(4).

Hazard Communication Program. Milwaukee, WI: National Funeral Directors Association; April 1988.

Organ and Tissue Procurement Manual. Pittsburgh, PA: Pittsburgh Transplant Foundation; 1987.

Pervier NC. *Textbook of Chemistry for Embalmers*. Minneapolis: University of Minnesota; 1961.

Resource Manual. Milwaukee, WI: National Funeral Directors Association; 1979.

Rules and regulations. *Fed Regist.* 1982;47(No. 186): 42301–42302.

Vital Statistics Registration Manual State of Ohio. Columbus, OH: Department of Health, Division of Vital Statistics; 1978.

2

Professional Performance Standards

Professional performance standards originate from a diverse group of federal, state, local, international, association, and voluntary sources. State boards of embalmers and funeral directors set minimum standards that dictate such areas of practice as the preparation room; personal practices within the preparation room; equipment required; attire to be worn; and who may be present during the preparation of a body. Local and state boards of health have often set standards of preparation regarding bodies dying from highly contagious diseases or embalming standards to be followed for bodies where disposition will be delayed or internment will be in aboveground mausoleums. Regulatory agencies set minimum standards of practice when bodies have been treated with radioactive isotopes. Medical societies and colleges set standards of preparation for bodies that will be used in their anatomy dissection programs. Foreign governments have set standards regarding the preparation of bodies being shipped into their countries, in particular those having died from highly infectious and contagious diseases; their rules generally include regulations regarding the containers in which these bodies are shipped into their countries. In years past, individual states had health laws governing the preparation of bodies being shipped between the states. Airlines and other common carriers today still have regulations concerning the containers in which bodies are shipped between the states. The Department of Defense has standards for the preparation

of members of the armed services, both viewable and nonviewable remains. These standards are contained in the contracts that the various armed services award to independent contractors who are charged with the preparation of servicemen and women in the states and abroad. Through more recent governmental agencies such as the Occupational Safety and Health Administration (OSHA) and the Centers for Disease Control and Prevention (CDC), work practices within the preparation room have undergone many changes. An indirect set of standards for embalming comes through the educational process of the embalmer. Combined, all of these standards help to provide a safeguard for the immediate environment of the embalmer; protection for the safety and health of the general public; and a uniformity of the preparation of bodies anywhere in the United States. In this chapter, we look at two sets of professional performance standards. The first is a current voluntary standard arrived at through a combination of standards from the basic course content in embalming, research by those who supply embalming chemicals, and finally standards required by the governmental agency OSHA. The second set of standards, from the Department of Defense, were in place prior to OSHA, but these rules still give us an excellent performance protocol for dealing with the preparation of viewable and nonviewable remains.

Each course in a college of mortuary science employs a basic course content. Now overseen by various committees of the American Board of Funeral Service Education, the basic course content in embalming is a foundation for uniform performance standards in the preparation of all bodies embalmed in the United States. This basic course content also allows the Conference of Funeral Service Examining Boards to administer a uniform objective examination to those candidates for a license. As an introduction to this chapter we are going to take an overview of the development of the basic course content in embalming, as it lays the foundation for professional performance standards.

Mortuary colleges, as we know them today, are relatively recent in origin. The development of mortuary education has followed the general pattern common to all professional fields. It emerged slowly from a period in which knowledge was transmitted from preceptor to student by means of observation and informal discussion, to its present academic status.

Following the American Civil War, when funeral homes first came into existence, the pioneers in funeral service experimented with materials, equipment, and methods for their use. There were no channels for wide distribution of the knowledge they gained through trial and error. Training was conducted solely by means of apprenticeship.

As the scope of funeral service expanded and as embalming came into wider use, commercial companies were organized to supply the needs of the embalmer and funeral director. Research was directed to developing better products, and this resulted in a rapid increase in knowledge of what today is termed *mortuary science*. During the latter decades of the 19th century, the establishment of trade journals made possible a wider distribution of this knowledge. These same companies employed skilled lecturers and demonstrators to instruct funeral directors in the use of these products and in improved methods of embalming. These early "classes," lasting from a few hours to a few days, provided the first formal vocational instruction.

As the public health and welfare aspects of funeral service became more widely recognized, state licensing laws were established. For the first time educational requirements were formulated and a definite course of training was legally prescribed. At about this same time educators established the first schools of embalming to train students in a relatively new art. Over the years, these pioneers in mortuary education expanded and improved the scope of training, often keeping far ahead of requirements prescribed by law and by licensing authorities.

A system for national accreditation of mortuary schools was first introduced in 1927 by the Conference of Funeral Service Examining Boards, a national association of state licensing boards. Higher standards governing qualifications of faculty, the curriculum, and teaching facilities were established and enforced. Details of the development of mortuary schools can be found in Part II of this textbook.

The National Council on Mortuary Education was established in 1942 by the National Funeral Directors Association and the National Association of Embalming Schools and Colleges. After World War II, with the termination of restrictions on assembly, a formal meeting was held in December of 1945 in Cleveland, Ohio. Officers for the Council were Chairman, Ralph Millard; Vice-Chairman, Jacob Van't Hof; and Secretary-Treasurer, R. P. MacFate. The Council was attended by 62 school administrators, faculty members, state board authorities, and various funeral service association officers. The program committee comprised John Eckles, Jacob Van't Hof, and Otto Margolis. This meeting gave a fresh impetus to progress toward educational competence and professional status in funeral service. In March of 1947 the First National Teacher's Institute was held in Cincinnati, Ohio. Forty-four representatives from 14 schools met to lay the foundation for the course content in Chemistry and Mortuary Administration. Charles O. Dhonau of the Cincinnati College of Embalming presided over the meeting. In November of 1947 the Second Teacher's Institute was held in Pittsburgh, Pennsylvania (Fig. 2–1). More than 75 individuals from 23 schools and associations were present. At this meeting the first course content for the curriculum in embalming was drafted. The committee on the basic course content in embalming consisted of R. H. Hannum (Cleveland), L. G. Frederick (Dallas), R. Victor Landig (Houston), J. E. Shea (Boston), and E. L. Heidenreich (Wisconsin). The formulation and analysis of the embalming basic course content was brought about through the efforts of mortuary colleges, state boards, state associations, and the profession in general. The task was difficult because it meant resolving many individualistic teaching procedures into one common, sound educational basis. Once the basic course content was established it was immediately recognized there would be an imperative need to review and update the curriculum every few years. Revision of the course content has continued over the years and is currently overseen by the American Board of Funeral Service Education. In their July 1994 meeting in Denver, Colorado, a glossary of terminology was appended to the basic course content in embalming. In a meeting in Denver as late as July of 1995, the basic course content in embalming was again reviewed, amended, and prepared for editing and input by the member schools of the American Board of Funeral Service Education. This basic course content is an example of a professional performance standard in the field of embalming in America.

The first professional performance standard is a re-

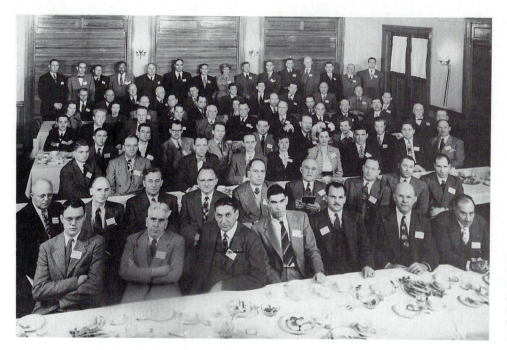

Figure 2–1. Educators from across the United States gathered for the Second Teachers Institute held in Pittsburgh, Pennsylvania, November 8 and 9, 1947. At this meeting the first curriculum in anatomy and embalming was established and the Mortician's Oath was adopted. *(Courtesy of the Pittsburgh Institute of Mortuary Science, Pittsburgh, Pennsylvania.)*

cent draft of minimum embalming standards drawn together from various sources. Primary drafters of this protocol were Gordon W. Rose, Ph.D., and Leandro Rendon, M.S. In the early 1970s, following the adoption of the Federal Trade Commission (FTC) Rule for Funeral Service, Rose and Rendon along with Robert N. Hockett began an in-depth investigation into the usefulness of embalming practices based on experimental data and confirmatory evaluations. Additional independent research was carried out by P. A. Burke and A. L. Scheffner of the Snell Laboratories. Their studies using available data, emphasizing those techniques and procedures that must be considered when establishing a set or profile of minimum standards for the practice of embalming, led to procedural recommendations based on laboratory evaluations that were realistic and defensible. By the late 1970s, several drafts of the performance standards had been published, demonstrating that by employment of proper embalming techniques, good preservation of the body could be established and effective sanitizing of the body could be accomplished.

In the summer of 1989 the Committee on Infectious Disease of the National Funeral Directors Association expanded the original Rendon and Rose document to include many of the work practice requirements of OSHA as they pertained to the embalmer. The document of *Public Health Precautionary Requirements and Standards—Funeral Service Practitioners* is an excellent

example of voluntary *embalming performance standards* or *minimum standards of practice*. In studying these practices it will be noted that there will be need to vary some of the recommendations. (For example, milder formaldehyde-based arterial solutions may be necessary to use at the start of the embalming process to clear blood discoloration and establish good vascular distribution of the arterial solution. Once this is accomplished stronger arterial solutions can be introduced.) Rendon states that "the voluntary adoption and profession-wide implementation of professional performance standards in embalming is a necessary first step to assure improved and standardized services to the public. The goal should be to make certain that when embalming is performed, a measure of uniformity of minimum professional skills is employed by all licensees. To achieve such a goal or set of goals, it is necessary to delineate those techniques and procedures that have been confirmed to be most effective. Such procedures should be adopted as the minimal standards to professional practice when embalming is to be performed." It is important to state that the minimum standards are just that—minimum. There will be individual situations where it will be necessary for the embalmer to modify practices to accomplish preservation and sanitation of the body and still achieve an appearance of the deceased acceptable for viewing by family and friends.

PUBLIC HEALTH PRECAUTIONARY REQUIREMENTS AND STANDARDS

I. Background

Prevention of the transmission of recognized classical and/or opportunistic pathogens from human remains to the embalmer, from the embalmer to his or her family, and to the families and friends of the deceased is a reasonable public health expectation.

Many of the infectious agents associated with medical and paramedical environments are classified as "opportunistic" pathogens or microbial agents considered to be of lower or reduced virulence. The increasing association of "opportunistic" pathogens with symptomatic infectious diseases has all but eliminated the reference to the category "nonpathogen."

The implementation of minimum professional practice standards in embalming is necessary to provide a standard of quality control and quality assurance in the preservation and disinfection of human remains. It is important that when embalming is performed, a significant measure of uniformity of professional skills will be employed by all funeral service practitioners.

Following somatic or functional death, normally structurally intact epithelial, facial, and other tissue barriers undergo a loss of structural integrity and permit the bodywide translocation and distribution of systemic microflora and create alternate body fluid and body tissue reservoir sites of host contamination.

During life, the body fluids or body secretions most frequently associated with the transmission of potentially infectious doses or densities are quite definable. After death, this is no longer true. All body fluids and body tissues may become reservoirs of infectious agents within a relatively short postmortem interval.

Cellular death may not be complete for up to 12 hours after somatic or functional death. During this postmortem interval, the viability and potential infectivity of bloodborne viruses, e.g., HIV and hepatitis B, may persist and the exiting of the agents from any body opening, natural or artificial, may occur.

Funeral service practitioners normally have more than casual contact with parenteral (including open wound) and mucous membrane exposure to blood and body tissues. Such individuals occupationally exposed to blood, body fluid, or tissues can be protected from the recognized risks of bloodborne agents such as HIV and HBV [hepatitis B virus] by imposing barriers in the form of engineering controls, work practices, in-service training, and protective equipment and attire.

II. Recommendations

It is recommended that every funeral service firm/facility in the United States adopt the following policies and guidelines for implementation: (1) public health guidelines; (2) personnel health precautions for the prevention of bloodborne microbial agent(s) and infections; (3) minimum standards for the embalming and disinfection of human remains. The recommendations and guidelines within each of the three categories described above are as follows.

1. Public Health Guidelines

A. Care of the Human Remains. Thoroughly cleanse and disinfect the body surface and natural or artificial body orifices/body openings with a suitable EPA-registered, hospital or health care facility-acceptable agent, e.g., tuberculocidal, germicidal detergent. The tuberculocidal germicidal detergent, e.g., a phenyl-phenol or a third-generation quaternary ammonium compound complex, should be an EPA-registered product offering confirmatory evidence of all label claims, including the recommended use dilution. The disinfected body surfaces should be thoroughly rinsed following a minimum of a 10-minute exposure interval.

Injection and drainage procedures should include (a) multisite injection and drainage procedures, (b) intermittent or restricted drainage, (c) the use of a 3.0% v/v formaldehyde-base arterial injection solution or a 2.0% glutaraldehyde-base solution, and (d) the use of 1 pint of concentrated cavity chemical per major or primary body cavity, e.g., abdominal, pelvic, and thoracic, or 1 pint of concentrated cavity chemical per 50 pounds of body weight.

B. The Embalmer (Universal Precautions). This category of barrier attire utilization and precautions has replaced the health care facility category of Blood and Body Fluid Precautions. The category requires the *minimum* barrier attire utilization of a whole body gown or apron and gloves. The wraparound, moisture-repellent or moistureproof gown or apron of rubber, plastic, or impregnated fabric is considered to be disposable or a single-use barrier attire item. The same is true for the gloves. Double rubber or plastic gloves are recommended for funeral service personnel (Figure 2–2).

This minimum standard of barrier attire protection is to be employed in the preparation of *all* human remains, no matter what the indicated cause of death reported. The risk of blood and body fluid exposure is significantly high for all funeral service personnel and frequently the infectious disease status of the deceased is unknown. Therefore, it is recommended that all persons performing postmortem procedures consider the use of additional barrier attire items such as protective eyewear, oral–nasal masks, and shoe and head covers.

Hands should be thoroughly scrubbed, using an EPA-registered* medicated liquid soap, before and after gloving. If a glove is penetrated by a sharp or the

---

*For example, *para*-Chloro-*meta*-xylenol (PCMX) or chlorhexidene gluconate (CHG) biocidal additive.

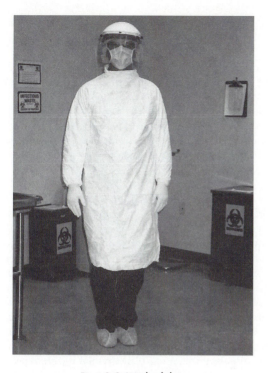

Figure 2–2. Attired embalmer.

uneven edge of a bone, the glove is to be removed and replaced as soon as possible.

All instruments employed during the embalming should be sterilized or disinfected prior to reuse. A high-level disinfecting liquid immersant may be employed in lieu of a steam sterilizer if the latter is not available. Chemical germicidal detergents registered with EPA as "cold chemical sterilants" can be used either for sterilization or for high-level disinfection, depending on the interval or contact.

C. Air Handling Within the Environment "at Risk". An efficient air supply and air exhaust system or an air purification system must be operative within the embalming environment. The air handling system should protect the embalmer from a hazardous airborne density of biologic particulates as well as from the accumulation of formaldehyde monomers exceeding 1.0 ppm, the permissible exposure limit or 8-hour time-weighted average (TWA) concentration. The TWA "action level" is 0.5 ppm of formaldehyde monomer concentration.

D. Terminal Disinfection and Decontamination. All instruments, horizontal surfaces such as floor, operating table, sink, and countertop, waste receptacles, and any other surface in direct or indirect contact with the preparation site must be cleansed and disinfected upon removal of the human remains from the preparation environment.

All instruments, including trocars and venous drainage tubes, must either be steam sterilized or immersed in a suitable cold chemical sterilant. Note: the

use of a hypochlorite, 1000 to 5000 ppm, may be used for the "spot" disinfection of body fluid spills on hard, nonporous surfaces. However, immediate rinsing is necessary to prevent the formation of BCME (bis-chloromethyl ether), a confirmed carcinogen, in the presence of formaldehyde monomers.

E. Solid Waste Management. Potentially infective, contaminated solid wastes associated with the preparation of human remains should be placed in "alert" colored plastic bags, e.g., red, the bag twist-closed and securely tied prior to ultimate disposition. Local codes permitting, bulk blood and suctioned/aspirated fluids may be carefully drained into the sanitary sewer system and vacuum breakers must be installed on all involved water lines to prevent the back-siphoning of contaminated liquids into potable water supply lines.

F. Hearse/First Call Vehicles. Cleanse and disinfect all mortuary cots or trays following exposure to the unembalmed human remains. Employ cleansed and disinfected cot or tray covers for each transfer of unembalmed human remains from the home or from the health care facility to the preparation room. Cleanse and sanitize the internal horizontal surfaces of the hearse/first call vehicle following the transfer of the remains to the preparation room.

G. Funeral Service Personnel Health Recommendations

1. Annual physical examination
2. Annual TB skin testing
3. Immunizations—annual influenza, single dose/single series Pneumovax, hepatitis B. Rubella vaccine is recommended for all women of pregnancy age if not protected and for all male employees because they can transmit to the female employee.

2. Personnel Health Precautions for Prevention of Bloodborne Agent(s) and Infections

A. Removal/Transfer of Human Remains

1. Removal personnel (licensees, resident trainees, nonlicensees, and nonresident trainees)—disposable whole-body barrier attire and plastic or rubber gloves.
2. Avoid contact with covering of remains at sites of body fluid or exudative contamination. Place the remains in an impervious plastic whole-body pouch and effect zipper closure.
3. Sanitize the transfer vehicle following the transfer of remains to the preparation room.

B. Transfer of the Remains to the Preparation Room, Using a Team of Two Employees. Transfer the pouched remains to the preparation room table, open pouch, and loosen body coverings. Allow the body coverings to fall into the pouch. Carefully position the remains from side to side for the careful removal of the pouch and contents. Dispose of the pouch and contents as contaminated solid wastes.

C. Terminal Disinfection

1. Disinfect all horizontal inanimate surfaces in direct or indirect contact with preparation site.
2. Sterilize or disinfect all instruments by cold chemical sterilizer immersion or by steam sterilization.
3. Remove all barrier attire items, place in plastic bag, and treat as contaminated solid wastes in terms of final disposition.
4. Scrub ungloved hands and wrists with a medicated liquid soap preparation, preferably one that is recommended as a health care personnel handwash.
5. Complete whole-body bathing or showering and shampooing prior to return to home or office.

3. Minimum Standards for the Embalming and Disinfection of Human Remains

The following professional profile of standards for embalming practices and procedures is based on laboratory evaluations and postembalming observations.

A. Multiple-Site Injection and Drainage. Multiple-site (two or more) injection and drainage procedures assure a more consistent distribution and ultimate diffusion of the disinfection and preservation chemicals to all receptive tissue sites, deep and superficial. This will more consistently provide public health protection as expected from the thorough preparation of human remains for ultimate disposition.

B. Rate of Flow of Arterial Injection Chemicals. A moderate rate of flow, 12 to 15 minutes per gallon of arterial injection solution, accompanied by a sufficient arterial injection pressure to maintain the desired rate of flow, 2 to 10 psi, are recommended for the assurance of distribution and diffusion of the arterial injection chemicals.

C. Intermittent or Restricted Drainage. This method of venous drainage should produce maximum preservation and disinfection. It is considered to be one of the most effective procedures for the assurance of adequate distribution of arterial injection solution(s). It is especially recommended following the removal of surface discolorations.

D. Total Volume of Arterial Injection Solution Employed. Consideration should be given to the use of a minimum of 3 to 4 gallons of arterial injection solution in adult remains weighing 125 to 175 pounds. Injection and drainage procedures may involve the removal of 4 to 6 quarts of body fluids. To properly restore the loss of body fluids and overcome the loss, through drainage, of arterial injection chemicals, it becomes necessary to employ the recommended volume of arterial injection solution, e.g., 1 gallon per 50 pounds

of body weight, exclusive of the primary injection solution(s) volume.

E. Use of Supplemental Injection Chemicals. The enhancement of the arterial distribution of the arterial injection solution may often require the use of supplemental additives, e.g., modifying and surface tension-reducing additives, water softeners, etc. The use of such additives may increase the efficacy of injection solution distribution as well as the efficacy of venous drainage.

F. Concentration (%) of Preservate/Disinfecting Chemicals in the Arterial Injection Solution. Laboratory investigative data indicate that the percent of formaldehyde v/v in the formaldehyde-base arterial injection solution should not be less than 2.0. Formaldehyde concentrations ranging from 2.3 to 3.0% v/v will inactivate resident bacterial densities 95% or more. Formaldehyde concentrations less than 2.0%, e.g., 1.0% v/v, may produce expected tissue fixation, but may not produce the desired level of microbial inactivation. Significant reduction in the endogenous microbial populations should always exceed 70% if public health expectations are to be fulfilled on a consistent basis.

Formaldehyde is categorized as an "intermediate" to a "high-level" chemical disinfectant when employed in concentrations ranging from 3.0 to 8.0% v/v. The recommended use of a minimum 2.0% v/v concentration of formaldehyde is based on this categorization as well as investigative data.

G. Cavity Chemical Utilization. Following the thorough treatment of the thoracic, abdominal, and pelvic cavities, including the aspiration of liquids and semisolids from nonautopsied remains, the injection of 1 pint (16 ounces) of undiluted cavity chemical into each of the three trocar-prepared cavities is recommended. In remains weighing in excess of 150 to 200 pounds, it is recommended that the embalmer use 1 pint of concentrated cavity chemical per 50 pounds of body weight. The weight of the body viscera may approximate 15% of the total body weight. The chemically targeted hollow and solid organ tissues require maximal chemical contact following the trocar penetration and separation to ensure the prevention of the microbial generation of putrefactive activity, including body opening purge.

III. Administration

The funeral home owner/manager/employer should establish formal policies and procedures to ensure that all job-related tasks that involve an inherent potential for mucous membrane or skin contact with blood, body fluids, or tissues, or a potential for spills or splashes of blood or body fluids, will require appropriate preventive/protective measures. These preventive measures would be applicable to licensed, nonlicensed, resident trainee, and nonresident trainee personnel. Engineering controls, work practices, and protective barrier attire are critical to minimize exposure to HBV, HIV, and other blood and body fluid transmitted microbial agents and to prevent infection(s). It is essential that the funeral home employee be fully aware of the reasons for the required preventive measures. Therefore, employee education programs must be implemented to assure familiarity with applicable work practices.

The employer should establish the following formal policies:

1. Develop and provide in-service training programs for all employees whose responsibilities include the direct or indirect exposure(s) to blood, body fluids, or tissues.
2. Document the attendance of employees at all scheduled and announced in-service training programs. The in-service training course content should include the approved Standard Operating Procedures (SOPs) for embalming practices and the required items of protective equipment and personnel barrier attire items.
3. Assure the convenient availability of all items of protective equipment and barrier attire items.
4. Surveillance of the workplace to ensure that the required work practices are being observed and that the protective barrier attire items and equipment are conveniently available and properly used.
5. Investigation of known or suspected parenteral exposures to body fluids or tissues to establish the conditions associated with the exposure and to improve training, work practices, or preventive equipment to prevent a recurrence.

IV. Training and Education

As recommended under the heading "Administration," the employer must establish an initial and periodic training program for all employees who may sustain direct or indirect exposure to blood, body fluids, or tissues. The employee must understand the following as a result of adequate in-service training:

1. Modes of transmission of HBV, HIV, and other blood and body fluid transmitted microbial agents.
2. The basis for the employment of the types of protective equipment and items of barrier attire.
3. The location of protective equipment and items of barrier attire, the procedures for the proper use of same and for the removal, decontamination, and disposition of contaminated barrier attire items or equipment.
4. The corrective actions necessary to disinfect blood and body fluid spills or splashes.
5. Concurrent and terminal disinfection and decontamination procedures. Disposable, puncture-resistant containers are to be employed for used needles, blades, etc.

V. Work Practices

1. Work practices should be developed on the assumption that all body fluids and tissues are infectious.
2. Provision must be made for the safe removal, handling, decontamination, and disposition of protective clothing items, equipment, soiled linens, etc.
3. Work practices and SOPs should provide guidance on procedures to follow in the event of spills or personal exposure to fluids or tissues.

VI. Personal Protective Equipment

A required minimum of choice of barrier attire items or protective equipment should be specified by the firm's SOPs. As more departments of public health require the reporting of infectious disease causes of death by category of precautions implemented by the health care facility, it becomes increasingly important for the funeral service firm to be aware of the infectious diseases included in a given category or patient isolation precautions. The following is a recommended listing of barrier attire items that should be employed for a reported category of health care patient isolation precautions:

Category-Specific Health Care Facility Precautions	Recommended Funeral Service Personnel Barrier Attire Precautions
1. Strict precautions	Masks (face covers), gowns, gloves (double plastic or rubber gloves are recommended), head covers, shoe covers, eye protectors
2. Contact precautions	Gowns, gloves, shoe covers
3. Respiratory precautions	Masks, gowns, gloves, head covers, shoe covers
4. Enteric precautions	Gowns, gloves, shoe covers
5. Blood and body fluid or **universal** precautions	Gowns, gloves, masks, head covers, shoe covers, eye protectors

VII. Medical

The employer should make available, at no cost to the employee, the voluntary HBV immunization for all employees whose responsibilities involve the direct or indirect exposure to blood, body fluids, or tissues. The employer should also provide for the monitoring, at the request of the employee, for HBV or HIV antibodies following known or suspected parenteral exposure to blood, body fluids, or tissues.

VIII. Record Keeping

The employer should require the completion of a case report for the preparation of all remains. Each case report should include (1) health care facility reporting of category of patient isolation precautions implemented, if applicable, (2) sites of injection and drainage employed, (3) volumes and concentrations of arterial injection and cavity treatment chemicals, (4) protective equipment and barrier attire items employed, (5) preembalming appearance and condition of the remains, and (6) any other observations or procedure relating to the public health status of the remains.

ARMED SERVICES SPECIFICATION CARE OF REMAINS OF DECEASED PERSONNEL

On September 15, 1979, a specification was published by the Department of Defense that establishes minimum standards for the care and handling of deceased personnel among the armed services. This is a uniform specification that is applicable to all branches of the military establishment. It became effective starting with fiscal year 1981. Complete preservation (embalming) and disinfection of remains and application of restorative art techniques and/or cosmetics are stressed.

5. Treatment of Remains

5.1. General: Frequently, final disposition of processed or re-processed remains may not be effected for a period of 10 days or more; may be transported over long distances; or be subjected to hot, humid conditions. At all times, the remains must be free of putrefaction and infectious agents. This requires the thorough disinfection and uniform preservation of all body tissues. Employment of continuous injection and intermittent drainage will enhance chemical distribution and penetration. Use of humectants (moisture retention chemicals) in the arterial injection solution will help to achieve greater tissue penetration, and to restore normal body moisture content.

5.1.1. Preembalming Procedures: The following basic steps shall be accomplished in the course of processing or re-processing of all viewable remains, and to the extent possible, nonviewable remains.

5.1.2. When possible, remains shall be bathed, male facial and scalp hair shall be washed and groomed . . . suitable hair preparations shall be accomplished on females. Fingernails shall be cleaned and trimmed. The mouth shall be securely closed to form a natural expression and proper attention given to the eyes to prevent wrinkling of the eyelids and a sunken appearance of the eyes. Cosmetics shall be applied only in the amount necessary to produce natural color and texture.

5.1.3. All lacerations, abrasions, incisions, excisions and burn wounds shall be sutured and/or sealed to prevent leakage. Swollen or distorted features shall be reduced to the normal contours enjoyed during life. Postmortem stains shall be chemically bleached by applying compresses and/or needle injection. On viewable areas, further treatment shall consist of the use of masking cosmetics to render stains nondetectable.

5.1.4. All body orifices shall be treated with a disinfectant, nonastringent chemical (generic categories such as phenylphenols and iodophors), and then packed with cotton. Bedsores, ulcerated, burned, and necrotic tissue shall be treated either by hypodermic injection, or pack application of deodorizing/preserving chemicals.

6. Preparation of Remains

6.1. General: The military services require that all remains be processed or reprocessed in a manner reflecting the highest standards of the funeral service profession. Each remains, viewable and nonviewable, requires variation in the embalming treatment to accomplish the optimum results. A recommended procedure to achieve these goals is the injection of the solution at a moderate rate. The addition of a humectant to the solutions is also helpful in reducing overdehydration effects.

6.1.1. Processing Nonviewable remains: In all instances, multisite injection and drainage technique shall be attempted. When arterial injection is possible, each gallon of arterial fluid shall have a minimum concentration of 5% by volume aldehyde or aldehyde derivative preservative agent(s). The total volume of arterial solution injected shall be not less than one gallon per 50 pounds of body weight. All body areas shall be further treated by means of a trocar using undiluted cavity chemicals having a 30 index (%) or greater. In addition, packs, special gel and/or dry sanitizers shall be used, as required, to assure preservation, prevent leakage, and eliminate all offensive odor. Cranial, thoracic, and abdominal cavities, when present, shall be relieved of gasses and distention. The cavities shall then be treated by injecting a minimum of 32 ounces of a concentrated cavity chemical, having a 30 index (%) or greater. When arterial injection and/or cavity treatment is impossible, all articulated and disarticulated anatomical portions shall be thoroughly disinfected and preserved via accessory chemical embalming techniques. Noninjectable intact remains and/or disarticulated anatomical portions shall be immersed or hypodermically injected with trocar and/or syringe and needle, using full strength cavity chemicals 30 index (%) or greater. Surface application of liquid, gel, or dry sanitizers and preservatives is also required to supplement primary needle and/or hypodermic injection techniques.

6.1.2. Processing Viewable Remains: A thorough preembalming case analysis shall be made in order to determine the best embalming techniques to be used to obtain optimum results. The technique of arterial injection and venous drainage is of utmost important as well as the need for adding humectants (moisture retention chemicals) to the arterial solution injected. Whenever possible, a six point arterial injection with multisite drainage shall be accomplished. The arterial chemical injection solution shall contain a 2 to 3% concentration, by volume, of aldehyde or aldehyde derivative preservative agent(s), with equal parts of a humectant chemical also being added to the injection solution. The thoracic, abdominal, and pelvic cavities shall be thoroughly aspirated and injected with full strength cavity chemicals having a 30 index (%) or greater, using a minimum of 16 ounces for each cavity. In addition, needle injections packs or other special treatment shall be accomplished, as required, to assure the preservation and disinfection of all body tissues including those associated with body cavities (organs). A lanolin-base (or comparable) massage cream shall be applied on the face and hands.

6.1.3. Autopsied Remains: If a partial or complete autopsy has been performed, a six point injection with multisite drainage shall be accomplished, using arterial chemical injection solutions as specified for processing viewable remains. Thoracic and abdominal walls shall be hypodermically injected using the same strength solution as injected arterially. On thoracic and/or abdominal autopsies, the viscera shall be removed and immersed in concentrated cavity chemical having a 30 index (%) or greater. When a cranial autopsy has been performed, the calvarium shall be replaced and securely stabilized. The scalp shall be replaced over the calvarium and neatly sutured to avoid an unnatural appearance and the hair shall be washed. The inner surfaces of the body cavities shall be given a liberal application of gel preservative, the organs replaced within the cavities in normal anatomical location and liberally covered with hardening compound.

6.1.4. Treatment of Scalp (Viewable Remains): When the scalp has been shaved because of medical treatment or surgery, processing or re-processing shall be accomplished as specified for viewable remains, after which the head shall then be wrapped with gauze or equivalent in a neat and professional manner.

6.1.5. Mutilated Hands Viewable Remains: When the hands are mutilated so that restoration is not possible, the hands shall be treated in a manner which shall render all tissue firm, dry, and thoroughly preserved. The hands will then be covered by either wrapping with gauze or equivalent in a neat and professional manner; or by placing surgical gloves on the hands followed by white (military) gloves.

6.1.6. Dressing Remains Including Intact Nonviewable: Remains shall be dressed in the clothing provided by the Contracting Officer. Nonviewable remains that cannot be dressed shall be wrapped in the rubber or polyethylene sheeting and blanket furnished by the Contracting Officer. Wrapping shall be accomplished as follows: A blanket, furnished by the Contracting Officer, shall be spread on the dressing table with opposing corners at the head and foot ends of the table. The blanket is then covered with a white cotton sheet followed by a sheet of polyethylene. Two strips of cotton are laid down the center of the plastic sheet and liberally sprinkled with hardening compound. The remains are then laid on the cotton strips, coated with hardening compound and covered with additional cotton strips. The polyethylene sheet is then wrapped around the remains. The white cotton sheet is then wrapped around the plastic sheathed remains followed by the blanket which shall have as few creases as possible, and be secured with large safety pins placed no more than eight inches apart.

6.1.7. Embalmer Evaluation: The embalmer (Contractor's Agent) processing or re-processing the remains shall critically evaluate the completed treatment to insure that any remains cared for under this contract are effectively disinfected, uniformly preserved and shall arrive at destination in a satisfactory condition. The Contracting Officer or designate will authorize delivery or shipment of remains when he is assured that the services and supplies furnished by the Contractor meet this specification. The Contractor shall state on a certificate (Preparation Room History) furnished by the Contracting Officer that the services and supplies meet this specification in its entirety.

7. Hygienic Practices

a. The Contractor shall employ protective, precautionary hygienic measures and techniques designed to accomplish concurrent and terminal disinfection and decontamination of the entire funeral service establishment of port of entry mortuary preparation room and shipping area environment. The application of appropriate in-use concentrations of chemical disinfectants (such as generic categories as phenylphenols or iodophors) to body surfaces and orifices, instruments, preparation room, floor, walls, and equipment surfaces and general sanitation of public visitation areas (as applicable) will help prevent the transmission of actual and potential pathogens to personnel.

b. Also recommended is the wearing of protective, surgical-type, oral–nasal masks designed to prevent the inhalation of infectious particles originating from the surface, orifices, and cavities of human remains.

The specification further requires that all supplies and technical procedures shall conform to standards and professional techniques acceptable to the funeral service industry. Arterial, cavity, and other embalming chemicals used in the treatment of all remains, under the specification, shall effect the maximum preservation and disinfection of all body tissue including those associated with body cavities (organs).

Any and all optional techniques available shall be used by embalmers to ensure complete and adequate treatment of remains.

Until this current specification was adopted, each branch of the military establishment had its own set of requirements for the care and handling of its deceased personnel. It is commendable that funeral licensees within the mortuary affairs programs of the Armed Services continue to update and upgrade professional responsibilities and obligations involved in serving the needs of the next of kin.

KEY CONCEPTS

1. Prepare a protocol for the pre-embalming sanitizing of the body after it has been transferred to the preparation table. (Include a protocol for clothing and jewelry.)
2. Prepare a protocol for the pre-embalming grooming.
3. What protocol of minimum standards would you require for your funeral or embalming establishment, in addition to those contained in this chapter?
4. Prepare a protocol for post-embalming grooming and cosmetic application.
5. Prepare a protocol to be followed by your establishment for the dressing and positioning of bodies within the casket.
6. Prepare a pre-embalming protocol for positioning of bodies.
7. Prepare a post-embalming protocol for the sanitizing of instruments, cleaning of the preparation room, and disposal of wastes.
8. Prepare a minimum standard protocol for attire to be worn by embalmers in the preparation room.
9. Prepare a minimum standard protocol of attire for persons doing cosmetics and hairdressing of an embalmed body.

BIBLIOGRAPHY

Armed Services specification care of remains of deceased personnel. In: *Champion Expanding Encyclopedia.* Springfield, OH: Champion Chemical Co.; 1980:No. 503.

First Annual Educational Conference in Casket and Sunnyside. New York, NY: The Casket; January 1946.

National Funeral Directors Association, Committee on Infectious Disease. *Summary of Guidelines Submitted to OSHA.* Milwaukee, WI: 1989.

Perspectives on embalming. In: *Champion Expanding Encyclopedia.* Springfield, OH: Champion Chemical Co; 1984:No. 552.

Public health guidelines. In: *Champion Expanding Encyclopedia.* Springfield, OH: Champion Chemical Co.; 1976:No. 465.

Rose GW, Rendon L. Embalming performance standards. In: *Champion Expanding Encyclopedia.* Springfield, OH: Champion Chemical Co.; 1989:No. 597.

Schools Stage First Teachers Institute in *Casket and Sunnyside.* New York; April 1947.

Twenty-Three Schools Represented at Second Teachers Institute. *American Funeral Director.* New York; Kates Boyleston Publications, Inc.; December 1947.

3

Environment and Personal Health Considerations

The art and the multidisciplinary science of embalming have historically encompassed the principles and practices of public health concern of preserving and disinfecting human remains. The epidemiological basis for this concern has been established and documented by several related studies.

The practitioner of embalming is professionally responsible of a *three-tiered spectrum:* (1) public health safety, (2) personal involvement dealing with the embalmer's immediate family, and (3) the community served by the embalmer.

The first level of responsible practice involves the maintenance of a work environment that is hygienically clean and safe. The embalmer must constantly be aware of the necessity for the use of (1) protective barrier attire, (2) disinfection and decontamination chemistry, and (3) practices and the identification of primary work environment reservoirs of actual and potential infectious disease hazards.

The "at risk" nature of preparing human remains for disposition demands the implementation of effective personal health and safety measures if funeral service is to offer acceptable standards of quality assurance and quality control. The community expects this.

FAULTY THEORIES

In recent years, critics of the practices of conventional and traditional funeralization involving embalming and in-state viewing have alleged that embalming is of little value in terms of accomplishing public health protection. Surprisingly, even individuals with educational and practical backgrounds in the physical and biological sciences argue that unembalmed remains are harmless and do not constitute reservoirs of classical or opportunistic pathogens. Several of the critics of embalming erroneously maintain that "germs die with the host," a most dangerous assumption on the part of anyone responsible for the handling and preparation of human remains.

An extensive review of literature pertinent to the public health hazards associated with human remains was conducted in 1968 by Maude R. Hinson,* a medical research librarian, and sponsored by the Embalming and Chemical Manufacturers Association. The review included abstracts of 88 bound references and 265 journal publications which repeatedly referred to the persistence and survival of pathogenic microbial agents in unem-

---

*See Selected Readings for the complete M. R. Hinson literature search.

balmed remains. The review also indicated that the absence of antemortem cellular and chemical body defense mechanisms contributes to increased virulence factors associated with postmortem microflora.

CONFIRMED STUDIES

Laboratory studies involving the postmortem microbiological evaluations of specimens procured from remains certified to have died from causes other than an infectious disease have confirmed that **unembalmed remains constitute an ideal environment for microbial growth and proliferation.**

The normally operative antemortem epithelial, fascial, and other tissue barriers which tend to maintain systemic and/or anatomic localization of host microflora during life may undergo:

1. Loss of structural integrity soon after somatic death. [This loss of structural, systemic compartmentalization of endogenous microflora characteristic of a given functional system (upper respiratory tract, genitourinary tract, gastrointestinal tract) contributes to the postmortem translocation and redistribution of host microflora on a hostwide basis.]
2. The reticuloendothelial system (RES), another nonselective barrier to antemortem translocation, contributes to the same phenomenon of microbial relocation after death.
3. The blood–brain barrier, an example of one of the antemortem anatomic defenses against microbial invasion of the central nervous system, becomes inoperative soon after death.

ENDOGENOUS INVASION

Endogenous invasion of cerebrospinal fluid by bacterial agents associated with the colon occurs within 4 to 6 hours of death. *The colon, designated as the postmortem origin of "indicator" organisms recovered from extraintestinal sampling sites, seems to be the primary source of many of the translocated microbial agents.* The isolation of "indicator" organisms as well as nonindicator organisms from such sampling sites as the left ventricle of the heart, the lungs, the urinary bladder, and the cisterna cerebellomedullaris indicates the extent to which microbial agents of low, moderate, and high virulence can translocate within a relatively brief postmortem interval of 4 to 8 hours.

The postmortem multiplication of systemic and translocated recoverable microbial agents may begin

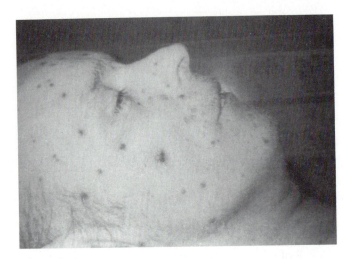

Figure 3–1. Secondary infection. Cause of death was listed as leukemia; however, the individual also exhibits the secondary infection of chicken pox.

within 4 hours of somatic death and reach peak densities of 3.0 to 3.5×10^6 organism per milliliter of body fluid or per gram of body tissue within a 24- to 30-hour postmortem interval.*

Postmortem factors contributing to the translocation of endogenous microflora include chemical and physical changes, movement and positional changes of the remains, passive recirculation of blood from contaminated body sites, thrombus fragmentation and relocation, and the inherent true mobility of many of the intestinal bacilli.

The relocated organisms may exit from body openings, natural and other, and become associated with adjacent animate and inanimate surfaces. They may also become airborne particulates in the form of aerosols (droplet infection particle) or dried particles (droplet nuclei) and constitute sources of body surface, either upper respiratory or other body site, contamination of living tissues.

LACK OF INFORMATION

A factor not to be ignored by the embalmer is the all too frequent lack of information related to deaths caused by reportable contagious or communicable infectious diseases. Throughout the United States there seems to be considerable inconsistency on the part of health care facilities (acute, general, and extended) to alert the receiving funeral director or funeral home that an infectious disease was the primary or a contributing cause of death (Fig. 3–1).

---

*See Selected Readings for the complete Rose and Hockett reprint.

those microbial agents measuring 5.0 to 100 micrometers in diameter.

(2) The air handling system should also prevent the accumulation of formaldehyde vapor and/or paraformaldehyde aerosol concentrations in the preparation room environment by creating a minimum of 6 air exchanges per hour. Formaldehyde concentrations exceeding 2.0 ppm constitute a potential health hazard to the embalmer. [See Fig. 3–2.]

4. **Terminal disinfection and decontamination**
   A. The Preparation Room
      (1) Cleanse and disinfect all instruments, the operating table surfaces, aspirating equipment and appurtenances, preparation room floor and wall surfaces, water faucet handles on sinks, door knobs, waste receptacles, etc. In cases of known or confirmed reportable infectious disease, contagious or communicable, and/or instances of gas gangrene, all instruments, including trocars and drainage tubes, should either be steam sterilized (autoclaved) or immersed in a suitable cold chemical sterilant, e.g., 2.0% acid–glutaraldehyde (Sonacide) or alkalinized (Cidex) glutaraldehyde, Bard–Parker solution (8.0% v/v formaldehyde in 70% ethanol or isopropanol), 400–500 ppm of an iodophor, 5000 ppm of hypochlorite solution, or other suitable disinfectant.
      (2) Incinerate all incinerable fabric or plastic body coverings, e.g., bandages, dressing, sheets, towels, or other patient-associated items placed in direct contact with the remains.
   B. The Funeral Coach/Service Vehicle(s)
      (1) Cleanse and sanitize the mortuary cot or

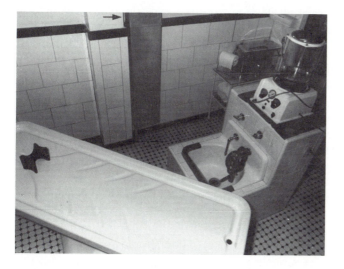

Figure 3–2. Note the exhaust duct aginst the back wall. It exhausts fumes from the floor level.

tray. Use freshly cleansed and sanitized cot or tray covers on each transfer of remains.

(2) Cleanse and sanitize the internal surfaces of the funeral coach/sanitize vehicle following each transfer of remains.
   C. The Embalmer(s)
      (1) Remove and dispose of gloves. Gloves are a single-use accessory and should not be considered reusable items. Scrub hands and forearms with a suitable medicated liquid soap or 200 ppm of an iodophor or other suitable germicide.
      (2) Shower-cleanse entire body surface, including the germicidal shampooing of the hair.

5. **General guidelines***
   A. Vacuum Breakers
      The potential hazards associated with biologic and chemical contaminants encountered within the preparation room environment must not be allowed to enter any network of plumbing cross-connections within the preparation room. Vacuum breakers must be installed in all involved water lines to prevent the back-siphoning of contaminated liquids into potable water supply lines.
   B. Physical Examination
      Funeral service personnel should receive a thorough medical/physical examination at least annually, and preferably biannually.
   C. Immunization
      Funeral service personnel should adhere to an effective program of preventive/prophylactic immunization schedules. All embalmers should follow the recommended booster periodicity for typhoid fever, influenza, tetanus, etc.
   D. Mantoux Skin Test for Tuberculosis
      All embalmers should be skin tested for tuberculosis on an annual basis until they convert from skin test negative to skin test positive. At the time of conversion, a chest x-ray should be performed. Thereafter, in the absence of symptoms, chest x-rays should be performed every two to three years.
   E. Rubella Vaccination
      All embalmers, male or female, should be vaccinated against German measles (rubella) if it is known that they do not possess protective antibody level against the virus. Women of pregnancy age may sustain a teratogenic effect from exposure to the virus during the first trimester of pregnancy; males may transmit the virus to susceptible females.
   F. Hepatitis B (Serum Hepatitis) Vaccination (Heptavax B)
      All embalmers not immune to hepatitis B should be vaccinated against it. Hepatitis B may be transmitted to the embalmer via any body

*See Selected Readings for complete CDC Universal Precautions.

fluid originating from the deceased victim of the viral disease. Embalmers sustaining accidental skin penetration during the preparation of a hepatitis A (infectious hepatitis) or hepatitis B (serum hepatitis) victim and are known to be susceptible, should promptly seek the administration of immunoglobulin (specific antibody preparations against the viral diseases).

G. Administration of Prophylactic Antibodies
   Embalmers involved in the preparation of known deaths related to bacterial meningitis (meningococcic meningitis) should contact a physician, clinic, or emergency center for the administration of preventive/prophylactic antibiotic(s).

H. Oral–Nasal Masks
   All embalmers involved in the preparations of known victims of systemic fungal infections, e.g., histoplasmosis, coccidioidomycosis, blastomycosis, or known victims of hepatitis B, AIDS (HIV), viral encephalitis, bacterial meningitis, etc., should always take the precaution of wearing an oral–nasal mask designed to entrap biologic particulates of minute diameters, 0.1 micrometer or greater.

At the present time, nearly 90% of clinical infections occur in four body sites: urinary tract, skin and subcutaneous tissue (wound), upper respiratory tract, and vascular system (bacteremia/septicemia). There are an increasing number of immunocompromised hosts whose susceptibility to infection may be two to three times greater than that of the average member of the community. The majority of infections originate from endogenous sources: hands, nasopharyngeal secretions, fomites, and the contaminated surfaces of preparation room equipment.

Airborne transmission may involve the etiologic agents of such infectious diseases as tuberculosis, whooping cough, measles, Legionnaires' disease, chicken pox, and fungal infections. Newly identified and recognized infectious agents and the mode(s) of transmission of the same can be anticipated. As the number of immunocompromised hosts, the "walking wounded," increases, the clinical presentations of infections and the causative agents involved will change. There will always be a constantly changing cast of microbial "actors" with new and different epidemiological costumery.

The best defense against the emergence of new pathogens and the environmental selection of increased microbial resistance to inactivation is to effectively interrupt the direct and indirect modes of transmission within the "at risk" environment.

The public health guidelines that should be a part of every funeral home's personal health policies should be accompanied by a set of minimum standards for the preparation of human remains for in-state viewing. The implementation of the following standards together with the previously listed public health guidelines will more consistently ensure the public health quality of our professional practices.

RECOMMENDED MINIMUM STANDARDS FOR THE EMBALMING OF HUMAN REMAINS

The voluntary adoption and implementation of minimum professional practice standards in embalming are a necessary first step in the provision of quality control and quality assurance in the preservation and disinfection of human remains. This is especially important in terms of providing more precise definitions of the public health values of embalming. It is to be highly recommended that when embalming is performed, a measure of uniformity of minimum professional skills be employed by all practitioners. The experimental studies completed to date confirm that **embalming is effective when the commercially available embalming chemicals are used in proper concentrations and in adequate total volumes, and are administered under conditions of proper techniques.**

The following professional profile of minimum standards of embalming practices is based on laboratory evaluations and postembalming observations.

Multiple-Site Injection and Drainage. Multiple-site (two or more) injection and drainage methodology ensures a more consistent distribution of the disinfection and preservation chemical solutions to all receptive tissue areas, both deep and superficial. Maximal chemical perfusion of receptive tissues is necessary to ensure the effectiveness of embalming. This more consistently provides the public health protection expected and eliminates any environmental impact hazards in earth interment.

Rate of Flow of Arterial Injection Chemicals. A moderate rate of flow (10–15 minutes per gallon) and sufficient injection pressure to maintain the moderate rate of flow (2–10 psi) are companion recommendations for the assurance of distribution and diffusion of the injection chemicals. Occasionally, it may be necessary to initiate and to maintain drainage. These conditions may be applicable to the first gallon of injection solution only, after which the moderate conditions should be employed. The injection pressure(s) should exceed vascular resistance and create moderate movement of the injection solution. Injection pressure(s) and rate(s) of flow should not, however, cause excessive short circuiting and loss of the injection solution or undesirable tissue distortion.

Use of Intermittent (Restricted) Drainage. One of the most effective methods of ensuring adequate distribution of the arterial injection solution is the use of intermittent drainage. It is especially recommended after surface discoloration has been removed, for example, after the first gallon of arterial injection solution has been injected. If proper drainage has been accomplished, this technique will not impede further drainage. Solutions under pressure tend to follow routes of least resistance. This method should produce maximum preservation and disinfection effects from the injected chemicals.

Total Volume of Arterial/Injection Solution Employed. Consideration should be given to employing a minimum of 3 to 4 gallons of arterial injection solution for the average adult weighing from 125 to 175 pounds. Injection and drainage techniques may involve the removal of 4 to 6 quarts of blood and body fluids. To properly restore the loss of body fluids and overcome the loss of preservative and disinfecting arterial injecting chemicals, especially in the use of continuous drainage, it is necessary to employ the total injection solution volume of 3 to 4 gallons, for example, 1 gallon per 50 pounds of body weight, exclusive of primary injection solution(s).* (By today's standards this rule would be better to read: inject 1 gallon of properly prepared arterial solution for every 40 pounds of body weight.)

Use of Supplemental Chemicals. The enhancement of the distribution of the injected disinfectant/preservative solution may often require the use of supplemental chemicals, for example, modifying and surface-active additives, primary injection chemicals, and water conditioners. The use of such additives may increase the efficacy of injection solution distribution and drainage.

Concentration (Percent) of Preservative/Disinfectant in the Injection Solution. Data from extensive laboratory evaluations indicate that the concentration of formaldehyde preservative/disinfectant in the arterial injection solution should never be less than 2.0% v/v. Formaldehyde in concentrations ranging from 2.3% to 3.0% v/v inactivates existing bacterial populations in excess of 95%. It is known that formaldehyde concentrations less than 2.0 to 3.0%

may produce tissue fixation, but may not reduce microbial densities (microbicidal effect) by more than 50%. Significant reductions should be a minimum of 70% or greater. Formaldehyde is classified as a "high-level" disinfectant when used in concentrations of 3.0 to 8.0% v/v. The recommended use of a 2.0% v/v concentration of formaldehyde in arterial injection solutions, and preferably a 3.0% v/v concentration, is based on investigative documentation.[†] It may be necessary to begin arterial fluid injections using a 1.25 to 1.50% v/v concentration for the first gallon or, often, until all intravascular discolorations are cleared and fluid is distributed through most body areas. The solution strengths can then be increased to 2.0 to 3.0% strength. Use of restricted cervical injection may also be necessary. This would allow for injection of the stronger arterial solutions into the trunk areas and the use of a milder arterial solution for the head and facial tissues. This may be necessary because many arterial fluids would produce too much facial dehydration when used at a 2.0 to 3.0% v/v concentration, and it may be difficult with some fluids to establish good distribution.

Use of Cavity Treatment Chemicals. Thorough and adequate treatment of the thoracic, abdominal, and pelvic cavities should include the aspiration of liquids and semisolids that can be aspirated from the nonautopsied remains and the injection of 1 pint (16 ounces) of concentrated cavity chemical into *each of the major cavities*. When body weight exceeds 200 pounds, it is recommended that the embalmer use 1 pint of concentrated cavity chemical per 50 pounds of body weight. The cavity treatment techniques employed should ensure maximal tissue contact as a result of pretreatment trocar separation and perforation of all organs in each of the three primary body cavities.

PERFORMANCE PROCEDURES

The preceding minimum standards of performance include disinfection and decontamination procedures that are important to the public health protection of the embalming practitioner, that is, concurrent disinfection of the remains, gloved hands of the embalmer, and all adjacent contact surfaces and the terminal disinfection of these and other direct and indirect contact sites in the preparation room.

---

*Preinjection fluids are those fluid formulations and compositions whose primary purpose of injection into the vascular system is vascular preparation. **Arterial fluids** are those compositions and fluid formulations whose primary purpose after injection into the vascular system is the preservation and disinfection of tissue. Herein, those concentrations are expressed in formaldehyde concentrations by volume as follows: low concentration—up to 1% formaldehyde; moderate concentration—1% to 2% formaldehyde; high concentration—2% formaldehyde or above. **Coinjection fluids** are those compositions and fluid formulations whose primary purpose is to accompany, supplement, and enhance the action of the other two fluids.

---

†It would take 12.8 ounces (or 13 ounces) of a 20-index fluid to make 1 gallon of a 2% solution or 18.7 ounces of a 20-index fluid to make a 3% solution. With a 30-index fluid, 8.5 ounces would be needed for a 2% solution or 12.5 ounces of concentrated fluid to make 1 gallon of 3% solution.

All items of attire, soiled clothing, health care gowns or pajamas, and postsurgical or skin and subcutaneous wound dressings should be immersed in a disinfectant solution or steam sterilized (autoclaved). Incineration of these items is no longer permitted.

The body surfaces of the remains should always be cleansed and sanitized and the body orifices treated with an appropriate disinfectant and packed with cotton previously saturated with disinfectant. Contaminated disposable items may be placed in a waste receptacle lined with an impervious, autoclavable plastic bag. The plastic bag with contaminated contents should not be transferred from the preparation room to a site of disposition until steam sterilization has been completed.

A professional framework of practical and reasonable minimum standards for the practice of embalming will contribute significantly to the accomplishment of our public health goals and obligations.

The recommended set of minimum standards for the preservation and disinfection of human remains should, when implemented, enhance the distribution of the arterial injection chemicals throughout the entire cardiovascular system. Protocols include (1) multisite injection and drainage, (2) restricted drainage, (3) adequate total volume of injection solution, and (4) the use of supplemental chemicals. The structural mediator of the delivery of the injection chemicals to receptive tissue sites is the fundamental and simplest division of the blood vascular system, the capillary. In this sense, arterial embalming might be referred to as *capillary embalming*. These simple endothelial tubes with an average diameter of 7 to 9 micrometers connect the terminal arterioles and the venules.

The surface area of the capillary network in the human body approaches 6000 square meters or 64,585 square feet. This vast membrane of over 1.5 acres is the permeable barrier that controls the delivery of preserving and disinfecting chemicals to deep and superficial body tissues. The closed circulatory system of humans normally contains 5 to 6 quarts of blood, 8.0% of the body weight, 85% of which is contained within the capillaries. Obviously, thorough perfusion of the soft tissue sites with appropriate concentrations of injection chemicals involves far more than filling the aorta and its primary branches. The long-term preservation and disinfection of human remains require the embalmer to use such standards of technique as to effectively transform routine "injection" into "capillary embalming."

RISKS OF INFECTION

Most embalmers, pathologists, and epidemiologists readily agree that human remains constitute an "at risk" reservoir of infectious agents and pose a continuing occupational health hazard. Although the public health significance of embalming has been adequately documented, recorded public health statistics confirming the high incidence of infections among embalmers are minimal. The lack of such confirmatory vital statistics has, unfortunately, discouraged appropriate recognition of embalming as a public health function and the "at risk" role of the embalmer by public health agencies–local, state, and national.

The increasing incidence of herpes simplex virus, hepatitis B virus, and the HIV or AIDS virus infections has caused many public agencies to reevaluate the potential infectious disease risks assumed by morticians, e.g., the Office of Biosafety, Centers for Disease Control, Atlanta, Georgia. Morticians, pathologists and anatomists are often unknowingly exposed to hepatitis B because the virus may remain dormant in carriers. Further, the hepatitis B virus in serum or plasma may be transmitted indirectly via inanimate environmental surfaces.

VIRAL HEPATITIS

Type	Transmission
Hepatitis A	Fecal–oral (enteric)
Hepatitis B	Parenteral (bloodborne) and sexual
Hepatitis C	Parenteral and sexual
Delta hepatitis	Parenteral and sexual
Hepatitis E	Fecal–oral
Non-A, non-E enterically transmitted	Fecal–oral
Non-A, non-E parenterally transmitted	Parenteral

The author is aware of a service embalmer who was hospitalized for hepatitis B and died. The postmortem diagnosis was infectious jaundice or leptospirosis, a spirochetal infection against which there are effective therapeutic antibiotics. In this instance, misdiagnosis needlessly took the life of an embalmer who sustained a needle penetration of the skin during embalming. Although the incidence of tuberculosis has declined in the United States, a study of 129 cases in which tuberculosis was considered to be the primary cause of death indicated that diagnosis did not occur until autopsy in 33% of the cases. Such retrospective diagnoses tend to underline the potential for transmission of infectious disease to the embalmer.

SANITATION SURVEY

A sanitation survey involving more than 2000 responding mortuary science licensees was conducted by the

Champion Chemical Company in 1975. More than 18% of the respondents indicated that they had sustained **one or more** serious infections during their careers in the funeral service profession.

Tuberculosis (14%), viral upper respiratory infections (44%), infectious hepatitis (13%), fungal infections (19%), bacterial septicemias (17%), and bacterial wound infections (14%) were the most frequently reported funeral service-associated infections. The incidence of infectious disease among funeral service licensees was two to three times higher than the incidence in the general population. The incidence of tuberculosis, infectious hepatitis, and fungal infections among pathologists is approximately 16%, slightly above the incidence associated with funeral service practitioners. The higher incidence in the funeral service profession may well be indicative of careless and/or negligent practices employed in the preparation of human remains.

Table 3–1 summarizes the basis for the protective measures recommended in the section entitled Public Health Guidelines. Methods of chemical and physical decontamination must be employed to eliminate "reservoirs" or infectious agents and to prepare preparation room surfaces, instruments, and equipment hygienically safe for reuse and the reexposure of the embalmer–host.

TABLE 3–1. BREAKING THE CYCLE OF TRANSMISSION OF INFECTIOUS AGENTS IN THE PREPARATION ROOM: PUBLIC HEALTH GUIDELINES FOR THE AT-RISK EMBALMER "HOST"

Portal of "Host" Entry	Infectious Agent
Skin or mucous membrane respiratory tract, alimentary tract, body openings—natural and/or artificial (abrasions, cuts, lacerations, wounds)	Bacteria, fungi (molds and yeasts), viruses, rickettsia, protozoa
Proper "barrier" attire	Personal health practices
Aseptic technique(s)	Personnel health policies
Handwashing, gloves	Environmental sanitation
Disinfection and decontamination	Disinfection and decontamination

Modes of Transmitting the Infectious Agent	Reservoirs of Infectious Agents in the Preparation Room
Direct contact (aerosol or droplet infection) and indirect contact (air, contaminated surfaces) and objects or fomites, body fluids and exudates, insects	Remains, equipment (e.g., hydroaspirators, trocars, razors), instruments, adjacent hard surfaces, air contaminated linens, bandages and dressings, solid and liquid wastes
Proper "barrier" attire	
Handwashing, gloves	
Proper disposition of wastes	
Effective air handling system	
Concurrent and terminal disinfection	

Note: Proper "barrier" attire may include whole-body covering, head cover, shoe covers, gloves, oral–nasal mask, and eye protection (safety glasses).

Chemical and physical decontamination is a very important weapon in the fight against infectious diseases, especially in environments exposed to a multitude of actual and potential pathogens. It should be emphasized that chemical and physical disinfection is no substitute for good housekeeping and practical cleaning procedures. The following terms are applicable to the function of environmental control, using methods of disinfection and sterilization:

Asepsis	Freedom from infection and from any form of life—sterility
Bactericidal	Destructive to bacteria
Bacteriostatic	Inhibiting the growth or multiplication of bacteria (no destruction of viability implied)
Cleaning	Removal of infectious agents by scrubbing and washing, as with hot water, soap, or suitable detergent
Disinfectant	An agent, usually chemical, applied to **inanimate** objects/surfaces for the purpose of destroying disease causing microbial agents, but usually not bacterial spores
Germicide	An agent, usually chemical, applied either to inanimate objects/surfaces **or living tissues** for the purpose of destroying disease-causing microbial agents, but usually not bacterial spores
Sanitizer	An agent, usually chemical, that possesses disinfecting properties when applied to a precleaned object/surface
Sterilization	A process that renders a substance free of all microorganisms

Primary disinfection is the application of disinfection and decontamination measures prior to embalming. **Concurrent disinfection** is the application of disinfection and decontamination measures during embalming of the body. **Terminal disinfection** is the application of disinfection and decontamination measures after completion of the preparation of the remains. Primary, concurrent, and terminal disinfection require the application of physical and chemical methods for the control of microbial contamination (Table 3–2).

"High," "intermediate," and "low" levels of antimicrobial activity are recognized for the proper disinfection of critical, semicritical, and noncritical environments and objects. As seen in Table 3–3, an essential property of a **high-level disinfectant** is effectiveness against bacterial spores; suitable reagents include aqueous 2.0% glutaraldehyde, 8.0% formaldehyde solution in 70.0% alcohol, 6.0 to 10.0% stabilized hydrogen peroxide, and ethylene oxide gas.

TABLE 3–2. CHEMICAL AND PHYSICAL METHODS FOR CONTROLLING MICROBIAL CONTAMINATION

Method of Decontamination	Temperature Requirement	Minimum Interval of Exposure (min)
		0 2 10 12 15 20 90 120 150 180
Sterilization: Complete destruction of all forms of microbial life	285°F (140°C)	⊢—⊣ (instant)
Saturated steam under pressure (autoclaving)	270°F (132°C)	⊢—⊣
	250°F (121°C)	⊢———⊣ 30 min for hepatitis viruses
Ethylene oxide gas	130°F (54°C)	2 to 12 h
Hot air, e.g., oven	320°F (160°C)	2 h or more or more
Chemical sporicide solution, e.g., 8.0% formaldehyde plus 70% isopropanol, glutaraldehyde[a]	Room temperature	3 to 12 h or more
Disinfection: killing of disease-producing microbial agents, but not resistant spores		
Boiling water or free-flowing steam	212°F (100°C)	⊢—⊣ or more, 30 min for hepatitis viruses
Chemical germicide solutions, e.g., iodophors, phenylphenols, quarternary ammonium compounds	Room temperature	⊢———⊣ or more
Sanitization: Chemicals aided by physical methods of soil removal	Maximum of 200°F (93°C)	⊢————⊣

[a]Recommended for high-level disinfection.
Modified from a chart copyrighted in 1967, Research and Development Section, American Sterilizer Co., Erie, PA.

Intermediate-level disinfectants do not necessarily kill large numbers of bacterial spores in a relatively short time, but they do inactivate the tubercle bacillus. These disinfectants are also effective against fungi as well as lipid and nonlipid medium-size and small viruses; examples include 0.5% iodine, 70 to 90% ethanol and isopropanol, chlorine compounds (free chlorine as derived from sodium or calcium hypochlorite), and some phenolic ("tamed" phenols) and iodophor-based disinfectants.

Low-level disinfectants cannot be relied on to destroy bacterial spores, the tubercle bacillus, or small nonlipid viruses. These disinfectants, such as quaternary ammonium compounds and mercurials, may be useful in actual practice because they can rapidly kill vegetative forms of bacteria and fungi as well as medium-size lipid-containing viruses. The disinfecting levels of iodophors ("tamed" iodines) and phenolic compounds may be classified as intermediate or low depending on the concentration employed (Table 3–4).

Noncritical items within the preparation room environment may include walls, floors, and furnishings.

Many embalmers rely on low-level disinfectants for application to such surfaces, used either alone or in addition to cleansing with detergent systems.

Blood, mucus, or feces, when present on items to be disinfected, may contribute to the failure of a given disinfectant or sterilization procedure. The organic contamination may occlude microbial agents and prevent penetration of the disinfection chemical(s). Or, the organic material may directly and rapidly inactivate certain disinfection chemicals such as chlorine- and iodine-based disinfectants and quaternary ammonium compounds.

TABLE 3–3. LEVELS OF DISINFECTION ACTIVITY

Level of Activity	Bacteria		Fungi	Viruses	
	Vegetative	Tubercle Bacillus	Spores	Lipid and Medium size	Nonlipid and Small
High	+	+	+	+	+ +
Intermediate	+	+	−	+	+ +
Low	+	−	−	+	+ −

+, Positive microbicidal effect; −, negative microbicidal effect.
From Block SS: *Disinfection, Sterilization, and Preservation.* 3rd ed. Philadelphia: Lea & Febiger; 1983, with permission.

TABLE 3–4. ACTIVITY LEVELS OF SELECTED MICROBICIDES

Liquid Microbicide[a]	Use Concentration	Activity Level
Glutaraldehyde, aqueous, e.g., Cidex, Sonacide, Sporicidin	2.0%	High
Formaldehyde + alcohol	8.0% + 70.0%	High
Stabilized hydrogen peroxide	6.0%–10.0%	High
Formaldehyde, aqueous	3.0%–8.0%	High to intermediate
Iodophors, e.g., Betadine, Wescodyne, HiSine, Iosan	75–200 ppm	Intermediate
Iodine + alcohol	0.5% + 70.0%	Intermediate
Chlorine compounds, e.g., sodium hypochlorite as in chlorine bleach	1000–5000 ppm	Intermediate
Phenolic compounds, aqueous, e.g., Amphyl Staphene, O-Syl	0.5–3.0%	Intermediate to low
Quaternary ammonium compunds, e.g., Phemoral, Zepharin Chloride, Diaparine Chloride	0.1–0.2% aqueous	Low
Mercurial compounds, organic and inorganic, e.g., Merthiolate, Mercurochrome, Metaphen	0.1–0.2%	Low

[a]Trade names of certain microbicides are given.
From Block SS: *Disinfection, Sterilization, and Preservation.* 3rd ed. Philadelphia: Lea & Febiger; 1983, with permission.

TABLE 3–5. ACCEPTABLE ANTIMICROBIAL PROCEDURES/EXPOSURE INTERVALS

Objects	Vegetative Bacteria and Fungi, Influenza Viruses Disinfection	Tubercle Bacilli, Enteroviruses Except Hepatitis Viruses, Vegetative Bacteria and Fungi, Influenza Viruses Disinfection	Bacterial and Fungal Spores, Hepatitis Viruses, Tubercle Bacilli, Enteroviruses, Vegetative Bacteria and Fungi, Influenza Viruses Sterilization
Smooth, hard surface objects	A —10 min D— 5 min E —10 min F —10 min H —10 min L — 5 min M— 5 min	B —10 min D —10 min G —10 min H —10 min L —10 min M —10 min	D —18 h J K L — 9 h M —10 h
Rubber tubing, rubber catheters	E —10 min F —10 min H —10 min	G —10 min H —10 min	J[a] K
Polyethylene tubing, polyethylene catheters	A —10 min E —10 min F —10 min H —10 min	B —10 min G —10 min H —10 min	D —18 h J[a] K L — 9 h M —10 h
Lensed instruments	E —10 min F —10 min H —10 min K M —10 min	K M —10 min	K
Hypodermic needles	Sterilization only	Sterilization only	J
Thermometers[b]	C —10 min K	C —10 min K	D —18 h L — 9 h M —10 h
Hinged instruments	A —20 min D —10 min E —20 min F —20 min H —20 min L —10 min M —10 min	B —30 min D —20 min G —30 min H —30 min L —20 min M —20 min	J K L — 9 h M —10 h
Floors, furniture, other appropriate room surfaces	E — 5 min F — 5 min H — 5 min I — 5 min	G — 5 min H — 5 min	Not necessary or practical

Key

A. Isopropyl alcohol (70–90%) plus 0.2% sodium nitrite to prevent corrosion

B. Ethyl alcohol (70–90%)

C. Isopropyl or ethyl alcohol plus 0.2% iodine

D. Formaldehyde (8%)–alcohol solution plus 0.2% sodium nitrite to prevent corrosion

E. Quaternary ammonium solutions (1 : 500 aq.) plus 0.2% sodium nitrite to prevent corrosion

F. Iodophor—75 ppm available iodine plus 0.2 sodium nitrite to prevent corrosion

G. Iodophor—450 ppm available iodine plus 0.2% sodium nitrite to prevent corrosion

H. Phenolic solutions (2% aq.) plus 0.5% sodium bicarbonate to prevent corrosion

I. Sodium hypochlorite (1 : 500 aq.—approx. 100 ppm)[a]

J. Heat sterilization } see manufacturers' recommendations

K. Ethylene oxide gas } or technical literature

L. Aqueous formalin (40%)

M. Activated glutaraldehyde (2% aq.)

[a]Investigate thermostability when indicated.

[b]Must be thoroughly wiped, preferably with tincture of soap, before disinfection or sterilization. Alcohol–iodine solution will remove markings on poor-grade thermometers.

Note: 1000 ppm of available chlorine is recommended for inactivation of hepatitis B virus and 5000 ppm for inactivation of HIV (AIDS). Thoroughly rinse all inanimate surfaces of any excess formalin prior to application of the hypochlorite disinfectant. Keene (1973) cautions that when formaldehyde reacts with hydrochloric acid, the compound bischloromethyl ether (BCME) may be formed. BCME is a highly toxic, carcinogenic compound.

This effect is correspondingly greater with weak concentrations and with low-level disinfectants than with strong concentrations and high-level disinfectants.

This emphasizes the necessity of thoroughly cleansing contaminated instruments such as trocars, hydroaspirators, and forceps prior to chemical disinfection. In fact, physical cleaning may be the most important step in a disinfection process, which, by definition, does not include the possible "overkill" factor of a sterilization procedure.

The chemical agents listed in Table 3–4 are categorized by type rather than by specific formulation. Whenever there is a choice between "cold" chemical sterilization (high-level activity) and sterilization by heat (autoclaving), the latter is preferable.

Specific recommendations, grouped by types of objects to be disinfected or sterilized, are presented in Table 3–5. The numbers designate the specific procedures that are acceptable in each situation; the key to the numbers is given at the bottom of the table; exposure times for each situation are included. It should be noted that certain chemical agents tend to cause some materials to corrode or rust; recommendations for prevention of corrosion are footnoted below the table.

CONCLUSION

The dictates of logic, reason, and research all demand that the dead human body be considered a source of pathogenic microorganisms. Embalmers are charged by the same dictates and by law with the responsibility to implement protective and thorough procedures to ensure that the potential for contagion through exposure to the body is minimized. This chapter has presented a set of public health guidelines and minimum standards that if followed by the embalmer, will accomplish this objective.

KEY TERMS AND CONCEPTS FOR STUDY AND DISCUSSION

1. Define the following terms:
   Capillary embalming
   Cisterna cerebellomedullaris
   Concurrent disinfection
   Disinfectant
   Droplet nucleus
   Germicide
   Iodophor
   Opportunistic pathogens
   Primary disinfection
   Protective barrier attire
   Terminal disinfection
   Translocation

2. At what concentration do airborne formaldehyde monomers constitute a potential health hazard to the embalmer?
3. Bacterial spores require high-level disinfectants for effective treatment. Name two other microbial agents of current public health importance that also require this level of activity for proper treatment.
4. What is the incidence of infectious diseases among funeral service personnel compared with the (a) general population and (b) pathologists?
5. Tuberculosis is an airborne respiratory infection. How is it possible for an embalmer to contract tuberculosis from human remains via the respiratory route of transmission?
6. Several critics of embalming maintain that "germs die with the host." Why is this an erroneous assumption?
7. Why are multiple-site injection and drainage preferable to single-site injection and drainage in the recommended minimum standard for embalming?
8. Specify three conditions that commercially available embalming chemicals must fulfill for the embalming process to be effective.
9. List the three areas of public health safety for which funeral service practitioners are professionally responsible.
10. Describe five methods for breaking the cycle of transmission of infectious agents in the preparation room.

BIBLIOGRAPHY

Benenson AS (ed). *Control of Communicable Diseases in Man.* 12th ed. Washington, DC: American Public Health Association; 1975.

Block SS. *Disinfection, Sterilization, and Preservation.* 3rd ed. Philadelphia: Lea & Febiger; 1983.

Burke PA, Sheffner AL. The antimicrobial activity of embalming and topical disinfectants on the microbial flora of human remains. *Health Lab Sci* 1976;13(2, October).

De Moulin GC, Paterson DG. Clinical relevance of postmortem microbiologic examination: A review. *Hum Pathol* 1985;16.

Finegold SM, Kirby WMM. Changing patterns of hospital infections: Implications for therapy. In: *Proceedings, 13th International Congress of Chemotherapy, Vienna, August 28 to September 2, 1983.*

Fuerst R. *Frobisher and Fuerst's Microbiology in Health and Disease.* 15th ed. Philadelphia: WB Saunders; 1983.

Hinson MR. *Final Report on Literature Search on the Infectious Nature of Dead Bodies for the Embalming Chemical Manufacturers Association.* Cambridge, MA: Embalming Chemical Manufacturers Association; 1968.

Hockett RN, Rendon L, Rose GW. In-use evaluation of glutaraldehyde as a preservative–disinfectant in embalming. In: *Abstracts of the Annual Meeting of the American Public Health Association.* Session 449, Contributed Papers: Microbiology–Immunology. Washington, DC: American Public Health Association; November 1973.

Isolation Techniques for Use in Hospitals. U.S. Department of Health, Education and Welfare, Public Health Service, DHEW Publication No. (HSM) 71-8043. Reprinted June 1973.

Junqueira LC, Carneiro. *Basic Histology.* 3rd ed. Los Altos, CA: Lange; 1980.

Keene BRT. *Chemistry in Britain,* Vol. 9, 1973.

McCurdy CW. *The Embalmer as Sanitarian: Embalming and Embalming Fluids.* Doctoral manuscript, University of Wooster, Wooster, OH; 1895.

Oviatt VR (Chief, Environmental Safety Branch, National Institutes of Health, Public Health Service, Bethesda, MD). Letter dated January 25, 1978.

Rose GW, Hockett RN. The microbiologic evaluation and enumeration of postmortem specimens from human remains. *Health Lab Sci* 1971;8(2, April):19.

Rose GW, Rendon L. Coping with the present and the future: Minimum standards for performance of embalming. In: *The National Reporter.* Evanston, IL: National Research and Information Center; 1979; vol 2, No. 9.

Rose GW, Wetzler TF. A public health view of embalming. In: *The Director.* Milwaukee, WI: National Funeral Directors Association; January 1969.

Sanitation survey results. In: *Champion Expanding Encyclopedia of Mortuary Practice.* No. 459. Springfield, OH: Champion Company; July–August 1975.

Teaching Outline for Occupational Safety and Health in the Funeral Service Profession. New York: Ad Hoc Committee, American Board of Funeral Service Education, Inc.; April 1977.

4

Technical Orientation of Embalming

Today's progressive, professional funeral home owner realizes that embalming is a vital, important part of the total service and that the preparation room is as important as any area in the building. Currently, most funeral service managers recognize that embalming is basic to present-day funeral practices and, therefore, believe that the preparation room should be given its fair and generous share of the operating and building budgets.

OBJECTIVES

The primary purpose of a well-designed and organized preparation room is to provide a safe and comfortable workplace. It should also be available to serve as a public relations tool if a community group wishes to tour the funeral establishment. Informational visitations need not stop with the opening of a new funeral home. Many organizations such as church groups and service clubs visit the funeral home and are gratified with the response and reactions they receive. A tour that does not include the preparation room can only serve to heighten unfounded suspicions and misconceptions concerning the embalming process.

In planning remodeling or new construction, emphasis should be placed on making the area functional and efficient. A layout that saves a few steps here and there can save many working hours in the course of a year. A door planned just barely wide enough to accommodate the removal cot can be a source of annoyance, inconvenience, and irritation long after the small extra cost of a slightly wider door is forgotten. Whether the owner/manager does his or her own embalming or hires a large staff, he or she naturally wants to provide a clean, comfortable, cheerful, and efficient workplace. If the workplace is unpleasant, unattractive, or inefficient, best efforts are not put forth in spite of good intentions. This psychology has been demonstrated repeatedly in classrooms, industrial plants, offices, and other work places.

HEALTH AND SAFETY STANDARDS

Today, with the abundance of scientific evidence on the infectious nature of the dead human body, and with the importance of embalming to protection of the public health, sanitation and ease of housekeeping should be major concerns in planning a preparation room. At one time, the simple installation of a sterilizer was all that was thought to be necessary. **A means of sterilizing instruments after each embalming is still essential in every preparation room,** but is far from the total answer. To fulfill professional obligations in this regard the embalmer must take other factors into account.

Funeral home facilities are governed by a variety of laws and regulations from federal, state, and local agencies because they are public places of business and employ workers in a workplace. A brief review of the major sources of regulations governing the preparation room environment follows, and throughout this chapter reference is made generally to standard requirements. Funeral service students learn many of the regulations governing employer/employee duties, responsibilities, and rights during the course of their funeral service education. Funeral home owners are advised to consult experts in the legal and construction fields to be certain that their facilities, planned or existing, conform to all local requirements.

SOURCES OF REGULATIONS

OSHA Requirements

The federal Occupational Safety and Health Administration (OSHA) prescribes in detail the physical and environmental requirements that employers must meet to provide a safe workplace. These requirements are enforced through workplace inspections, warnings, and citations. In the event of failure to correct continual noncompliance or serious violations, substantial fines are levied. A well-known example is the Hazard Communication Standard.

Lesser known requirements have to do with the necessity for an adjacent shower and locker facility, electrical grounding, ramp and stair-step angles and heights, and a host of other areas of concern to the worker. Caution should be exercised to be certain that **all** OSHA requirements are being met in the workplace.

Four areas of OSHA directly impact the funeral service practitioner: (1) OSHA General Rule, (2) Hazard Communication Standard, (3) Formaldehyde Standard, (4) Bloodborne Pathogen Standard.

"Right to Know" Laws

An emerging area of legislation on the local and state levels is "right to know" legislation. This is directed at employers and requires them to post information warning employees of chemical that may be hazardous or harmful to their health and well-being. Firms in locales that have enacted such legislation may have to meet these requirements as well as those of OSHA.

Building Permits

All construction of any magnitude requires that a building permit be obtained from local authorities. The application procedures usually require that detailed plans and specifications be submitted regarding plumbing, electrical, and other construction materials so as to ensure that all materials and construction meet certain minimum

standards. Although the materials and methods recommended in this chapter generally conform to most building code requirements, a competent architect, contractor, or both should be consulted prior to permit application in a particular locale.

State Codes and Local Ordinances

State boards of health and mortuary science have enacted regulations governing the minimum standards for preparation rooms. *Two examples demonstrate such minimum standards.* The State Board of Funeral Directors of Pennsylvania and the Board of Embalmers and Funeral Directors of Ohio have published the following rules and regulations dealing with the facilities and equipment requirements for the preparation or embalming room:

Pennsylvania

The preparation room shall be constructed solely for the purpose of scientifically preparing human remains and shall contain the following facilities and equipment for the purpose of preventing disease and properly disposing of waste material arising out of the embalming process:

1. A sink with running water and sewage connections and possessing a two-inch capacity drain pipe.
2. A metal or porcelain-covered operating or embalming table.
3. A metal cabinet or metal or glass shelves or a material impervious to water and stain.
4. A waste container with cover.
5. A first-aid kit placed in a conspicuous place.
6. Surgical instruments and apparatus for the preparation of embalming of a body. Aspirator must be a nonbackflow type or have a nonbackflow valve in the line.
7. Walls which are airtight and covered in their entirety by tile, plaster, composition board, or similar material. With the exception of tile, all of those materials must be finished with enamel or some other smooth, hard, waterproof material.
8. Airtight ceiling.
9. A floor which must be entirely of concrete with glazed surface or tile or wood flooring covered with linoleum or material of similar composition so as to be impervious to water.
10. Outside ventilation which may be provided by screened windows or transoms or, in lieu thereof, by an eight-inch pipe leading to the exterior of the building and otherwise constructed so as to conform to the highest health standards.
11. Solid doors which are painted or enameled and windows which are screened.
12. Sterilizer, chemical or otherwise.
13. Flushing facilities to flush injurious corrosive materials from the eyes or body
    (a) The facilities, which must be accessible, op-

erable, and near the work area, are to be either:

    (1) An eye bubble or eye shower, or both, available from safety equipment suppliers; or

    (2) A four-foot length of ¾-inch hose attached to simple quick opening valve.

  (b) Clean cold water must be available for either of the facilities listed in subparagraph (i) of this paragraph and must not exceed 25 pounds pressure.

  (c) Portable eye washers are permitted if of a type approved by OSHA.

14. Protective wearing apparel as follows:

  (a) Rubber gloves or other type impervious to the chemical being handled.

  (b) Goggles.

  (c) Suitable clothing or apron, rubber or other material impervious to the chemicals being handled.

Ohio

The minimal requirements for the preparation or embalming room shall be as follows:

1. Sanitary floor (cement or tile preferred).
2. All instruments and appliances used in the embalming of a dead human body shall be thoroughly cleansed and sterilized by boiling or immersion for ten minutes in a one percent solution of chlorinated soda or an equivalent disinfectant immediately at the conclusion of each individual case.
3. Running hot and cold water with a lavatory sink for personal hygiene.
4. Exhaust fan and intake vent, permanently installed and operable with the capacity to change the air in the room four times each hour.
5. Sanitary plumbing connected with sewer, cesspool, septic tank, or other department of health approved system.
6. Porcelain, stainless steel, metal-lined or fiberglass operating table.
7. All opening windows and outside doors shall be adequately screened and shielded from outside viewing.
8. All hydroaspirators shall be equipped with at least one air breaker.
9. Containers for refuse, trash and soiled linens shall be adequately covered or sealed at all times.
10. First-aid kit and eyewash.
11. The embalming or preparation room shall be strictly private. A "private" sign shall be posted on the door(s) entering the preparation room. No one shall be allowed therein while the body is being embalmed except the licensed embalmers, apprentices and other authorized persons and officials in discharge of their duties.
12. All waste materials, refuse, used bandages and cotton shall be destroyed by reducing to ashes by

incineration, or shall be buried in a licensed landfill.

13. Every person, while engaged in actually embalming a dead human body, shall be attired in a clean and sanitary smock or gown covering the person from the neck to below the knees and shall, while so engaged, wear impervious rubber gloves.

14. All bodies in the preparation room should be treated with proper care and dignity and should be properly covered at all times.

Extensive planning and consultation are required in advance of any construction in the funeral home in general and the preparation room in particular. Funeral home owners, as business people serving the public and employing people in the workplace, have special obligations that must be met. Add to these the public health aspects of the embalming operation and environment, and it should be clear that extraordinary care in construction and design in the embalming laboratory are in the best interests of all concerned.

LOCATIONS

Basement

The basement is often where space is most readily available, although frequently this is not the most desirable site. Ceiling height is the most common difficulty in this area because of overhead pipes as well as heating and air conditioning ducts. Often there is little that can be done to remedy the situation with reasonable cost. Sometimes, pipes and ducts may be diverted, run between floor joists, or sometimes concealed in wall cabinets. Lighting fixtures may also be kept from lessening head room if they are recessed between floor joists.

Plumbing can present vexing questions if sewer drains are substantially above floor level. A sump pump in this circumstance may be the only answer, but it should be remembered that sump pump becomes inoperative during a power failure. There are other plumbing considerations, too, which will be discussed later. Ventilation and air conditioning are more costly in basement areas. Stairs can be a considerable inconvenience—even a hazard. An elevator or lift or a ramp may offer a solution here.

A wet basement might be the greatest single deterrent to using this area. One should be certain beyond all doubt that the water problem can be completely corrected by interior or exterior waterproofing of the walls, relocation of dry wells, grading away from the building, or some other means before any construction is begun and especially before any flooring is laid. Normal dampness is rather easily handled by a dehumidifier, and it is essential that this be done.

First or Second Floor

The first floor is usually the most logical and least costly location of a preparation room if ample space is available. Most of the basement problems are eliminated and certain advantages accrue automatically. Climbing stairs, building a ramp, or installing an elevator becomes unnecessary. Natural daylight is normally available to create more pleasant working conditions; however, other considerations now arise. Access to the room should be from a nonpublic area. If the room is adjacent to a public area such as the selection room, adequate soundproofing is extremely important. If this is impractical or impossible, a flashing light should be installed in the preparation room to alert staff members that a family is in the next room. Odor control and proper exhaust venting must be provided. Those who work in a funeral home become accustomed to certain odors that would be obvious and objectionable to a visitor.

If the installation of an elevator is feasible in a two-story building, the second floor may well be the best of the several alternatives. More natural light is available, and ventilation is less expensive and more effective. Normally, a second floor room is completely removed from the public areas. here again, sound levels must be considered. Plumbing may be nonexistent in the immediate area, but totally new plumbing may be reasonable considering the other advantages to be gained.

PREPARATION ROOM SIZE

The size requirement of the preparation room is also of critical importance in determining the location. A room that is too large can necessitate extra steps and encourage use of the surplus space for storage. Many problems can be forestalled by partitioning a part of the area for planned storage. Allow adequate work space but keep all equipment, instruments, and supplies readily accessible.

The firm that conducts as many as 100 funerals annually should find one permanent table ample. A folding table that may be stored in a closed when not in use will serve in an emergency and can double as a dressing table when required. An area 120 to 150 square feet for this room should be considered a minimum. This should allow for ample cabinets and counterspace, assuming the room is not an unusual shape and that it does not have more than one or two doors opening into it. When locating plumbing for the table, keep in mind the need to allow ample passage for the removal cot and for a casket, if casketing is to be done in the preparation room. Doors and corridors leading to the room must also be of ample width, especially if turning corners is required.

A firm anticipating 100 to 150 funerals per year should try to provide a bit larger area if at all possible.

One table would normally still be adequate, but the extra folding table is essential.

A firm contemplating 150 to 350 funerals should provide a minimum area of approximately 400 square feet and two completely equipped tables. A firm doing a larger volume should seriously consider a separate dressing room where hairdressing and cosmetizing may be done.

PHYSICAL DESIGN

Discuss the requirements with an architect on a new building or when remodeling. Show the architect the existing equipment and describe the movement made in the room. Consider plumbing needs. Plumbing costs should not always be the overriding determining factor.

Maneuverability within the finished room is tremendously important. When the tentative location for the table(s) is set, mentally go through the motions of getting the removal cot and the casket into the room. Once the general plan seems satisfactory, draw the room to scale with all equipment in place and think again about all the movements that must take place in the finished room.

Storage Cabinets

Next, consider storage cabinets. Although space should be provided for working quantities of supplies, the preparation room should not double as a storeroom. Ready-made base cabinets are generally 24 inches deep. Obviously, these would normally be the least costly. Depending on the size and shape of the room, however, custom cabinets may be a necessity. They could be 18 or 12 inches deep, if space is very limited. If the space is such that cabinet depth is not a problem but counter length is limited, it might be desirable to use a stock 24-inch cabinet and hold it out from the wall to permit a 30-inch deep countertop. The vacant space behind the cabinets might be used for water pipes or electrical wiring.

The Doorway

Unless an architect is made aware that caskets will be taken through the door, she or he might well specify a conventional 30-inch door. **A 3-foot opening should be an absolute minimum. The narrower the corridor or passageway from which the room is to be entered, the wider the door should be to permit turning.** In addition to width, the direction in which the door opens is very significant. If a normally hung door might create problems, perhaps a "pocket" or recessed sliding door might be the answer. Should there be a structural reason that this is not practical, double-hinged doors folding to the right or left may be required.

Table Arrangements

There are virtually as many table arrangements as there are sizes and shapes of rooms; however, two are the most common and popular.

Conventional Parallel Table Plan. The conventional parallel table plan is a perfectly functional layout, although it may not be the best choice because the exhaust system, depending on where it is placed, may draw odors past the embalmers. With this plan, caution must be taken against making the waste sink a part of the cabinet line. This makes the sink and surrounding areas more difficult to clean. Instead, mount the sink on the face of the base cabinets or on the floor, leaving some clearance between the sink and cabinet.

Better yet is the "island" cabinet (Fig. 4–1), which gives the embalmer freedom to pass completely around the table without stepping over hoses and electric cords. No part of the wall storage cabinets is obstructed. In fact, a drum of hardening compound or similar item may be stored in the base of the "island." All plumbing connections are within the cabinet and readily accessible if a problem should arise.

Two-Table Room Arrangement. If a sufficiently large square or rectangular room is available, the two-table room arrangement is preferred. It provides two completely separate work areas, allows maximum flexibility in movement within the room, and generally does not interfere with doors.

FLOORING

Now that the location of the preparation room in the building and the layout of the room itself have been considered, perhaps the first specific aspect of the room that should be discussed is the floor.

The floor must withstand very heavy traffic and considerable static weight. If selected carelessly it can harbor infectious organisms, cause anything on wheels to roll toward low spots, cause glare, and create difficult working conditions or perhaps require recovering or even structural repair more quickly than it should. The architect must be made fully aware of the weights this floor will hold and, therefore, the amount of structural support necessary.

Basement Preparation Room

It is essential that the proper base be laid for any cement floor. There should be a thick stone bed covered by vinyl vapor barrier sheeting underneath the cement. A small ditch should be constructed around the outside, with ample leach lines to feed into the ditch in case water does start to collect. The cost of a small sump pump might well be worthwhile. Located in an out-of-the-way spot, it would pick up and discharge any water accumulation. Building codes should be consulted.

If the new floor is to be tiled, be sure to consider the curing time. The alkalines in uncured cement will affect the tile adhesive. When tiling an old cement floor, hollows and cracks in the cement must be filled and the floor leveled before proceeding. There are cementing com-

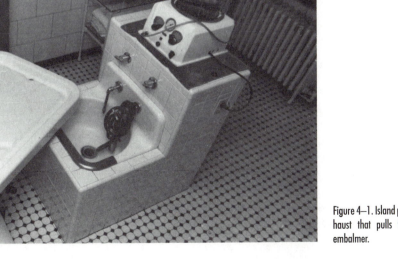

Figure 4–1. Island preparation design. Note the duct for exhaust that pulls fumes to the floor, away from the embalmer.

pounds on the market that have four times the compressive strength of ordinary concrete. These compounds cure rapidly, are highly resistant to chemicals, and are impervious to moisture and temperature extremes. They are applied with a trowel in any thickness desired and adhere to wood, concrete, brick, steel, and aluminum.

If the preparation room is located in a basement with a cement floor, it is best to cover it with something as standing on cement is uncomfortable. Building a wood floor over the cement is a common answer to this problem. If the wood floor were built directly on top of the concrete, moisture would cause it to rot. Therefore, various methods are used to raise the wood floor and leave an air space between it and the concrete. In addition to preventing rot, the space acts as an excellent sound absorber.

It is also important to have enough floor joists and a thick enough wood subfloor to support the heavy concentrated weight the floor will bear. Try to anticipate locations for desired electrical and plumbing lines before closing up the floor.

First or Second Floor Preparation Room

When building a preparation room on the first or second floor, the architect should again be cautioned about the loads that the floor must support. An embalming table can weigh 300 or 400 pounds and that, plus the weight of a subject, could create a low spot on an insufficiently supported floor. The floor's sinking, in turn, can cause cracking of tiles or other floor coverings. Over a span of 12 feet a normal floor (without a bearing wall) could use 2×10-inch timbers on 16-inch centers for floor joists; however, a preparation room with 2×12-inch timbers on 12-inch centers is preferred. Alternatively, to keep timber height uniform with that of adjoining rooms, the 2×10-inch on 16-inch centers should be doubled.

FLOOR COVERING

Terrazo Floor

A terrazo floor is one sort that might be considered for this application. It is a natural polished floor that is very durable and easy to maintain. Terrazo is very hard and, therefore, tiring to stand on for extended periods. Also, it is slippery when wet. This problem can be overcome with the use of rubber mats.

Clay and Ceramic Tile

Clay and ceramic tile are both excellent choices. The size of such tiles makes a very important difference. The large 4×4-inch tiles with a slight roundness on the top make a natural recess or ditch for the grout fill as well as for dirt and accumulated wax. Some 1×1-inch tiles are also rounded and create the same difficulties. There are, however, flat 1×1-inch tiles and these are good. Any cleaning implement, from a hand sponge to an electric scrub brush machine, will make contact at all points and leave the floor completely clean. Remember that liquids will be spilled occasionally. A floor of glazed ceramic tiles would become slippery and such tiles should be avoided.

Vinyl Tile

Vinyl tile is, for good reason, probably the type of flooring most commonly chosen. It is very resilient so it is comfortable to stand on for several hours. It is attractive and sold in many colors and patterns so it can easily be color coordinated with any room. The three basic types of vinyl flooring are no-waxing sheet vinyl, homogeneous vinyl tile, and vinyl-asbestos tile.

Asphalt Tile

Asphalt tile has been around for a long time. Made of resin asphalt compounds and asbestos fibers, it is very hard and brittle. Of all tile floors it is the least expensive per square foot. It is easy to install, too! However, it must be used on cement or on an exceptionally strong floor that will not "work" (move) at all. Asphalt tile becomes increasingly brittle with age and new tiles will not have the aged appearance of those around them, making repaired areas very visible. This type of floor needs to be well waxed to ensure long life in the preparation room.

Epoxy

Another kind of floor covering is epoxy. It is usually used directly over a cement floor. A layer of epoxy is spread over the floor and then chips of color (supplied with the epoxy) are often sprinkled onto it. When the epoxy sets, several coats of clear plastic are applied. The number of coats (and the quality of the particular brand chosen) determine the durability of the floor. There are several types on the market. Epoxy coverings can also be used over old tile, wood, and other types of floors, but preparation of the old surface must be extremely thorough. Finally, these preparations can also be used on all surfaces. Epoxy floors are seamless so it is an easy surface to disinfect.

Paint

Paint, of course, is the least expensive floor covering of all. But it will not stand up under wear and it is especially susceptible to damage from chemicals, so spillage is a real problem. If a floor is to be tiled, all the paint must be sanded off to obtain good bond for the tile.

WINDOWS, DOORS, AND CEILINGS

Windows, doors, and ceilings all function to some degree to control sound, light (Fig. 4–2), and odors.

The first factor influencing the selection of a window is the location of the preparation room in the building. Local climate and the direction of prevailing winds should also be considered. If the preparation room is built in the basement there will probably be a need to augment the natural ventilation available with some system of forced air. Aside from the obvious odor problems, the natural summer dampness in most parts of the country is a problem in a basement. Windows can be an available source for fresh incoming air when mechanical exhaust systems are running.

Privacy must always be ensured in the preparation room. In a basement location, frosted glass is usually necessary. Wire reinforcement in the glass is often essential in city areas because of vandalism. Frosted jalousie windows afford privacy while permitting air flow and can be a good choice. The inverted awning-type window ensures privacy when the window is open.

Look for windows associated with the fewest maintenance problems. Below (or even just above) ground level, a wooden sash is likely to swell in dampness and create opening and closing problems. Keeping paint on damp wood (to prevent rot) also requires frequent attention; steel, aluminum, or vinyl sashes should be used here instead. If a basement window is below grade and drainage around the window is poor, a well can be dug and a plexiglass bubble placed over the window and well to keep snow or rain from accumulating.

There are other considerations in selecting windows for first and upper floors. Movements within the room should not be visible as silhouettes or shadows on the window. When work must be done at night, heavy drapes are suggested as well as rolling floor screens or folding screens. At street level, windows can be protected from view by shrubbery or a louvered fence. Use inside or outside the building of materials that substantially decrease the volume of air flow possible through the windows should be avoided. Access to fresh air is important.

Select windows for quality. There is a little maintenance with good windows but cheaper ones can be very

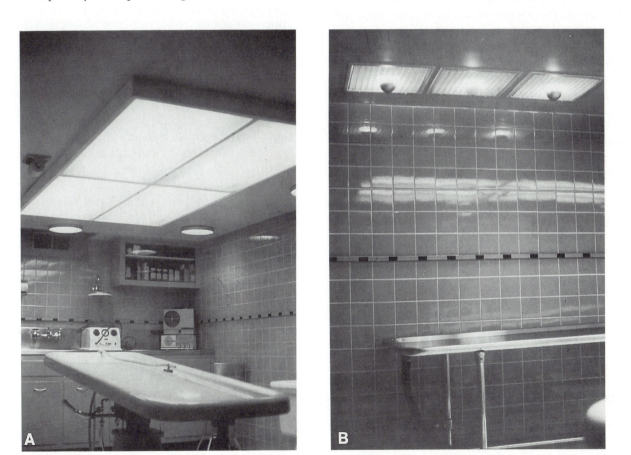

Figure 4–2. Preparation room lights. **A.** Adequate lighting. Note the number of electrical outlets available. **B.** Adjustable cosmetic lights.

irritating. They warp, bind, rattle, and leak. Unlike poor-grade windows, good-quality wood, metal, and vinyl frames are dimensionally stable. Good windows also prevent heat loss.

One of the best sources of light if architecture permits is the glass block wall; however, additional windows then become necessary for ventilation. If the preparation room is located on the top floor and is wedged between other buildings, restricting light and air flow from regular windows, plastic dome skylights should be considered. This sort of window also allows full use of wall space. Ventilation is aided as warm air rises rapidly to the ceiling and through the skylight under most weather conditions.

Doors

The doors in the preparation room should be of the same high quality as the windows. These doors will get a heavy flow of traffic and must not warp, bind, catch poorly, or need to be slammed shut. Prehung doors are an excellent choice because they are of good quality and also save time in installation. To some extent the size of the entrance and the area to which that entrance leads determine the type of door needed. If the door leads to an adjoining garage, the insurance company or building code will probably call for a metal-covered door. In selection of an interior door, choices include doors with solid cores, hollow cores, solid fresco cores, solid wood staved cores, solid wood flake cores, or lead shield cores. All these types are available with different odor and sound control properties. Be sure that the door selected is able to stand up to heat, moisture, scuffs, and stains.

Busy doors should always have push plates and kick plates to save on wear and tear. Flat-surface doors are best with regard to sanitation. Ridges and crevices in old-style doors are hard to clean well and are, therefore, bacterial breeding grounds. Old doors may be renovated and flush-surfaced by simply laminating them with any of the variety of materials available for this purpose. Advise the architect that all doors must be wide enough so that a stretcher or casket can easily pass through, and that the stretcher or casket may need to be turned at various angles to move it into or from a hallway or around some wall or other obstacle on one side of the door or the other. This warning has been previously mentioned but bears repeating. **Improper door size is one of the most common errors in preparation room planning.**

Ceilings

Ceilings can present a real problem, especially in renovation than in new construction, and, in particular, if the preparation room is in the basement. Frequently, the basement location means a low ceiling made lower by water pipes, heating ducts, and electrical lines. If consid-eration is being given to renovate such a ceiling to better insulate for sound, for the sake of appearance or for sanitation reasons, it must first be determined if there is sufficient height below the pipes, ducts, and electrical lines to construct a ceiling. If there is not enough height in the room or a room is being designed for a new building, be sure that at least 4 inches of sound insulation material is used, and the contractor allows complete and easy access to all pipes, valves, and electrical connections.

New "hung" or suspended ceilings can be an excellent choice if sufficient height is available. The large tiles provide easy access to everything above. These tiles are available in many materials. Repainting or even replacing old ceiling tiles is a fairly inexpensive way to brighten up the room every few years.

Many suspended ceilings are available as complete systems, incorporating light fixtures and ventilation systems as well as the tile. Such systems, which disperse air through large areas of the ceiling, are especially suited to delivering large quantities of air at considerable temperature differentials with minimal draft and noise. Most of these systems require at least $15\frac{1}{2}$ inches of hanging height.

Johns–Manville offers acoustical tile specially treated with antibacterial finish and bacteriostatic core. Tests have shown that the finish reduces bacterial population on the surface by 90% in 6 hours, and the bacteriostatic core does not support bacterial proliferation.

For ceilings full of pipes or ducts, remember to clean the tops of these regularly with a good disinfectant. Infectious organisms often rest on such areas, and a breeze from a door or window can dislodge these organisms. If they fall on a host who provides the proper conditions, the organisms may proliferate.

Many funeral homes are created from old residences, and this usually means plaster ceilings. If the ceiling is in good condition a coat of paint will make it look excellent again. If the plaster is at all loose, do not add ceiling material to it. Pull off the old ceiling, or at least all that is loose. Fur out the old base to align the new ceiling correctly.

The material of the various suspended ceilings should be checked for fire-retardant qualities. Ratings are given by most manufacturers in their date booklets.

Simple painting may not be sufficient to save an old ceiling, but the "hung" ceiling may not be a good choice because of height limitations. The assortment of ceiling material is large, and the selection depends on the amount of money available for the project. A new ceiling of $\frac{3}{8}$-inch plasterboard properly nailed with the new, better-gripping plasterboard nails and correctly taped can give years of service. Use of the new acrylic enamel paint would make it an easy ceiling to wash. **A white ceiling is a must. It gives the advantage of reflected light, and as accumulation of dirt is readily apparent on white, it is easy to make sure the ceiling is kept clean and sanitary.**

Another good ceiling material is one of the high-gloss finish hardboards. Marlite is a good example. These are usually available in 12 × 12- and 12 × 16-inch blocks. They also come in 4 × 8-feet sheets. The thickness is usually only about ¼ inch. The small squares are easy to install and have tongue-and-groove edges for easy alignment. These boards can be glued in place. Try to avoid unnecessarily deep grooves between sections in the ceiling because they can collect dirt and serve as a possible breeding ground for bacteria. The 4 × 8-feet Marlite hardboards come with matching joint moldings. Good-quality chrome finish moldings stand up well. Poor-quality chrome moldings will "pit" (form small spots of rust) as a result of temperature variations and moisture.

Walls

As with ceilings, walls should be selected with careful concern for the ease with which they can be kept sanitary (Fig. 4–3). Late in 1974, California enacted new regulations specifying sanitary requirements not only for preparation rooms but also for storage rooms (where bodies are held awaiting disposition). If a new wall is to be created, the material and method of construction are, in part, determined by the sort of room that will be on

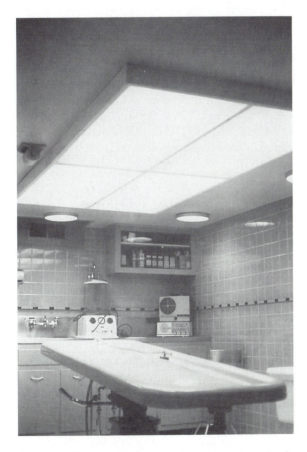

Figure 4–3. Walls tiled from the floor to the ceiling. The ceiling is soundproof.

the other side. If that room is to be used by the public (as an arrangement or smoking room), then the wall must be insulated against noise and odor. Planning for a series of cabinets along such a wall is ideal in that they can serve as the needed insulation. If there must be electrical or plumbing lines in this wall, perhaps cabinets can be built out in front of these. Never plan an employee bedroom or kitchen next to a preparation room. Control of odor and bacteria is a constant worry. There are plans for setups such as this, but they should not be seriously considered.

A possible covering or finish for any wall of concrete is glazed masonry block. This comes in many sizes, styles, and colors and is easy to keep clean. The contractor must see to it that the mason keeps the grout joints smooth and close to flush with the tile surfaces for ease of cleaning. A poured concrete wall can be spray-painted after imperfections are plastered. Many plain and multicolored epoxy paints are available for use over any concrete surface. These surfaces should be finished with a clear glaze.

Modern adhesives make it possible to use ceramic tile on wallboard, which creates an excellent-looking and durable wall. When dry wallboard is used by itself it should be taped and surfaced carefully and sealed with good washable enamel. Plasterboard will absorb moisture, so it must be kept an inch or two from the floor and a cove base used. In a basement or damp area, set plasterboard considerably away from the outer wall. Moisture rots the outer paper and causes the plaster to soften and disintegrate.

Marlite wall board is used extensively and is available in many colors with matching moldings. Marlite is one of the easiest walls to maintain as are formica-surfaced cabinets. Formica has to be glued to a solid base like plywood or particle board. The thickness of the board is dependent on stud spacing and anchoring techniques used. It is always good to make panels in this type of wall removable for easy access to wiring and other equipment located inside the wall.

Many choose to use tile of some sort only part of the way up the wall and paint or wallpaper above that. This is fine provided that good, washable paint or paper is used. A flexible vinyl floor covering can also be used on a wall if there is a solid base surface to which it may be glued. In short, as long as the selection is durable and able to be cleaned thoroughly, the wall is a question of taste and budget.

Sound Insulation

Sound insulation should not be overlooked. If the room is below, above, or adjacent to public areas the sounds of instruments dropping or machines in operation will certainly be unwelcome in those areas. Many companies make special-density cellulose fiber structural board that can be used in ceilings, walls, and floors to deaden sound. The use of such material in preparation room construction is highly recommended.

PLUMBING

As with all facets of preparation room planning, to avoid later difficulties with plumbing, work closely with the architect and describe all the work that goes on in the area so that all fixtures, waste lines, and other equipment can be properly located. In case of blockages, all cleanout points in waste lines should be conveniently accessible. After the room is constructed, changes are often difficult. For example, feed lines are generally buried in floors and walls (Fig. 4–4). Addition of a fixture not initially planned will probably not be easy.

Water pipe is like electrical service wire in that the larger the diameter of the pipe or wire, the more water or current will flow through it. Today, copper is usually used for water pipe because it does not easily corrode or rust. The size of pipe used to bring the water in from the street is determined by the size and use of the building. Another very convenient material to work with is polyvinyl chloride (PVC) for both supply and drain. It is

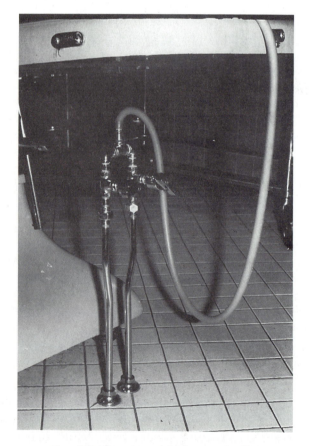

Figure 4–4. A floor water supply for the preparation table.

approved by many communities for residential use, but restrictions may be enforced for commercial applications. To avoid excessive commercial water rates when a residence is planned in the building, it might be well to have a separate water meter installed to measure the water consumption in the residence.

The feed line after the water meter is normally $\frac{3}{4}$ to 1 inch in diameter. It then decreases to $\frac{1}{2}$ inch as it feeds into the individual fixtures in the building. The supply lines to the preparation room should be at least $\frac{3}{4}$ inch in diameter. This size allows enough volume to operate waste sink flushometers properly and creates a good vacuum in a hydroaspirator. Some embalmers find that the vacuum is not great enough in their aspirators unless they run both hot and cold water through a dual mixing faucet. This lack of suction could be the result of very small feed pipes or old, galvanized pipes. These pipes corrode and the buildup on their internal walls restricts flow and, therefore, reduces vacuum.

> A good reason to have removable panels and ceiling tiles in strategic areas (so that access to plumbing and electrical wiring is convenient) is that of changing municipal codes. If there is a question of compliance with a plumbing code, it will be possible to make changes without ripping out the walls.

The second major plumbing consideration deals with codes. Having discussed bringing in an adequate water supply, the subject of disposal of waste water must be considered. How wastes are handled is a major concern. Codes and regulations change as knowledge of good sanitation procedures increases. In some areas the water table is very high and good filtration is needed or life is endangered by feeding harmful bacteria back into the drinking water.

Backflow

Backflow is the unwanted reverse flow of liquids in a piping system. It can be caused by back-siphonage, back-pressure, or a combination of both. Back-siphonage is due to a vacuum or partial vacuum in the water supply system. It is caused by *ordinary gravity*—when water supply is lost and a fixture that is elevated is opened, allowing air into the system, water will (by gravity) reverse flow; *undersized piping*—high-velocity water traveling through undersized piping can cause an aspirator effect and draw water out of branch pipes causing a partial vacuum and a reverse flow; and *vacuum*—pumping water from the supply system creates a pressure drop or a negative pressure in the system, or a break in the main or excessive usage at a lower level in the system can also be a cause.

Many water departments now require a backflow prevention (one-way) valve at the point at which the wa-

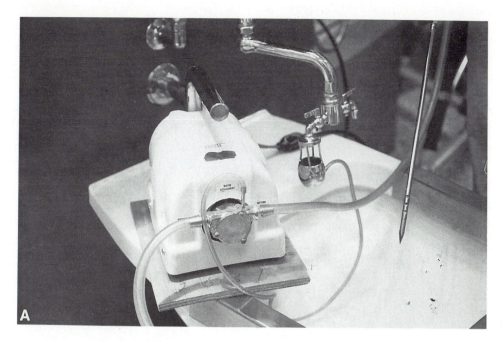

Figure 4–5. **A.** Electric aspirator.

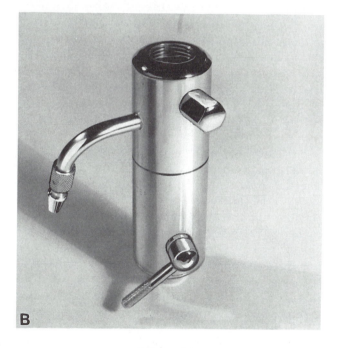

B. Hydroaspirator.

ter enters the funeral home from the street. Several types are available. Favored is the installation of these devices where the water enters the preparation room (not just the funeral home) on both hot and cold lines. In this way the public within the funeral home, as well as the community, are protected from accidentally contaminated water.

Incredible concentrations of bacteria of various types exist on and within every subject brought into the preparation room, so the need for precautionary measures is obvious. In early 1970, the state of Connecticut

started a program requiring the use of blackflow prevention devices. Since then, additions to these regulations now require special faucets to be used with hydroaspirators, which must be equipped with vacuum breakers. These faucets are made for industrial use as in commercial laundries. The fixture is dull in finish and has a vacuum breaker built into the top of the spout.

Electric Aspirator. The trocar is attached via the hose on the right side of the impeller casing. The hose coming off the left side leads directly to the top of the flush sink. The small tube off the top of the impeller casing draws water from the bulb that is attached to the water faucet. The water faucet attachment has two water supplies—one to the bulb to keep the impeller lubricated when no aspirant is flowing through the trocar, and one off the opposite side (with an attached hose) for water to be supplied for other purposes. The impeller casing has three screws that allow for removal of the impeller for replacement or drying (Fig. 4–5A).

Hydroaspirator. The hydroaspirator is attached to a water faucet over a flush sink. A clear plastic hose connects the aspirator and trocar. The level near the bottom of the aspirator allows for clean water flow from the hose or for aspiration (suction) if the lever is vertically aligned with the aspirator (Fig. 4–5B).

Vacuum Breakers. Two vacuum breakers are shown at two levels: The lower one is the top half of the aspiration unit and is directly attached to the water faucet. The second one is higher and is seen behind the clear plastic hose in line with the plumbing pipes. The hydroaspirator is a part of a counter installation of aspirator and two water lines. The larger open pipe nearest the counter is the aspirator

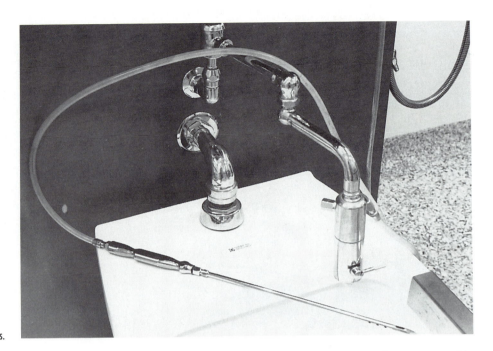

Figure 4–6. Vacuum breakers.

unit. The vacuum breaker is shown to the right side and at a higher level than the hose attachment. The hose is attached in line via a hydraulic connector and can easily be removed for cleaning and disinfection. The handle on the right side controls the water flow; it is the water flowing through the unit that creates the suction (Fig. 4–6; also see Fig. 4–8A).

One consideration is to put vacuum breakers into the hot and cold supply lines for the preparation room rather than on each faucet. A siphon-breaking device or backflow preventer is a rather simple mechanism that is attached to a threaded faucet before the hydroaspirator is mounted. It combines a check valve and air vents. When water forces open the check valve, the air vents are automatically closed. If water pressure drops, the check valve closes automatically and the air vents are opened, preventing any backflow into the supply line. The air vents break any built up vacuum. This inexpensive but effective device is available through most preparation room suppliers.

Backflow and siphonage are very real hazards in funeral homes, especially if the volume and pressure of the water coming entering the building are not great enough to adequately supply all outlets in the building. For example, if the pressure is barely adequate for aspiration, flushing a toilet or starting a washing machine can cause such a drop in pressure at the aspirator faucet that a vacuum results, drawing waste materials into the waterline.

Because of the serious nature of backflow problems, OSHA has addressed the problem nationally, whereas many states have yet to do so. Subpart J of the Occupational Safety and Health Act pertains to general environmental controls. Paragraph 1910.141(b)(2)(ii) contains the following statement: "Construction of non-potable water systems carrying any other nonpotable substance shall be such as to prevent backflow or back siphonage into a potable water system."*

Some manufacturers claim that their backflow valves work when installed in the drain line at a point lower than the level at which that drain pipe ultimately empties. This sort of installation is very undesirable, however, and is most often not in compliance with sanitary codes.

In discussing placement of hydroaspirators, it is important to remember that the aspirator should not be attached to a faucet in a sink in such a way that it is below the top of the sink walls (Fig. 4–7). This means that the operator cannot see the aspirator. The sink drain's runoff may not be as fast as the inflow of water from the faucet. With the aspirator deep in the sink or below the rim, the vents will be covered with water. If, for example a toilet is flushed elsewhere in the system, backflow will result. The aspirator, therefore, should be at least 2 inches above the rim of the sink. Another problem with hydroaspirators can occur during aspiration of tissue particles. These can become lodged in the aspirator throat and block it, causing the operator to inject water into the body via the trocar.

Drains

No discussion of preparation room plumbing needs would be complete without a thorough discussion of drains. In planning the location of drains, remember that the drain pipe must have a downward slope of $\frac{1}{4}$ inch over every foot of length from point of entry into the room to

---

*This revision was published in *Fed Regist.* 1973;38:10930.

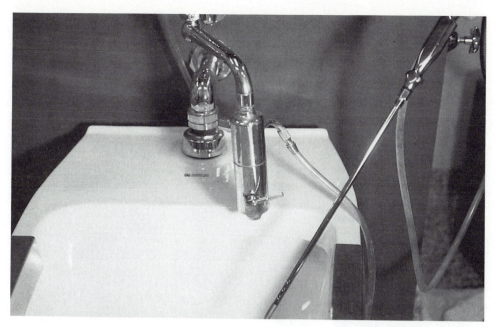

Figure 4–7. Hydroaspiration in a visible position.

the point of exit. Commercial sealed sump pumps can be installed to lift wastes. Also, where codes allow, flush-up toilets may be used (Fig. 4–8A). Such toilets need a minimum of 40 pounds psi of pressure sustained at 4 gallons per minute for a 10-foot lift. Many basement preparation rooms use small electric pumps to lift drainage water. Any unit of this type should have frequent checks to make sure the collecting pot is being thoroughly rinsed.

A central floor drain surrounded by a slope is inconvenient. Church trucks and cots can wobble, roll, and cause damage. A floor drain in an out-of-the-way corner surrounded by a small area of slope avoids these problems (Fig. 4–8B). Waste drains must be vented to flow properly. A drain in a basement floor, in an area with a high water table, must have a one-way flap installed to prevent backup. Also, in areas where sewers are not available and septic tanks are used, remember to check codes to determine minimum distances between septic tank systems and wells for water.

Water Supply

Most codes require hot as well as cold water in the preparation room. Certain states even set a minimum temperature requirement of 130° or 145°. The need for hot water in the preparation room is easy to understand. OSHA requires that all steam and hot water pipes be insulated when it is possible for an employee to come in contact with the pipes. It is not always convenient to insulate. One possible alternative for pipes leading to freestanding sinks is to enclose them in a cabinet.

Convenient water service to the embalming table, the embalming machine, and the sinks can save much time and many steps. The table is the work center. Water can be fed to it either from an overhead supply or directly from service sinks. If the table is permanently located, a supply line can be placed under the head area, coming up from the floor or dropping from the ceiling. The overhead service is really handy for washing the remains and shampooing and rinsing the hair.

Sinks

There are many alternatives from which to choose in selecting a waste sink for the embalming table (Figs. 4–7 and 4–8AB). Room size and expense are two factors to be weighed. A sink that permits good floor maintenance should be selected. Flushable sinks, whether floor-standing or wall-hung, are the most sanitary. The flush valve incorporates a vacuum breaker. A minimum of 20 pounds psi is required at the valve while flushing.

Hand sinks should be located conveniently for the operator and need not be too large. Remembering the need for sanitation, controls should be selected that do not require handling of faucets, which will collect untold numbers of bacteria. There are controls for knee operations, foot operation, and elbow or forearm operation. A gooseneck faucet facilitates the filling of large bottles and pails (Fig. 4–9AB).

Sinks can have surfaces of china, enamel on pressed steel, or stainless steel. Enamel on pressed steel chips easily but is least expensive to replace. Stainless steel is popular but harder to keep clean looking. A bottle or instrument dropped in a stainless sink makes an awful racket! Flush-surface hand sinks in countertops are even easier to maintain than wall-mounted ones. If plans call

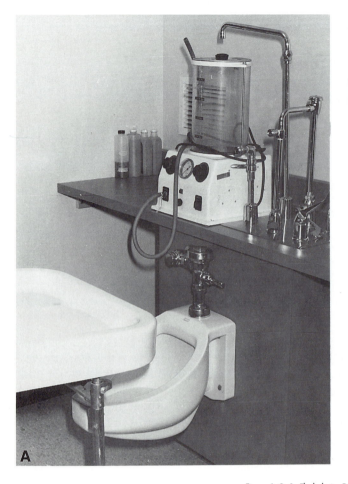
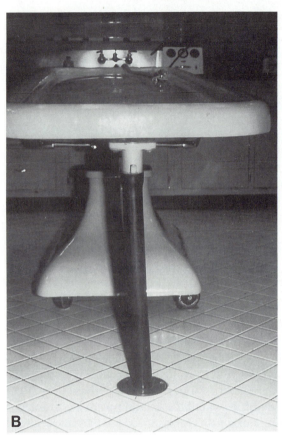

Figure 4–8. **A.** Flush drain. **B.** Floor drain.

for a separate dressing room, the cosmetician and hair-dresser should have their own sink.

VENTILATION

The subjects of ventilation and operator exposure to air-borne microbes are often relegated from the position of potential health hazard to a position secondary to the threat of direct physical contact with pathogens from the body itself. Because of this, teaching and funeral home management policy directives often emphasize the need for protective gloves, garb, and cleaning, while ignoring the necessity to monitor and limit the inhalation of disease organisms in the preparation room. No discussion of the embalming environment is complete without a thorough and cautionary discourse on the subject of ventilation and the necessity to protect the embalmer. Adequate ventilation is an essential key to Tier I of the three-tiered spectrum of public health and safety—personal protection of the embalmer, especially through the

maintenance of a work environment that is hygienically clean and *safe*.

Formaldehyde

In recent years, many individuals have become convinced that formaldehyde is a proven carcinogen. In fact, there is a much larger body of research indicating the opposite. Extensive studies have been conducted, both within the funeral service field and among those who work with formaldehyde in all fields, that indicate strongly that there is no adverse health effect from lifelong exposures at levels usually encountered in the workplace. Such were the findings reported in *Proportionate Mortality Among New York Embalmers* by Dr. Walrath of the National Cancer Institute. (This paper was presented to the Chemical Industry Institute of Toxicology in 1981.) Another study, *The Effects of Occupational Exposure on the Respiratory Health of West Virginia Morticians* by Levine, Dal Colrso, Blunden, and Batigelli, is available through The Formaldehyde Institute, 1330 Connecticut Avenue, NW, Washington, DC 20036. The most important, broad-based paper was done for the National

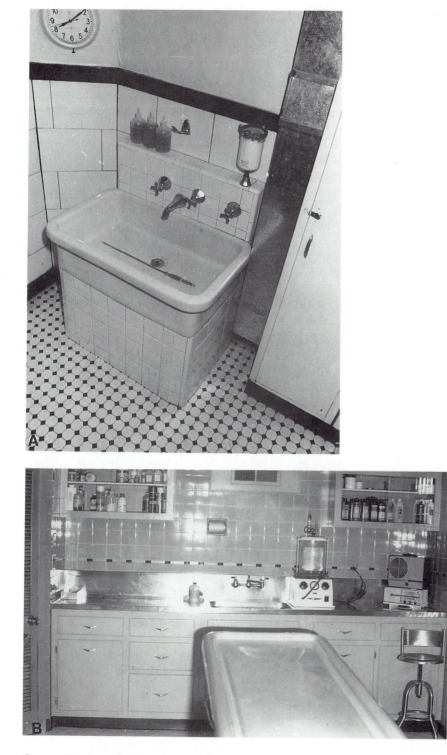

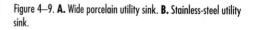

Figure 4–9. **A.** Wide porcelain utility sink. **B.** Stainless-steel utility sink.

Cancer Institute by Dr. Aaron Blair in 1986 and is entitled *Mortality Among Industrial Workers Exposed to Formaldehyde.* The paper is based on a study of 26,000 workers who were occupationally exposed to formaldehyde. The author writes: "The data provides little evidence that mortality from cancer is associated with formaldehyde exposures at levels experienced by workers in this study." (This paper is available through the National Cancer Institute, 3607 Landow Building, Bethesda, MD 20205.)

There are two very real problems with formaldehyde. First, it is irritating to work with if encountered in levels above the 1 ppm currently allowed by OSHA. For this reason alone, proper ventilation is an absolute necessity. It is well known that formaldehyde has been proven to cause a form of nasal cancer in rats not known to occur in human beings. What often is not known is that these rats were subjected for long periods to concentrations that no human being could or would voluntarily withstand even momentarily. These rats were exposed to 15 ppm 6 hours a day, 5 days a week, for 16 months. At one embalming chemical manufacturing facility, formaldehyde-sensitive instruments have measured readings no higher than 4.5 ppm, and such readings occur after spills. At 4.5 ppm, it is *very* uncomfortable.

The following passage from a report for the National Institute for Occupational Safety and Health (NIOSH) validates the need for ventilation in terms of user irritation:

> *Formaldehyde*—HCHO, a colorless, pungent gas produced commercially by the catalytic oxidation of methyl alcohol. The current legal (OSHA) permissible exposure limit is set at 0.75 ppm for an 8-hour time-weighted average (TWA).

The second problem is that formaldehyde gas may cause severe irritation to the mucous membrane of the respiratory tract and eyes. The gas has recently been proven carcinogenic in animals.* Morrill reported sensory irritation (itching of eyes, dry and sore throat, increased thirst, and disturbed sleep) in paper process workers at 0.9–1.6 ppm formaldehyde. Bourne and Seferian reported from another occupational setting intense irritation of eyes, nose, and throat at levels ranging from 0.13 to 0.45 ppm. More recent studies by Kerfoot and Mooney and Moore and Ogrodnik† conducted in funeral homes indicate that concentrations from 0.25 to 1.39 ppm evoke numerous complaints of upper respiratory tract and eye irritation and headache among embalmers. Schoenber and Mitchell report that acute exposure to formaldehyde phenolic resin vapors at levels around 0.4 to 0.8 ppm causes lacrimation and irritation of the upper as well as the lower respiratory tract.

Taking this into account, NIOSH has recommended a 30-minute ceiling of 1.0 ppm. The levels at which serious inflammation of the bronchi and lower respiratory tract would occur in humans are unknown; inhalation of high levels, however, has caused chemical pneumonitis, pulmonary edema, and death.

In humans, concentrations of 2 to 3 ppm have caused mild tingling sensations in the eyes, nose, and posterior pharnyx. At 4 to 5 ppm, the discomfort increases rapidly, and some mild lacrimation occurs in most people. This level can be tolerated for perhaps 10 to 30 minutes by some persons. After 30 minutes, discomfort becomes quite pronounced. Concentrations of 10 ppm can be withstood only a few minutes, and profuse lacrimation occurs in all subjects, even those acclimated to lower levels.

Very little is known about the effects of long-term exposure to low levels of formaldehyde; however, several instances of "occupational asthma" caused by formalin have been reported, even in persons who were not known to be atopic. Although there remains the question whether the illness represents a true hypersensitivity reaction or an acute chemical pneumonitis provoked by formalin, progressive dyspnea and chest tightness accompanied by attacks of wheezing and productive cough seem to be the common features. All these symptoms return to normal within hours or days of withdrawal, depending on the exposure dose.

It is not surprising that many state boards of mortuary science are now prescribing through rule and regulation a minimal number of room air changes per hour in the preparation room. The *Public Health Guidelines* recommended a ventilation system "creating a minimum of six air changes per hour, preferably more" in the preparation room environment. Further, the federal government recommends a minimum of 12 room changes per hour for autopsy rooms.

Emerging technology and thought in the design and construction of preparation rooms reflect the recognition that because formaldehyde is heavier than air, exhaust systems located at or near floor level, when combined with the introduction of uncontaminated air from the ceiling level, are an efficient method of ventilation. In addition, such systems have the added advantage of drawing fumes and contaminants down and away from the operator's face during the embalming procedure. There are, nevertheless, several alternate and more conventional methods of ventilating a preparation room that are satisfactory. **The key to the creation of an embalming environment protective of the embalmer's health and comfort is air flow and adequacy of ventilation.**

Anything so crucial to the comfort and safety of those working in the preparation room warrants careful consideration. The number and location of windows and doors are obviously components of the total ventilation system. Cross-ventilation (which requires windows on opposite walls) is highly desirable and should be designed into every preparation room if at all possible.

If there is sufficient height in the room to install a hung ceiling, install one that will dispense air through large areas in the ceilings. These have the ability to deliver large quantities of air at considerable temperature differentials with minimal draft and noise.

Many preparation rooms are equipped with the familiar kitchen exhaust hood. When it is installed over the waste sink at a height of about 4 feet, air is drawn out

---

*According to Riccobono, who heads a task force on formaldehyde for the American Textile Manufacturers Institute. Reported without detail.
†See Selected Readings for complete Kerfoot–Mooney Study and Moore–Ogrodnik study.

slightly above table level. Because the hood is located over the waste sink, unpleasant odors are kept away from the operator. In many places, the embalmer must stand between the exhaust fan and the source of the odor. This is uncomfortable as these odors pass by the face; it is also dangerously unsanitary. In choosing the location of the exhaust, care should always be taken so that air flows AWAY from the operator. Calculations should also be obtained from a ventilation engineer to determine the number of room air changes per hour created by the system. See Figure 4–1; the ventilation duct opens at floor level.

The grill on the exhaust fan, and on all other grills in the room, should be easily removable for cleaning. Grills are often loaded with dust "kitties," and this environment is a perfect site for proliferation of bacteria. Be careful when planning an exhaust vent that goes directly from the preparation room to the roof. The architect may not realize that such a vent, located too near a roof-mounted air conditioner, could cause foul odors and pathogens to return through the air conditioner's intake vent.

Basement preparation rooms are the toughest to ventilate properly. One major problem in some areas of the country is the stagnant, humid air that can make a basement very unpleasant during the summer. Mold can start developing unless a dehumidifier is installed. Then, the water from the machine must be emptied periodically, unless it can be linked directly to a drain. Without a dehumidifier other problems can occur. Any of the various types of absorbent embalming powders can become thick and lumpy or harden completely if left uncovered. Linens, too, can absorb moisture and feel clammy.

The possibility of drafts creating dehydration should be considered carefully in laying out the preparation room. Several new preparation rooms have required expensive redesign and reinstallation of ventilation systems because the first few cases embalmed were so seriously dehydrated by drafts.

Air Conditioning

Today, most people planning a new preparation room will air condition it. Although there are many different air conditioning units to choose from, the size of the room in cubic feet and the desired number of room air changes per hour determine the size of the unit needed. If the entire funeral home is air conditioned by the same unit, there must be independent controls for the preparation room. Odors must not reach the main air flow serving the funeral home. Many times, a separate preparation room "zone," controlled manually, is recommended.

The wall or window unit is also adaptable for cooling the preparation room. Such units pull in cool fresh air from outdoors. If properly balanced with the exhaust system, a "once through" ventilation system can be created and used during the embalming operation.

In summary, ventilation experts can use the guidelines recommended to create a system of ventilation, either ongoing or manually controlled, that will provide for adequate ventilation of the embalming environment.

PREPARATION ROOM EQUIPMENT

Tables

Embalming tables are available with stainless-steel or porcelain tops and case iron, steel, or aluminum bases. These bases may have a hydraulic or ratchet-type raising, lowering, or tilting mechanism. They all have a drain channel around each side, with a drain hole at the foot end. Most stainless-steel tables have wheels, whereas the porcelain tables have a swivel-action base (Fig. 4–10). Porcelain tables may be undercoated to reduce the noise of instruments laid on the table surface.

At the completion of the embalming, the body may be transferred from the embalming table to a dressing table. Dressing tables usually have a laminated plastic top and an aluminum frame. The frame usually has wheels, is adjustable in height, and perhaps can fold in the middle. There is no drain channel or hole in a dressing table as in the embalming table.

Injection Apparatus

Today, almost all arterial embalming is done using electric machines for the injection of arterial solution. To be complete, however, several older mechanical methods are considered in this discussion. These devices are generally used today when the electronic machines are not working or when there is an electrical failure. Basically, six devices can be used to inject arterial solution: (1) gravity, (2) bulb syringe, (3) combination of gravity and bulb syringe, (4) hand pump, (5) air pressure machine, and (6) centrifugal pump.

Gravity Injection (Historical). Of the six methods of injection the simplest is the use of the gravity percolator (Fig. 4–11). Fluid is simply poured into a large glass percolator which has a delivery hose attached to the bottom of the bowl. The device is then elevated above the body and the fluid flows into the arterial system. Approximately one-half (0.43) pound of pressure is developed for each foot of height the device is raised above the injection point (for every 28 inches of height, one pound of pressure is created). Years ago, when this method of injection was popular, the percolators held several gallons of fluid. The percolators sold today generally hold a gallon or less of fluid. This creates a need for constant refilling. Because of height restrictions in most preparation rooms pressure is limited with gravity injection. The most frequent uses for this form of injection are as a substitute for mechanical

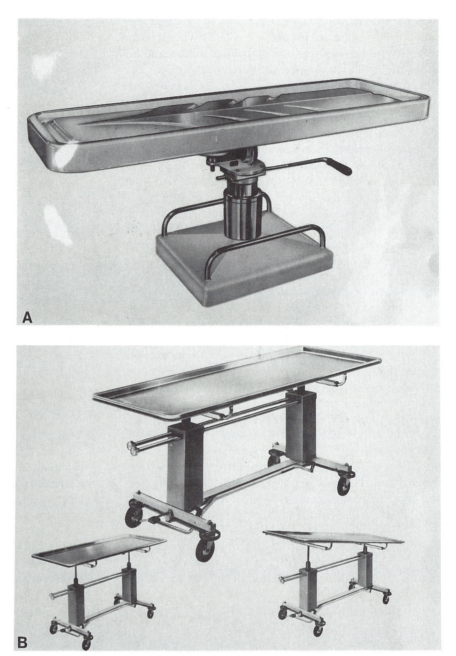

Figure 4–10. **A.** Hydraulic porcelain preparation table. Note the elevated central portion and ribs to drain fluids away from the body. **B.** Metal preparation table.

injectors when they are not working or when there is an electrical power failure and in the embalming of bodies for dissection in medical schools. The advantage of this method of embalming is that it provides a slow, steady method of injection that allows the body to accept the embalming solution at a slower but much more thorough rate. Too often, mechanical injectors rapidly force fluid into the body, and much of the fluid rushes through the vascular system with little time for absorption and is lost in the form of drainage.

Bulb Syringe (Historical). This hand-held and -operated device consists of a rubber bulb with hoses attached to ei-

ther end. A one-way valve in the device allows for this pump to operate. One hose is dropped into a container of embalming solution. Fluid flows into the bulb when the device is squeezed and continues out through the second delivery hose and into the body. It is important to remember that fluid actually passes through the bulb syringe. A body can be injected quite rapidly with this device when it is combined with the gravity percolator. Pressures created are unknown and the operator, when working alone, must use one hand constantly to operate the device. This method of injection can be used today, like the gravity percolator, when the mechanical equipment fails. The tank of the mechanical embalming machine can be used as the source for the mixing and storage of the embalming solution. In this manner the embalmer can be aware of the volume of fluid injected. As pressures build in the body during injection the operator finds the bulb syringe more and more difficult to squeeze (Fig. 4–12A).

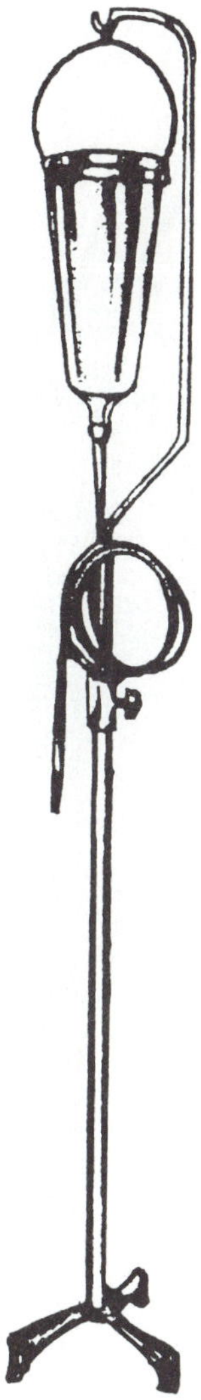

Combination Gravity and Bulb Syringe (Historical). In this method of injection the delivery hose from the gravity percolator connects to the bulb syringe. The body can be embalmed by the gravity method, but pressures and rate of flow can be increased periodically by squeezing on the bulb syringe. The reason for adding the bulb syringe to the gravity device is to overcome the limited ceiling height that can limit the pressure created by the gravity system.

Hand Pump (Historical). This hand-held device is a pump that not only creates pressure but can also be adopted to create a vacuum for aspiration. Unlike the bulb syringe, arterial fluid does NOT flow through the hand pump. Fluid is placed in a jar and the lid is sealed into position. Air pumped by the hand pump enters through the hose leading from the hand pump to the jar. A delivery hose, which drops to the bottom of the jar, then carries the fluid out of the jar and into the body. By attaching the air hose to the other nozzle of the hand pump, air can be withdrawn from the jar and, thus, a vacuum created. A trocar can be attached to the delivery hose and the system of hand pump and jar used for aspiration (Fig. 4–12B, C).

The pressure of injection is unknown. The containers are generally small (about a half gallon) and must be constantly refilled. As with the bulb syringe, the operator must constantly use one hand to operate the hand pump. Also, like the bulb syringe, any resistance to the flow of fluid in the body will be noticed by the difficulty in operating the hand pump. There always exists the pos-

Figure 4–11. Gravity injector.

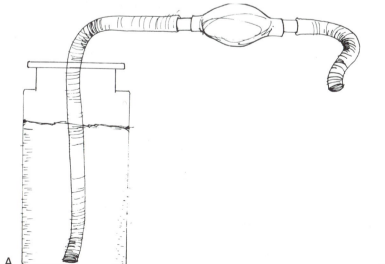

A

Figure 4–12. **A.** Bulb syringe. (*Continued*)

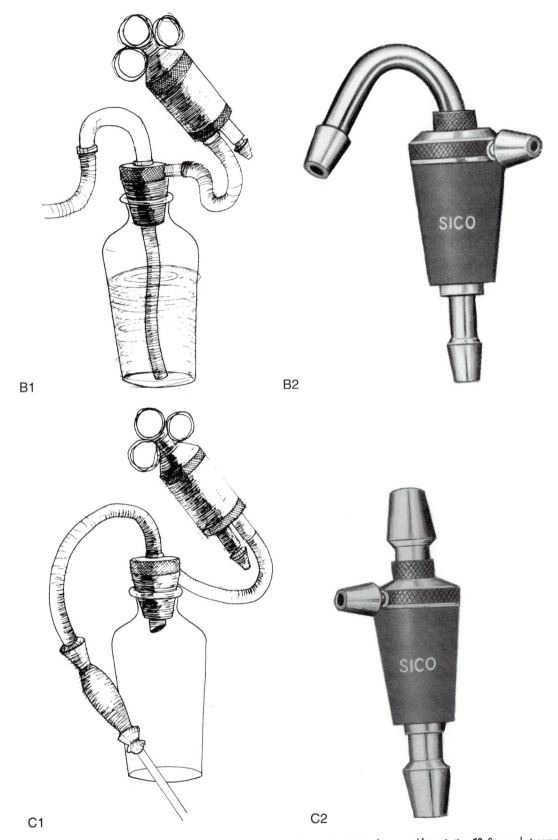

B1

B2

C1

C2

Figure 4–12 (*Continued*). **B1.** Hand pump used for injection. **B2.** Gooseneck stopper used for injection. **C1.** Hand pump used for aspiration. **C2.** Gooseneck stopper used for aspiration.

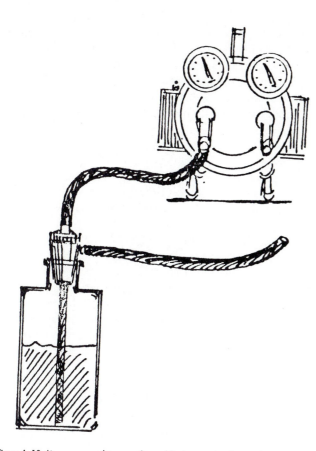

Figure 4–13. Air pressure machines may be used for injection (as illustrated) or aspiration.

sibility that the glass jar may explode or implode. It is easy, if a careful check is not kept on this operation, to inject air into the body. Like the devices previously described, this is used when the mechanical apparatus is inoperable.

Air Pressure Machine.

The air pressure machine (Fig. 4–13) operates just like the hand pump, but because it is motorized, it relieves the embalmer from having to physically operate the device. The air pressure machine, like the hand pump, can be adopted to aspiration. Embalming solution and aspirated materials DO NOT flow through the machine. The machine provides only air pressure or a vacuum. The delivery hose from the machine is attached to a glass jar or metal pressure tank. The jar is the source of arterial solution, the container into which aspirated materials will collect. This device can be very dangerous and pressures must be carefully observed. With the mechanical air pump the bottles can easily explode.

When these machines were popular as injection devices, special metal shields could be purchased that were placed around the bottles to protect the operator. Care must be taken to observe when arterial solution has about run out of the bottle, for air can easily be injected into the body. These machines do provide a steady pressure

and one that can be regulated. Because of the small volume of the bottles a great amount of time can be wasted refilling fluid containers. In use of this type of machine, note the following:

1. Fill the glass bottle with the solution to be injected.
2. Place the rubber gooseneck adaptor in the bottle.
3. Connect the flexible tube from the injection control on the motor to the gooseneck.
4. Connect a second flexible tube from the gooseneck to the arterial tube. When the motor is turned on and the pressure is set, the motor forces air into the bottle through one connection on the gooseneck and forces fluid through the gooseneck and out the other connection.

In use of the air pressure machine for aspiration, the flexible tube from the gooseneck to the motor is attached to the suction valve rather than the injection valve, and the other connection in the gooseneck is attached to a flexible tube connected to the trocar. When the machine is turned on it creates a vacuum in the bottle. This vacuum causes a suction to be created in the trocar, allowing the body to be aspirated.

Centrifugal Pump.

Because the centrifugal pump is the most widely accepted method of injecting arterial solution today, a more extensive explanation is given for this mechanical pump (Fig. 4–14). The centrifugal pump em-

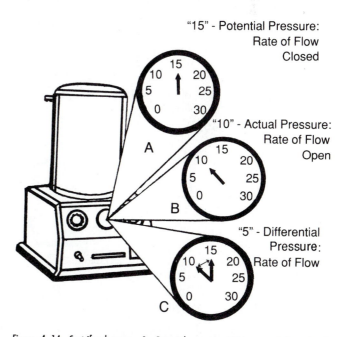

Figure 4–14. Centrifugal pump. **A.** Potential pressure (15), rate of flow closed. **B.** Actual pressure (10), rate of flow open. **C.** Differential pressure (5) or rate of flow.

balming machine is a self-contained device. Over the years a wide variety of machines, each with special features, have been available. Some even contain a separate system similar to an air pressure machine for aspiration. Most of these machines have large-volume tanks, a few of which hold as much as $3\frac{1}{2}$ gallons of fluid. With the motorized force pump a constant preset pressure can be maintained in addition to the preset rate of flow of arterial fluid into the body. It is always recommended that pressure be adjusted prior to injection of arterial fluid into the body. The rate of flow can be determined as the arterial injection begins.

During the embalming it may become necessary to reset pressure and rate of flow to establish a good distribution of the embalming solution. The pressure ranges in the motorized force pump can be very great. Some ma-

chines are capable of producing up to 200 pounds of pressure. In some machines the motorized centrifugal pump runs at a constant speed. In others, the speed can be varied, and in yet other machines two separate motors operating at different speeds are available. Many of these machines can produce a pulsating injection of fluid into the body.

Several terms must be explained at this point. *Pressure* is the force required to distribute the embalming solution throughout the body. The *rate of flow* is the amount of embalming solution that enters the body in a given period and is measured in ounces per minute. *Potential pressure* is the pressure reading on the gauge in the centrifugal machine, indicating the pressure in the delivery line of the machine with the rate-of-flow valve closed or the arterial tubing clamped shut. **Differential pressure** is the difference between the potential pressure reading and the actual pressure reading; this is an indicator of the *rate of flow*. **Actual pressure** is the reading on the pressure gauge on the centrifugal pump when the rate-of-flow valve is open and the arterial solution is entering the body.

In the example described in Figure 4–14, with the rate-of-flow valve CLOSED, the potential pressure is 15 pounds psi. The differential pressure is 5 and the actual pressure when the rate of flow valve is open is 10. If it were open until the gauge dropped to 5 actual pounds, the differential would be 10, or it can be said that the rate of flow would be twice as fast as the previous setting. The differential reading indicates the amount of resistance in the body, in the arterial cannula, and in the tube running from the machine to the cannula. The differential is also an important indicator of the rate of flow. Flow-rate gauges may also be added to the centrifugal machine.

There has been much misunderstanding in regard to the pressure that may exist inside the body as a result of the injection of solution. The mere fact that a pressure gauge reading on the device used for injection indicates a given pressure at which the fluid is leaving the machine does not necessarily mean that this pressure exists within the body. To determine what the pressure reading on the gauge really means, take a look at the schematic diagrams (Figs. 4–15, 4–16), showing the internal structure of an embalming machine, with four different flow paths shown as "filled" tubes (solid black) numbered from 1 to 4.

Liquid flows from the "well" beneath the tank to the pump from which it follows either path 1 or 2 or both paths (Fig. 4–15). Path 1 represents the bypass flow from the pump back to the tank. As the pump functions at a steady and continuous capacity, it is necessary to provide such bypass when injection of fluid at a slow rate is desired. Otherwise, the full force of the pump pressure could not be controlled to permit such low injection rates. Path

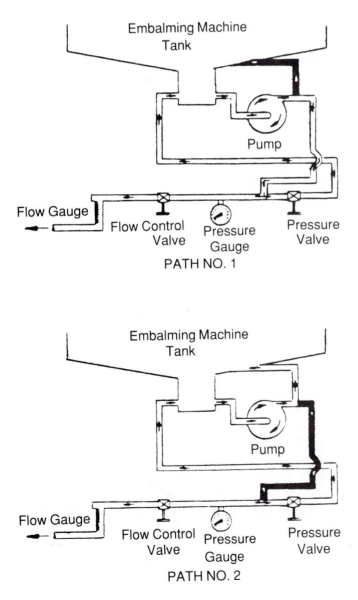

Figure 4–15. Pressure paths 1 and 2.

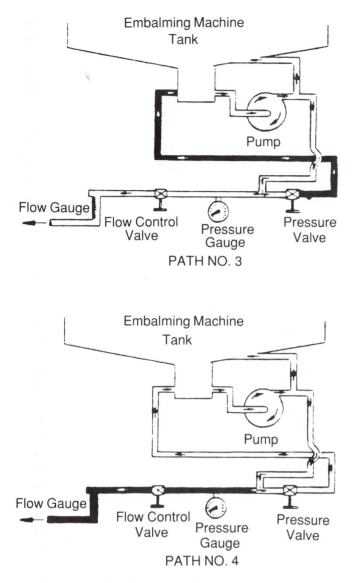

Figure 4–16. Pressure paths 3 and 4.

2 is the flow from the pump to the intermediate line just prior to the outlet line.

The intermediate line contains the rate-of-flow control valve and the pressure control valve. As may be surmised, the pressure control valve determines how much fluid will be returned to the tank via path 3 (Fig. 4–16), which constitutes a second bypass in the system. If, for example, a maximum pressure is set at the pressure valve control, very little, if any, liquid will flow through path 3. The needle valve in the pressure control valve actually cuts off fluid flow to that bypass and so the fluid is forced, then, to flow on to the outlet.

As the fluid proceeds to the outlet, the rate-of-flow control valve will determine how much will be delivered to the arterial tube outlet indicated by path 4. When the rate-of-flow control valve is drastically reduced so that only a small trickle of fluid is delivered, then high pressures can readily be registered on the pressure gauge. This does not mean, as can be readily realized, that the fluid is leaving the arterial tube under THAT much pressure!

In other words, with liquid flow paths 3 and 4 cut off by reducing the rate of flow and cutting off the bypass of fluid beyond the pressure control valve (causing high pressures to be registered), fluid can then leave the pump in large quantities only through path 1, which is the bypass back to the tank. It should be remembered that regardless of the amount of pressure being used or how fast the rate of flow might be, the pump ALWAYS operates at the same speed and its output is ALWAYS the same. With this knowledge in mind, safety features in the nature of the bypass are included in pressure machines. The pressure reading on the gauge merely indicates the amount of resistance being offered to the flow of the liquid WITHIN the confines of the machine. Continual use of "high" pressure places a heavy load on the motor and pump and, most often, this is not necessary.

INSTRUMENTATION

An embalming chemical supply catalog lists several hundred instruments, most of which come in a variety of sizes and modifications. For this reason the list seems so long. Actually, very few instruments are needed in the preparation of the unautopsied or autopsied body. Most of the instruments have several uses and this helps to limit the number needed. Unlike a surgical procedure, embalming is not performed under sterile conditions, so instruments can be reused during the embalming process. Most instruments are constructed of steel and plated with nickel or chrome for protection against rust or chemical agents. They are chemically treated to be heat resistant and durable.

General Instruments

Aneurysm Needle. A blunt instrument (Fig. 4–17), the aneurysm needle is used for tissue dissection for the location and elevation of arteries and veins. The aneurysm

Figure 4–17. Aneurysm needle.

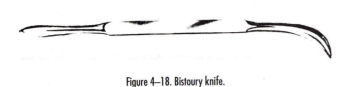

Figure 4–18. Bistoury knife.

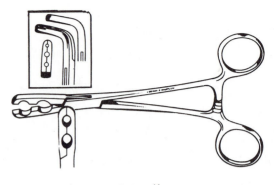

Figure 4–20. Arterial hemostat.

needle has an "eye" in the hook portion of the instrument, which could be used for passing ligatures around a vessel. An *aneurysm hook* is similar but has a sharp pointed tip. Most embalmers prefer to work with the blunt instrument.

Bistoury Knife. The bistoury knife is a curved cutting instrument that cuts from the inside outward (Fig. 4–18). Some embalmers prefer this type of instrument for opening arteries and veins. It can also be used for the excision of tissues.

Hemostat (Locking Forceps). A wide variety of hemostats are available. The hemostat can be used to clamp leaking vessels. A modification is the arterial hemostat, which is used to hold the arterial tube in an artery. The ends of hemostats may be curved or straight, serrated or smooth, or plain or rat-toothed. *Dressing forceps* are very long hemostats. They can be used for packing orifices or handling con-taminated bandage dressings (Figs. 4–19 to 4–21).

Scalpel. The scalpel is a sharp cutting instrument used for making incisions (Fig. 4–22). It can be purchased with a permanent blade, or the handles can be purchased and disposable blades used.

Scissors. Scissors are used for cutting. Like the bistoury knife and scalpel, scissors can also be used to open arteries and veins (Fig. 4–23). There is an *arterial scissor* (Fig. 4–23D) manufactured for opening vessels. Scissors vary in length, and their tips may be straight or curved, or pointed or blunt. The blunt side should be used against the skin surface of the body. *Bandage scissors* (Fig. 4–23E) have a very large blunt end to help protect the skin from being cut.

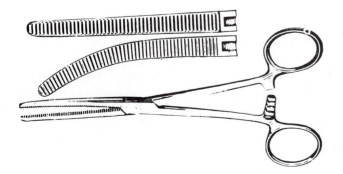

Figure 4–19. Serrated edges.

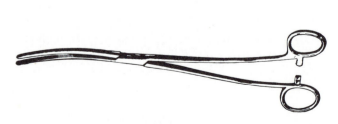

Figure 4–21. Dressing forceps.

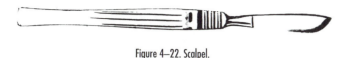

Figure 4–22. Scalpel.

Separator. The separator is used to keep vessels elevated above the incision. This instrument can be made of hard rubber, bone, or metal. Often, the handle of an aneurysm needle is designed to function as a separator (Fig. 4–24).

Suture Needles. A variety of suture needles are available (Fig. 4–25). The large *postmortem needles* (Fig. 4–25A, B) are used to close autopsy incisions as well as incisions

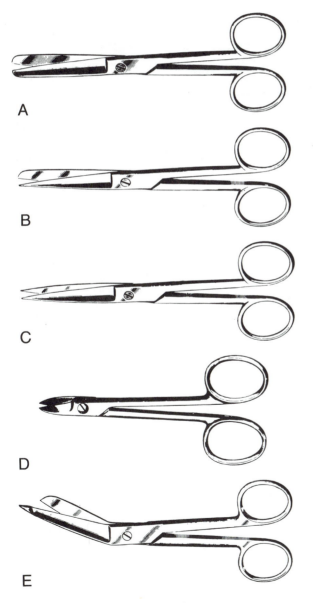

A

B

C

D

E

Figure 4–23. Various types of scissors.

made to raise vessels for injection. These needles are curved or double curved. The ⅜-inch *circle needle* is used for more delicate suturing. The needle eye may be the patented type called a "spring eye" for "self"-threading. The edges can be smooth or cutting (Fig. 4–25C). The half-curved *Loopuypt needle* (Fig. 4–25E) is designed to better grip the instrument.

Spring Forceps. The spring forceps is an instrument used for grasping and holding tissues. The limbs may be straight, curved, or angular (Fig. 4–26). Angular spring forceps are used as a drainage instrument, generally in the internal jugular vein. The tips of forceps may be serrated, smooth, or rat-toothed. Most embalmers use several types and lengths of spring forceps. This instrument is available in a large variety of lengths.

Suture Thread. Suture thread is sold by the twist or cord, 3 cord being thinner than 5 or 7 cord. Suture thread is also available in nylon, cotton, and linen. Some embalmers prefer that it be waxed. Dental floss can also be used for suturing.

Injection Instruments

Arterial Tubes. There are many types, lengths, and sizes of arterial injection tubes: those small enough for injection of infants and distal arteries, such as the radial and ulnar arteries in the adult, and those large enough for injection of the large carotid arteries. Carotid tubes are short and very large in diameter. The hub of an arterial tube can be *threaded* (Fig. 4–27A), to which a stopcock can be attached, or a *slip-type,* to which the delivery hose from the machine can be directly attached. The tube itself can be curved or straight. Luer-Lok (Fig. 4–27C) arterial tubes were developed for high-pressure injection. These tubes attach to a connector on the delivery hose much the same as a hypodermic needle attaches to a syringe.

Stopcock. The stopcock is used to attach the delivery hose from the injection device to the arterial tube (Fig. 4–28A). Luer-Lok stopcocks are used for arterial tubes with Luer-Lok attachments (Fig. 4–28B). The stopcock can be used to maintain and stop the flow of fluid into the arterial tube.

Y Tube. The Y tube was developed for the embalming of autopsied bodies. It allows the embalmer to embalm both legs or arms or sides of the head at the same time (Fig. 4–29). Double "Y" tubes have been developed that allow for injection of four body regions at the same time.

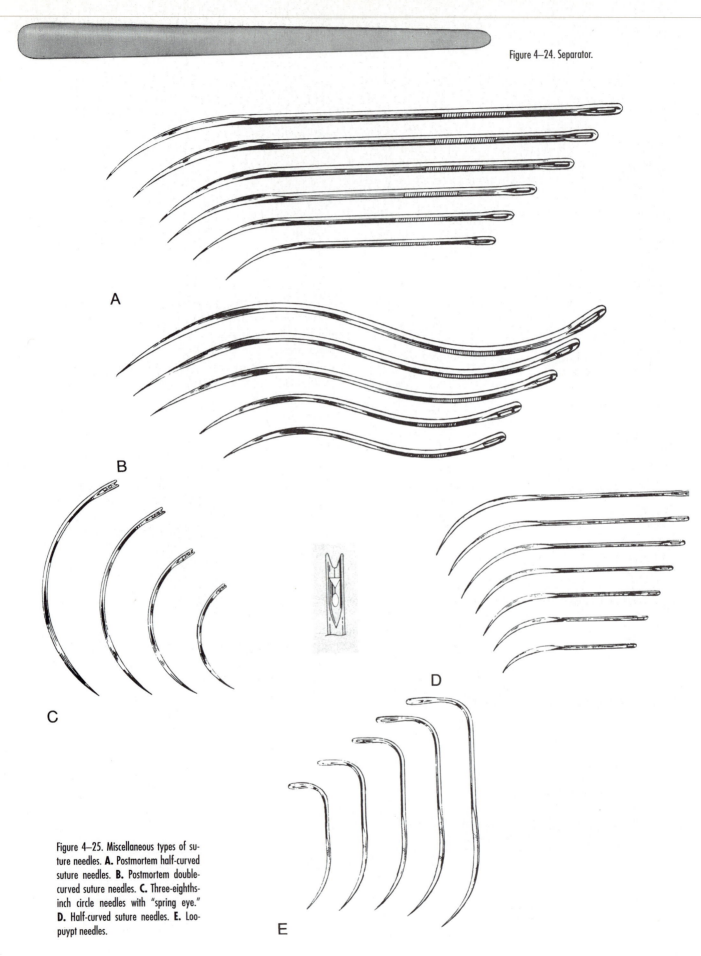

Figure 4–24. Separator.

A

B

C

D

E

Figure 4–25. Miscellaneous types of suture needles. **A.** Postmortem half-curved suture needles. **B.** Postmortem double-curved suture needles. **C.** Three-eighths-inch circle needles with "spring eye." **D.** Half-curved suture needles. **E.** Loopuypt needles.

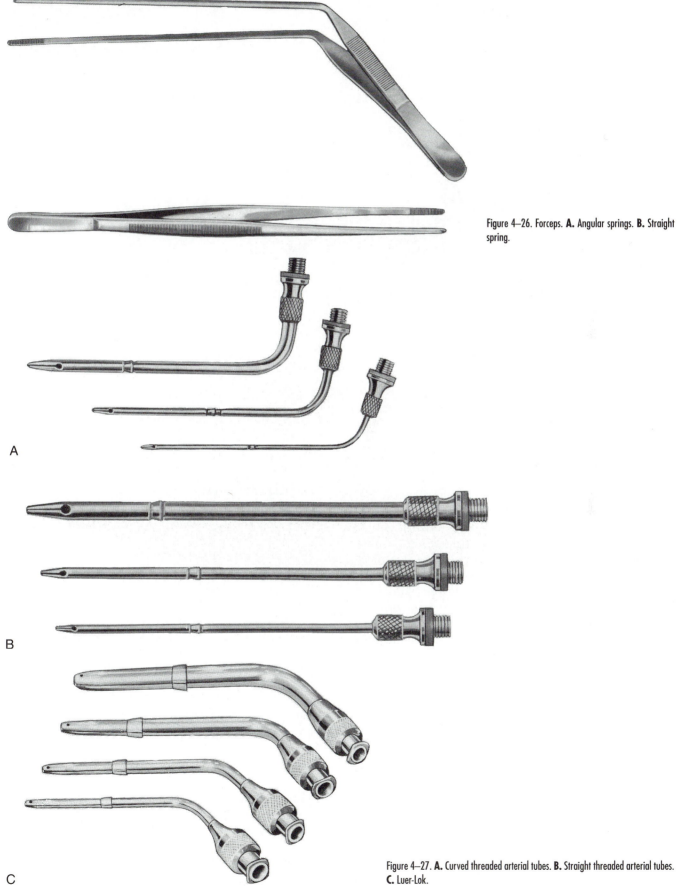

Figure 4–26. Forceps. **A.** Angular springs. **B.** Straight spring.

Figure 4–27. **A.** Curved threaded arterial tubes. **B.** Straight threaded arterial tubes. **C.** Luer-Lok.

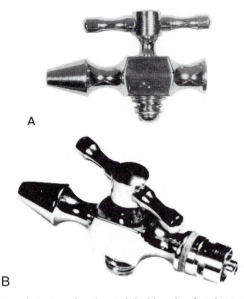

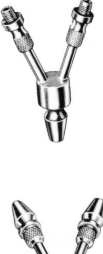

Figure 4–28. Stopcocks. **A.** Stopcock used to attach the delivery hose from the injection device to the arterial tube. **B.** Luer-Lok stopcock used for arterial tubes with Luer-Lok attachments.

Figure 4–29. A Y tube used for embalming autopsied bodies.

Drainage Instruments

Drain Tube. The drain tube is a metal cylinder with a cleaning rod designed to be inserted into a vein (Fig. 4–30). Drain tubes are always inserted TOWARD the heart. They help to keep the vein expanded and can be closed to build circulatory pressure. The stirring rod can be used to fragment large clots. There are many sizes. Jugular drain tubes are generally very large in diameter and short; axillary drain tubes are often slightly curved; infant drain tubes can be used for small vessels such as the femoral and iliac in the infant. A hose can easily be attached to the drainage outlet so the blood drained can easily be controlled or collected and disinfected.

Iliac Drain Tube The iliac drain tube is a long drain tube designed to be inserted into the external iliac vein and the tip is directed into the right atrium of the heart (Fig. 4–31). These tubes may be soft rubber, plastic, or metal.

Grooved Director. The grooved director is used to expand a vein to help guide a drain tube or drainage device such as angular spring forceps into a vein for a drainage (Fig. 4–32).

Aspirating Instruments

Autopsy Aspirator. An autopsy aspirator has many openings so as to be "nonclogging." It is used to aspirate blood and arterial fluid from the cavities of autopsied bodies (Fig. 4–33).

Hydroaspirator. The hydroaspirator is an aspirating device that creates a vacuum when water is run through the mechanism (Fig. 4–34). Most are equipped with a vacuum breaker so aspirated material flowing through the device does not enter the water supply should there occur a sudden drop in water pressure.

Nasal Tube Aspirator. The nasal tube aspirator attaches to the aspirating hose. It is designed to be inserted into the nostril or throat for limited aspiration of the nasal passage or the throat (Fig. 4–35).

Trocar. The trocar is a long hollow needle. The length and the diameter of this instrument are quite variable (Fig. 4–36). The points are threaded so they may be changed when dull. The handle may be threaded or have a slip hub. Infant trocars are short and small in diameter. They

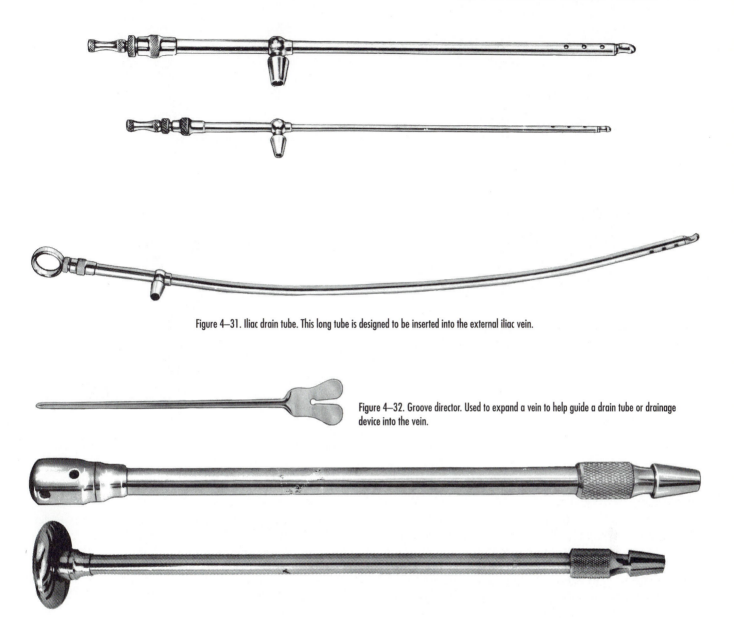

Figure 4–31. Iliac drain tube. This long tube is designed to be inserted into the external iliac vein.

Figure 4–32. Groove director. Used to expand a vein to help guide a drain tube or drainage device into the vein.

Figure 4–33. Autopsy aspirator. The many openings guard against clogging during aspiration of either blood or arterial fluid from the cavities of autopsied bodies.

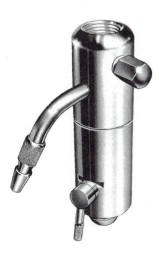

Figure 4–34. Hydroaspirator. This aspirating device creates a vacuum when water is run through the mechanism.

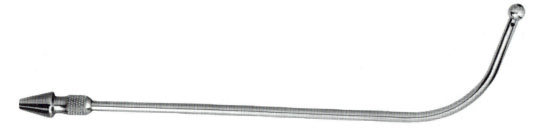

Figure 4–35. Nasal tube aspirator. Attaches to the aspirating hose. Designed for nasal insertion.

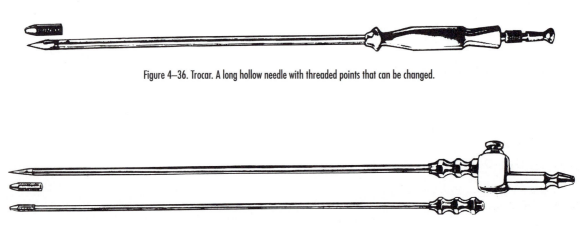

Figure 4–36. Trocar. A long hollow needle with threaded points that can be changed.

Figure 4–37. Hypovalve trocar. Designed for hypodermic treatments. Used for injection, not aspiration.

may also be used for hypodermic injection treatments. The standard trocar is used to aspirate and inject body cavities.

Hypovalve Trocar. The hypovalve trocar is designed for hypodermic treatments (Fig. 4–37). It is *not* used for aspiration but rather for injection.

Cavity Fluid Injector. The cavity fluid injector screws onto the cavity fluid bottles. When the device is inverted, cavity fluid flows through the trocar into the body cavities (Fig. 4–38).

Trocar Button. A threaded plastic screw used for closing trocar punctures, the trocar button may also be used to close small punctures, surgical drain openings, and intravenous line punctures (Fig. 4–39).

Trocar Button Applicator. The trocar button applicator is used to insert the trocar button (Fig. 4–40).

Feature Setting Devices

Eyecaps. Eyecaps are plastic disks inserted under the eyelids. They keep the eyelids closed and prevent the eyes from sinking into the orbit (Fig. 4–41).

Mouth Formers. Mouth formers are plastic or metal devices used to replace the teeth when the natural teeth or dentures are absent (Fig. 4–42).

Needle Injector. A needle injector is used to insert a "barb" into the mandible and maxilla to hold the lower jaw in a closed position (Fig. 4–43).

Positioning Devices

Positioning devices enable the embalmer to properly position the head, arms, hands, and feet of the deceased. Most are constructed of metal, hard rubber, or plastic. Embalmers often employ specially cut blocks of wood to elevate shoulders, arms, and feet. These devices should be properly painted with a water-resistant paint so they can be cleaned after each use.

Head Rests. Head rests can be used to elevate the head and neck. They can also be used to support the arms and raise the feet. A head rest can also be placed under the thigh area to help steady bodies with severe spinal curvature or an arthritic condition (Fig. 4–44).

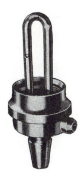

Figure 4–38. Cavity fluid injector. Screws onto cavity fluid bottles.

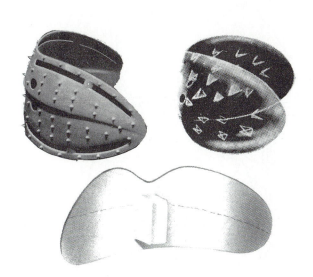

Figure 4–42. Mouth formers.

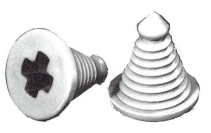

Figure 4–39. Trocar button. Threaded plastic screw used for closing trocar punctures.

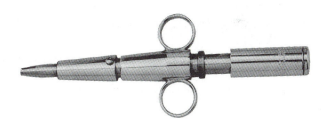

Figure 4–43. Needle injector.

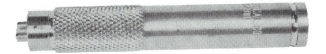

Figure 4–40. Trocar button applicator. Used to insert the trocar button.

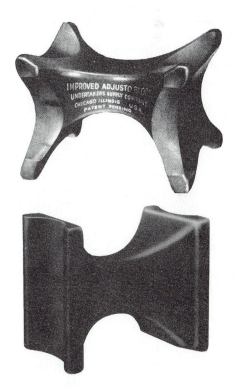

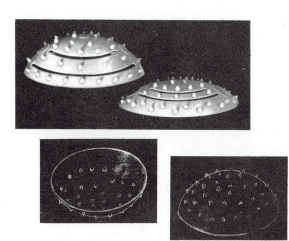

Figure 4–41. Eyecaps.

Figure 4–44. Headrests.

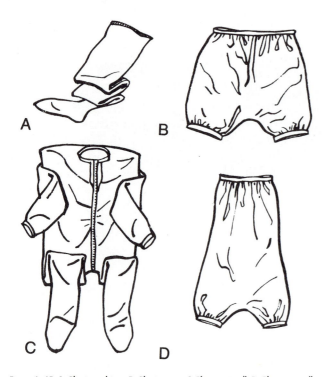

Figure 4–45. A. Plastic stockings. **B.** Plastic pants. **C.** Plastic unionall. **D.** Plastic coveralls.

Arm and Hand Rests. Arm and hand rests consist of two curved metal arm holders attached by an adjustable strap. The strap rests across the body while the arms are secured in the arm holder. It is designed to fit bodies of different size and retain both arms and hands in a desirable position.

Shoulder, Body, and Foot Rests. Rests of plastic or metal blocks are used to raise shoulders, feet, or buttocks off the table.

PLASTIC UNDERGARMENTS

Plastic undergarments are a necessity. These garments can be used to protect clothing from conditions such as ulcerations, gangrene, or burnt tissue. Plastic garments help to control leakage from the autopsied body or the condition of edema. Powdered deodorants and preservatives may be placed within the garment to help control these conditions. The coverall covers the trunk of the body from the upper thigh to the armpit. The unionall covers the entire body except for the hands, neck, and head areas (Fig. 4–45).

CONCLUSION

This chapter has emphasized that the preparation room is an essential part of the physical facility known as the "funeral home." It has evolved with technology and with the recognition of the central role that embalming and public health concerns play in American funerary behavior. In addition, an attempt has been made to provide advice and counsel that might be helpful to funeral service practitioners and architects in planning renovations or new construction of the preparation environment. Finally, the necessity to design and construct a facility that facilitates rather than hinders achievement of the objectives of embalming, not the least of which is the personal health and protection of embalming personnel and the general public, is stressed.

KEY TERMS AND CONCEPTS FOR STUDY AND DISCUSSION

1. Define the following terms:
   autopsy aspirator
   bistoury
   grooved director
   hydroaspirator
   pressure
   rate of flow
   serrated edge/smooth edge
   slip hub/threaded hub
   unionall
   vacuum breaker
2. Discuss the disadvantages of a basement preparation room.
3. Discuss the proper locations for an exhaust system in the preparation room.
4. How does the hand pump differ from the bulb syringe.
5. With reference to the centrifugal injection machine explain the terms potential pressure, actual pressure, and differential pressure.
6. Review the statutes, rules, and regulations your state has concerning the preparation room.

BIBLIOGRAPHY

Bourne H, Seferian S. Formaldehyde in wrinkle-proof apparel processes: Tears for my lady. *Ind Med Surg* 1959;28:232.

Hendrick DJ, Lane DJ. Occupational formalin asthma. *Br J Ind Med* 1977;34:11.

Johnson P. NIOSH Health Hazard Evaluation Determination Report HE 79-146-670, March 1980.

Kerfoot E, Mooney T. Formaldehyde and paraformaldehyde study in funeral homes. *Am Ind Hyg Assoc J* 1975;36:533.

Moore LL, Ogrodnik EC. Occupational exposure to formaldehyde in mortuaries. *J Environ Health* 1986;49(1):32–35.

Morrill E. Formaldehyde exposure from paper process solved by air sampling and current studies. *Air Cond Heat Vent* 1961;58:94.

Porter JAH. Acute respiratory distress following formalin inhalation. *Lancet* 1975;2:876.

Proctor NH, Hughes JP. *Chemical Hazards of the Workplace*. Philadelphia: JB Lippincott; 1978:272.

Riccobono PX. *Current Report: Bureau of National Affairs*. October 1979:471.

Sakula A. Formalin asthma in hospital laboratory staff. *Lancet* 1975;2:876.

Schoenber J, Mitchell C. Airway disease caused by phenolic (phenol–formaldehyde) resin exposure. *Arch Environ Health* 1975;30:575.

U.S. Department of Labor. *Occupational Safety and Health Standards (OSHA) for General Industry.* January 1978.

USDHEW/PHS/HRA. *Minimum Requirements of Construction and Equipment for Hospitals and Medical Facilities.* National Technical Information Service, DHEW Publication No. (HRA) 74-4000, September 1974.

5

Death—Agonal and Preembalming Changes

DEATH

Death is a process and not a moment in time. During the process there is a series of physical and chemical changes, starting before the medico-legal time of death and continuing afterward. . . . In the sequence of death there is a point of irreversibility that can generally be diagnosed by physicians. When this point is reached, nothing more can be done to restore intelligent life.

Older criteria defined death as that moment in time when the heart or lungs had irreversibly ceased to function. In light of current scientific knowledge and instrumentation, these two vital functions can now be mechanically sustained and, thus, new criteria must be established in defining death. These criteria must take the brain into account and, therefore, the definition can be shifted to state that a person is not dead when the heart stops, but rather when the brain stops.

The dying of an individual may be either slow or quick. The speed depends on the age, physical constitution, environment, and cause of death. The body actually dies in steps, but with today's medical advances it is possible to prolong these steps. The agonal period can be extended from minutes to hours, days, or years. This is the primary reason embalmers see body conditions totally different from those they did 20 years ago. The ag-

onal period has been greatly increased; thus disease processes are permitted to progress to degrees not seen in the past. When death does occur, we may see extreme emaciation, extensive skin discoloration, large amounts of edema, organ failure (such as liver and kidneys), and atrophied musculature and tissues, which have broken down and easily separate from the body. Secondary infections can also add to the problems created by the disease processes.

Currently, the state laws concerning the definition of death fall into three categories: (Showalter, 1982) "(1) those with alternative definitions, (2) those that consider brain death function only if artificial means of support prevent determination of death by the traditional means, and (3) those that ignore the traditional standards and refer to brain death only."

States using the alternative definitions can define death as that time at which the patient either sustains irreversible cessation of spontaneous circulation and respiration or has irreversible cessation of spontaneous brain function. Some argue that this approach appears to hold the misconception that there are two types of death when, in reality, death is death. The second category uses the definition of brain death but specifies the circumstance in which this should be applied. The third way in which states have defined death is to use solely the definition of brain death. Some states exclusively apply the brain death definition, whereas others do not prevent the use of other medical standards (Ryan, 1982).

There was an attempt to create a uniform definition of death for all the states. In 1979, the President's Commission for the Study of Ethical Problems in Medicine and Biomedical and Behavioral Research was established by Congress. The Commission proposed a model statute which was endorsed by the American Medical Association, the American Bar Association, and the National Conference of Commissioners on Uniform State Laws in 1980. The statute is the Uniform Determination of Death Act and reads as follows:

1. Determination of Death—An individual who has sustained either (1) irreversible cessation of circulatory and respiratory functions or (2) irreversible cessation of all functions of the entire brain, including the brain stem, is dead. A determination of death must be made in accordance with accepted medical standards.
2. Uniformity of Construction and Application—This Act shall be applied and construed to effectuate its general purpose to make uniform the law with respect to the subject of this Act among states enacting it.

A few states have begun to adopt this Act as their own current legal definition of death. This definition also permits the determination of death to be made according to "accepted medical standards." As newer and improved methods for determining death are discovered, these may be used by the medical community.

Spitz and Fisher (1980) point out that other definitions of death must be added. After a person is legally dead, individual muscle fibers and other cells may continue to live varying amounts of time. Because of this phenomenon, the death of the person as a whole has come to be referred to as somatic death and the ultimate death of all of the cells of the body is described as cellular death.

EARLY SIGNS OF DEATH

Signs of death are those manifestations by which it may be recognized in the body. These changes occur at about the time of death or within a few minutes of death. Their importance lies in the fact that they can be used to determine if death has, in fact, occurred. Such signs of death include:

1. Cessation of respiration
2. Cessation of circulation
3. Pallor of the skin
4. Muscular flaccidity
5. Contact flattening and pallor of the tissues in contact with an object

6. Eye changes
    a. Clouding of the cornea ⎫
    b. Loss of luster of the conjunctiva ⎬ all brought about by dehydration of the eye
    c. Flattening of the eyeball ⎭
    d. Pupil dilation and no muscle response to light

LATER SIGNS OF DEATH

During the first several hours some of the noticeable changes will include:

1. Postmortem lividity
2. Rigor mortis
3. Algor mortis
4. Decomposition (this is the most positive sign of death)

TESTS OF DEATH

A test of death is any procedure used to prove a sign of death. The expert tests are generally administered by a properly trained individual.

1. Stethoscope—used to detect audible sounds of circulation or breathing
2. Ophthalmoscope—used to examine the eye to detect circulation in the capillaries; tests the response
3. Electroencephlogram (EEG)—used to detect brain activity
4. Electrocardiogram (ECG, EKG)—used to detect heart activity
5. Auditory brain stem response (ABR)—measures activity in the brain stem, an area that controls heart and respiratory function

INEXPERT TESTS

Inexpert tests can be as simple as placing a saucer of water on the chest to detect any ripples of the water that might suggest cardiac or respiratory activity.

1. Ligature test—A finger is ligated with string or a rubber band; if it becomes swollen and discolored this is a sign of circulation.
2. Ammonia injection test—A very small amount of ammonia is injected subcutaneously; if there is a reddish reaction this indicates life is present.
3. Pulse—Digital pressure can be applied to the radial artery or the common carotid artery to feel for a pulse beat.
4. Placing the ear over the chest cavity—Heart or respiratory sounds can be heard in this manner.

Some states still require that two tests of death be administered prior to embalming. These old statutes came about around 1919 when so many persons died during the influenza epidemics in the United States.

TYPES AND STAGES OF DEATH

There are two types of death: somatic and cellular. Somatic death is defined as the death of the whole organism. It proceeds in an orderly progression from clinical death to brain death, then to biological death, and, finally, to postmortem cellular death. The series of events culminating in somatic death can be referred to as the mechanisms of death. These are different from the cause of death. The cause of death initiates the events that lead to death (stroke, myocardial infarction, infectious disease). There are three mechanisms that lead to the actual death and immediately bring about a life-threatening situation. These mechanisms revolve around the brain, the circulatory system, and the respiratory system.

Somatic death has historically been recognized by the failure of one of the following three organs that constitute the "tripod of life": (1) syncope—stoppage of circulation by disease or injury, (2) asphyxia or apnea—stoppage of respiration by disease or injury, (3) coma—stoppage of brain function by disease or injury. Failure of any one of these organs will bring about the loss of integration of the body systems. This will almost immediately begin the stages of somatic death. Recent medical advances have made the progression of the stages of death difficult to establish. It is now possible to keep the body alive by artificial support. Death of the brain is now the crucial factor in determining when a patient is biologically dead.

The following chart presents the order of occurrence leading up to death as well as the antemortem cellular death, the death of individual cells during life. Necrobiosis is the physiological, or natural, death of cells as they complete their life cycles. Necrosis is the pathological death of body cells as a result of disease processes. Gangrene and decubitus ulcerations are two examples frequently encountered in embalming.

ANTEMORTEM PERIOD

Cellular Death
Necrobiosis
Necrosis

STAGES OF DEATH

Agonal period
Somatic death
Clinical death
Brain death
Biological death
Postmortem cellular death

Clinical death (legal death) occurs when spontaneous respiration and heartbeat irreversibly cease. If resuscitative steps are begun at the moment of clinical death, life may be fully restored. Clinical death will be established within 5 to 6 minutes maximum after the stoppage of respiration or circulation. This is a reversible phase of somatic death.

Just as the body dies in steps, so does the brain. Brain death could also be referred to as functional death. In time, all body cells will die of oxygen starvation (anoxia). The first part of the brain to die (after the 5 or 6 minutes) is the cerebral cortex. The midbrain dies next, followed by the brain stem. It is possible to have death of the higher brain centers (the cerebrum) without damage to the brain stem. In this condition, even though the patient is unconscious, the heart and respiratory system may function for years.

After death of the brain, biological death occurs. This is the irreversible phase of somatic death. Biological death represents the cessation of the simple life processes of the various organs and tissues of the body. At this point, spontaneous respiration and circulation cannot be restored. Now, the death of individual cells begins.

Postmortem cellular death (or molecular death) will vary depending on metabolic activity of the cells. The more highly specialized the cells of the body are and the more active the body cells are, the faster these cells react to a decrease in oxygen or nutrients. As all cells die from oxygen starvation (anoxia), those less specialized and those richly supplied with oxygen at the time of somatic death continue to live in the body a number of hours after somatic death, as shown in these examples:

Cells in the brain and nervous system	5 minutes
Muscle cells	3 hours
Cornea cells	6 hours
Blood cells	6 hours

In preparing a body that has been dead for a short period, almost every embalmer has seen a twitching of fingers or a rippling of skeletal muscles. Admittedly, this is a very rare happening today with the many delays caused by hospital protocols and removal of the body. When the reaction is noted it is simply the contraction and relaxation of muscle cells in response to the stimulus of the embalming fluid. Do not be mistaken that there is any type of "life" to the body. These are isolated muscle cells that have not yet depleted their oxygen supply.

AGONAL PERIOD

The agonal period is that period just prior to somatic death, and some of the changes that can occur in that period may have significance in the embalming process. As previously stated, the agonal period has been greatly increased by medical science. The result, however, is that the disease processes have more time to act on the body organs and tissues. There may be an increase in secondary infections over long agonal periods. Many body changes occur that would never be seen if the agonal period had not been extended. These prolonged agonal periods along with the extensive use of drug therapy have had a dramatic effect on the postmortem conditions of all bodies embalmed today where there has been institutionalization of the individual for a period prior to death.

Two thermal changes can occur during the agonal period: **Agonal algor** is a cooling or lowering of the body temperature just prior to death. This is often seen in the death of elderly patients, especially when death occurs slowly. The metabolism has slowed in these individuals and, no doubt, the circulatory system has slowed. Lowering the body temperature is, of course, an advantage from the standpoint of embalming complications. Lower temperature slows the onset of rigor mortis and decomposition.

Agonal fever is an increase of the body temperature just prior to death. This is often seen in persons with infections, toxemias, or certain types of poisoning. Frequently elevated temperature can stimulate microbial growth. Likewise, elevated temperatures help to stimulate rigor mortis and decomposition after somatic death.

Agonal Circulatory Changes

Agonal Hypostasis. During the period just prior to death, a slowing of the functioning of the circulatory system can bring about a settling of blood into the dependent body tissues. Blood in these capillaries can begin to clump, and during the embalming process removal of this blood may be difficult.

Agonal Coagulation. Any slowing of the circulatory system can bring about clotting and congealing of blood elements. This condition can, of course, make the embalming process very difficult if the clotting and congealing are extensive.

Agonal Capillary Expansion. In an attempt to get more oxygen to the tissues and cells, the pores of the capillaries expand. In addition, the small muscles that allow blood to flow into the capillary beds expand. This change brings about the elevated moisture in the tissues. If these channels remain wide open after death, swelling of the tissues would be more likely during arterial injection.

Agonal Moisture Changes

Agonal Edema. Because of the capillary expansion prior to death, there is an increase in moisture in the tissues and in the body cavities. A good example is agonal pulmonary edema frequently seen at the autopsy of an individual whose death was caused by trauma. Even though the agonal period lasted only minutes, the tissues of the lungs are found to be quite moist. This reaction by the body brought about by capillary expansion is an attempt to get more oxygen to the body tissues. From the embalming standpoint any increase in tissue moisture helps to speed the decomposition process. In addition, increased tissue moisture increases the need for preservative. Keep in mind that organs in the thoracic and abdominal cavities are affected by agonal edema, and any elevation in moisture in an organ such as the lungs also helps to speed decomposition of these organs.

Agonal Dehydration. In some lingering deaths there can be a great loss of body moisture during the agonal period. This can bring about a thickening of the blood and dehydration of the mucous membranes.

Agonal Translocation of Microbes and Bacteremia. With expansion of the capillary system of the body, there now exists a good possibility that the microbes that normally inhabit a particular area of the body, such as the gastrointestinal tract, will find a passage into the circulatory system and travel throughout the body. This process really begins to take effect after death, when the natural defenses of the body no longer operate. Translocation of microbes can accelerate the decomposition process after death. In addition, it now becomes necessary for the embalmer to be certain the fluids injected are of sufficient strength to sanitize the tissues and of sufficient volume to reach all the tissues. This agonal process (and even postmortem process) is one that does not easily exhibit itself except when gas-forming microbes are present in the tissues after death. It is important to embalm every body as if all the tissues contained saphrophytic and gas-forming microbial agents.

The most dramatic organism that could translocate and cause very definite postmortem problems is *Clostridium perfringens*. This tissue gas-producing anaerobic bacillus is responsible for true tissue gas. Its presence throughout the body after death can bring about immediate embalming and preservation problems. Within just 1 or 2 hours of death, if this organism is present in the tissues, it can produce gases that distend the tissues to the point where viewing the body might be impossible. Of all the agonal changes, this translocation problem with this specific microbe is the most important to the embalmer.

THE POSTMORTEM CHANGES

In the period between death and embalming, the body undergoes a number of physical and chemical changes. The embalming of the body interrupts these changes and, in some cases (such as dehydration), even reverses the changes. The longer the time between death and embalming, the more changes will occur, and some changes such as decomposition may have such an effect on the body tissues that the embalming process will not be successful.

These postmortem changes are classified into two groups: physical and chemical changes. Many of these changes are very dependent on one another. The physical changes are brought about by the physical forces of nature, resulting in a change in the state of the body or body tissues, but products with new chemical compositions are not formed. For example, after death, the blood, because of gravity, slowly gravitates to the dependent tissues of the body. No new product is formed; the liquid blood has merely moved to the lower areas of the body. A chemical change is one brought about by chemical activity. As a result, new substances are formed, for example, postmortem stain. The hemoglobin molecule breaks down, releasing the pigmented portion of the hemoglobin, which easily passes into the tissue spaces to stain the tissues.

In making a preembalming *analysis* of the body the embalmer examines the effects of four factors concerning the body: (1) general body condition, (2) effects of disease on the body, (3) effects of drug therapy on the body, (4) postmortem changes.

In examining the body the embalmer is concerned about weight, age, state of nutrition, effects of disease such as tumors, discoloration, moisture content of the tissues, discoloration caused by renal or liver failure, nitrogenous waste buildup in the tissues, and, finally, postmortem changes such as the degree of rigor mortis, signs that decomposition has begun, and blood discoloration or stains. All these factors taken together help to determine the embalming technique to be used. Often, the postmortem changes have the greatest influence on the embalming technique (Fig. 5–1).

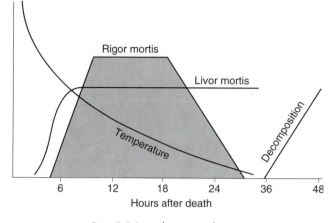

Figure 5–1. Principal postmortem changes.

Table 5–1 lists the classic changes that have been defined in embalming literature over the years. They are classified as a physical or chemical change and a brief description of each change is given.

POSTMORTEM PHYSICAL CHANGES

Postmortem physical changes include algor mortis, hypostasis, livor mortis, dehydration, and increase in the viscosity of the blood. The changes are brought about by the stoppage of blood circulation, gravity, and surface evaporation.

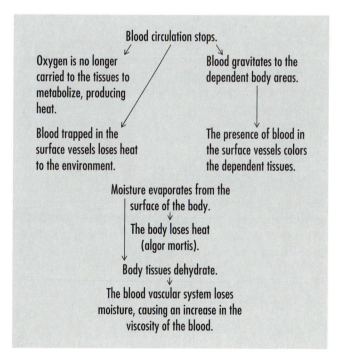

TABLE 5–1. POSTMORTEM PHYSICAL AND CHEMICAL CHANGES

Postmortem Change	Characteristics of Origin	Description
Algor mortis	Physical	Cooling of the body to the temperature of the surrounding environment
Dehydration	Physical	Loss of moisture from the surface of the body to the surrounding atmosphere
Hypostasis	Physical	Gravitation of the blood and body fluids to the dependent areas of the body
Livor mortis	Physical	Postmortem intravascular blood discoloration brought about by the presence of blood in the dependent surface vessels of the body
Increase in blood viscosity	Physical	Thickening of the blood after death caused primarily by loss of the liquid portion of the blood to the tissue spaces
Postmortem caloricity	Chemical	Temporary rise in body temperature after death
Hydrolysis	Chemical	Ability of water to split compounds and to enter itself into the products formed
Change in the pH of the body	Chemical	Change in body tissues from slightly alkaline in life (pH 7.38–7.40) to more alkaline immediately after death (pH 6.0–5.0) to alkaline (basic) during decomposition
Rigor mortis	Chemical	Temporary postmortem stiffening of all the body muscles by natural body processes (Rigor will pass naturally in a variable length of time by natural body processes.)
Postmortem stain	Chemical	Extravascular color change brought about by hemolysis (Liberated heme seeps through the capillary walls and into the body tissues; the stain cannot be removed by arterial injection and venous drainage.)
Decomposition	Chemical	Separation of compounds into simpler substances by the action of bacterial and/or autolytic enzymes

In discussing postmortem changes emphasis should be placed on the effects the process or condition has on the embalming of the blood, as this is the primary purpose for including these changes in this text.

Algor Mortis

Algor mortis is a postmortem cooling of the body. The body cools to the temperature of the surrounding environment. Normal body temperature is 98.6°F, and there is usually a slight rise in body temperature after death due to the stoppage of circulation, respiration, and execretion. It takes time for the body to cool to the temperature of the surrounding environment. In the first few hours after death the body usually cools faster. Then, cooling slows as the body temperature reaches that of the environment. For years, forensic pathologists have tried to establish a method for determining how long a person had been dead by using the temperature of the body organs. This temperature is taken with a rectal thermometer or by making a small opening under the liver and inserting a thermometer. *The internal organs cool much slower than the surface tissues of the body. For this reason putrefactive and autolytic decomposition may begin early in the visceral organs.*

Even in some bodies removed from refrigeration, the abdominal cavity can be distended with gases as a result of decomposition changes. The wall of the abdomen can be green in the lower right quadrant, or the outline of the large intestine may be seen because of a color change on the abdominal wall. Many variables influence the onset and speed of algor mortis. The following is a list of some considerations, but more can be added:

I. Intrinsic Factors
  1. Size of the body: Larger persons cool slowly; thin persons cool faster.
  2. Body weight: Corpulence and adipose tissue help insulate a body and slow cooling.
  3. Cause of death: Febrile diseases elevate temperature and slow the onset of algor; wasting diseases can speed the onset.
  4. Age of the individual: A child or infant cools much faster than an adult.
II. Extrinsic Factors
  1. Body coverings: The amount of clothing or body covering slows the onset of algor.
  2. Environment: Placing a body in a refrigeration unit after death speeds algor; death in a house without air conditioning during the summer months slows algor.

It is easy to see how difficult a formula would be that uses algor mortis as a criterion for establishing the time of death. Attempting to establish a time by the cooling of the body has value only up to approximately 12 hours from the time of death. Of importance to the embalming process is the fact that cooling of the body as quickly as possible (through refrigeration after death) helps to slow the very important processes that make the embalming much more difficult (Fig. 5–2).

Cooling of the body slows the onset of rigor mortis, slows the onset of decomposition, and helps to keep the blood in a liquid state. This aids in the removal or drainage of the blood.

On the other hand, there is a disadvantage with bodies that have been refrigerated and the blood kept in a liquid state. These bodies are usually found to have a greater degree of liver mortis discoloration. Refrigeration cooling also speeds the establishment of postmortem staining of the body. Refrigerated bodies often take on a hue similar to that of embalmed bodies in which there is a cosmetic dye in the fluid. The pink hue is produced by the hemolysis of red blood cells trapped in the capillar-

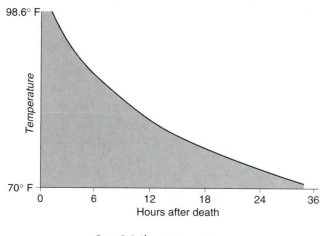

Figure 5–2. Algor mortis versus time.

ies of the superficial tissues. In other words, refrigerated bodies often look as if they were already embalmed. That color of the body, accompanied by the stiffening caused by the refrigeration and rigor mortis, can give a false sign of embalmed tissue. Care must be taken in embalming refrigerated bodies to use additional amounts of dye with the fluid to trace the presence of this fluid.

Hypostasis

Postmortem hypostasis is a settling of blood into the dependent tissues of the body. This settling brings about the discoloration described as livor mortis. After time passes, the blood begins to break down and the hemoglobin portion passes through the walls of the capillaries and stains the tissues. The discoloration is postmortem stain. It is extravascular and cannot be removed by arterial fluid injection and subsequent blood drainage.

The dependent part of the body is the lowest part of the body, so depending on the body position after death any portion of the body could become the dependent portion. For example, if a body dies in the supine position (on its back), the tissues of the back of the body (trunk, neck, legs, etc.) are the lowest and blood will gravitate into these areas. Likewise, if a person were to die in a slumped position, it is easy to see that the head could be the dependent part of the body. With the victim of a hanging, the lower extremities are the more dependent body areas.

The thinner the blood (low viscosity), the faster hypostasis occurs. For persons who die from diseases for which they were treated with medications that thin the blood, the process occurs faster. For persons who die from conditions in which the blood is thickened (high viscosity), the process is longer.

Hypostasis can begin prior to death if there is a slowing of the heart and the circulation. *Remember that it is the movement of the blood that creates the intravascular discoloration of livor mortis.* In refrigerated bodies,

the blood tends to remain very liquid. Therefore, a more rapid postmortem hypostasis of the blood is expected, as is movement of a greater volume of blood into the dependent tissues. This is why, in refrigerated bodies, there is often a very intense blood discoloration of the tissues.

If the hospital places the body on a flat cart to remove and store it without any support or elevation of the head, the head actually becomes dependent relative to the heart. The blood begins to gravitate into the tissues of the neck and face. This, of course, leads to discoloration of these tissues. In bodies from which the eyes are to be removed, it is important to keep the head elevated. Otherwise, there can be considerable leakage of blood from the eye orbit during and after eye enucleation.

As a rule the head of the body should be elevated at all times. This is important to remember in moving a body. The head should always be elevated when carrying the body and a pillow or support should be used in transporting the body. Likewise, if the body is to be refrigerated prior to embalming, be certain the shoulders and head are elevated. Even after embalming and aspirating the body, it is possible for blood that was not drained to mix with the arterial solution already injected and to gravitate into dependent body areas. This is another important reason to keep the head elevated at all times prior to casketing, especially if the body is being shipped to another funeral home. Many times, graying of the face and neck is noticed with shipped bodies. This is due to gravitation of the blood that remained in the body after embalming and that moved into the neck and face because the head and shoulders were not properly elevated in the shipping container.

As previously written, postmortem hypostasis refers to the movement of blood into the dependent body tissues. It should be remembered, however, that other liquids in the body likewise gravitate into the dependent tissue areas. A good example is seen in bodies dead with skeletal edema present. Even during life the edema has a tendency to gravitate if the individual has been confined to bed. After death, the gravitation of the edema becomes quite marked. This is noted in the hands if they have been placed at the sides of the body, and in the lower trunk and back regions as well as in the backs of the legs and thighs. In these dependent areas, a large amount of moisture is present in the tissues whether it be blood, interstitial fluid, or edema. Because of the increased moisture in these dependent tissues these areas can be expected to be the locations where bacterial activity could be very high. Often, gases of decomposition present in the facial tissues will have originated from bacteria located in these dependent areas. Increased moisture increases the preservative demand for these body regions. Care should be taken during the arterial embalming of all bodies to be certain that the dependent tissues are massaged and manipulated to attract as much fluid as possible into these areas.

Where the dependent areas of the body are in contact with the embalming table or positioning devices, extravascular pressure is applied to the vascular system (Fig. 5–3). As a result, it may be very difficult to establish good distribution through the tissues that are in contact with the table or positioning devices.

If the embalmer feels there are inadequate amounts of embalming solution in these regions after the arterial injection, a solution of preservation chemical (such as very strong arterial fluid or diluted cavity fluid) can be directly injected into these areas via an infant trocar to thoroughly saturate the tissues with preservative chemicals.

Gravitation of liquids will later include arterial solution. After arterial treatment there will be some movement of arterial solution through the tissue spaces and circulatory system into the dependent areas of the body. This gravitation of arterial solution must NOT be relied on to ensure preservation of these dependent tissues, which usually have a high moisture content.

There is a very valuable side to postmortem hypostasis from an embalming standpoint. The settling of blood into the dependent tissues can possibly serve to expand the small vessels and capillary networks. This expansion assists in attracting the flow of arterial solution into these regions. For example, if the hands of the body are dropped over the sides of the embalming table or laid at the side of the body, fluid will be noted in the tissues of the hands shortly after injection. This can also be seen with bodies where the hands are placed over the abdomen at the start of the embalming but little or no solution enters the arms and hands during arterial injection. If the operator lays the hands down over the sides of the embalming table during the later phases of the arterial injection, arterial solution quite often enters these tissues. When beginning to embalm an unautopsied body, place the hands down over the sides of the embalming table. This encourages hypostasis of the blood into the areas of the hands and expands the vessels at the same time. It also encourages the flow of arterial solution into these dependent areas.

Livor Mortis

Livor mortis is a postmortem intravascular blood discoloration produced as a result of hypostasis of the blood. This postmortem physical change is also called **postmortem lividity** or **cadaveric lividity.** After circulation of the blood has stopped, the blood tends to gravitate into the large veins of the trunk, the venae cava and the major veins. The blood gradually continues to gravitate into the veins and venules and capillaries of the dependent body regions, producing the discoloration of livor mortis. Livor can be seen as dull reddish patches approximately 20 to 30 minutes after death. The discoloration is well established by 6 to 10 hours after death (Fig. 5–4). Once the condition is well established the skin can take on a deep reddish-blue appearance.

There will be instances when antemortem hypostasis of the blood occurs as a result of a slowing of the circulatory system prior to death. In these bodies, the livor mortis will be noticed immediately after death. Two factors play an important role in the degree of intensity of livor mortis: blood volume and blood viscosity. Where hemorrhage has occurred (as in trauma) or when diseases or medications have resulted in internal bleeding, the intensity or degree of the livor mortis would be decreased. Embalmers will note in their work some bodies that have been dead for several hours and exhibit little or no livor discoloration. The viscosity of the blood is responsible for the degree of livor.

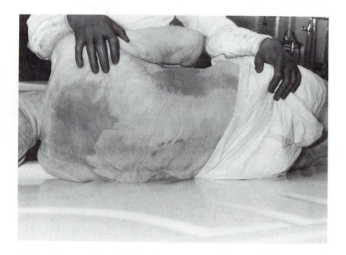

Figure 5–3. Dark areas show livor mortis and postmortem stain. The light-colored area on the back shows contact pallor where the body rested against the table.

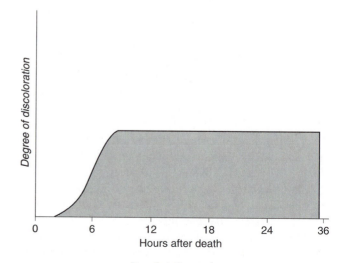

Figure 5–4. Livor mortis.

Two good examples are bodies that have been treated with blood thinners and bodies that have been refrigerated immediately after death. In both instances the blood may exhibit a thinner (low) viscosity. Thus, the livor will establish itself sooner after death and, depending on the viscosity and volume of blood in the body, will probably be very intense.

Livor mortis is an *intravascular blood discoloration.* The blood is still present in the small vessels and capillaries. This is important for the embalmer; because it is intravascular, the discoloration of livor mortis can be removed by arterial injection and subsequent drainage of the contents of the blood vascular system. In a simple test used to determine if the discolorations is livor mortis and intravascular, digital pressure is applied to the tissue by pinching or pushing on a body area. If the area pinched returns to normal skin color, the discoloration is intravascular and can be removed. Use of too strong an arterial solution may help to set the livor mortis discoloration. This was the reason that years ago preinjection fluids were developed, to help clear the blood discoloration prior to injection of the preservative solution. If the preinjection fluid is not used, the arterial solution may be kept mild until the livor mortis condition is cleared. This is important if the discoloration is present in the facial tissues. Frequently, livor is seen in the facial tissues, especially when the body has been laid flat without elevation of the head. If a strong solution is needed a co-injection chemical could be used with this solution to help control the action of the arterial fluid. This will assist in the clearing of the intravascular blood discoloration.

With regard to drainage of bodies in which livor mortis is present, another recommendation is to use concurrent (or continuous) drainage until the discolorations are cleared, especially in those regions that will be seen by the public (face, neck, hands, and arms). After clearing of the livor, use restricted drainage techniques such as intermittent or alternate drainage. If livor does not clear from an area it may be because the artery supplying this area with embalming solution is blocked. Direct injection of the discolored area may be necessary. (Intermittent drainage may possibly help for it will prevent the short circuiting of arterial solution and force the solution into these high-resistance tissues.) If the area of livor mortis is tested and DOES NOT clear when pinched, it can be assumed that enough time has elapsed for the discoloration now to be a postmortem stain. This condition will be described later as the next step after discoloration of livor mortis.

Postmortem stain is an extravascular condition and cannot be removed by arterial injection and blood drainage. Livor and stain occur in the same tissue areas. For this reason, some of the discoloration many times can be removed. The portion that was stain (usually lighter and redder) will remain. After embalming, the stain mixes with the formaldehyde and, in time, the tissues may become gray.

The presence of livor mortis can also be of value to the embalmer. When the condition exists and only a short time has elapsed between death and embalming, this is a good indicator that the blood is in a liquid state and drainage can be expected to be good. This is often confirmed when the vein that is to be used for drainage is opened and a large amount of blood drains PRIOR to the start of arterial injection. A second advantage of livor is that when the livor begins to clear *by itself* during arterial injection and not as the result of elevation or massage, this is a good sign of arterial solution distribution in the area where the livor is clearing.

As postmortem hypostasis draws the blood into the dependent tissues resulting in the discoloration of livor mortis, and after a certain period or when any condition exists that brings about hemolysis of the red blood cells and the resultant stain, it is easy to understand why it is so important to *always* keep the head elevated. To repeat, the head should be elevated in transporting the body and both the head and shoulders must be kept elevated during the embalming and dressing of the body.

Because livor mortis is intravascular, when livor is present as an intense condition in the neck and facial tissues, it can be often cleared by elevating the shoulders and head. During the setting of the features, bathing of the face, shaving, and so forth, much of the discoloration can be drained from the tissues just by gravitation prior to the injection of arterial solution. Some embalmers elevate the head and shoulders and then wait a short period, giving the livor condition an opportunity to clear. The head and shoulders should remain elevated, for any blood (even after embalming and cavity treatment) that gravitates back into the facial tissues would mix with the formaldehyde present and bring about a graying of the tissues. Table 5–2 summarizes embalming considerations and blood discolorations.

Dehydration

Dehydration is the loss of water from body tissues and fluids by surface evaporation. When dry, especially warmed, air is allowed to pass over the body in a very short period, the loss of moisture from the body can be noted on the exposed surfaces. There are two basic factors at work in postmortem loss of body moisture: surface evaporation and gravitation or hypostasis of the blood and body fluids.

Surface Evaporation. Surface evaporation results from the passage of dry air over the surfaces of the body. When a person dies fully clothed, as time passes the mucous membranes of the eyes and mouth begin to darken. Areas of the face such as the forehead and cheekbones take on a

TABLE 5–2. EMBALMING CONSIDERATIONS AND BLOOD DISCOLORATIONS

Antemortem Hypostasis	Postmortem Hypostasis	Time → Livor mortis	Time → Postmortem Stain	Embalming → Formaldehyde Gray
Occurs prior to death or during the agonal period	Begins at death	Seen as soon as blood fills superficial vessels; beings approximately 20 minutes after death; depends on p.m./a.m. hypostasis	Normally occurs about 6 hours after death; cause of death and blood chemistry vary rate	Occurs after embalming
Intravascular	Intravascular	Intravascular	Extravascular	Intravascular or extravascular
Movement of blood to dependent tissues[a]	Movement of blood to dependent tissues[a]	p.m. blood discoloration as a result of p.m./a.m. hypostasis	p.m. blood discoloration as a result of hemolysis	Embalming discoloration
a.m. physical change	p.m. physical change	p.m. physical change	p.m. chemical change	—
	Speed depends on blood viscosity	Color varies with blood volume and viscosity and amount of O_2 in blood	May occur prior to, during, or after arterial fluid injection	Seen after arterial fluid injection
Antemortem	Postmortem	Postmortem	Postmortem	Postmortem
—	—	Pressed on skin clears	Pressed on skin does NOT clear	Seen as a gray stain
—	—	Removed by blood drainage	Not removed by blood drainage	Methemoglobin HCHO + blood
—	Arterial injection stops progress	Arterial injection (mild) clears/with drainage	Strong solutions bleach and "set" livor as stain	—
	Speeded by cooling of body, low blood viscosity	Speeded by cooling, blood "thinners," low blood viscosity, CO deaths	Speeded by cooling, rapid red blood cell hemolysis, CO deaths	Speeded by poor drainage

p.m. postmortem; a.m. antemortem.
[a]Dependent body area varies with body position.

yellow to brown discoloration. If the tissues are touched they feel tight and hard.

A body placed in a hospital or morgue refrigeration unit also loses water to the cold air being circulated around it. It is interesting to note that when the body is naked and wrapped in a cotton sheet and refrigerated for a time, the entire surface of the body exhibits the effects of dehydration. Today, however, most hospitals and coroners' offices wrap bodies in plastic sheeting or place the body in a large plastic, zippered pouch. In this case, the body is quite often covered with a great amount of moist condensation. Even though the plastic might slow the dehydration process it also traps moisture on the body surface.

Gravitation or Hypostasis of the Blood and Body Fluids.
This gradual, physical movement of the body liquids out of the higher body regions and into the lower body areas helps to dehydrate the portions of the body from which the fluid is gravitating. At the same time, this gravitation temporarily adds moisture to the more dependent tissues. It is very important for the embalmer to know that in bodies with skeletal edema, liquid in the tissues will indeed gravitate to the dependent body areas such as the posterior areas of the shoulders, trunk, buttocks, and backs of the thighs and legs. The gravitation of edema then continues by passage through the body skin. This is why it is so important in the preparation of bodies with large amounts of skeletal edema to be certain hypodermic treatment has been applied to the dependent trunk areas. In addition, plastic garments such as coveralls, unionalls, and plastic stockings should be used.

Dehydration of the body after death can be explained by taking the two processes of surface evaporation and gravitation of body fluids and combining them with a third factor, imbibition. After death, the cells of the body have the ability to pull surrounding moisture into themselves. This "pulling action" draws moisture from the capillaries. The liquid portion of the contents of the blood vascular system has a tendency to be drawn into the tissue spaces by the process of imbibition. This, combined with surface evaporation, gradually drains the circulatory system of its liquid portion of the blood and lymphatic fluids. In addition, a major portion of the liquids of the blood vascular system gravitates into the dependent body areas.

Imagine that the entire blood–lymphatic system of the body is contained in a tube. This tube is contained in a large cylinder which represents the body tissues. As the liquid is pulled out of this "inside tube" by imbibition, it travels through the tissues of the cylinder and eventually, if the conditions are right, is given up by surface evaporation to the surrounding air (Fig. 5–5). If the body is embalmed while the moisture content of the tissues is still high, this moisture can serve as a secondary dilution for the arterial solution. This condition, in which the moisture content of the tissues is elevated postmortem, is called **postmortem edema**. It is a temporary condition, but while it is present the tissues will feel soft and "mushy." This condition is generally seen in bodies that have been refrigerated several days. Given time, dehydration can progress to the point where the body is completely desiccated and, thus, preserved. Is this not a condition similar to that brought about by the process of mummification? It must be remembered that dehydration can and will continue after the body has been embalmed. The embalming process itself can bring about a great amount of dehydration.

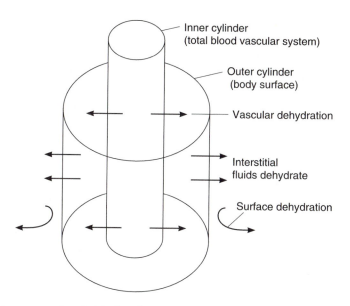

Figure 5–5. Total vascular system and the effects of dehydration.

- Inner cylinder (total blood vascular system)
- Outer cylinder (body surface)
- Vascular dehydration
- Interstitial fluids dehydrate
- Surface dehydration

There are other embalming considerations with respect to dehydration. As liquid is lost from the blood vascular system the viscosity of the blood increases. Blood cells have a tendency to stick together. This clumping of blood cells after death is referred to as "sludge." Blood drainage, therefore, can be difficult to establish.

Dehydration will bring about surface discolorations ranging from a yellow into the browns and, finally, black. Dehydrated tissues cannot be bleached. It is possible in rare instances to moisturize the skin by arterial injection. In addition, by the application of moisturizing creams to the surface of the dehydrated tissue, it is possible to restore some tissue moisture and remove some discoloration. These conditions generally require cosmetic treatment, opaque cosmetics being employed to hide the discoloration.

In addition to being very hard to the touch and discolored, dehydrated tissue is also shriveled and wrinkled. Eyelids, lips, the tip of the nose, and the fingers easily show this wrinkled and shriveled condition. The use of tissue builders after embalming seldom helps restore these dehydrated regions. Some embalmers make it a practice to inject some tissue builder into the fingers as a postembalming restorative measure on every body embalmed. This technique ensures that there will not be any postembalming dehydration of the fingers.

Note that there are "natural lines" in the lips. These lines are vertical. In fact, they are called the "vertical lines of the lip." The large lines of the lips created by dehydration are horizontal.

Dehydration is a postmortem physical change that occurs before embalming but can also be increased by embalming and can continue after embalming. This subject is dealt with from a clinical standpoint in Chapter 21.

Increase in Blood Viscosity

Viscosity refers to the thickness of a liquid. The blood is composed of two portions: a "solid" portion made up of the various groups of blood cells, and a "liquid" portion in which the cells are suspended. After death the blood has a tendency to increase in viscosity and thicken. This thickening is brought about by the dehydration of the body. As the tissues lose moisture to the surrounding air, the liquid portion of the blood begins to move through the capillary walls into the tissue spaces. Given enough time and the proper conditions this liquid could leave the body by surface evaporation. The remaining blood begins to thicken as a result of a gradual loss of the liquid or serum portion of the blood.

As a result of this thickening the blood cells begin to stick together, and if this occurs in the arterial system, the agglutinated blood will eventually clog small arteries during arterial injection. On the venous side, blood drainage will be difficult. Not only is dehydration responsible for the thickening of the blood, but gravity alone tends to "drain off" the liquid portion of the blood, leaving behind a more viscous blood.

If this blood thickening occurs fast enough it will diminish the degree of discoloration created by livor mortis, for the blood will not move as fast into the dependent tissues. What generally happens is the blood settles into the dependent tissues first; then the blood increases in viscosity, so the livor mortis and later postmortem stain are already established.

Table 5–3 summarizes the embalming significance of the postmortem physical changes.

POSTMORTEM CHEMICAL CHANGES

The postmortem chemical changes include **postmortem caloricity, postmortem stain, shift in pH, rigor mortis, decomposition, and hydrolysis.** These changes all involve or are a result of definite chemical reactions in which new products are formed in the dead human body. Unlike the physical changes, which center around such physical factors as gravitation, radiation of heat, an evaporation, the chemical changes are more complex.

Oxygen Debt

Metabolism is defined as the sum total of all the chemical reactions that occur within a cell. In the living body metabolism is most dependent on the respiratory and the circulatory systems. Oxygen is brought into the body through the respiratory system, and wastes from cell metabolism are removed from the body by the respiratory system. The system that carries the oxygen to the cells and wastes away from the tissues and cells is the circulatory system. There are two phases to metabolism: a

TABLE 5–3. EMBALMING SIGNIFICANCE OF THE POSTMORTEM PHYSICAL CHANGES

Algor mortis	Slows the onset of rigor mortis and decomposition
	Helps to keep blood in a liquid stage
	Can increase the degree of livor mortis and postmortem stain
Hypostasis	Responsible for livor mortis (Hemolysis can later cause postmorten stain.)
	Increases tissue moisture in dependent tissues
Livor mortis	Discoloration can vary from slight reddish hue to almost black; depends on blood volume and viscosity
	Intravascular; can be cleared
	Can be "set" as a stain if excessively strong uncoordinated embalming solution is injected
	Can help to expand the capillaries; this can help distribute the fluid, i.e., lower hands over the embalming table *before the start* of the embalming
	If it clears by itself during arterial injection, can be used as a sign of fluid distribution
	May be gravitated or massaged from an area
Dehydration	Increases blood viscosity
	Can create a "temporary" postmortem edema in the tissues
	Darkens skin surface; cannot be bleached
	Causes wrinkling and shriveling of features
	If extreme enough, can retard decomposition
	If extreme enough, can preserve the body
Increase in blood viscosity	Thickened blood and coagulation; intravascular or increased resistance
	Difficult blood removal; difficult arterial solution distribution

building phase called **anabolism** and a breakdown phase that releases heat and energy called **catabolism.**

After death the circulatory and respiratory systems no longer function. Oxygen, however, will be trapped in many of the cells of the body. Because oxygen is still present in the tissues, metabolism continues until the oxygen is depleted. In examining the postmortem chemical changes it is noted that oxygen (respiration) and circulation are two vital elements in the chemical changes that occur after death.

The trapped oxygen allows metabolism to continue, which produces body heat. Because the circulatory and respiratory systems no longer function there will be a slight rise in body temperature after death—**postmortem caloricity.** In the living body with an abundant supply of oxygen, glycogen (carbohydrates) stored in the muscles and tissues is broken down to pyruvic acid. The pyruvic acid is then converted to carbon dioxide, water, and energy. It is the energy formed that helps to keep a large supply of adenosine triphosphate (ATP) in the muscle tissues. After death, however, as the oxygen in the cells is used up, more lactic acid is formed than pyruvic acid. Now, the ATP cannot be resynthesized, so it gradually is depleted. The depletion of ATP causes the filaments of the muscle cells to combine as rigid links. This rigidity of the muscle is described as **rigor mortis.** It has been previously noted that the pH of the muscle tissues changes because of the buildup of lactic acid, so a few hours after death there is a *shift in pH* from slightly alkaline (7.38

in living tissues) to acid. This shift in pH to a slightly acid medium causes the process of AUTOLYSIS to begin. This is a form of **decomposition.**

The acid medium is also responsible for gradual rupture of the red blood cells (hemolysis), which causes **postmortem stain.** This stain can be thought of as a form of decomposition, for it is caused by the breakdown of the hemoglobin portion of the red blood cell. As decomposition progresses and the proteins of the body begin to decompose, there is a gradual shift in pH from the acid pH produced by the decomposition of the body carbohydrates to a basic pH brought about by a breakdown of the body proteins.

The order of decomposition of the body compounds (*generally stated*) is carbohydrates → proteins → fats → hard proteins → bone.

Postmortem Caloricity

Postmortem caloricity is a rise in body temperature after death. This rise in temperature after death occurs in all bodies. It is most noticeable, however, when the body was functioning in a healthy manner prior to death. This is especially true where there was vigorous physical activity prior to death. Cellular metabolism continues in the body after somatic death until the entire oxygen supply in the tissues is used. This oxidation reaction by the cells of the body releases heat and energy.

After somatic death the heat becomes trapped in the tissues, for the normal pathways of heat loss—circulation, respiration, and excretion—are no longer functioning. Thus, the body exhibits a slight rise in temperature. It has been estimated that in the average 160-pound body, the glycogenolysis that occurs is capable of raising the body temperature approximately 3.6°F. It must be remembered that this temperature rise also takes place in the body cavities (and viscera), which, because of their depth, take longer to cool. The trapped heat within the cavities can speed other chemical changes. In addition, if the body is clothed heat loss is slowed; if the environment is warm the loss of heat is slow; and if the body temperature was elevated prior to death from febrile disease the temperature loss is slow.

The body cools faster if little or no clothing was worn, the body itself is thin and not obese, there is movement of air over the body, the body was immersed in cool water rather than exposed to air, and the environmental temperature is low.

Many factors enter into the loss of heat from the body. Two of the other chemical postmortem changes that are speeded by the presence of heat are decomposition and rigor mortis. Both of these changes are adverse to thorough and effective embalming. By speeding these two chemical processes of rigor and decomposition, all the complications they have in the embalming process now affect the embalming of the body. Again, as a rule, the sooner after death the body can be prepared the better the results of the embalming process.

Postmortem Stain

Postmortem stain is an extravascular blood discoloration brought about by the hemolysis of blood. After death, the blood gravitates into the vessels of the dependent areas of the body, termed postmortem hypostasis (a postmortem physical change). The gravitation of the blood creates another postmortem physical change, a discoloration called livor mortis. After livor mortis, the red blood cells begin to break down. The breakdown or hemolysis of red blood cells begins approximately 6 to 10 hours after death. The onset of hemolysis occurs faster in some bodies, most frequently in persons who died from carbon monoxide poisoning or in bodies that have been refrigerated.

The red blood cell contains several million hemoglobin molecules per cell. Hemolysis releases the hemoglobin, which rapidly decomposes into globin and heme (Fig. 5–6). The heme then passes through the walls and pores of the capillaries and moves into the tissue spaces. Once in the tissue spaces the discoloration is permanently fixed, because it is now extravascular. During arterial injection and subsequent drainage, the livor mortis discoloration is cleared from the tissues, but left behind is a reddish color—the postmortem stain.

As already explained, if blood discoloration or livor and postmortem stain exist prior to embalming they can be differentiated by pressing against the darkened tissues. The area pressed on clears to normal skin color if the discoloration is livor mortis. If the discoloration is a stain, very little clearing of the area is noted. Remember that both stain and livor occur in the same tissue areas. The stain is a result of a time change and the decomposition of red blood cells. Also remember that this condition is NOT caused by the presence of blood in the tissues after death. It is, rather, the presence of the protein portion of the hemoglobin molecule in the tissues.

Postmortem stain, like all blood discolorations, may be bleached by formaldehyde. The presence of stain usually means that the body has been dead for a time and it is assumed that the embalmer will prepare the body using a stronger-than-average arterial solution. The stronger arterial solution helps to bleach the stained tissue. Dye added to the solution helps to hide the discoloration of the stain. Later, however, the stain will have a tendency to turn gray as a result of the mixing of formaldehyde with heme, but fluid dye will help to hide the graying. In addition, some embalmers use an external pack of a bleaching fluid or autopsy gel not only to bleach stained areas when they are present in visible areas (such as the face and hands), but to assist in ensuring that the tissues are well preserved.

The color changes of livor mortis and stain also occur in the tissues of the viscera. From a forensic stand-

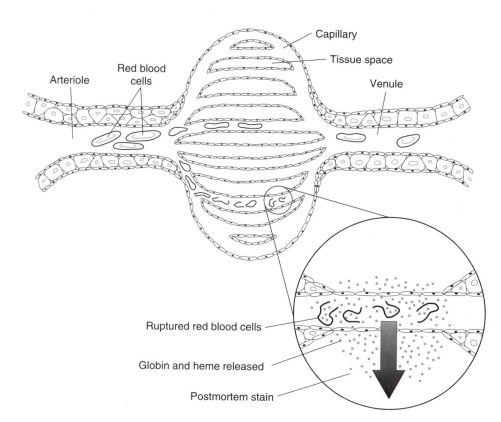

Figure 5–6. Release of globin and heme.

point postmortem stain indicates a time lapse between death and the presence of the stain. In addition, the location of the stain helps to determine the position of the body after death.

In refrigerated bodies the stain can be quite pronounced. Forced cooling of the body helps to keep the blood in a liquid state, thus rapidly establishing the livor mortis. Refrigeration also seems to speed hemolysis of red blood cells so that the staining problem is quite frequently seen in refrigerated bodies. An interesting fact to note, in embalming bodies that have been refrigerated for some period, is that quite often the superficial tissues have a pinkish hue prior to embalming. The coloring resembles that of the embalmed body in which fluid dye has been employed. Actually, the pink discoloration is a result of the failure of blood to drain from the superficial capillaries. The red blood cells have undergone hemolysis and the resultant faint pink discoloration is actually postmortem stain.

The embalmer should pay particular attention to this pink discoloration, for it would be quite easy to mistake this discoloration for the distribution of arterial solution. The refrigerated body is often in a state of rigor and the tissues can feel quite firm to the touch as if the firming had been caused by the reaction from the embalming fluid. These are all observations the embalmer should note in making a case analysis.

Shift in Body pH

Postmortem changes in body tissue pH are the third postmortem chemical change. pH is a measure of the strength of an acid or a base. The scale ranges from 0 to 14, with 7 considered neutral. Acidity is from 0 to 7, the closer to zero the stronger the acid. Alkalinity (or basicity) is from 7 to 14, the higher the number the stronger the base. The normal pH of blood and tissue fluids is slightly alkaline, about 7.38 to 7.40. After death there is a drop in the pH of blood and tissue fluids into the acid range, which begins about 3 hours after death. The body remains acid during the rigor mortis cycle; then gradually, as the decomposition process advances and the rigor mortis passes, the body tissues acquire an alkaline pH.

The pH scale shows the pH ranges for alkaline and acid strengths. The normal pH of the tissues and blood is approximately 7.38–7.40. This same pH is the best pH for the reaction between the body tissues and the arterial embalming solution. Most embalming fluids have a slightly alkaline pH. A group of chemicals called buffers are used to control embalming fluid pH and tissue pH.

During life the carbohydrates (glycogen) stored in the liver and muscles are broken down to pyruvic and lactic acid by the oxygen present. Normally, this pyruvic acid is oxidized to carbon dioxide, water, and energy. The energy, in turn, is used to build up the ATP of the

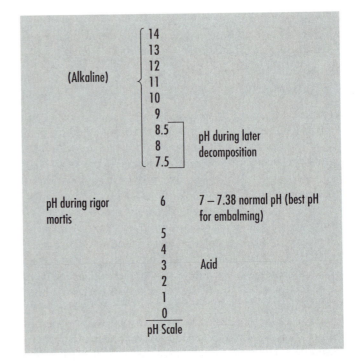

body by converting adenosine diphosphate (ADP) and adenosine monophosphate (AMP) to ATP. The oxygen present in life prevents the buildup of lactic acid by oxidizing it to carbon dioxide and water. After death occurs, the oxygen is gradually used up, and now the lactic acid is not inhibited and begins to accumulate in the muscle tissues. This buildup of acid occurs during the first hours after death (approximately the first 3 hours). This cycle is closely and directly related to the cycle of rigor mortis. The pH will drop to an acid level of approximately 6.0 and has even been recorded as low as 5.5.

As a result of the acid buildup in the tissues the conditions become right for the breakdown of the soft proteins of the body. Later, as the protein breaks down, there is a gradual buildup in the tissues of nitrogen products such as ammonia and amines. The ammonia, which is basic, neutralizes the acids present in the tissues from carbohydrate breakdown. As the body contains much more protein than carbohydrates, the ammonia products gradually begin to build to a point where the pH of the tissues becomes basic (or alkaline). During decomposition the tissues are found to have an alkaline pH.

Embalming bodies in a state of decomposition requires much stronger fluids and arterial solutions. Ammonia, of course, acts to neutralize formaldehyde. Because there is so much ammonia in the tissues during decomposition, it is easily seen that these bodies have a higher preservative demand.

Rigor Mortis

Rigor mortis is a postmortem stiffening of the body muscles by natural body processes. This condition affects only the muscles, and usually all of the muscles of the body are affected. Once the condition passes it does not recur. Immediately after death, the muscles are very relaxed. This is called **primary flaccidity.** (If embalming occurs during this period, body proteins will react well with the preservative and produce firm tissues.) The body muscles gradually become very firm; this is the actual stage of rigor mortis. When a body is embalmed during this period, it is difficult to establish good distribution of the arterial solution.

As the proteins of the muscles are tightly bound together there is little reaction with the preservative. Within 36 to 72 hours of death, the rigor passes in the unembalmed body. This stage is called **secondary flaccidity.** In this stage, preservative demand increases as a result of the breakdown of muscle protein (Fig. 5–7).

During the rigor cycle, a change in tissue pH also occurs. After death the body is slightly alkaline. The tissues gradually become acid. This low pH occurs when the muscles are in a state of rigor. As the muscle proteins decompose, rigor passes and the tissues become alkaline because of the formation of alkaline products by the decomposition of muscle proteins. For some time, it was thought that the shift in pH caused rigor mortis. Now it is understood that it is the inability of the body to resynthesize ATP that causes the muscle proteins to lock together and form an insoluble protein.

Rigor mortis marks the end of muscle cell life. It can generally be observed in the average body 2 to 4 hours after death. During rigor all the muscle fibers contract. This is why rigor is so much stronger than normal muscle contraction. Muscles in rigor do not decompose. The acid present inhibits bacterial activity. Autolysis gradually occurs, and in time, the muscle protein shows evidence of decomposition.

Rigor appears to begin in the involuntary muscles of the eye, then moves to the face, neck, upper extremities, trunk, and lower extremities. It appears to pass from the body in the same order as its onset. Rigor tends to be retained in the digits and the jaw. The phenomenon is speeded by heat and is more intense in the healthy well-developed body. In emaciated bodies in which muscles have atrophied, the condition is less intense. If the condition rapidly occurs it rapidly passes; if it slowly occurs it will slowly pass.

Cold stiffening of the tissues resembles rigor. At 40°F, the body fats solidify, giving the tissues a firmness similar to that of mild rigor. Muscles in badly burnt bodies shorten, causing flexing of the body joints. This flexing is due to the heat rather than to rigor mortis. A third condition that can resemble rigor is the cadaveric spasm, which occurs most often in accidental deaths. It is a very firm fixation of the muscles.

After death, there is a gradual depletion (or decomposition) of ATP. ATP is an organic molecule that stores and releases energy for use in cellular processes. After death oxygen is no longer supplied to the cells. As a result ATP is depleted. Anaerobic respiration begins after death in the oxygen-starved tissues. Carbohydrates (glycogen stored in the muscles and liver) are broken down to produce a small amount of energy, so some ATP is formed; however, pyruvic acid is also formed. In the absence of oxygen the pyruvic acid is reduced to lactic acid. The inability of the body to build ATP results in the formation of rigor complexes. The rigor complexes are, in turn, responsible for the gradual stiffening of the muscles after death. For this reason it is easily seen why persons who die as a result of exhausting diseases or who die during strenuous exercise rapidly develop rigor: the oxygen in the tissues is greatly reduced.

> After death, chemical deterioration in muscle fibers permits Ca^{2+} to leak out of the sarcoplasmic reticulum. The Ca^{2+} binds to troponin and triggers sliding of the filaments. ATP synthesis has ceased, however, so the myosin cross-bridges cannot detach from actin. The resulting condition, in which muscles are in a state of rigidity (cannot contract or stretch), is called *rigor mortis* (rigidity of death). Rigor mortis lasts about 24 hours but disappears after another 12 hours as tissues begin to degenerate. [Tortora, 1993]

Rigor can be forcibly reduced by flexing, bending, rotating, and massaging the joints and muscles. Once broken, or passed off by natural processes, rigor does not recur. Some problems are associated with embalming bodies in rigor:

1. There may be difficulty in establishing good position of the body.
2. The jaw may be tightly closed and difficult to open.
3. Rigor can imitate (give a false sign of) preserved tissue.

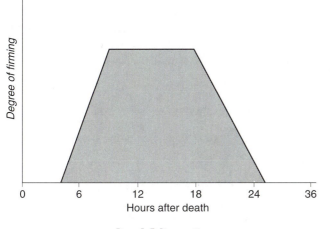

Figure 5–7. Rigor mortis.

4. Distribution of arterial solution is poor; tissues are swollen and cause extravascular resistance to fluid distribution and blood drainage.
5. The precapillary sphincters can contract and prevent fluid from flowing into the capillary beds.
6. After the passage of rigor, tissue demand for preservative increases.
7. The acid pH does not provide a good medium for reaction with the preservative.

Hydrolysis

Hydrolysis means cleavage with water, a reaction in which water is one of the reactants and compounds are often broken down. In the hydrolysis of proteins, the addition of water accompanied by the action of enzymes results in the breakdown of proteins into amino acids.

The process of hydrolysis requires water to break apart, a catalyst, and heat. Hydrolysis has been called the single most important factor in the initiation of decomposition. It is most important to remember that water chemically reacts with the body substrates to break them down, and hydrolysis is a chemical reaction.

During the process of hydrolysis water is split into its constituents, the hydrogen ion (H^+) and the hydroxyl ion (OH^-). The process requires the presence of a catalyst, a substance that influences the rate of a chemical reaction. Although it affects the rate of the reaction, the catalyst, itself, does not become a part of the products of the reaction. The autolytic enzymes present in the cell act as the catalysts. After death, tissues become slightly acid. This shift in pH causes the lysosomes within the cells to rupture. Lysosomes are cell inclusions that contain digestive enzymes. In the presence of water, the released enzymes begin to digest the carbohydrates, fats, and proteins of the cell. The end products of the hydrolysis of proteins are amino acids. Carbohydrates are reduced to monosaccharides (simple sugars) and fats are reduced to fatty acids and glycerine.

As autolysis (hydrolysis) of proteins proceeds, the resultant product makes more and more sites available for union with the preservative. It can be stated then that autolysis (hydrolysis) greatly increases the preservative demand of the body tissues. This process is speeded by heat and slowed by a cold environment. The mild acid pH also stimulates hydrolysis. As the process continues, more and more nitrogen end products are produced. This causes the pH to shift to an alkaline condition. The alkaline (or basic) condition now provides an excellent medium for bacterial growth. With this growth of bacteria the process of putrefaction greatly increases.

Decomposition

Proteins. The three major biochemicals are proteins, carbohydrates, and lipids. Proteins are most important from the viewpoints of structure and function. Structurally, proteins are the principal constituents of connective tissue, tendons, cartilage, ligaments, skin, hair, and nails. Proteins also have dynamic functions. They are responsible for body movements in the form of contractile proteins found in muscles. Proteins regulate physiological processes in the form of certain hormones. They also control the rates of all chemical reactions in the human body, as biological catalysts, enzymes, are proteins. A protective role is found in the work of these proteins known as antibodies. Proteins also have a transport role as part of hemoglobin, the compound that carries oxygen from the lungs to the tissues, is a protein.

The proteins are also the most important type of biochemical to the embalmer. The chemical reactions that occur during the embalming process achieve preservation and disinfection of human remains by crosslinking proteins, both the proteins of the human remains and the proteins of microorganisms.

Proteins are very large molecules. All proteins contain the elements carbon, hydrogen, oxygen, and nitrogen. Some proteins contain sulfur and, in small amounts, copper, iodine, iron, manganese, magnesium, phosphorus, and zinc. Proteins are defined as polymers of amino acids. A polymer is a large molecule composed of many similar units. The basic unit of proteins is the amino acid. Twenty amino acids are the building blocks of proteins. The general formula for any amino acid is

$$H_2N - \overset{\overset{\displaystyle R}{|}}{\underset{\underset{\displaystyle H}{|}}{C}} - \overset{\overset{\displaystyle O}{\|}}{C} - OH$$

The "R" in the representation is a side chain. The chemical composition of the R group is the distinguishing factor that gives an individual amino acid its identity. Two amino acids join together in a synthesis reaction, which involves the splitting off of the constituents of water from the amino acids:

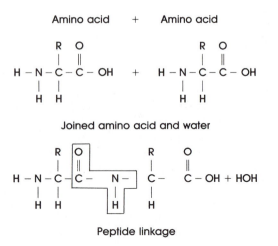

Peptide linkage

The chemical bond that links together the two amino acids is called a peptide bond or peptide linkage. This bond is blocked off in the scheme. Both ends of the structure are able, likewise, to join to other amino acid molecules. In this way, many amino acids link together to form a large polymer, a protein, of amino acids.

It is possible to decompose the dipeptide (two amino acids joined together) and any protein either in a laboratory situation or in human remains. In the laboratory, the breakdown requires addition of some inorganic acid or base and heat. In human tissue, the reaction is under the control of biological catalysts (enzymes) called proteases. In either case, the reaction is the reverse of the synthesis reaction previously diagrammed.

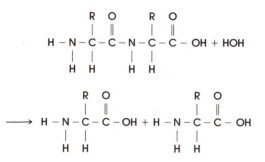

External agents such as heat and catalysts are also needed for the biochemical decomposition. This type of decomposition reaction is hydrolysis.

The major type of protein decomposition occurring after death is putrefaction, an anaerobic process brought about by the action of enzymes.

> The proteolytic enzymes (protein-splitting enzymes, proteinases) produced by bacteria split complex proteins into proteoses, peptones, polypeptides, amino acids, ammonia, and free nitrogen. Protein decomposition is known as *putrefaction*. Some authorities restrict the term "putrefaction" to the decomposition of proteins by anaerobic bacteria, which results in the formation of hydrogen sulfide and other foul-smelling decomposition products, and they use the term *decay* for the decomposition of proteins by aerobic bacteria. The latter does not result in the formation of malodorous decomposition products. [Smith, 1980, p. 68]

Hydrolysis is the first chemical reaction in the putrefactive process. During hydrolysis, large protein molecules are broken down by water into smaller fragments called proteoses, peptones, and polypeptides. These intermediates are a good food source for bacteria, which increase dramatically during putrefaction. As degradation continues, the final products are amino acids.

These amino acids undergo further chemical changes. Amines, carbon dioxide, and water are some of the products. Amines are organic compounds that are considered to be derivatives of ammonia. They contain

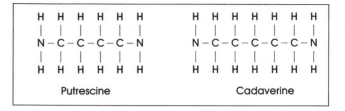

Figure 5–8. Decomposition products of amino acids.

at least one nitrogen, and chemically are basic or alkaline substances. Many have foul odors. Two amines are putrescine and cadaverine. Their chemical structures are drawn in Figure 5–8. They are commonly called ptomaines.

The word *ptomaine* is derived from the Greek word *ptoma* meaning "corpse." The amino acid tryptophan produces two other amines, indole (C_8H_7N) and skatole (C_9H_9N). See Figure 5–9 for the structural formulas of these compounds. They contribute to the characteristic odor of feces.

Putrefaction continues by the breakdown of the amines. Complete decomposition of putrescine and cadaverine yields ammonia, which is also alkaline, carbon dioxide, and water. The formation of ammonia during proteolysis has significance with respect to the chemicals used in the embalming process. Formaldehyde reacts with ammonia to produce hexamethylenetetraamine, also called urotropin:

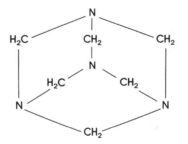

If extensive putrefaction occurs prior to embalming, the presence of ammonia causes a higher-than-normal preservative demand.

Other odoriferous products formed during putrefaction are gaseous hydrogen sulfide, mercaptans, and gaseous hydrogen phosphide. The sources of the first two

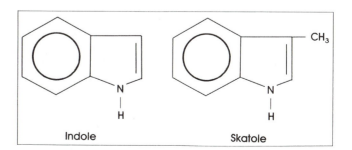

Figure 5–9. Decomposition products of the amino acid tryptophan.

are sulfur-containing amino acids. Hydrogen sulfide smells like rotten eggs. A garliclike odor characterizes hydrogen phosphide. Two other gases that are by-products of these reactions are methane and hydrogen. Both are odorless.

Protein breakdown may also occur in an aerobic environment. This process, referred to as decay, consists of those chemical reactions that oxidize proteins to compounds that do not have foul odors. Oxidation of amino acids produce ammonia and organic acids called carboxylic acids.

During protein decay, all the previously described processes occur simultaneously (Fig. 5–10).

Table 5–4 summarizes the postmortem chemical changes and their embalming significance.

Carbohydrates. The carbohydrates, the second class of biochemicals, also decompose after death. Bacteria and enzymes play a role in initiating and controlling the chemical reactions. The storage form of carbohydrate in the human body is glycogen, a polymer that is hydrolyzed to many molecules of glucose. Intermediate products of the breakdown of glucose by a process called fermentation are organic acids, one example of which is acetic acid (*Note: fermentation is the bacterial decomposition of carbohydrates under aerobic conditions.*) The production of acid does not alter the overall alkaline environment of the decaying remains, as the basic products of putrefaction neutralize the effects of the acids. The final products of the breakdown of carbohydrates are carbon dioxide and water. It is not the function of any of the chemicals of embalming fluids to retard the decomposition of carbohydrates.

Lipids. As is true of the proteins and carbohydrates, hydrolysis reactions cause the decomposition of lipids. In the presence of enzymes called lipases, lipids are broken down into glycerol and long-chain organic acids called fatty acids. Because these products do not have the pu-

TABLE 5–4. POSTMORTEM CHEMICAL CHANGES AND THEIR EMBALMING SIGNIFICANCE

Rigor mortis	Extravascular resistance
	Difficult positioning
	Difficult-to-pose features
	Tissues easily distensible on injection
	False sign of preservation
	Little absorption of preservative
	Firming difficult to achieve after passage
	Increases in demand of the body for preservative
	Minimal decomposition if any
	pH changes not conducive to good fluid reaction
Decomposition	Poor distribution of embalming solution
	Tissues easily distensible during injection
	Increased demand for preservative
	Possible presence of color changes, odors, skin-slip, gases in cavities and tissues, and purge
Postmortem stain	Extravascular discoloration that cannot be removed, but may be bleached
	Increased demand for preservative
	False sign of arterial solution distribution
	Possible graying of affected tissues after embalming
	Indicates delay between death and preparation
Postmortem caloricity	Increases rigor mortis cycle
	Speeds decomposition cycle
Shift in pH	Interferes with fluid reactions
	May create "splotching" of fluid dyes
Hydrolysis	Sets off the decomposition cycle

trid odors characteristic of decaying proteins, lipid decomposition is not as important to the embalmer as protein decomposition. There is, nonetheless, one source of odor from lipid material. Microorganisms can cause fatty material, especially in a moist environment, to become rancid, producing short-carbon-chain organic acids with unpleasant odors. The role of embalming with respect to lipid decomposition is to inhibit proliferation of microorganisms.

To the embalmer, one interesting compound associated with lipids is **adipocere,** commonly called grave wax. It is soft, whitish, crumbly or greasy material formed in the soft tissues. It is thought to consist mainly of fatty acids formed by the hydrolysis and hydrogenation of body fats and has a sweetish, rancid smell. Adipocere can occur in any body fat including that of the liver. It first begins in the superficial fat. In children, all the body fat can be converted to adipocere. As it is a relatively permanent substance its formation can preserve the surface features for years.

The presence of moisture is necessary for the formation of adipocere, and warmth will speed the formation. Once adipocere starts to form putrefaction is retarded, for the acids formed along with the dehydration that occurs in these tissues combine to halt the bacterial activity. Formation of adipocere extracts moisture from the tissues. This produces a certain degree of mummification. It is felt that adipocere formation starts within days of death. It becomes visible in about 3 months.

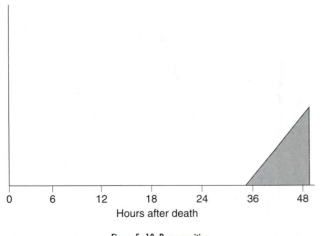

Figure 5–10. Decomposition.

In summary, the three major biochemical compounds are hydrolyzed after death to simpler substances. Associated with many of these degradation products, especially those of the proteins, are putrid odors. Microorganisms and enzymes have key roles in controlling the rates of decomposition chemical reactions.

CATALYSTS

In previous discussions of the types of decomposition reactions, it was shown that heat and catalysts were needed in addition to the reactants for decomposition to occur. In every chemical reaction, intermediate in time to the reactants and the products, there is a transition state. This arrangement, which represents breakage of the chemical bonds of the reactants and formation of the chemical bonds of the products, is higher in energy than either the reactants or the products and must be achieved for the reaction to occur.

In many laboratory situations, the transition state is formed by heating the reactants. One way to form products from reactants is to add a catalyst, which provides an alternate pathway for the reaction. Therefore, the energy of the transition state in a catalyzed reaction is less than that in an uncatalyzed reaction. The catalysts of biochemical reactions are enzymes.

Chemically, enzymes are proteins. As proteins, the actions of enzymes are influenced by such conditions as temperature and hydrogen ion activity (the pH) of a solution. A characteristic of proteins is that they take on shapes that they must maintain to participate in reactions. In the case of enzymes, their shapes must be complementary to those of their substrates, which are the reactants of the chemical changes catalyzed by the enzymes. For a protein in aqueous solution, the shape is such that the parts of the protein that are not soluble in water are oriented toward the inside of the three-dimensional configuration of the molecule, while the water-soluble parts are on the outside of the protein where they can be in contact with water. The overall shape of a protein is maintained by various forces that are generally electrostatic in nature and classified as chemical bonds. The hydrogen bond is the prominent type of bond found in proteins. It is an attractive interaction between a slightly negative oxygen and a slightly positive hydrogen:

$$\overset{S-}{>C=O} \ \text{-----} \ \overset{S+}{H-N<}$$

Addition of heat to a protein may break some of these bonds and alter the normal shape of the molecule, thereby inactivating it. Anyone who has ever cooked an egg has observed the change in the physical appearance of the protein egg albumin induced by the application of heat.

Every enzyme has an optimum temperature. The activity range for most enzymes is 10° to 50°C, with the optimum temperature for enzymes in the body being close to 37°C. Below 10°C, the activity of enzymes is reduced to a very slow rate or may cease. Enzymes generally can be reactivated by increasing temperature. Above 50°C, the enzyme protein is denatured and coagulates.

The enzymes that regulate the decomposition reactions of human remains are influenced by temperature. After death, there usually is a rise in temperature above normal body temperature known as postmortem caloricity. This elevation occurs because the heat that is produced by chemical reactions that are still occurring in the body cannot be removed from the body by normal mechanisms. Neither respiration, circulation, nor perspiration continues after death. Also, loss of heat by radiation is not as effective as during life. After a certain period, the heat-producing oxidation reactions slow down and eventually stop. Consequently, the body gradually cools to the temperature of its surroundings (algor mortis). The closer this temperature is to the optimum temperature of the decomposition enzymes, the faster is the rate of decomposition.

Provided the surrounding temperature is not so high as to denature the enzymes, it is generally observed that decomposition is favored by higher temperatures. Actually, the optimum temperature for decomposition is a balance between the rise in activity of an enzyme with temperature and the denaturation of the protein by heat. This balance is illustrated in Figure 5–11.

In the region of the graph in which the temperature increases to the optimum temperature A, the rate of the reaction increases as it is easier for the reactants to reach the transition state. From temperature A to temperature B, competition is occurring between the effect of increasing temperature on attainment of the transition state and the increasing denaturation of the enzyme. Finally, beyond temperature B, the enzyme is completely denatured, so no reaction can occur.

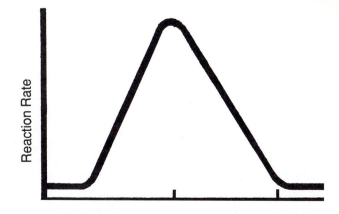

Figure 5–11. Effect of temperature on the reaction rate of an enzyme-catalyzed reaction.

The activity of a protein is also influenced by pH. The pH scale indicates the relationship between acidic and basic substances in a solution. A pH of 7 indicates neutrality, which means equal amounts of acidic (H^+, hydrogen) and basic (OH^-, hydroxide) ions are present in solution. At pH values less than 7, there is a larger amount of H^+ ions than OH^- ions; conversely, at pH values greater than 7, the OH^- ions are in excess. The pH controls the state of ionization of a protein in an aqueous solution. As some enzymes must be in a specific state of ionization to interact with their substrates, changes in pH can alter the ability of an enzyme to function. In addition, a large change in acidity or in alkalinity (basicity) may disrupt the hydrogen bonds that are necessary to maintain the proper shape of an enzyme.

Every enzyme has an optimum pH. For the majority of digestive enzymes such as proteases, lipases, and amylases, the optimum pH is slightly alkaline. An exception is pepsin, a protease of the stomach, which has an acidic optimum pH of 1.5. After death, the pH of the tissues changes from about 7.4 to acidic. One cause of this phenomenon is the buildup of lactic acid, a product of cellular respiration, which continues for some time after death in an environment lacking oxygen. The acidic pH favors the action of some microorganisms in the body and causes rupture of membranes surrounding organelles called lysosomes (see Autolysis). As decomposition proceeds, the pH switches back to alkaline as basic decomposition products form. With the return to alkalinity, the action of the decomposition enzymes with this type of optimum pH is accelerated.

AUTOLYSIS

In human remains the enzymes of decomposition have two different sources, saphrophytic bacteria and lysosomes. These bacteria are normal residents of the human digestive tract. After death, they translocate and increase in number by using dead organic matter for their nutrition. Aerobic bacteria may also enter the body through the respiratory tract. They deplete the tissues of oxygen, producing chemical conditions favorable for anaerobic organisms, most of which originate in the intestinal tract.

In addition to bacterially caused decompositions, living cells have their own self-destruct mechanisms. During life, organelles called lysosomes contain the digestive enzymes of a cell. As previously mentioned, as the pH changes from alkaline to acidic, the membranes surrounding the lysosomes rupture. As the cells' own digestive enzymes are released, they digest the surrounding cellular material. This process is called **autolysis**, which means cell self-decomposition. The products of autolysis are amino acids, sugars, fatty acids, and glycerol. These substances are sources of food and energy for microorganisms. Therefore, autolysis also favors microbial destructive action on human remains.

SIGNS OF DECOMPOSITION

There are five cardinal signs of decomposition. It should be pointed out that not all of these signs may be present even though decomposition is occurring. Decomposition proceeds at different rates in various body areas. The following orders of decomposition demonstrate this fact:

1. Order of body decomposition
   A. Cells
   B. Tissues
   C. Organs

Cells, tissues, and organs that contain high levels of moisture and autolytic and bacterial enzymes break down before similar structures that contain less water and autolytic and bacterial enzymes.

2. Order of tissue decomposition
   A. Soft tissues
   B. Firm tissues
   C. Hard tissues

The vascular system is one of the last organ systems to decompose. Even in advanced decomposition it would be possible to inject some preservative chemicals in an attempt to slow the decomposition and control the odor.

> When the body is considered as a whole there are five cardinal signs of decomposition:
>
> 1. Color changes
> 2. Odor
> 3. Desquamation
> 4. Gases
> 5. Purge

Color Change. The first external color change that occurs in the unembalmed body is a greenish discoloration over the right lower quadrant of the abdomen. This discoloration is caused by the combination of hydrogen sulfide (a product of putrefaction) with hemoglobin from the blood. In many bodies this discoloration follows the surface outline of the large intestine, which is located just beneath the abdominal wall. The abdomen as a whole gradually discolors and the chest, neck, and upper thighs are affected in time (Fig. 5–12).

The blood trapped in the superficial vessels gradually breaks down, staining the surrounding tissues. The outline of the veins on the surface of the skin is easily de-

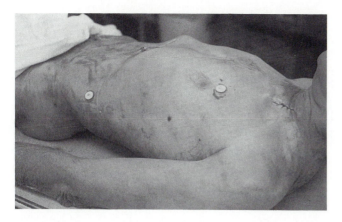

Figure 5–12. Partial decomposition. Both hypodermic and arterial embalming treatments were used. Note the discolorations.

tected. This purplish-brown discoloration of the superficial veins is most pronounced in the veins of the shoulder, upper chest, lower abdomen, and groin. An early discoloration that occurs as a result of the hemolysis or breakdown of red blood cells is postmortem stain. This staining of the tissues is extravascular and cannot be removed by arterial solution injection and blood drainage.

Odor. As the protein materials of the body decompose putrefactive odors become apparent. This odor is caused by foul-smelling amines, mercaptans, and hydrogen sulfide. The preservative solution reacts with these compounds to form odorless compounds.

Desquamation (Skin-Slip). The outer layers of the skin weaken because the deeper skin layers are undergoing autolysis. Hydrolysis of collagen and elastin causes the superficial skin to be pulled away easily from the deeper skin layers. When the skin is pulled away a shiny, pink moist surface is exposed. Gradually, this moist area dehydrates, turns brown, and is slightly firm to the touch. If the loosened skin is not touched, which causes the skin to slip away over a period, large blisters can form. The blisters, which may increase to 3 to 6 inches in diameter, contain a watery blood-stained fluid having a putrid odor.

Gases. As decomposition progresses, gases form in the viscera, generally starting in the stomach and intestines. Later, gases form in the body tissues. The gas causes the abdominal cavity to swell, and later the body tissues become distended. When pushed on, the gas crepitates. It can be felt and heard moving through the tissue when pressure is applied. Weakened areas such as the eyelids, scrotum, and breasts easily distend with gases. In time, eyelids, cheeks, and lips distend and the tongue protrudes.

Purge. The result of the pressure from the gas formed in

the abdomen is postmortem evacuation of the contents of the stomach, lungs, or rectum from a body orifice. The purge from the stomach generally is a foul-smelling liquid described as "coffee grounds." The purge material is acid in pH, for it contains a large amount of hydrochloric acid, and any blood present appears brown. Purge from the lungs is generally described as frothy, and if blood appears in this purge it may retain its red color. The stomach and lung purge may exit from the mouth or the nose.

DISINFECTION AND PRESERVATION BY EMBALMING

Two of the purposes of the embalming process are disinfection and preservation of human remains. These processes are achieved by the chemicals in embalming fluids. The actions of these chemicals can be summarized as three over-all effects. First, they inactivate the action chemical groups of proteins and amino acids. This inactivation inhibits the decomposition of the protein. Second, they inactivate enzymes. These enzymes are those produced by putrefactive bacteria and the autolytic enzymes produced by the digestive organelles of cells. Third, they kill microorganisms. This is accomplished in two ways. Inactivation of the chemical groups of the structural proteins of human remains deprives bacteria of their primary source of nutrition. Furthermore, the structural proteins of the bacteria are denatured by the preservative chemicals. This denaturation, which kills the bacteria, disinfects the remains and eliminates one of the sources of the enzymes of decomposition.

CROSSLINKING REACTIONS

As a result of the interactions between preservative chemicals and the tissues of human remains, proteins are crosslinked. These proteins include the structural proteins of the remains, the enzymes native to the remains, the enzymes produced by putrefactive bacteria, and the proteins of microorganisms. Commonly used crosslinking agents are formaldehyde and glutaraldehyde (Fig. 5–13).

Crosslinking occurs by chemical reactions between the aldehyde and nitrogen atoms of the protein. Nitrogen may occur in the structure of a protein in imino groups, in amino groups, and in peptide linkages (Fig. 5–14).

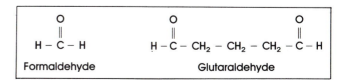

Figure 5–13. Crosslinking agents.

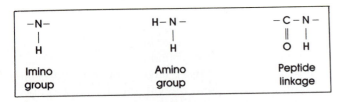

Figure 5–14. Nitrogen-containing groups on proteins.

The amino acids proline, hydroxyproline, tryptophan, arginine, and histidine contain the imino group (Fig. 5–15). Two of these groups react with formaldehyde:

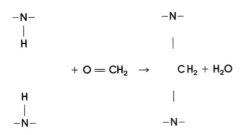

If two residues of any of the imino group-containing amino acids are in two protein chains such linkage may occur. A similar reaction occurs between amino groups and formaldehyde. At the end of every protein chain is an amino group. Also, the amino acids lysine, arginine, and glutamine have an additional amino group in their structures (Fig. 5–16).

The reaction between formaldehyde and two amino groups is

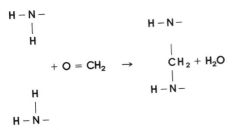

This process, like the reaction with the imino group, joins two protein chains.

A third crosslinking reaction is the interaction of a molecule of formaldehyde with two peptide bonds:

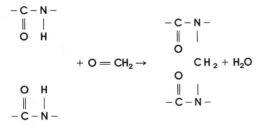

This reaction occurs at multiple sites between two protein chains, as every protein contains many peptide bonds, one between every two amino acids.

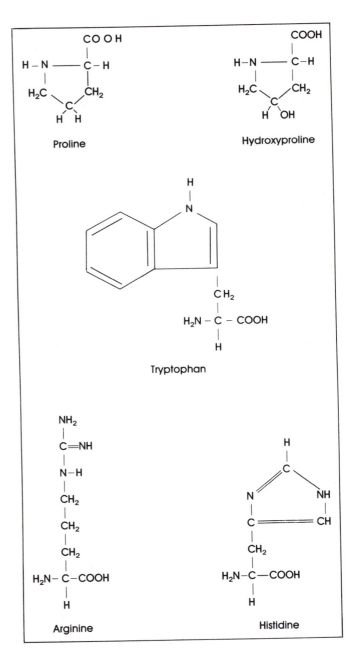

Figure 5–15. Amino acids that contain imino groups.

Because water is a product of all of these crosslinking reactions, embalming with formaldehyde dehydrates the embalmed tissue, hence the need for humectants (water-attracting agents) in embalming fluids. A second consequence of the production of water is the possibility of reversal of the reactions by large amounts of water. Such reversal can be observed several hours after the embalming of an edematous limb. There exists, through the process of hydrolysis, the potential for the "embalmed" tissue to become "unembalmed."

Pervier (1961) summarizes the reactions between formaldehyde and body proteins in the following statement which answers the question "How does embalming work?"

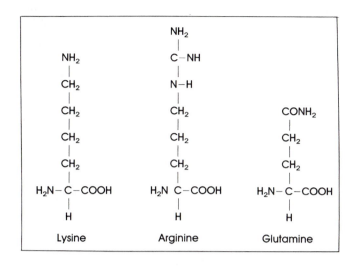

Figure 5–16. Amino acids that contain additional amino groups.

Embalming destroys somewhat the colloidal nature of the proteins, neutralizes the active centers of the molecules and establishes many chemical crosslinkages that were not there before between adjacent protein molecules. The net result is the conversion of protein into a high molecular, crosslinked lattice work of inert solid materials that can no longer serve as food for bacteria or as a substrate for enzyme action. The inert structures have lost their ability to retain water and their stability is maintained by the presence of a little uncombined formaldehyde.

KEY TERMS AND CONCEPTS FOR STUDY AND DISCUSSION

1. Define the following terms:
   Agonal period
   Antemortem
   Autolysis
   Death
   Decay
   Enzyme
   Expert test of death
   Extrinsic factors
   Intrinsic factors
   Lysosome
   Postmortem chemical changes
   Postmortem physical changes
   Protein
   Putrefaction
   Signs of decomposition
2. Discuss several of the agonal changes that can influence the embalming of the body.
3. What factors can speed or slow the establishments of liver mortis?
4. Discuss the signs of decomposition.
5. Discuss the problems rigor mortis can create for the embalmer.
6. Discuss the pH changes that occur in the dead human body after death.
7. How does formaldehyde embalm (or preserve) the dead human body?

REFERENCES

Arnow EL. *Introduction to Physiological and Pathological Chemistry.* St. Louis, MO: CV Mosby; 1976.

Camps FE (ed). *Gradwohl's Legal Medicine.* Baltimore, MD: Williams & Wilkins; 1968.

DeSpelder LA, Strickland AL. *The Last Dance.* Palo Alto, CA: Mayfield; 1983.

Dorn JM, Hopkins, BM. *Thanatochemistry, A Survey of General, Organic, and Biochemistry for Funeral Service Professionals.* Reston, VA: Reston; 1985.

Evans WED. *The Chemistry of Death.* Springfield, IL: Charles C Thomas; 1963.

Gregory DR. Death—A new definition. *Leg Med* 1981; 2(4):491–500.

Hendin D. *Death as a Fact of Life.* New York: WW Norton; 1973.

Hole JW. *Essentials of Human Anatomy and Physiology.* 2nd ed. Dubuque, IA: William C Brown; 1986.

Los JM, Roeleveld LF, Wetsema BJC. Pulse polarography. Part X. Formaldehyde hydration in aqueous acetate and phosphate buffer solutions. *J Electroanal Chem* 1977;75:819–837.

Pervier NC. *A Textbook of Chemistry for Embalmers.* Minneapolis: University of Minnesota; 1961.

Redding RA. Physiology of dying. In Wass H (ed): *DYING Facing the Facts.* New York: Hemisphere/ McGraw-Hill; 1979.

Ryan PL. The Uniform Determination Death Act: An effective solution to the problem of defining death. *Washington Lee Law Rev* 1982;39:1511–1531.

Showalter J. "Determining death: The legal and theological aspects of brain-related criteria. *Catholic Lawyer* 1982;27(Spring):112–128.

Sleichter GM. *A Study of the Combining Activity of Formaldehyde with Tissues.* Thesis submitted in partial fulfillment of the requirements for master's degree, University of Cincinnati; 1939.

Smith AL. *Microbiology and Pathology.* 6th ed. St. Louis, MO: CV Mosby; 1980.

Spitz WU, Fisher RS. *Medicolegal investigation of death: Guidelines for the application of pathology to crime investigation.* Springfield, IL: Charles C Thomas; 1980.

Tortora GJ. *Principles of Human Anatomy.* 7th ed. New York: Harper & Row; 1993.

6

Embalming Chemicals

This chapter looks at the eight groups of chemicals and their ingredients that are used to compose the various embalming fluids*:

1. Preservatives
2. Germicides
3. Modifying agents (including buffers, humectants, water conditions, and inorganic salts)
4. Anticoagulants
5. Surfactants
6. Dyes
7. Perfuming agents
8. Vehicles

These groups of chemicals are combined in various ways to produce the embalming fluids and accessory and supplemental chemicals employed in the preparation of the dead human body:

■ Preservative arterial fluids
■ Preinjection (primary injection) fluids
■ Co-injection fluids (antidehydrant chemicals, water-corrective chemicals, restorative chemicals)
■ Cavity fluids

---

*Much of this chapter was prepared by Leandro Rendon, Director of Chemical Research and Educational Programs, The Champion Company, Springfield, Ohio.

■ Arterial fluid dyes
■ Autopsy gels
■ Cautery agents

The eight groups of chemicals are combined in a standard bottle of arterial fluid (solution): Most of these chemicals overcome the adverse effects of preservatives on the tissues of the body during the embalming process.

There are *disadvantages* to the use of formaldehyde as a preservative in embalming fluids: it rapidly coagulates the blood, converts the tissues to a gray hue when it mixes with blood not removed from the body, fixes discolorations, dehydrates the tissues, constricts the capillaries, deteriorates with age, can be oxidized to formic acid, and can be decomposed to alcohol and formic acid in a strong alkaline pH.

The advantages of formaldehyde as a preservative in embalming fluids outweigh the disadvantages.

By examining the use of the various groups of chemicals, the adverse effects of formaldehyde can be controlled. There are *advantages* to the use of formaldehyde: it is inexpensive; it is bactericidal and inhibits the growth of yeasts and molds; it can rapidly destroy autolytic enzymes; it rapidly acts on the body proteins and converts them to insoluble resins that stop body decomposition; only a small percentage of formaldehyde is needed to act on a large amount of protein; it produces rapid fixation, which aids in positioning the dead human body and also indicates that preservation is taking place; and it deodorizes the body amines formed during putrefaction.

ESTABLISHMENT OF MINIMUM STANDARDS

After the turn of the century (approximately 1906), when formaldehyde became a widely used ingredient in embalming fluids, various state health departments required that a minimum standard of formaldehyde be used to embalm bodies to render them sanitized. This established a standard amount of formaldehyde to incorporate into the formulations. At that time a minimum amount of embalming solution was to be used in the preparation of bodies dead from noninfectious diseases as well as those dead from infectious and contagious diseases. The minimum standard established was not less than the following: 1 gallon of 14% of a 40% solution of formaldehyde for every 100 pounds of body weight for "normal cases" and 1 gallon of this same strength for every 75 pounds of body weight for infectious and contagious disease cases.

In these early years the manufacturers of embalming fluid sold it with the water already added. (The fluid was sold by the half-gallon ready for injection.) Later, because of the costs involved in bottling, packing, and shipping, it was decided to omit as much of the water as possible and sell the concentrated solution in pint bottles. To maintain the required minimum standards established by state laws, each pint bottle had to contain at least 8.96 ounces of 40% formaldehyde and the same proportion of other chemical ingredients. It must be kept in mind that formaldehyde acts harshly on body tissues, does not distribute or diffuse well, dehydrates, and darkens and grays body tissues. The use of strong embalming solutions (approximately 5.75%) was enforced in the years immediately following the influenza pandemics of 1918 and 1919. To overcome the adverse effects of formaldehyde on the body, a variety of supplemental fluids, such as blood solvents (later known as preinjection solutions), were developed; coinjection and jaundice fluids were developed and in use as early as 1910. It would not be until the development of penetrating agents and machine injection in the mid- to late 1930s that milder arterial solutions would be employed, the standard until the early 1970s would be 1 to 1.5% solution strength. This was quite sufficient to produce firming. It was not until the early 1970s that research demonstrated that a minimum of at least a 2% formaldehyde-based arterial solution was necessary to sanitize body tissues effectively. In the near future it is expected that formaldehyde and phenol-based preservative fluids will be replaced with fluids containing preservatives and sanitizing elements that do not have the adverse effects of the preservatives currently in use.

Formaldehyde can deteriorate and become formic acid. Likewise, it can polymerize and remove itself from an aqueous solution by forming insoluble paraformaldehyde. Groups of chemicals are added to the arterial fluid concentrate to control the adverse effects of the formaldehyde, to maintain its stability, and to lengthen its shelf life.

In explaining the various embalming fluids on the market today and the categories of chemicals that make up these embalming fluids, the following definitions are used: **embalming fluid**—the concentrated chemical composition sold by the manufacturer; and **primary dilution**—the "in-use" solution of embalming chemicals formed when the concentrated embalming fluid is diluted in the tank of the embalming machine with water and any other additive chemicals for injection into the body. (This is also referred to as the embalming solution.)

GENERAL CHEMICAL PRINCIPLES OF EMBALMING FLUIDS

An important point to keep in mind is that commercial embalming fluids are composed of various chemicals and that the same chemicals, when used in different concentrations, may produce different effects. This means each individual chemical ingredient has a specific function to perform and it reacts according to its own concentration, distribution, diffusion, and individual activity.

Among the main chemicals common to almost all embalming preservative solutions are formaldehyde and methyl alcohol. The remaining ingredients used in embalming solutions vary immensely.

Just as important as the need to replace equipment at frequent intervals and to maintain the proper facilities with which to manufacture and compound chemical solutions is the need to improve on and make changes in the general nature of formulations. These changes are occasioned by developments in the technical fields. Suppliers make use of such developments and adapt them into existing products or design new products containing them. This factor makes it unlikely that two different "brands" of fluid will have similar composition. The continuing investigations and studies conducted by the technical staffs of fluid manufacturers who maintain research laboratories also often result in attention being devoted to some particular compound that produces an innovative effect when blended with special ingredients.

Years ago, because of the similar chemical makeup of the fluids, it was possible in many instances to take the label off one firm's product and place it on another. The user could not readily distinguish the difference in the fluids from the embalming results obtained! Today, the many commercially available chemical preservative solutions differ with respect to the following factors: pH of the solution; type of buffer materials used to maintain pH; grade of formalin used; type of alcohol; wetting agents (anionic, nonionic, or cationic); anticlotting agents; modifiers; physical features such as specific gravity and surface tension; and so on.

In brief, the "20-index" fluid made by one manufacturer today can be expected to be chemically different in composition and even to produce different embalming results from that produced by another firm.

There is no general agreement on what constitutes a "standard" embalming fluid. Embalming personnel show varying preferences in the type of results they desire. Some require a fast-acting fluid with little or no internal cosmetic effect, whereas others desire such a fluid to produce an internal cosmetic effect. In other instances, a mild to moderately firming fluid that produces a noticeable coloring is preferred. An important factor for consideration is the effect of pathological conditions on the fluid injected and vice versa. The chemical preservation solution may produce different results when applied to different cases.

BRIEF SUMMARY OF CHEMICAL COMPONENTS

The ingredients that might be found in the majority of embalming fluids can be classified according to the specific purposes for which they are used (Fig. 6–1).

Preservatives

Preservatives, which inactivate saprophytic bacteria, render the medium on which such bacteria thrive unsuitable for nutrition. They arrest decomposition by altering enzymes and lysins of the body as well as convert the decomposable tissues into a form much less susceptible to decomposition. Formalin, as the commercial source of

formaldehyde, is the most commonly used chemical for this purpose. Other examples are paraformaldehyde, formaldehyde condensation products or formaldehyde "donors," "light" aldehydes, glyoxal, glutaraldehyde, phenol, phenolic derivatives, and lower alcohols (see pp. 113–117).

Germicides

Germicides are employed in embalming fluids to kill microorganisms or to render them inactive. This can be accomplished in two ways: (1) the chemical acts directly on the protein of which the microbe is composed or (2) the chemical acts on the protein material from which it derives its nourishment.

These chemicals kill or render incapable of reproduction the disease-causing microorganisms. As these microbes are made of proteins and the enzymes that they make are protein in nature, most of the preservative chemicals act as germicides. Phenol and phenolic derivatives are germicidal. Glutaraldehyde in an alkaline pH is particularly effective. Quaternary ammonium compounds such as Roccal and Zephiran Chloride are good examples of germicides incorporated into cavity fluids.

An important purpose of embalming is the sanitizing of the tissues of the body. Germicides are incorporated into **arterial fluid, some coinjection fluids, cavity fluids,** and **surface disinfectants.** The embalmer uses the surface disinfectants to sanitize the nasal and oral cavities as well as the surface of the body and, in the case of an autopsied body, the surface walls of the abdominal, thoracic, pelvic, and cranial cavities (see pp. 117–118).

Modifying Agents

Modifying agents influence the chemical reactions produced by the preservative solution and function in em-

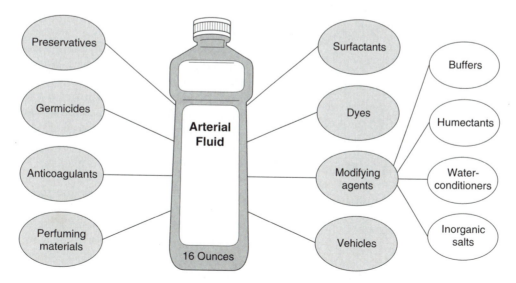

Figure 6–1. Ingredients that may be found in the majority of embalming fluids.

balming fluids to control the action of the main preservative agents. Modifying agents are chemicals for which there may be greatly varying demands predicated on the type of embalming, the environment, and the embalming fluid to be used. Because of special needs, embalmers may wish to greatly increase the concentration of one or more ingredients in a given embalming fluid (see pp. 118–119).

Humectants. A humectant can be used to moisturize tissues as well as to dehydrate tissues. These chemicals increase the capability of embalmed tissues to retain moisture. These would be added to dilute solutions when the body predisposes to dehydration. They also function to control and delay the firming and/or drying action of the preservative ingredients. Examples include glycerin, sorbitol, emulsifiable oils, and lanolin (see p. 118).

Buffers. Buffers effect the stabilization of the acid–base balance within embalming solutions and embalmed tissues. Many of the chemicals used as anticoagulants serve as buffer pairs to control the pH. Examples include borates, citrates, carbonates, monodisodium phosphate, and ethylenediaminetetraacetic acid (EDTA) salts (see p. 119).

Water Conditioners (Water Softeners). Water conditioners are added to the water used to dilute arterial embalming fluids when it is known that the water contains such minerals that it would be classified as "hard" water. When added in sufficient concentration they reduce the water used in preparing the embalming solution to "zero" (or nearly so) hardness. Water conditioners contain high concentrations of sequestering or chelating chemicals that might not be compatible with the other ingredients in embalming fluids over a long shelf life and so *must be packaged in separate formulations.* The amount of this type of chemical incorporated into regular arterial formulations is insufficient for "water conditioning" purposes. Examples include carbonates, borates, and trisodium phosphate (see pp. 119–120).

Inorganic Salts. Inorganic salts should be included under the heading of "modifying agents." These salts are actually found in a number of the other categories of the chemicals that constitute an arterial fluid. They can be found in buffers, preservatives, germicides, water conditioners, and anticoagulants. The salts play an important role in determining the osmotic qualities of the embalming solution. The osmotic force of the solution is responsible for its diffusing qualities (see p. 119).

Anticoagulants

Anticoagulants retard the tendency of blood to become more viscous by natural postmortem processes or prevent adverse reactions between blood and other embalming chemicals. The anticoagulants may be the principal ingredients of a nonpreservative, preinjection fluid, or coinjection fluid. They maintain blood in a liquid state and, thus, facilitate the removal of blood from the circulatory system. The chemicals employed for this purpose can also function as water softeners or water conditioners. When added in sufficient concentration, they will reduce the water used in preparing the embalming solution to zero hardness (or nearly so). In such concentrations they may not be compatible with other ingredients in arterial fluids over a long shelf life, and so must be formulated as separate compositions. Examples of anticoagulants are citrates, phosphates, oxalates, borates, and EDTA (see pp. 120–121).

Surfactants

Wetting agents, surface tension reducers, penetrating agents, surface-active agents, and emulsifying agents—all surfactants—reduce the molecular cohesion of a liquid and thereby enable it to flow through smaller apertures. This class of compounds is used to promote diffusion of the preservative elements through the capillary walls to saturate the tissues uniformly. They also help to distribute the coloring agents uniformly for internal cosmetic purposes. The presence of surfactants in the chemical solution aids in the displacement of body liquids from body tissue so that the injected preservative chemical elements may readily replace the volume previously occupied by body liquids (blood and tissue fluids). Examples include sulfonated oils (alkyl sulfonates), polyethylene glycol ethers, alkyl aryl polyether alcohols, alkyl aryl polyether sulfonates, alkyl aryl polyethyl sulfates, alkyl diethyl benzylammonium chloride, and sodium lauryl sulfate (see pp. 121–123).

Dyes

Dyes are substances that on being dissolved, impart a definite color to the solvent. They are classified with respect to their capacity to impart permanent color to the tissues of the body into which they are injected as ACTIVE (staining) and INACTIVE (nonstaining). Active dyes are usually a blend of dyes, mainly coal-tar derivatives, and they have an internal cosmetic effect. Red dyes of various shades and degrees of intensity are usually blended in an attempt to restore a natural color to the tissues. The coloring materials blended for the purpose specified may range from those that impart a straw or amber color to those that emit a brilliant shade of red. The coloring materials selected for use in any given embalming fluid formulation depend to a great extent on the pH of the solution. Examples include eosin, erythrosine, ponceau, fluorescein, amaranth, and carmine (see pp. 123–124).

Reodorants (Perfuming and Masking Agents)

Reodorants have the ability to displace an unpleasant odor or to convert an unpleasant odor into a more pleasant one. Their primary function is to enhance the odor of the embalming solution. This class of chemicals is usually selected not only for its power in covering harsh chemicals, but also because of its pleasant odor and antiseptic value. Actually, the use of these chemicals in embalming fluid is not intended to cover the harshness of formaldehyde. It is, rather, to give the product a more pleasing odor. The materials generally used are those that are water soluble and are derived from essential oils. Most of the reodorants used are floral compounds, which have been found to more successfully mitigate the irritating fumes associated with embalming formulations. Examples include methyl salicylate (oil of wintergreen), benzaldehyde, and many related higher aldehydes (see pp. 124–125).

Vehicles

Vehicles serve as the solvents for the many ingredients incorporated into an embalming fluid. Most embalming formulations consist of a mixture of alcohols, glycerine-like materials, water, and possibly glycols, which function to keep the ingredients of the formulation in proper chemical and physical balance. It is necessary that vehicles also provide some stability to the formulation. In specially designed formulations it is possible that a special solvent may be added as a part of the innovation to dissolve or keep in solution any special additive materials in the product. Later, the concentrated chemical is further diluted by the solvent water (see p. 125).

PRESERVATIVES

Generally speaking, the chemical compounds classified under "preservative ingredients" are the agents in the chemical preservative solution that cause the proteins to change in nature. Such compounds change a protein from a state in which it is easily decomposed to a state in which it will endure and not undergo putrefaction. In June 1988, the *New York Times* reported that it is now felt that it is the "unfolding of the proteins by formaldehyde with the result that the long strings of protein then intertwine into a network that hardens. This result is the *fixed protein.*" The type of action may be described as a "cooking" action in which the nature of the protein is changed, as occurs when a raw egg is fried. In that particular instance, the heat causes the albumin to change from a water white to a dull white.

What are some of the materials that are regarded as the main active preservative ingredients in modern-day embalming fluid preparations? The chemical compound employed is selected because of its chemical reactive properties that change the basic nature of the protein molecule.

Aldehydes, for example, react with the amino radicals of the protein structure to form a new compound in which the aldehyde radical adds on to the protein structure and water is released. The following formula represents a simple explanation of the action of the aldehyde on the amino part of the protein structure:

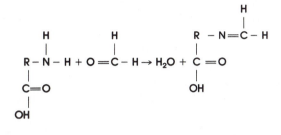

The amount of aldehyde that is taken up by the protein structures depends on such factors as initial concentration of aldehydes, pH value of the solution, effect of certain chemical compounds on aldehyde uptake, temperature, and conditions of tissue.

Formaldehyde and Formaldehyde-Type Preservatives

Formalin. Formalin is the commercial source of formaldehyde. Formaldehyde solutions containing 37% by weight formaldehyde gas absorbed in water, or in water and methyl alcohol, are known as formalin. The solution has a density slightly above that of water and contains approximately 40 grams of formaldehyde per 100 cubic centimeters. Therefore, commercial formaldehyde solution (i.e., "formalin") is described as containing "40% formaldehyde by volume." The NF (formerly USP) grade of formalin contains an average of 7% methyl alcohol, 37% minimum–37.3% maximum formaldehyde, and the remainder water. The alcohol present in the solution helps to stabilize the formaldehyde so that it will not precipitate and settle to the bottom as a powdery sediment (paraformaldehyde) at ordinary temperatures.

The regular product of commerce is a 37% by weight (40% by volume) formaldehyde gas in water solution. There are available, however, certain solutions that contain 40, 55, and even 70% formaldehyde in alcohol. The last two concentrations mentioned are subject to precipitation, and at cool temperatures the formaldehyde tends to fall out of solution very readily and form a fine powdery sediment at the bottom of the container. The sediment that settles to the bottom is actually **paraformaldehyde,** a solid form of formaldehyde. The formaldehyde that drops out of solution to the bottom of the container is not available for chemical reaction and results in a weaker concentration of formaldehyde in the top layers of the solution than at the bottom. In other words, the concentration of formaldehyde throughout the solution is not uniform.

A "formaldehyde solution" is any solution that contains formaldehyde. The NF or USP grade of formalin, on the other hand, is a formaldehyde solution consisting of 40% formaldehyde gas by volume or 37% formaldehyde gas by weight. In view of the various grades and types of formalin solutions now commercially available, it is important to designate the grade of formalin being used to state the percentage of formaldehyde gas present.

For many years the word *index* was generally understood to be the percentage strength of concentrated embalming fluid, and referred to the amount of absolute formaldehyde gas by volume present. It should be understood that the reference was to formaldehyde gas and not to formalin, which is the 40% (by volume) solution of formaldehyde. The Embalming Chemical Manufacturers Association and the schools and colleges of mortuary science have generally agreed on the following definition of index: "An embalming fluid will be said to have formaldehyde index, N, when 100 milliliters of fluid, at normal room temperature, contain N grams of formaldehyde gas." Thus, a 20-index product contains 20 grams of formaldehyde gas per 100 milliliters of concentrated fluid. The word *index,* therefore, identifies only the absolute formaldehyde gas present in any given product. It is **not** a measure of the total aldehyde concentration present. *Index refers only to the amount of formaldehyde gas present* (see p. 000).

Formaldehyde is a colorless gas at ordinary temperatures and has a strong, irritating pungent odor. **It is very soluble in water and is extremely reactive.** Because of its chemical nature, which makes it highly reactive, formaldehyde cannot be properly masked without affecting its chemical structure. In other words, to mask the odor of formaldehyde completely, it is necessary to neutralize it, and in such cases, the formaldehyde could not be available for preservation in embalming.

The chemistry of formaldehyde is a very specialized and complicated field of study, and F. J. Walker (1964) of DuPont published a book on the subject. This compound has been studied quite extensively and has been found to be **a very powerful germicide.** It destroys putrefactive organisms when carried by a proper vehicle that permits it to penetrate these organisms. It preserves tissues by forming new chemical compounds with the tissues. The new compounds that are formed are stable and unfit as food for organisms. An interesting comparison has been used effectively:

> The buttons on your coat, the barrel of your fountain pen, the comb on your dresser, and many other things you may commonly use are made of formaldehyde and phenol or carbolic acid, as it is commonly known.

Either formaldehyde or carbolic acid would injure you severely if taken into your mouth. You may, however, with impunity hold a button from your coat in your mouth because it differs definitely from either of its component ingredients. In other words, it is a resin.

This statement describes exactly the action of formaldehyde on albuminous materials. New resins are formed that are neither formaldehyde nor albumin. These resins may be hard resins, soft resins, or semihard resins, depending on the control chemicals (modifying or plasticizing materials) used in combination with the formaldehyde.

Formaldehyde acts quickly on the particular area with which it is in contact. The more formaldehyde there is in a certain area, the greater the action on the tissues in that area. The closer the tissue to the formaldehyde, the greater the action on it. This action takes up more formaldehyde than may be needed for preservation, possibly leaving little or no formaldehyde for the more remote tissue areas.

To use an analogy, the preceding action of formaldehyde on tissue may be compared with the action of a sponge in water. The sponge absorbs or takes up water depending on how much water there is to begin with and also depending on how long the sponge is permitted to remain in contact with the water.

If an embalming solution is hurried through the circulatory system as the result of too much pressure and excessive drainage, some tissue area will receive little or no formaldehyde. This, in turn, causes "soft spots" to develop. Such areas result when tissue does not receive a sufficient amount of formaldehyde to preserve it. There is also the possibility that a localized tissue area, because of some pathological condition, may be undergoing decomposition. Thus, the free amines may absorb more than the usual share of formaldehyde so that little formaldehyde is left for the remote parts. This situation is further exacerbated when an average of only 2 gallons of solution is injected. In such a case it is possible that an insufficient amount of formaldehyde is used to achieve thorough preservation of the body tissues.

Paraformaldehyde. Paraformaldehyde is described as a polymer of formaldehyde. It is a white, powdery solid containing from 85 to 99% formaldehyde. The NF grade of paraformaldehyde contains 95% formaldehyde. Paraformaldehyde is generally prepared from water solutions of formaldehyde by processes involving evaporation and distillation until concentration to a point at which solidification or precipitation take place. This form of formaldehyde is used where powdered preparations are involved such as in hardening compounds or other powered preparations used for "dusting" the body walls and viscera.

Trioxane. Another polymer of formaldehyde is trioxane, a colorless crystalline material with a rather pleasant odor resembling that of chloroform. This material is sometimes incorporated into formulations to act as an accessory preservative along with formates. It is rather costly when compared with other forms of formaldehyde and, therefore, is too expensive to warrant its extensive use for embalming purposes.

Other Aldehydes. Some of the other lower or "light" aldehydes have been proposed for use in embalming preparations and some are occasionally found in modern embalming fluids. Examples of these are acetaldehyde, propionaldehyde, and pyruvic aldehyde. Among the higher aldehydes, furfural and benzaldehyde may be listed. The important requirement of an aldehyde is that it possess denaturing and crosslinking properties that enable it to produce a firm tissue.

Condensation Products (Formaldehyde "Donor" Compounds, Formaldehyde Reaction Products). Aliphatic nitrohydroxy compounds are formed as the result of a condensation reaction between nitroparaffins (nitromethane, nitroethane, etc.) and certain aldehydes. Compounds of this type, in the presence of the proper catalyst (such as potassium carbonate), give off formaldehyde at a slow rate. When in solution, such formaldehyde condensation products exhibit an acid pH and need the alkali catalyst to release the formaldehyde.

Another type of formaldehyde "donor" compound is the methylol derivatives of hydantoin. These also liberate formaldehyde at a slow rate. Both types are used in low-odor or "fumeless" products. These complex organic substances make it possible to formulate fluids that are pleasant to use, as they do not give off noxious, irritating fumes. The formaldehyde is released after being distributed to all soft tissue areas where the usual preservative action is exerted. The disadvantage in using such materials is twofold: they have a slow reaction rate and are very expensive.

Dialdehydes

Another group of chemicals that are also aldehydes is the dialdehyde (two functional aldehyde groups in the molecule) class of chemical compounds. As far back as 1941, several firms in this industry investigated the possibility of using the then-known dialdehyde compounds available on a commercial scale. The principal dialdehyde and probably the only one available at that time in large commercial quantities and at an economical price that made its use in embalming formulations feasible was **glyoxal,** the lowest member of the dialdehydes. On November 2, 1943, a patent was granted relating to the use of glyoxal in embalming fluid formulations.

Glyoxal. Glyoxal is available commercially as a 30% yellowish, aqueous solution containing small amounts of ethylene glycol, glycolic acid, formic acid, and formaldehyde. It is also available as a special 40% clear solution. Because it contains a chromophore group, glyoxal solution tends to stain tissue yellow. This feature limits the use of glyoxal mainly to cavity fluid formulations, especially because its optimal pH range of activity is about 9 to 10.

Glutaraldehyde. In the early 1950s, a method was developed that made it possible to manufacture the five-carbon, straight-chain dialdehyde glutaraldehyde in commercial quantities. Glutaraldehyde was first employed as an embalming and fixative agent in early 1955 and was subsequently patented for use in embalming preparations. Commercially, it is supplied as a stable 25% aqueous solution that has a mild odor and a light color. Glutaraldehyde reacts through crosslinking to insolubilize both protein and polyhydroxy compounds. The pH of the commercial solution is 3.0 to 4.0 and the specific gravity is 1.058 to 1.068.

An interesting feature of glutaraldehyde is that unlike other aldehydes, it is capable of reacting with protein structures over a wide pH range. This is an important advantage for an aldehyde in embalming, because after death, tissue pH varies in different parts of the body and as time elapses between death and embalming.

Both glyoxal and glutaraldehyde are liquids, whereas formaldehyde is a gas. The following structural formulas serve to acquaint the reader with some of the aldehydes that have been mentioned:

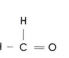

Formaldehyde

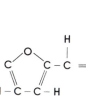

Furfural, 2-Furaldehyde

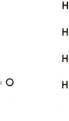

Glutaraldehyde

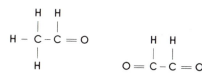

Acetaldehyde

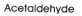

Glyoxal

In combining with proteins and tissue, glutaraldehyde changes the nature of the proteins, makes them unsuitable as food for bacteria, and makes them resistant to decomposition changes. At the same time less moisture is removed from the tissues as the result of the chemical reaction between glutaraldehyde and proteins than when formaldehyde is used. In addition, glutaraldehyde has been found to be many times more effective as a disinfectant than formaldehyde.

Other Preservative Agents

Other preservative agents generally used in combination with formaldehyde include the lower alcohols and the phenol (carbolic acid) compounds. The latter materials are usually selected on the basis of solubility, penetrability, compatibility, and stability. Some of the newer preservative ingredients include certain aromatic esters and formaldehyde reaction products. They react with proteins in a similar manner as formaldehyde to form insoluble resin, the main difference being in the rate of reaction. Formaldehyde firms tissue at a faster rate.

Methanol (Methyl Alcohol, CH₃OH). Generally, the synthetic grade of methanol is used and it is 99.85% pure. Methanol is used in embalming formulations for six reasons:

1. It is an outstanding preservative that destroys many organisms and precipitates albumins.
2. It is a good solvent for other chemicals not readily soluble in water alone, for example, derivatives of phenol.
3. It is an excellent penetrator of the tissues and it also exerts some bleaching action.
4. Methanol is a stabilizer of formaldehyde. It prevents the formaldehyde from changing to the powdered form.
5. Methanol serves as a diluent or vehicle for other ingredients of the formulation.
6. Investigations have indicated that methanol is more toxic to bacteria than grain alcohol (ethanol or ethyl alcohol).

Methanol and the lower alcohols have a dehydrating effect on protein structure. As methanol has the greatest precipitating effect of the lower alcohols and aids in removing body liquids, it is used more extensively in embalming fluids than either ethyl or isopropyl alcohol.

Phenol (Carbolic Acid, C₆H₅OH). Phenol is one of the most commonly found ingredients in both arterial and cavity fluids manufactured in the "early" days of the fluid industry. Today, it is used chiefly in cavity fluid formulations. Phenol is a coal-tar derivative that is a colorless crystalline solid. On exposure to strong light and metallic contamination, it becomes dark and assumes a dark amber or reddish brown appearance when in solution. Such change in color is due mainly to oxidation. The potency of phenol is not impaired to any great extent when such change occurs.

Phenol is very rapidly absorbed by protein structures and penetrates the skin very readily. Phenol and phenolic derivatives are good germicides. In addition, they assist formaldehyde in forming insoluble resins with albumins. Generally, their use in embalming fluids is confined to cavity fluids because they tend to produce a "putty gray" tissue. Formulations containing these compounds are often used as bleaching agents to lighten discolorations on the skin surface. The solution either is applied as an external pack or is injected subcutaneously with a hypodermic syringe.

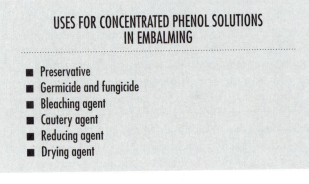

USES FOR CONCENTRATED PHENOL SOLUTIONS IN EMBALMING

- Preservative
- Germicide and fungicide
- Bleaching agent
- Cautery agent
- Reducing agent
- Drying agent

(Care should always be taken when working with phenol to protect skin and eyes.)

It is unfortunate that the most powerful germicides among the phenols are not water soluble. Some of the halogenated phenols found in embalming formulations include orthophenyl phenol, *para*-chlormetacresol, dichloro-*ortho*-phenyl phenol, tribromothymol, and other sodium salts of these and other phenol-related chemicals.

Sometimes the expression *triple-base fluid* is heard. This refers to a fluid containing phenol, alcohol, and formaldehyde. A "double-base" fluid presumably is one containing formaldehyde and alcohol, or formaldehyde and phenol, or alcohol and phenol. Commercial fluids almost always contain phenols in combination with formaldehyde and alcohol. The presence of the latter two compounds improves the bacteria-killing power of phenols. Phenols generally do not produce readily detectable firmness of tissue such as that produced by aldehydes.

Quaternary Ammonium Compounds. These materials are used chiefly for their germicidal and deodorizing qualities. They consist of mixtures of alkyl radicals from C₈H₁₇ to C₁₈H₃₇, that is, high-molecular-weight alkyl dimethyl benzylammonium chlorides. Aqueous solutions are usually neutral (pH 7). These compounds are not compatible with the wetting agents used in arterial fluids nor with many of the coloring materials incorporated into such fluids. Consequently, their use is restricted to cavity fluids and specialty formulations used for cold sterilization of instruments, linens, gowns, clothing, and other items; cleaning agents for moldproofing remains; deodorant sprays; and so on. Two of the best known "quats" are Roccal and Zephiran Chloride.

Salts. Various salts have been used in embalming products since the early days of embalming. Among the more commonly used compounds are potassium acetate, sodium nitrate and nitrate, and some salts of aluminum. The salts of the heavy metals are not used, as after 1906, many of the states prohibited their use in embalming compositions.

Germicides

Obviously, the ingredients used as preservatives also function as germicides. In addition, such chemicals as phenol, the quaternary ammonium compounds (Chloride), and glutaraldehyde are used as surface disinfectants and in embalming fluid solutions.

MODIFYING AGENTS

Modifying agents control the rate of action of the main preservative ingredients of embalming formulations. Many preservative ingredients, when used alone, exert adverse effects that interfere with good embalming results. For example, formaldehyde (when used alone) is so harsh an astringent that it sears the walls of the small capillaries and prevents diffusion of the preservation solution to remote soft tissue areas. It is necessary to control the rate of fixation so that the firming action is delayed long enough to permit thorough saturation of tissue cells. When the hardening effect of the aldehyde is delayed, the more uniform distribution of the coloring or staining agent is made possible. Buffers, antidehydrants, water conditioners, and inorganic salts usually control the rate of chemical action, modify the adverse color reaction produced by the preservative ingredient in the tissues, and control capillary restriction or other undesirable results produced by the preservative materials.

1. *Buffers:* agents that serve to control the acid–base balance of fluid and tissues
2. *Humectants* (antidehydrants): agents that help to control tissue moisture balance
3. *Inorganic salts:* agents that help control the osmotic qualities of the embalming solution

4. *Water conditioners:* chemicals that increase the compatibility of the water used to dilute the concentrated embalming fluid.

It should be pointed out that many chemicals in the preceding list serve similar functions. Many buffers can also act as water conditioners and anticoagulants. In addition, some of these chemicals are also inorganic salts and contribute to the osmotic qualities of the embalming solution. Even humectants can play a role in the osmotic quality of an embalming solution. Because certain chemicals have multiple uses in embalming solutions, specific chemicals appear under different headings. For example, in a discussion of the anticoagulants, buffers are also reviewed.

Buffers

Buffers are employed in embalming fluids to stabilize the acid–base balance of the fluid. These pH stabilizers not only help to maintain the acid–base balance of the fluid, but, in addition, assist in stabilizing the pH of the tissues where the embalming fluid reacts with the cellular proteins. **Keep in mind that the tissues of the body after death contain varying levels of acids or bases.** Normal body pH is about 7.38 to 7.4 after death, and through the rigor mortis cycle the tissues will have an acid pH as a result of carbohydrate breakdown. After the rigor cycle the tissues become basic as a result of protein breakdown. These reactions are not uniform throughout the body, so tissues will vary in pH depending on rigor mortis and decomposition cycles. In addition, the cause of death can influence tissue pH. Buffers play a very important role in providing good pH medium for the reaction of preservative with body proteins.

Alkaline Compounds

Certain alkalies are commonly employed to modify the action of formaldehyde. They "neutralize" the formalin used in making the fluid.

Borates. In a report released by the Public Health Service in 1915, it was found that **borax** (sodium borate) was a good, efficient neutralizer of formalin, providing a desired degree of alkalinity that rendered formalin stable for long periods. It has been found to reduce the hardening and graying actions of formaldehyde. Depending on the specific type for formulation and other ingredients present, boric acid may also be employed in embalming formulations. Formulations containing a well-balanced mixture of borates have been found to keep formaldehyde fairly stable beyond 2 years. The loss in formaldehyde strength in such instances is insignificant.

Carbonates. Sodium carbonate is used alone or in combination with borates to modify the action of formaldehyde on tissue. Magnesium carbonate is also used sometimes and may be added to the formalin prior to combination with the other ingredients in a formulation. This procedure is said to neutralize formalin and maintain it at pH 7. From all indications it would appear that carbonates are not as efficient as borates in preventing deterioration of formalin over long periods.

In a *Report and Review of Research in Embalming and Embalming Fluids* by the Minnesota State Department of Health, N. C. Pervier and F. Lloyd Hansen of the University of Minnesota studied the tissue reaction to injections of formaldehyde at various pH values. These investigators found that addition of a strong base, such as sodium hydroxide, improved tissue coloring; however, the high concentration of sodium hydroxide used caused deterioration of the preservative. When they injected formaldehyde solutions containing 1, 2, and 3% acid (HCl), the tissue tended to assume a putty-gray coloration.

The investigations of these two workers confirmed the findings of the U.S. Hygienic Laboratories reported some 50 years ago. Today, most arterial fluids are found to be **slightly alkaline** (with a pH of 7.2–7.4), whereas cavity fluids tend to be **acidic in nature.**

Humectants (Antidehydrants/Polyhydric Compounds)

Humectants are described as having a coating action; they wrap around the formaldehyde molecule and thus keep the formaldehyde from making direct contact with albuminous material until the tissues are thoroughly saturated and bathed with the preservative solution. The formaldehyde is under shackles for a time, and as it travels through the capillaries and to the tissue cells it gradually sheds its shackles and, on release, acts on the albuminous material. The addition of polyhydric compounds to embalming fluids assists in making the tissue more flexible and rubbery. In some instances such materials are also called plasticizing agents because of their pliable effects. These compounds include glycerin, sorbitol, glycols, and other polyhydric alcohols. Cosmetic oils, lanolin, and its derivatives are also used for their emollient properties.

Glycerine. A by-product of the manufacture of soap, glycerine is a member of the large family of alcohols. It has been produced synthetically from petroleum products. Although glycerine is not itself a germicide and has no preservative qualities, it does increase the germ-killing power of other chemicals, probably because it is an excellent solvent for disinfecting chemicals; its good solu-

bility makes it an efficient carrier for the chemicals. Glycerine is a good lubricator, is a good solvent for other compounds, and is hygroscopic, which means it has affinity for moisture. If retained in the tissues, it helps to prevent overdrying.

Sorbitol Glycols. Sorbitol is probably used more extensively today in embalming fluids than is glycerine. Chemically, it has a straight chain of six carbon atoms and six hydroxyl groups, whereas glycerine has three carbon atoms and three hydroxyl groups in its structure. Commercially, sorbitol is generally available as a 70% aqueous solution. An important characteristic of sorbitol is that it loses water at a slower rate than glycerine, and consequently, for controlling the rate of moisture loss, it is more efficient than glycerine. One disadvantage of sorbitol solutions is that at very low temperatures, sorbitol tends to drop out of solution. Different types of glycols (mainly propylene, ethylene, and diethylene) are also found in embalming preparations. Sometimes, these materials are used alone with formaldehyde; in other instances, they may be incorporated into a formulation already containing either glycerine, sorbitol, or both.

Ethylene glycol is a colorless, syrupy liquid with very little odor. It is quite readily soluble in water. Because of its hygroscopic properties it is used as a moisture-retaining and softening material.

Propylene glycol is reported to be superior to glycerine as a general solvent and inhibitor of mold growth. Like ethylene glycol, it is colorless, odorless, and completely soluble in water.

Emulsified Oils. Many materials have been investigated for their emollient characteristics. Materials such as lanolin and silicon are not in themselves water soluble, but certain fractions or derivatives are used that can easily be dispersed in aqueous solutions. It is the purpose of these materials in embalming fluid to mitigate the drying effect of the preservative agents. Highly penetrative oils of the oleate and palmitate types are also employed to help reduce the drying effect of aldehydes. Use of such materials requires an emulsion system that is able to maintain the formulation in a stable and uniform state over a long period.

Gums—Vegetable and Synthetic

The use of vegetable and synthetic gums is generally prompted by the need to restore moisture to tissue or to maintain the normal appearance of tissue when the subject is to be held for a period prior to burial. These materials, when added to water, swell and retain the moisture as the gum molecule is distributed to the soft tissue areas. Because of their molecular size, the gums, on taking up moisture, are actually trapped in the capillary bed and aid both in restoring moisture to the area and in filling out the tissues to overcome the emaciated appearance.

As these materials are large molecular entities they are generally added to the arterial embalming solution after the initial injection has been made and all surface discolorations have been cleared. Use of such compounds prior to complete removal of blood from the tissues may interfere with proper distribution of the injected preservative solution.

Examples of vegetable gums include **karaya** and **tragacanth.** The synthetic gums are generally cellulosic compounds of varying composition.

Inorganic Salts

The inorganic salts used in embalming fluids serve a variety of functions. They can act as buffers, anticoagulants, preservatives, germicides, and water conditioners. Their use is quite simple in that they can be dissolved in the limited space of the 16-ounce standard bottle of concentrated embalming fluid. By controlling the amount of inorganic salts used, the fluid remains balanced, as some of the salts do not "settle out" of the concentrated fluid. An obvious role for salts in any solution is their ability to control the osmotic qualities. This is true in embalming fluid. Once the embalming solution reaches the capillary beds it is very important that the solution be able to pass through the microscopic pores of the capillaries and thus enter the tissue spaces. It is a role of the inorganic salts to maintain an osmotic quality of the embalming solution that helps to draw fluid from the capillaries into the tissue spaces. Likewise, special fluids are used on bodies whose tissues are saturated with edema. These "special-purpose" fluids, when mixed according to the manufacturer's directions, actually draw the excess tissue moisture (edema) from the tissues back into the capillaries, from which it can then be removed by the drainage process. It is the osmotic qualities of those "special-purpose" fluids that bring about the dehydration of these bodies (see Chapter 21).

Water Conditioners

The products known as water "softeners" or water "conditioners" are used for one or all of four reasons.

First, such products are intended to be used as aids to improve drainage by keeping blood in a liquid state during the embalming operation and softening the framework of clotted material so that it readily breaks up into smaller pieces.

Second, by reducing "hard" water to zero hardness, such materials make it possible for the arterial fluid to function under better conditions. The interfering "hardness" chemicals such as calcium and iron actually prevent the preservative chemicals present in arterial fluids from performing their intended function of penetrating soft tissues to achieve preservation.

Third, experience and experimental work have indicated that the dyes used in embalming fluids produce the best internal cosmetic effect under slightly alkaline conditions. The arterial fluids cannot be compounded to stay on the alkaline side of the pH scale because aldehydes, especially formaldehyde, undergo breakdown and lose strength when kept under alkaline conditions for long periods. Consequently, the alkaline conditions must be created at the time the solution is going to be used. During such short periods, alkaline pH does not adversely affect the preservative chemicals. Addition of water softeners ("clot-dispersing products") to the embalming solution prepared for injection produces a most desirable alkaline condition. Such materials enhance the coloring properties and action of dyes by increasing their intensity.

Fourth, recent investigations have definitely shown that most aldehydes (and formaldehyde in particular) function better as fixative or firming agents under slightly alkaline conditions. But, as pointed out in the preceding paragraph, aldehydes cannot remain under alkaline conditions more than a couple of weeks (even less) without losing their effectiveness. Therefore, the alkaline conditions must be created more or less "on the spot" at the time the fluid is used. This is where the specially designed additive products come into play. Greater firmness is attained by progressive action where such materials are used along with the arterial fluid.

Often, it is claimed that a certain arterial fluid contains all of the materials necessary to reduce to zero hardness the water used in preparing the embalming solution. Because of the preservative materials that must be incorporated into the arterial fluid formulation (in addition to wetting agents, modifiers, coloring agents, perfuming materials, etc.), however, there is a limit to the amount of anticlotting and water-softening compounds that can be added to the formula. If sufficient amounts of such compounds were to be added to the regular arterial fluids to achieve the results expected from and produced by "water softeners," the chemical and physical balance of the formulation would be adversely affected. And what happens when the chemical and physical balance of the arterial fluid is adversely affected?

- There may be interference with proper penetration and diffusion of the preservative solution.
- There may be interference with the drainage qualities of the embalming solution.

■ By disruption of the chemical balance of the solution, addition of the extra amounts of anticlotting and water-softening chemicals to the arterial fluid formula could cause a gradual reduction of the formaldehyde strength of the fluid.

Consequently, embalming fluid manufacturers supply, as separate accessory products, "water softeners and conditioners" that are added to the embalming solution prepared for injection. This procedure enables the embalmer to use as much material as the case may require for proper and effective water- and clot-softening action.

The compounds in this class of embalming chemicals include those usually found in buffer systems. As has been pointed out previously, the degree of acidity or alkalinity of the medium in which a chemical reaction takes place influences, to a great extent, the chemical reaction that takes place between compounds and substances. During life, blood and body tissues have a pH of 7.4. After death, however, tissue pH varies greatly. Also, the pH of the body tissues at the time of embalming depends on the time that has lapsed since death. An embalming formulation containing the proper buffer mixture will perform uniformly because the buffer mixture will neutralize excess acidity or alkalinity and, thus, facilitate the action in a given pH range.

It is also necessary to maintain an embalming formulation at a given pH if it is to be retained for a long shelf life. Some chemicals that are used are stable only in certain pH ranges and so buffer agents must be employed to keep constant the acid–base balance of the solution. This ensures against deterioration and breakdown of the chemical compounds. For example, earlier it was stated that formaldehyde is not stable at high pH, that is, under alkaline conditions, over long periods. When embalming fluid is compounded, the manufacturer must try to anticipate the shelf life of the product so that the fluid is as effective the day it is used as the day it was compounded. A formaldehyde index on a fluid bottle label is maintained only through the proper chemical balance of the formulation, which also includes proper acid–base control of the solution.

Another important factor to keep in mind is that as the prepared embalming solution diffuses through the circulatory system, it comes into contact with tissues that may well be at different pH values. The acid–base balance of the tissues should also be so controlled and maintained by the buffer so that the fluid performs under the best pH conditions.

Many preservative chemicals when used alone exert bad effects that interfere with the achievement of good embalming results. For example, formaldehyde when used alone is so harsh and astringent that it sears the walls of the small capillaries and prevents diffusion of the preservative solution to remote soft tissue areas. Consequently, it is necessary to control the action of the formaldehyde so that the fixation of tissue (firming action) is delayed sufficiently to permit thorough bathing of tissue cells. By delaying the hardening action of formaldehyde, uniform distribution of the coloring or staining agent is also possible. It can be said that these modifying agents also enhance the internal cosmetic effect.

Many years ago, the U.S. Hygienic Laboratories found that formaldehyde, when present in an acid solution or used at acid pH, tends to promote rapid bleaching of muscular tissue to an ashen gray. This observation suggested the use of alkaline materials in combination with formaldehyde for embalming formulations. Many alkalies, however, have a deteriorating effect on formaldehyde, especially over prolonged periods (longer than 2 weeks).

ANTICOAGULANTS (ANTICLOTTING AGENTS)

Anticoagulants are an important component of embalming fluids, especially arterial fluids, because they are used to maintain blood in a liquid state and thereby make it easy to remove from the circulatory system.

When blood collects in the capillary bed in the dependent parts of the body after death, it has a tendency to thicken and clot very easily. In some cases, as in death from pneumonia, the blood tends to clot more readily. The volume of circulating blood tends to decrease when high fever precedes death, and the blood becomes more viscous and clots more readily after circulation stops.

It is therefore necessary to include, in an embalming fluid, chemicals that maintain blood in a liquid state so that it is easily displaced from the body. Such chemicals inhibit or stop the clotting of blood. Claims are often made that such materials also "liquefy" clotted blood, but it is not likely that this happens.

The ingredients that are used for this purpose must be chemically compatible with, or inert toward, other intimately blended ingredients of the formulation. The materials that are employed as anticoagulants also function as "water softeners" or "water conditioners"; however, products specially designed for that purpose are commercially available and are sold for use as additives or accessory chemicals with the arterial solution.

Citrates

Sodium citrate, a white, odorless, crystalline or granular material, is often used for its anticoagulant as well as its water conditioning properties in embalming fluid. This compound inactivates calcium in the blood as well as in the water supply. Without calcium, blood coagulation does not occur.

Oxalates

Another calcium precipitant, sodium oxalate, a white crystalline powder, is sometimes used but not as extensively as the citrates.

Borates

Borates are the compounds most extensively found in embalming formulations. In addition to its function as a stabilizer of formaldehyde, sodium borate also serves to prevent or reduce coagulation. Sodium borate (borax, sodium tetraborate, or pyroborate) is a white crystalline powder that is readily soluble in a mixture of water and glycerine. Boric acid is a white powder that is often used in combination with borax.

Ethylenediaminetetraacetic Acid

The sodium salts of EDTA are very effective sequestering or chelating agents, which means that they very readily combine with calcium ions to prevent blood coagulation and also to remove hardness chemicals from the water supply. Generally, these materials are not found in arterial fluids. These agents are quite alkaline and are not compatible with the other ingredients in embalming fluids over a long shelf life. Such materials are used most advantageously as separate formulations, that is, in the form of supplemental or accessory chemicals that are added to the embalming solution at the time of use.

Other Materials

Among the other compounds often used as anticlotting materials are magnesium sulfate (Epsom Salts), sodium chloride, sodium sulfate, and sodium phosphates. At one time or another these compounds have been recommended for use in capillary wash solutions, and some are still used in arterial fluid formulations. This class of chemicals also contains some of the materials employed in buffer systems to maintain a constant pH in a fluid formulation. These are used in combination with those mentioned earlier.

SURFACTANTS

Probably one of the greatest developments that has occurred in the chemistry and physics of embalming since the discovery of formaldehyde is the principle of removing body liquids by lowering their surface tension. It is necessary, before complete circulation may take place in the body, to remove the liquid that is held in the capillaries. Capillary attraction, or the force that attracts and holds liquid in the capillary tubes, is the result of surface tension. If the surface tension of the liquid in these tiny tubes is lowered, the liquid easily loosens and flows out.

Much has been said and written about the important role and use of surfactants (*surface-active agents, tension breakers, tension reducers*) in embalming formulations. Actually, there is no industry that has not investigated these compounds and found them adaptable for a variety of uses. The chemical structure of surfactants is rather complex: one part of the molecule has a strong attraction or affinity for water, whereas the other part of the molecule dislikes water. This latter part of the molecule has an affinity for nonaqueous liquids. Such a complicated molecular makeup functions to lower or reduce the surface tension of the solution to which the surfactant is added. In a water-and-oil mixture the surfactant destroys the surface tension of the components so that the oily mixture is more easily dispersible in water. Other materials are made "water soluble" in a similar manner.

It should also be called to mind that each cell in the soft tissues of the body is surrounded by a film of body liquid mostly water in composition. For easy, rapid penetration of the cell, this surface film must be dispersed. Such chemical substances, then, are used in embalming fluids for three reasons.

First, by lowering the surface tension of the preservative solution (the embalming solution), surfactants aid or cause the embalming solution to flow more readily and rapidly through the capillaries so that ALL of the millions of tissue cells are literally bathed by the embalming solution and, thus, thoroughly preserved. Naturally, the technique of injecting the solution and draining employed by the embalmer can assist or handicap the function of the surfactant. The process of moving the solution through the body being embalmed is a technique that should be planned and controlled by the embalmer to ensure that a sufficient amount of preservative chemicals is uniformly distributed throughout the body. It is also important that some of the normal moisture lost during embalming be replaced to safeguard against overdehydration.

Second, by reducing the capillary attraction (which is a phenomenon of surface tension) of blood and body liquids, surfactants cause the almost immediate clearing of blood from the capillaries. Surface tension is reduced, and the liquid more readily moves and flows out the capillary bed and through the venous drainage system. **As two things cannot occupy the same space at the same time, the capillaries must be emptied of blood before injected solution can flow through them to reach the tis-**

sues of the body. Only the solutions that pass by osmosis through the capillary walls into the intercellular spaces have any chance of being absorbed by the tissue cells. The embalmer must help the solution reach the tissues by employing the necessary physical manipulation such as massage and intermittent or restricted type of drainage.

Third, by increasing the ability of the solution to filter through the semipermeable capillary walls in a uniform manner, it is possible to incorporate coloring agents into the solution and obtain a normal appearance internally (Fig. 6–2).

The preceding concepts have been incorporated into the manufacture of embalming fluids since the early 1930s. Industrial investigators have found that the uniform penetration of the tissues by the embalming solution is necessary to obtain positive, long-lasting preservation.

Surface Tension and Embalming Solutions

Solids, liquids, and gases are all made up of molecules arranged in characteristic patterns depending on the material being studied. These molecules have an affinity or attraction for one another. Again, depending on the materials under study, this degree of molecular attraction differs. For example, the attractive force is greater between water molecules than it is between alcohol molecules. At 20°C, the surface tension of water is 72.75 dynes per centimeter, and for methyl alcohol it is 22.61 dynes per centimeter. (*Note: a dyne is the force required to accelerate a 1-gram mass 1 centimeter per second.*) Thus, water has a surface tension value more than three times that of methyl alcohol and penetrates much more slowly. In other words, **the lower the surface tension value, the faster the rate of penetration by the liquid substance.**

The surface tension of water is lowered by the addition of surfactants. Wetting or penetrating chemicals tend to destroy the bonds or attractive forces that normally exist between water molecules so that they seemingly break away from each other. The net effect of such physiochemical action is to cause liquids to diffuse and penetrate more readily through cellular tissue.

Surface tension is also defined as the contractive force that causes liquids to assume the shape in which they have the least surface, that is, a sphere. Wetting agents reduce or destroy this contractive force so that the liquid film becomes "wetter."

In embalming solutions, the addition of surfactants in proper concentrations produces better penetration of the preservative chemicals in a more uniform manner. This enables the preservative solution to more readily displace the body fluids from all cellular tissue and replace them to achieve the embalming function. Also, coloring agents are uniformly distributed through the use of surfactants. The even diffusion of such agents throughout the soft tissues results in a more lifelike color and appearance.

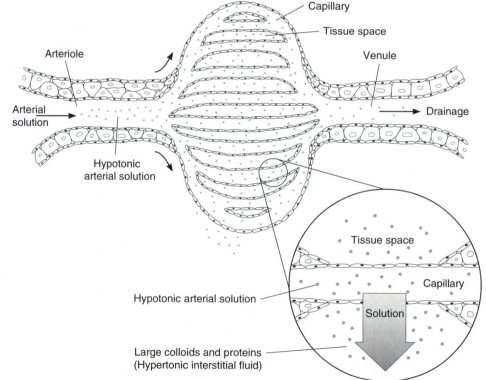

Figure 6–2. Movement of arterial solution from the capillaries into the tissue spaces.

Surface tension changes with variations in temperature. As the temperature rises, the surface tension value of a solution decreases. In embalming, this means that if warm water is used to prepare the solutions for injection, the resultant solution may be expected to penetrate more rapidly because of the lowered surface tension value. Also keep in mind that the chemical reaction between the preservative chemicals and the tissues will take place more rapidly as the result of using warm water. The fixative or firming action will occur faster than usual.

Surfactants also increase the germicidal activity of chemical solutions. It is believed that this is due to an increased speed of penetration into the bacterial cells as a result of the lowering of the surface tension of the solution.

Surfactants and Surface Tension

From the preceding discussion it might appear that the embalmer could easily make his or her embalming technique more efficient by simply adding an extra surfactant to the embalming solution. This is not true. This class of chemical compounds is extremely temperamental and sensitive. Surfactants function best in very low concentrations and must be carefully selected by experienced chemists with respect to the other ingredients present in the formulation. It is necessary to determine compatibilities between all the components of an embalming fluid and the surfactant, and the amount of surfactant to use to produce a properly well-balanced chemical formula. Addition of extra surfactant to an embalming solution may result in excessive drainage as well as oversaturation of tissue.

The following considerations, which must be thoroughly explored by the chemist in evaluating specific applications for any given surfactant, serve to illustrate the complex nature of such chemicals. The discussion is by no means complete.

Surface-active agents are generally classified into three groups: anionic, cationic, and nonionic. In brief, **if the surfactant molecule tends to ionize, then it is either anionic or cationic. If it does not ionize in solution, it is nonionic.**

Surfactants such as soap, alkyl sulfonates, alkyl aryl sulfonates, salts of sulfated alcohols, and oils are *anionic*. These compounds are compatible with other anionic and nonionic agents. They are not normally compatible with and are frequently precipitated from solutions by cationic materials and by certain inorganic cations such as aluminum, calcium, and magnesium.

Nonionic surfactants do not ionize in solution, but owe their surface activity and water solubility or dispersibility to nonionized polar groups within the molecule, such as hydroxyl or ether linkages. Ethylene oxide condensation products with amides and fatty acids be-

long in this group (specific examples are the Atlas "Tweens" and "Spans").

In actual chemical formulating practice, the result to be achieved by the end product must be kept in mind in deciding the type of surfactant to employ. Most generally, a blend of such materials is incorporated into embalming fluids to achieve the results mentioned at the beginning of this discussion.

Preliminary selection of the proper surfactant or blend of surfactants is usually based on the following factors: specific application, pH of solution to which it is added (acid, alkaline, or neutral), physical form of surfactant (liquid, gel, flake, or powder), nature of other ingredients in the formulation, concentration to use. The surfactant that works most satisfactorily in one brand of products may not function well or at all in another brand. As most of the water used in preparing embalming solutions tends to be "hard," it is customary among embalming fluid manufacturers to select surfactants that are not readily affected by "hardness" chemicals in the water.

DYES (COLORING AGENTS)

The coloring materials used in modern embalming fluids generally are employed for the purpose of producing an internal cosmetic effect that closely simulates the natural coloring of tissues. Such materials have high staining qualities and as they diffuse to the superficial tissue areas from the circulatory system, they impart color to the tissue. Usually, a blend of coloring materials, ranging from straw or amber to brilliant red, is used. The type of dye used depends to great extent on the pH of the arterial fluid. Dyes that color tissues are called **active dyes**. Those that merely lend color to the fluid in the bottle are **inactive dyes**.

Types of Coloring Agents

Coloring materials may be placed into two classes.

Natural coloring agents are vegetable colors such as cudbear, carmine, and cochineal. **Cudbear** is a purplish-red powder prepared from lichens by maceration in dilute ammonia and caustic soda and fermentation. **Carmine** is an aluminum lake of the pigment from cochineal. **Cochineal** is a red-coloring matter consisting of the dried bodies of the female insects of *Coccus cacti*. The coloring principle is carminic acid, $C_{17}H_{18}O_{10}$. This class of dyes is not generally incorporated into modern solutions.

Synthetic coloring agents are the coloring materials used in modern fluids and are mainly coal-tar derivatives. They are economical to use and are the most permanent if they are compatible chemically with the other ingredients in the fluid. Many different types and shades are available under rather confusing diversified commercial names and chemical nomenclature. For better solubility, most of the coal-tar dyes are supplied in sodium or potassium salts of the synthetic coloring matter. These materials then may be said to be dyes of alkali metal salts that have been reacted with coal-tar compounds. Several dyes are available:

- **Eosin:** known as tetrabromofluorescein, $C_{20}H_8Br_4O_5$; red crystalline powder
- **Erythrosine:** brown powder that forms cherry red solutions in water; known chemically as the sodium salt of iodeosin, $C_{20}H_6I_4Na_2O_5$
- **Ponceau:** dark red powder that is soluble in water and acid solutions; forms a cherry red solution and is a naphthol disulfonate compound
- **Amaranth:** coal-tar azo dye that forms a dark red-brown color in water but is only slightly soluble in alcohol.

Other synthetic dyes include croceine scarlet, rhodamine, rose bengal, acid fuchsin, and toluidine red.

Coloring Materials in Embalming Fluids

Coloring materials in use today in embalming fluids belong to a group known as biological stains, as such materials are used in clinical laboratories to stain different types of tissue for study under the microscope. The coloring agents used in fluids must be stable in the presence of formaldehyde, must be water soluble, should impart a natural flesh color to the tissues, and should have high tinctorial or staining qualities so that small amounts can produce the desired color. This last requirement is important because arterial fluids are diluted before use.

The coal-tar dyes possess the requirements of a coloring agent for use in embalming fluids. Molecularly they are fine enough to diffuse evenly and uniformly through tissue cells. As soon as surfactants (wetting agents) began to be used in embalming solutions, it was found possible to add staining materials to the formulations because wetting agents diffused the dye very effectively. The specific material that is to be used in any given formulation must be carefully selected, as some dyes produce different coloring effects at different pH values and different extents of dilution.

Natural-color materials such as the vegetable dyes are considered too unstable for use in embalming fluids. Some have good color-fast features but do not diffuse evenly because of their large molecular structures.

The "older" embalming fluids contained coloring materials mainly for the purpose of identification. They did not produce staining effects as do those in use today.

Such old fluids did contain salts known as nitrates, which caused a localized breakdown of red blood cells. As the contents of such cells spilled out, the hemoglobin, which is the coloring matter of blood, remained in the intracellular spaces and produced a color effect. One chemical theory states that the nitrate salts are converted to nitroso compounds which combine with a portion of the hemoglobin molecule, resulting in a permanent color.

Such salts are not generally used today because newer chemicals have replaced them and also because they required a slow type of action. The high-drainage-type chemical solutions in use now are made possible by replacing the older chemical compounds with modern ones that are faster acting and that produce even, uniform embalming results.

PERFUMING MATERIALS (MASKING AGENTS, DEODORANTS)

Generally, reodorants or perfuming agents are selected not only for their power in covering harsh chemicals but also for the pleasant odor they impart to a solution. By blending special synthetic essential oils with the harsh preservative chemicals in a formulation, the harshness or "raw" odor of the solution is reduced and replaced to some extent by a more pleasing scent. No attempt is made, however, to mask completely the fumes of formaldehyde. Any attempt to mask formaldehyde generally results in neutralization or destruction of the active chemical.

Floral compounds such as wisteria, rose, and lilac types, along with nondescript essential oils and aromatic esters, are used quite extensively in embalming formulations because of their "heavy" note. This property makes it possible to cover objectionable fumes during brief exposures. Such materials are made water soluble through the medium of nonionic-type surfactants.

If the formulation does not contain a high concentration of formaldehyde or other irritating chemicals, it is possible to use synthetic compounds that give off odors resembling spices (clove, cinnamon), fruit (strawberry, peach, etc.), mint (spearmint, peppermint, menthol), and many other "notes" designed by the essential oil chemist. Sassafras, oil of wintergreen (methyl salicylate), and benzaldehyde have been among some of the more commonly used materials for this purpose.

Occasionally, use is made of high concentrations of perfuming and masking agents in chemical solutions in an attempt to hide high concentrations of formaldehyde, especially in so-called "fumeless" fluids. Usually, the scent of the perfuming agent is immediately detected, while the presence of the formaldehyde remains in the background. The individual finally becomes aware of the formaldehyde as a result of a pinching sensation in the nose; the delayed awareness manifests in the form of an explosive effect with a resultant shortness of breath. The individual does not realize how much fumes are present until too late! Unfortunately, there are products still advertised as "fumeless" or "odorless" when, in reality, they are not. The true low-odor type of product is based on the use of "donor" compounds that release the aldehyde when contact is made with tissue so that a minimum amount of gas is released to bother the user.

The essential oils used in embalming fluids are selected on the basis of their stability in the presence of preservative chemicals and their ability to remain in solution when water is added. Some essential oils possess antiseptic properties but this usually is not why they are used in embalming formulations.

VEHICLES (DILUENTS)

The active preservatives and other ingredients in the formulation must be dissolved in a common solvent. As water is an essential component of tissue, its use in embalming solutions facilitates the diffusion and penetration of the active preservative constituents of fluids. The vehicle (sometimes called "carrier") must be a solvent or mixture of solvents that keeps the active ingredients in a stable and uniform state during transport through the circulatory system to all parts of the body.

To maintain the proper density and osmotic activity, that is, the proper chemical and physical balance of the formula, the vehicle or diluent may include glycerine, sorbitol, glycols, or alcohols in addition to water. Quite often, a special solvent may be used as part of an innovation to dissolve or keep in solution any special "new" ingredient in the product.

KEY TERMS AND CONCEPTS FOR DISCUSSION

1. Define the following terms:
   Anticoagulant
   Arterial fluid
   Arterial solution
   Buffer
   Cavity fluid
   Cosmetic fluid
   Dye
   Germicide
   Humectant
   Index
   Noncosmetic fluid
   Penetrating agent
   Perfuming agent
   Preservative
   Primary dilution
   Secondary dilution
   Surfactant
   Vehicle
2. List the uses for methanol in arterial fluids.
3. Describe embalming treatments using phenol.

BIBLIOGRAPHY

Dorn JM, Hopkins BM. *Thanatochemistry, A Survey of General, Organic, and Biochemistry for Funeral Service Professionals.* Reston, VA: Reston; 1985.

Eckles College of Mortuary Science Inc. *Modern Mortuary Science.* 4th ed. Philadelphia: Westbrook; 1958:206.

Encyclopedia of Industrial Chemical Analysis. Vol. 12: *Embalming Chemicals.* New York: John Wiley & Sons; 1971.

General chemical principles of embalming fluids. In: *Expanding Encyclopedia of Mortuary Practice,* Nos. 365–371. Springfield, OH: Champion Co.; 1966.

Walker J. *Formaldehyde.* 3rd ed. ACS Monograph No. 159. New York: Reinhold; 1964.

7

Use of Embalming Chemicals

The preceding chapter looked at the ingredients that constitute embalming fluids. This chapter examines the use of the various embalming fluids, including arterial fluids, coinjection fluids, preinjection (primary injection) fluids, water-corrective fluids, dyes, humectants, cavity fluids, autopsy gels, and cautery chemicals. The various factors that must be considered in selection and preparation of an arterial fluid are discussed. It is shown that many types of these fluids are available. *The embalmer selects the various chemicals he or she wishes to employ in the preparation room.*

Almost every funeral home will purchase at least one preservative arterial fluid and one type of cavity fluid. From that starting point, many types of fluids can be added to the shelf. There are a variety of arterial and coinjection fluids. **It is possible to embalm a body using preservative arterial fluid for injection and a cavity fluid for treatment of the cavities. All other fluids, such as preinjection and coinjection fluids, humectants, water conditioners, and fluid dyes, can be used to complement and enhance the embalming operation.** The selection and use of these chemicals become the personal preference of the embalmer.

In addition to a basic preservative arterial fluid, many embalmers prefer to keep on hand some of the special-purpose arterial fluids. Many funeral homes purchase a high-index arterial fluid for use when there has been a delay between death and preparation or when pathological conditions make firming of the body difficult. In addition, many funeral homes like to have available a jaundice fluid for preparation of those bodies exhibiting this discoloration.

DEFINITION OF EMBALMING FLUID

In 1928, Professor Charles O. Dhonau, dean of the Cincinnati College of Embalming, defined embalming fluid. He did not define the fluid itself as much as explaining how the fluid reaches the cells of the body. He further explained how the fluid works and what it does to bring about sanitation, preservation, and restoration of the tissues of the body. **This definition is as relevant today as it was more than 60 years ago and it serves well to explain the entire process of embalming:**

It is a chemical substance
which when given physical application (or injection)
at the right time
at the right temperature
in the right quantity
of the right quality, strength, dilution, concentration
so as to receive a complete distribution in arteries, capillaries, veins
will diffuse (spread from) from the capillaries
to the lymph spaces and to the intercellular spaces
and to the cellular tissues

to unite with the cellular substances
so as to normalize their water content
restore their colors
and so fix and preserve them that they will be preserved against organized (bacterial) and unorganized (enzymatic) decompositions
and will be preserved against other kinds of changes such as in water content; oxidation; from soil chemicals
just so long as the after-care provides the necessary means to protect
what has been embalmed.

A part which has been embalmed will not discolor from any cause within several weeks; it will not become blood discolored; or show dehydration changes; or show greenish colors from protein decompositions; or become malodorous from protein decompositions by proteolytic bacterial enzymes by which spore forming anaerobes, seeking (bound) oxygen, break up compounds containing it and release odorous gasses such as hydrogen sulphide; or become gas distended from the gaseous decomposition of proteins or carbohydrates (tissue gas); nor will the tissues soften and finally liquefy through the work of organized or unorganized ferments; nor will the tissues of the body pass through the cycle of changes which at the end converts the hundred or more body compounds into water, nitrogen, methane and carbon dioxide, as a result of all the oxidations through which decompositions proceed. A part which has not been properly embalmed should be thought of by the embalmer as an *an unsolved embalming problem,* to which he has contributed either by lack of understanding, by carelessness or by both.*

GENERAL PRECAUTIONS IN THE USE OF CHEMICALS

The embalmer handles a variety of chemicals, disinfectants, and sanitizing agents during preparation of the body and the terminal disinfection after the embalming. Care should be taken in the handling of all these chemicals, even such seemingly harmless products as talcum and drying powder used in cosmetic treatment of the body.

Some general guidelines apply to the handling of embalming chemicals:

1. *Wear gloves when working with embalming chemicals.* Some individuals can develop a sensitivity to chemical agents in embalming fluids. These sensitivities can cause skin irritations and eruption similar to allergic reactions. Formaldehyde has a tendency to dry the hand of the embalmer. This drying (after several days) can lead to cracking of the skin. Broken skin is

an avenue for the entrance of pathogenic microbial agents. Formaldehyde is also an irritant to the skin and, if concentrated enough such as in cavity fluids, can cause an inflammation of the skin.

2. *If chemicals are splashed or spilled onto the skin, flush these areas with cold running water.*

3. *Wear eye protection when handling embalming chemicals.* Eyeglasses, a face shield, or some type of protective eye covering should be used at all times. Formaldehyde, if splashed into the eye, is a severe irritant. Flush immediately with cool running water. An embalmer working with a chemical containing phenol (carbolic acid), or with concentrated phenol, should be certain that his or her eyes and skin are protected. Phenol can cause severe burns. **Whenever this chemical is accidentally splashed into the open eye, seek medical help immediately.**

4. *Wear protective clothing during embalming.* Many embalming fluids contain dyes that leave permanent stains on clothing.

5. *When using chemicals be certain that ventilation systems are in operation and, if necessary, wear a mask.* Formaldehyde fumes can be quite irritating and exposure to these fumes should be kept to a minimum. Care should also be taken in the handling of solvents used in mortuary cosmetology. Whenever embalming powders or cosmetic powders are in use, be certain rooms are well ventilated. Particulate from these powders is respirable and many of the small particulates in these powders are not exhaled, but retained in the lungs.

6. *Dilute any spillage immediately with cool water and clean.* Formaldehyde can be neutralized by applying a small amount of household ammonia to the spill. Any sponges or rags used in cleaning these spills should be flushed with cold water. If necessary, leave the room until the fumes decrease to a level at which working in the room to clean up the spill can be tolerated.

7. *Do NOT use formaldehyde-based chemicals as an antiseptic.* These chemicals are NOT for use on living tissue.

8. *Keep chemical data sheets available as well as chemical manufacturers' first-aid information.*

9. *Be certain bottles that are destroyed have been flushed out with water.*

10. *Keep machine tanks and fluid bottles covered and capped at all times to help reduce fumes.*

11. *Be certain formaldehyde is removed as much as possible before working with disinfectants such as sodium hypochlorite (laundry bleach).*

*From Dhonau O. *Defining Embalming Fluid.* File 100. Cincinnati, OH: Cincinnati College of Mortuary Science; 1928, with permission.

Combination of formaldehyde with these chemicals can produce gases that have proven to be dangerous.

12. *Pour fluid into a filled tank rather than filling after fluid is in the tank (Fig. 7–1).*

PRESERVATIVE ARTERIAL FLUIDS

Preservative arterial fluid is the concentrated embalming fluid that contains the eight groups of chemicals: (1) preservatives, (2) germicides, (3) anticoagulants, (4) vehicles, (5) surfactants, (6) dyes, (7) perfuming agents, (8) modifying agents. The vehicle water is used to dilute these fluids. It is added by the embalmer to create the embalming solution. In addition, supplemental fluids may be added to boost one or more of the chemicals.

1. Index Classification
   A. Low: those fluids with a formaldehyde index in the range 10–18
   B. Medium: those fluids with a formaldehyde index in the range 19–27
   C. High: those fluids with a formaldehyde index in the range 28–36

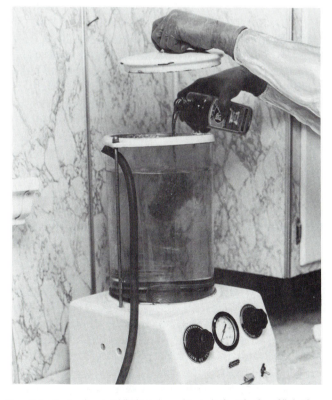

Figure 7–1. Pouring the arterial fluid into the machine tank after it has been filled with water reduces formaldehyde exposure. Keep the machines covered by using the lid.

2. Cosmetic Classification
   A. Cosmetic: those fluids that contain an active dye that colors the tissues
   B. Noncosmetic: those fluids that contain little or no active dye and do not color the tissues
3. Firming Speed
   A. Fast-acting: those fluids buffered to firm tissues rapidly
   B. Slow-firming: those fluids buffered to firm body tissues slowly
4. Degree of firmness
   A. Soft-firming: those fluids that are buffered and contain chemicals to control the preservative reaction to produce very little firming of the tissues
   B. Mild-firming: those fluids that are buffered and contain chemicals to control the preservative reaction to produce a medium firming of the tissues
   C. Hard-firming: those fluids that are buffered and contain chemicals to control the preservative reaction to produce very definite and hard firming of the tissues
5. Moisturizing Qualities
   A. Humectants: those fluids that contain large amounts of chemicals that act to add and retain tissue moisture
   B. Nonhumectants: those fluids that do not contain antidehydrant chemicals
6. Special-purpose arterial fluids
   A. Jaundice fluids: those fluids compounded to cover or remove the discoloration of jaundice
   B. High-index special-purpose fluids: a group of chemicals with indexes usually greater than 30, used in the preparation of extreme cases, such as bodies with edema, those dead from renal failure, and bodies dead for a long time
   a. Dehydrating: fluids compounded to bring about dehydration of the body tissues
   b. Nondehydrating: fluids compounded to contain large amounts of preservatives but controlled so as not to dehydrate tissues
   C. Tissue gas fluids: fluids designed to arrest and control the causative agent of tissue gas
   D. Fluids for infants and children: fluids designed for the delicate tissues of infants and babies

Remember that all the chemicals in this classification are designed to preserve and sanitize the body. Eight major chemical manufacturers manufacture 86 different types of preservative arterial fluids.

A look at other arterial fluids shows that these are used for specific reasons and, in and of themselves, do not embalm the body.

SUPPLEMENTAL FLUIDS

Preinjection (Primary Injection) Fluids. Preinjection fluids are fluids injected before the preservative arterial solution. They aid in blood removal and prepare the tissues for the preservative arterial solution.

Coinjection Fluids. Coinjection fluids are added to preservative arterial solutions to form a homogenous mixture. They serve to boost most of the arterial fluid chemicals with the exception of dyes and preservatives.

Standard coinjection fluids are designed to boost the penetrating and distributing qualities of the arterial fluid and to help modify and control the reaction of the preservatives. *Internal bleach and stain removers* are designed to bleach such blood discolorations as ecchymoses and postmortem stains. *Tissue gas coinjection fluids* are germicidal and act on the microbes responsible for tissue gas formation. *Edema-corrective coinjection fluids* enhance the dehydrating effect of the arterial fluid and aid in drying tissues that are edematous. *Germicide boosters* increase the germicidal effects of the arterial fluid and are used in routine embalming as well as in the treatment of bodies dead from infectious and contagious disease.

Water (Conditioning)-Corrective Fluids. These supplemental fluids are added to the arterial solutions to overcome the adverse effects of various chemicals that might be contained in the water.

Dyes. Active dyes are added to arterial solution. Some companies require only a few drops of these dyes. Other manufacturers require addition of several ounces to bring about the desired color in the tissue. Both pink tints and suntan tints are available.

Antidehydrants. Antidehydrants are added to the arterial solution to increase the antidehydrating effects of the arterial fluid.

Table 7–1 summarizes the various *arterial chemicals* used in embalming.

The eight categories of embalming chemicals can be combined in various ways to create three other widely employed embalming chemicals: cavity fluids; surface bleaches, cauteries, and reducing agents; and preservative (autopsy) gels.

Cavity Fluids. Cavity fluids are employed for three reasons: (1) they are injected via the trocar into body cavities; (2) they are injected by hypodermic into areas of the body that have not been reached by arterial injection; and (3) surface packs are added to bleach to preserve areas not reached by arterial injection or as a supplement treatment for areas requiring further drying and bleaching.

TABLE 7–1. CLASSIFICATION OF FLUIDS

Arterial Fluid[a] (Preservative)	Supplemental Fluid
Index	Preinjection
Low	Coinjection
Medium	Standard
High	Germicide booster
Nonformaldehyde	Edema-corrective
Color	Tissue gas
Cosmetic	Internal bleach
Reds	
Suntan	
Noncosmetic	Humectant
Firming speed	Restorative
Fast	Water-corrective
Slow	
Firmness	
Low	Dyes
Medium	Pink tints
Strong	Suntan tints
Antidehydrant	
Humectant	
Nonhumectant	
Special purpose	
Jaundice	
High index	
Dehydrating	
Nondehydrating	
Tissue Gas	
Infants	

[a] Aldehyde based fluids.

Cautery Chemicals. Cautery chemicals are very strong solutions containing basically phenol (carbolic acid). They are used as surface compresses and can be injected via a hypodermic for bleaching blood discolorations, reducing swollen tissues, and drying and cauterizing tissues. Care must be exercised in the handling of these chemicals, for the acid can severely burn the skin and lend permanent harm to the corneal tissue of the eye. In handling these chemicals it is imperative that some form of eye protection be used.

Preservative Gels. The last group of chemicals, preservatives, is a relatively new group. They were first sold as emollient (preservative) creams. During the past 25 years these preservatives have been improved and now have a long shelf life and the ability to penetrate deeply. They are employed as surface preservatives. Their viscosity varies. Some are in the form of very thick gels; others can easily be spread with a brush. The group includes **surface preservatives**, germicides, bleaches, and deodorizers. They are used for treatment of the viscera in autopsies, preservation of trunk walls in autopsies, treatment of surface lesions, and treatment of tissue areas not reached by arterial injection. They are applied by brushing on the surface or by using external compresses.

ARTERIAL FLUID DILUTION

The dilution of arterial fluid prepared by the embalmer is called the **primary dilution.** In preparing the primary dilution the best guide is the instructions on the fluid bottle. Generally, the label gives dilutions for three body conditions: "normal" bodies, edematous bodies, and dehydrated bodies. Some labels contain dilutions for special purposes such as bodies dead for long periods, bodies dead from renal failure, or preparation of infants. Note a typical fluid label:

	Dilutions
Normal bodies	7 ounces to 1 gallon of water
Emaciated bodies	4 ounces to 1 gallon of water
Dropsical or severe bodies	Up to 10 ounces per gallon of water
Dilution	Cold water or body temperature

Dilutions may be increased or decreased to suit the embalmer's technique and problem. In addition, most labels give the formaldehyde content, which is called the "index." Index is defined as *the amount of formaldehyde measured in grams, dissolved in 100 milliliters of water.*

The preceding label stated that the fluid has an index of 25. Today, fluid manufacturers recommend that a 2% strength primary dilution of arterial fluid be used to properly sanitize the body. The strength of the "average" embalming solution would be in the range 1.5 to 2.0% strength. To determine the strength of a primary dilution of arterial fluid a very simple linear equation can be employed. This formula has four factors:

$$\text{Index} \times \text{amount of fluid} = \text{strength of solution} \times \text{total volume}$$

$$c \times v = c' \times v'$$

To prepare a 2.0% arterial solution using the 25-index fluid just discussed, it is necessary to know how much fluid is needed to make 1-gallon solution of 2% strength:

$$25 \times x = 2.0\% \times 128 \text{ ounces of total } solution$$

$$25x = 256$$

$$x = \frac{256}{25}$$

$$x = 10.2 \text{ ounces of arterial fluid}$$

Approximately 10 ounces of arterial fluid and 118 ounces of water would be needed to make 1 gallon of 2.0% strength arterial solution.

Using the label directions, determine the strength of the arterial solution when 7 ounces of fluid and 1 full gallon of water are used.

$$25 \times 7 = x \times 135 \text{ (128 ounces of water and 7}$$
$$\text{ounces of fluid)}$$

$$175 = 135x$$

$$x = \frac{175}{135}$$

or approximately 1.29% or 1.3% strength (Table 7–2).

pH of the Arterial Solution

The pH of the arterial solution is determined by the fluid manufacturer. This is not an element of the fluid that the embalmer determines. Most arterial fluids are buffered to be slightly alkaline in pH, approximately 7.2 to 7.4. At this pH the fluid reaction is stable, dyes in the fluid work well, and the tissues do not exhibit a tendency to turn gray.

If the embalmer selects an arterial fluid buffered at acid pH, usually these fluids are labeled as "fast-acting" fluids. In addition to the fast reaction of the fluid with body tissues, the bodies tend to become slightly grayed several hours after arterial injection.

One word of caution concerning fast-acting arterial fluids: The embalmer must be certain that a sufficient volume of fluid has been injected. As these fluids result in rapid firming of the body, there is a tendency to run an insufficient amount of solution. After surface blood discoloration has been cleared, it would be wise to use intermittent drainage. Running a sufficient quantity of fluid and making every effort to RETAIN as much fluid as possible within the body should help ensure that a sufficient amount of arterial solution is needed.

Arterial Fluid Temperature

Again, the best instructions to follow in diluting arterial fluid are the manufacturer's recommendations. Most companies state on the label the temperature of water to employ. Most fluids are diluted with room temperature water. Only in special cases, such as in the treatment of tissue gas, is it recommended that fluids be diluted with warm water. When in doubt, use water at room temperature to dilute the fluid.

SOME PROPERTIES OF CHEMICAL SOLUTIONS: EFFECTS ON EMBALMING

Certain physical factors influence the results produced by any chemical. These factors play a role in governing the reactions between the tissues and the preservative chemical ingredients. As the type and amount of chemical substances in a solution are changed, a number of properties of the solution can be controlled.

Density/Specific Gravity

Certain solid chemical substances commonly known as "salts" play an important part in determining the char-

TABLE 7–2. PREPARATION OF VARIOUS-PERCENTAGE ALDEHYDE "IN-USE"SOLUTIONS[a]

Concentrate per Gallon (oz)	% Aldehyde in Concentrate				
	Index = 15	Index = 20	Index = 25	Index = 30	Index = 35
4	0.47	0.625	0.78	0.94	1.10
5	0.59	0.78	0.98	1.17	1.38
6	0.70	0.94	1.17	1.41	1.64
7	0.82	1.10	1.37	1.64	1.91
8	0.93	1.25	1.56	1.88	2.19
9	1.05	1.41	1.76	2.11	2.46
10	1.17	1.56	1.95	2.34	2.73
11	1.29	1.72	2.15	2.59	3.01
12	1.41	1.86	2.34	2.81	3.28
13	1.52	2.03	2.54	3.05	3.55
14	1.64	2.19	2.73	3.28	3.83
15	1.76	2.34	2.93	3.52	4.10
16	1.88	2.50	3.13	3.75	4.38
17	1.99	2.66	3.32	3.98	4.65
18	2.11	2.81	3.52	4.22	4.92
19	2.23	2.97	3.71	4.45	5.20
20	2.34	3.13	3.91	4.69	5.47
21	2.46	3.28	4.10	4.92	5.74
22	2.58	3.44	4.30	5.16	6.02
23	2.70	3.59	4.49	5.39	6.29
24	2.81	3.75	4.69	5.63	6.56
25	2.93	3.91	4.88	5.86	6.84
26	3.05	4.06	5.08	6.09	7.11
27	3.16	4.22	5.27	6.33	7.38
28	3.28	4.38	5.47	6.56	7.66
29	3.40	4.53	5.66	6.80	7.92
30	3.52	4.69	5.86	7.03	8.20

[a]Ounces × index divided by 128 (oz/gal) equals % aldehyde in solution.
Courtesy of Champion Co., Springfield, OH.

acteristics of the different embalming fluids and in controlling, to a large extent, the reactions between the cellular tissues and the chemical solution. If a "salt" is added to a liquid, a solution results. For example, common table salt is the "solute" and water the "solvent" when these are combined. After the salt has completely dissolved in the water and is thoroughly mixed by agitation, the result is a "true" solution. Naturally, if the solute does not dissolve completely in the solvent, a true solution does not exist.

The more "solute" added to the "solvent," the more concentrated the solution becomes. In other words, the strength of the solution actually indicates how much "solute" is present. The amount of "solute" in a solution has a direct effect on the density of the solution.

Density is defined as weight per unit volume and is expressed in such terms as grams per cubic centimeter or pounds per cubic foot. Thus, it is seen how density relates to the concentration of the solute in the solution. Often it is desirable to compare the weight of a given volume of a substance with an equal volume of water. This ratio is called **specific gravity.** A substance is said to have a specific gravity of 1.5; this means that compared with an equal volume of water, the substance weighs 1.5 times the weight of water. Again, as with density, the specific gravity of a solution varies with concentration.

In solutions used in medicine, the density or salt concentration of a solution is frequently compared with that of the blood. If a solution contains less of a dissolved substance than is found in the blood, it is said to be **hypotonic.** If it contains a greater quantity of a dissolved substance than is found in the blood, then it is said to be **hypertonic.**

During embalming, blood and other body liquids are being displaced and replaced with the chemical preservative solution, which eventually changes the nature of tissue. Such change resists decomposition. The penetration of such solution into all soft tissue areas should be thorough to achieve complete preservation and produce the best results.

It has been found that a solution that is slightly hypotonic to the blood and body fluids produces the best embalming results. A review of the scientific principle involved will show why this is so.

In the accompanying diagram, **A** is a membranous bag such as from a section of animal intestine that is "semipermeable," that is, permeable to some materials but not to others. The bag contains a 10% salt solution. If the bag is immersed in a container, **B** is observed to increase.

This serves to prove that water has passed into the bag. Now, it will be interesting to reduce this observation to a simple explanation.

The distilled water, being "hypotonic" (i.e., of *less* density), passes to the inside of the bag, which contains the more highly concentrated solution (i.e., of *higher* density). The solution in bag **A,** then, is "hypertonic" to the distilled water. What is the importance of all this to the embalming operation and to embalming fluids?

It is known that a solution will penetrate to the side or region containing the more "dense" solution; this fact is used in compounding fluids and in establishing the proper concentrations to use in embalming. When diluted according to the recommended usage, the resultant solution is slightly *"hypotonic"* to blood and body liquids. If less of the concentrated fluid is used, then the resultant solution may be more "hypotonic" than desired for proper embalming results. The tissues tend to become "waterlogged," which eventually results in "skin-slip" because of the lack of sufficient preservative material.

On the other hand, if too much concentrated fluid is used, according to the preceding principle, a "hypertonic" solution results, and it will have the effect of removing too much moisture. This, of course, causes

overdehydration. In some instances, the embalmer may want to make use of this principle to remove excess moisture from tissue areas, such as in dropsical or edematous cases. The "special" fluids designed for such purposes incorporate this principle.

Briefly, then, an embalming solution **less dense** (i.e., "hypotonic") than the tissue liquids will flow rapidly through the capillary walls into the soft tissue areas. If the solution is designed so that it has a **greater density** (i.e., "hypertonic") than the tissue liquids, it will draw tissue liquid through the capillary wall into the circulatory system and away from the soft tissue areas.

Osmotic Qualities

For the average or "normal" body in which there is no edema and no dehydration, the arterial solution should be *hypotonic* in its osmotic composition. This is generally achieved by following the manufacturers' dilutions. When the solution is *hypotonic* to the body tissues, the fluid moves from the capillary vessels into the tissue spaces. If these solutions were hypertonic, tissue fluids would move from the tissue space into the capillary vessels, thus causing dehydration and lack of arterial fluid in the tissues.

There are instances when *hypertonic* solutions are desired. This type of solution is generally used when embalming bodies with skeletal edema. These solutions help to move the excess water from the tissue into the capillary vessels. From there the water can be removed through drainage. Some embalmers add Epsom Salts to the arterial solutions to create these hypertonic dehydrating solutions. The high-index special-purpose fluids, when diluted in a certain manner, create dehydrating *hypertonic* solutions.

Quantity

Consider this example of different bodies that required special attention:

> Two bodies weighing 110 pounds—one a healthy teenager killed in an automobile accident, the other a 65 year-old adult who died of a wasting disease (e.g., cancer; in good health the individual weighed 190 pounds). Should the embalmer proceed to embalm the two in the same manner using the same chemicals, same concentrations, same total solution volume, and so forth? This situation might be used to introduce the concept of "preembalming" considerations.

The total volume of arterial fluid injected is determined by a number of factors. These factors should be noted in making the case analysis. Over the years a fairly safe rule to follow has been to **inject 1 gallon of properly selected and diluted arterial fluid for every 50 pounds of body weight.** Again, the embalmer must determine if a suffi-

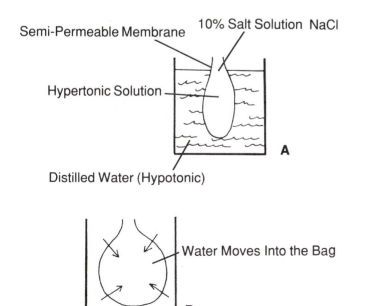

Semi-Permeable Membrane   10% Salt Solution NaCl

Hypertonic Solution

Distilled Water (Hypotonic)

A

Water Moves Into the Bag

B

cient quantity of fluid has been injected and if the fluid has been injected at a proper strength. Autopsied bodies have been prepared in which up to 3 or more gallons of solution has been injected into one leg. It is always wise to embalm the body on the assumption that the disposition will be delayed. Another thought is to prepare the body in such a manner that it is "overembalmed." Today, because large doses of medication are used, the following factors must be considered:

- Effect of the drug on the preservative solution
- Damage the drug has done to the body proteins
- Damage to specific organs such as the liver and the kidneys, causing retention of wastes such as ammonia and urea in the tissues
- Damage to the cell membrane—a possible condition in which it is difficult for fluids to pass through the cell membranes

Consider these points in determining the strength and amount of fluid to inject:

- Time between death and preparation
- Time between preparation and disposition
- Moisture content of the body
- Renal failure and the buildup of nitrogenous wastes in the body
- Liver failure and the buildup of toxic wastes in the body tissues
- Weight of the body
- Amount of adipose tissue versus muscular tissues accounting for body weight
- Protein levels of the body
- Progress of the postmortem physical and chemical changes, especially the stages of decomposition and rigor mortis
- Nature of death—sudden heart attack versus "wasting disease," use of life-support systems for many weeks
- Chemotherapy and medications given the individual

USE OF PREINJECTION FLUID

A preinjection fluid is injected into the body before the preservative arterial solution is injected. These fluids were first used because the early arterial fluids were so strong and harsh that they caused difficulty in clearing the blood from the capillaries and veins. The preinjection fluid (also called a primary injection fluid or capillary wash) was designed to clear the blood vascular system of the blood prior to injection of the preservative solution.

Today, arterial fluids contain a number of modifying agents that allow the arterial solutions to distribute and diffuse uniformly. Many embalmers, however, still feel the necessity to flush the vascular system with a preinjection solution. This helps to clear blood discolorations, adjusts the pH of the tissues, reduces blood coagulation, and, thus, improves draining. Two factors are necessary to obtain the best results with this chemical: (1) a sufficient quantity should be injected and (2) some time should be allowed for the chemical to work properly.

It has been suggested that at least 1 gallon should be injected and that the chemical should be allowed to sit 20 to 30 minutes before the preservative solution is injected. Most embalmers, however, inject approximately a quarter to one-half gallon of solution and immediately inject the preservative solution. In theory, any amount of preinjection fluid would enter the vessels *before* the preservative arterial solution. A quarter to one-half gallon of this solution would, no doubt, fill the empty arterial system, in the average-size body. Instructions will give dilutions for the use of the chemical and should be followed, for these fluids have little or no preservative and it is possible to waterlog the tissues and cells with this solution.

Some preinjection fluids contain small amounts of preservatives. For this reason, some embalmers use these chemicals to embalm infants and children. *In this text it is felt these fluids should NOT be used to embalm children; rather, standard preservative arterial fluid should be used for the preparation of infants and children.* The embalmer may wish to use a preinjection solution only to assist in preparing the circulatory system for the preservative arterial solution.

Preinjection treatment is generally used only on unautopsied bodies, not for treatment on autopsied bodies in which each body area is separately injected. Note also that preinjection fluids contain little or no active dye to color the tissues. Many embalmers also prefer to inject this solution with the drainage kept open.

In embalming bodies where there has been any great time delay between death and embalming or where the embalmer feels circulation may be difficult to establish, preinjection fluids should be avoided, or, if used, the embalmer should inject a minimal amount. A preinjection fluid loosens clots in the venous system and, thus, makes them easier to remove. This, in turn, improves blood drainage. If there is any clotting in the arterial system, preinjection fluids can loosen these arterial clots. They will be carried by the fluid to smaller arteries where they can easily block circulation channels.

Preinjection fluid works best when it is used on bodies that are still warm and when the embalmer feels circulation will be very good. An embalmer who feels circulation may be difficult to establish and arterial clotting may be present should avoid the use of a preinjection fluid. Because embalming is usually delayed with bodies dying in large hospitals, less preinjection fluid is being used today.

The following sample has been compiled from several different fluid company catalogs and contains descriptions of different preinjection fluids. It will help the student, in particular, to understand the purpose of these fluids.

Sample: Preinjection Fluids

KLM promotes drainage and capillary circulation. *Many bodies present the challenge of a highly complex residual body chemistry. The extent and identification of this chemistry are not always known.* KLM is proven to be the embalmer's best and most direct approach to the control of adverse residual body chemistry. KLM is unmatched in its scope for body conditioning, and its use prevents complications.

PQR is very fine primary injection fluid. It conditions the arterial system and expands the small arterioles and venules to make the subsequent arterial injections more effective and complete. Research has shown that an alkaline condition of the tissues is desirable to retain their natural color (acid brings on an ashen gray appearance), and yet, a strongly alkaline solution tends to waterlog the body.

The bonus feature of PQR is a *touch of preservative* effect. It has been found that a low index of formaldehyde in a *slightly alkaline* primary injection fluid is the complete answer, actually making the tissues more receptive to later contact with preservative chemicals. *One of PQR's most important functions is to establish the proper pH in the circulatory system and adjacent tissues to promote constantly uniform results in all cases.*

XYZ is a positive and dependable aid in *keeping the blood liquid and free flowing.* Its heavy specific gravity provides the driving force to keep the blood moving, while at the same time *strengthening and lubricating the capillary walls.* It is excellent for clearing discolorations caused by bruising and other injuries.

TUV acts with trigger-fast speed to dilute thick heavy blood and relieve the vascular congestion that acts as a barrier to arterial and capillary circulation. Smooth in it action, TUV slips quickly through the capillary walls to allow for an easier and more voluminous fluid passage. All of the *dark heavy blood is washed from the capillaries and veins,* preventing any possibility of the flushing or putty gray that so frequently mars embalming results. The widespread effect in the rapid disappearance of surface discolorations and the *greatly stimulated drainage* can be easily seen.

TUV contains efficient nonhardening preservatives that eliminate all danger of *waterlogging* the tissues but, at the same time, cannot possibly burn, harm or dehydrate the most tender body. TUV is osmotically balanced to ensure retention of the correct amount of tissue moisture and to maintain naturalness for the maximum period. TUV not only liquifies and removes heavy blood but it *reoxygenates both the blood and tissue cell as well.* The normal pink cast of the blood and tissues is restored by a natural process homologous to that which exists during life. *For a most satisfactory embalming termination the embalmer must have a proper beginning.* No arterial preparation can accomplish the best results unless the capillary system has been completely cleared of blood and the vessels expanded for maximum capacity.

USE OF COINJECTION FLUIDS

Most coinjection fluids are compatible with the majority of arterial fluids. An arterial fluid and a coinjection fluid should combine to form a homogenous solution that can be distributed and diffused throughout the body. As for the amount to use, remember that the manufacturers' labels are the best guide.

Most coinjection fluids are used in an amount equal to the amount of concentrated arterial fluid. Or, half as much coinjection fluid as concentrated arterial solution is used. Generally, the amount of coinjection fluid should never exceed the amount of concentrated arterial fluid. When too much coinjection is used (plus the use of water softeners), the fluid has a tendency to distribute unevenly and the dyes have a tendency to "blotch."

When in doubt, a good rule is to **use equal amounts of coinjection fluid and concentrated arterial fluid.**

When should a coinjection fluid be used? This chemical, unlike a preinjection chemical, can be employed with every preparation. It assists in distributing and diffusing the arterial solution and helps to control and enhance the arterial fluid. In some special conditions, embalmers use the coinjection fluid as the dilutent vehicle, for example, in the technique of "rapid tissue fixation." Some individuals also practice waterless embalming. In this process, the coinjection fluid takes the place of water in the arterial solution.

Sample: Coinjection Fluids

FGH *acts with all arterial fluids.* A few ounces added to the arterial solution will ensure the creation of an unparalleled naturalness and will practically eliminate the possibility of dehydration and feature shrinkage, no matter how long the interval between the embalming and interment. *Distribution and diffusion will be increased to a pronounced degree,* drainage will be more copious, preservation will be more permanent, and the skin will have the same velvety freshness it had in life. FGH is indispensable in every operation in which a standard arterial fluid is used, and especially so in emaciated subjects, infants and the aged—bodies usually susceptible to formaldehyde action—and in all situations where pathological or climatic conditions necessitate the use of a stronger than normal arterial solution.

FGH diffuses unhindered through the capillary walls and all internal membranes to enter every tissue cell and combine with the cellular protoplasm. It creates a permanent waxy moisture-retaining shield, the presence of which can be detected by the velvety texture of the skin.

ABC suppresses reactivation of calcium ion substances and disperses fibrin threads, which are the bonding agents in clots. ABC reduces agglutinated blood and, in addition, washes obstructions from the capillaries, strengthening and lubricating their walls. ABC helps to clear discolorations and *amplifies the preserving action of the arterial fluid.*

DEF is a *dual-purpose fluid* for addition to each arterial injection. In action, it *softens and lubricates blood clots*. At the same time it conditions and *reduces water hardness to zero,* with an overall improvement in embalming results. It is not a blood solvent, nor is it a preservative. It does, however, contribute importantly to the solution of any drainage problem. *It breaks down clots so they may be removed by way of the drain tube.*

(To date there is no known chemical that can be used effectively to dissolve a blood clot totally without having, at the same time, an adverse effect on the circulatory system.)

USE OF ADDED DYES IN ARTERIAL SOLUTIONS

Dye is used in arterial solutions for several reasons. Inactive dye merely colors the arterial fluid. In this manner the embalmer knows that the concentrated fluid has been added to the water in the tank. Active dyes serve several functions:

1. They act as a tracer so the location of the arterial fluid can be noted in areas of the body—a sign of arterial fluid distribution.
2. They help restore the natural color of the skin, which changes when blood is drained from the tissues.
3. They help to prevent the body from darkening as a result of reaction with the blood, which remains within the body after the embalming.

There are actually two ways which additional dyes are used with arterial solutions: In the first, dye is added to all of the solution injected. In the second, the embalmer adds the dye to the final gallon that is injected. There are two main objections to the use of additional dye throughout the embalming operation: (1) the tissues will be over-

stained and create a cosmetic problem, and (2) the embalmer, seeing the dye in the superficial tissue, may tend to underembalm the body.

The amount of dye to add again depends on the fluid manufacturer. Follow the directions on the label; then add or cut back to suit individual preference. For some dyes, only several drops are required per gallon; for other dyes, several ounces are required.

USE OF HUMECTANTS IN ARTERIAL SOLUTIONS

The separately purchased humectant (antidehydrant) is really a coinjection fluid. The reason for this is quite simple! The humectant is added and injected along with the arterial fluid. Some embalmers use humectants only when the body is dehydrated. Others add extra humectant to all arterial solutions when embalming a body with normal moisture to prevent dehydration. The amount of humectant added to each gallon of solution should follow the manufacturer's directions.

It should be pointed out that most humectants are colloids, and these viscous colloid mixtures, when injected into the arterial system, have a tendency to draw moisture *out of the tissues* and into the capillaries. If additional humectants are used and solutions are injected into the body with continuous drainage, evidence can be seen of dehydration in such areas as the lips, fingers, and backs of the hands. Most embalmers, when adding humectants to the arterial solution, use intermittent drainage. In this manner the humectant is held in the capillaries and tissue spaces and does not draw moisture from the tissues.

For a severely emaciated body, some embalmers add a large amount of humectant to the final gallon injected. In addition, they close off the drainage, causing the facial tissues to distend and restoring them to their natural contour. If this technique is employed, a close watch must be kept on the facial features, for gross distention of such areas as the tissues around the eyes can create more problems.

CAVITY FLUID

As the name indicates, cavity fluid is injected into the body cavities. Routinely, cavity fluid is injected into the thoracic, abdominal, and pelvic cavities. In some special cases the cranial cavity can also be treated by injecting some fluid via a large needle or infant trocar into the cranial cavity.

For the average body, 32 ounces (or two bottles) of cavity fluid is distributed via the trocar over the viscera of the thoracic, abdominal, and pelvic cavities.

The principal ingredient of these fluids is formaldehyde. Obviously, there is little need for dyes, anticoagulants, and humectants in these fluids.

Cavity fluid *preserves, disinfects,* and *deodorizes* organs of the cavities, contents of the hollow viscera, and walls of the cavities. There are, however, other uses for cavity fluids:

■ May be used to preserve viscera removed at an autopsy
■ May be used as a surface compress to help treat tissues not reached by arterial profusion
■ May be injected via hypodermic needle or trocar into tissues that lack sufficient arterial preservation
■ May be used as a surface compress on lesions and pathological conditions to dry and deodorize
■ (Some cavity fluids) may be used as an arterial fluid in the preparation of difficult cases such as advanced decomposition, tissue gas, and jaundice. (Use only those cavity chemicals recommended by the manufacturer for arterial injection; not all cavity chemicals can be injected arterially.)
■ May be used as a surface treatment for gangrenous and dropsical limbs to help dry and preserve the tissues
■ May be used to bleach blood discolorations
■ May be used to dry tissues when excisions have been performed
■ May be used for surface preservation of fetal remains

FUMELESS CAVITY AND ARTERIAL FLUIDS

As formaldehyde is the principal ingredient of most cavity fluids, these chemicals can be very difficult to work with because of the pungent odor produced by formaldehyde. Fumeless fluids, particularly cavity fluids, are produced by many manufacturers. There are three ways in which fumeless fluids can be produced: (1) cover the formaldehyde with a deodorant; (2) substitute other preservatives for formaldehyde (a good example would be the use of phenol); (3) use formaldehyde donor compounds (these compounds do not release the formaldehyde until it is in contact with the tissues). A problem with the first method, perfuming of the formaldehyde, is that the embalmer can breathe these fumes with little irritation at the time, but later notices that large amounts of formaldehyde have been inhaled. The second method is good and is used by many manufacturers, but other preservatives lack the penetrating qualities of formaldehyde. The last method is used mainly in the production of arterial fluids. Its cost is prohibitive in the formulation of most cavity fluids.

ACCESSORY EMBALMING CHEMICALS

Accessory chemicals are chemicals used to treat the dead human body for purposes other than arterial embalming or cavity treatment and include autopsy gels, concentrated cautery chemicals, hardening compounds, concentrated preservative powder, concentrated deodorant powder, concentrated disinfectant powder, mold-preventive agents, powdered sealing agents, cream or "putty" sealing agents, and surface sealing agents.

Autopsy (Surface) Gels

Years ago a product called "formal creams" was manufactured for surface or osmotic embalming. Each company had a different name for these emollient creams. Compared with the gels used today, they were very inferior. In the late 1960s, chemical companies began to produce a gel or jellylike surface preservative. These preservative gels are available in two viscosities: a gel that is thin and can be poured, and a more viscous gel that can easily be applied by brush to the skin surface. Not only are these gels easy to work with, but their penetrating abilities and preservative qualities far exceed those of the older formal creams. Autopsy gels are used in several ways:

■ May be poured over the viscera returned from an autopsy in the plastic bag in which the viscera have been placed
■ May be applied to the surface of viscera in partial autopsies
■ May be used as a preservative in the orbital area after enucleation
■ May be applied to walls of cavities and surfaces such as the cranial cavity and calvarium in autopsied bodies
■ May be applied as a surface preservative to pathological conditions such as decubitus ulcerations and gangrenous or necrotic areas; may be applied as disinfectant and as an odor reducer
■ May be applied to surface areas of the body that the embalmer feels have received insufficient arterial fluid
■ May help to bleach discolored areas such as ecchymoses and postmortem stains
■ May help preserve, cauterize, and deodorize burnt areas
■ May be used to pack the anal orifice and colostomy opening

Autopsy gels are designed as surface or osmotic preservatives. Some manufacturers claim that their product can penetrate several inches beneath the skin. These gels not only preserve tissues but bleach blood and decomposition discolorations. In addition, they help to eliminate odors in such pathological conditions as gangrene or decubitus ulcerations.

As with most preservative chemicals, care should be taken to use these gels in a well-ventilated embalming room. The embalmer may wish to wear a mask as protection from the fumes. When the gels are applied to an external surface they should be covered with cotton or plastic. This improves the effectiveness of the gel in addition to reducing the fumes.

Each manufacturer recommends the length of time the gels should remain on a surface to be most effective. Several hours would be a good rule. The embalmer can check from time to time on the working action of the gel. When the gels are applied to necrotic areas (as on the legs), plastic stockings should be placed on the body, and the gel should not be removed. The same would be true for application over decubitus ulcerations. The compresses should be left in place and plastic garments such as pants or coveralls should be placed on the body.

Cautery Chemicals

Although some may not classify cautery chemicals under the heading of embalming, but rather under the heading of restorative art, they very much belong to the group of chemicals used during or immediately after embalming.

Cautery chemicals are liquids that are basically phenol (carbolic acid). Many of those sold through embalming manufacturers contain about 2 to 5% phenol, whereas those solutions prepared by a pharmacy can be as strong as 70% or more carbolic acid.

It should be emphasized that whenever these chemicals are used, the embalmer *must* wear eye protection. Unlike most embalming chemicals that irritate the eyes, carbolic acid can actually burn and scar eye tissue. In addition, it is recommended that rubber gloves be worn in handling phenol.

Phenol can be applied to areas where the skin has been removed, for example, abrasions, skin slip, blisters that have been opened, and burned areas. Phenol is a rapid-acting cautery agent and dries these areas in minutes. Phenol can also be used as a surface bleach or can be injected subcutaneously and bleach from underneath the skin. It is a good germicide; it can be injected into swollen areas such as black eyes or hematoma and allowed to remain for a time. Then the area is massaged. Some of the phenol is forced from the area along with some of the liquids responsible for the swelling. In other words, phenol is a reducing and constricting agent.

Phenol has many applications during the embalming operation. It can be used as a cautery agent for searing raw tissue, a surface bleach, an internal bleach, a reducing and constricting agent, and a germicidal agent.

Hardening Compounds

Hardening compounds are blends of powdered chemicals. They dry moist tissue by dehydrating it. In addition,

some hardening compounds also contain powdered preservatives, disinfectants, and deodorants. The primary use of this embalming chemical is in treatment of the cavities of the autopsied body. The powdered compound can also be used to treat the visceral organs returned after an autopsy. Hardening compound is often used in the plastic garments placed on bodies with burned tissue, decubitus ulcerations, or edema. Some of the chemicals used in these compounds are plaster of Paris (a hardening agent); paraformaldehyde; aluminum chloride and alum dehydrating, disinfectant, and preservative agents; wood powder (wood flour—very fine sawdust), and whiting and clays (moisture-absorbing chemicals).

Chemical manufacturers have made an effort to develop "dustless" hardening compounds for the safety of the embalmer. When embalming powders are used, the room should be well ventilated and a mask and goggles should be worn. Every effort should be made to reduce the inhalation of any particulate. Consult the Kerfoot studies in Selected Readings for the dangers caused by embalming powders.

The hardening compounds are not as effective preservatives and disinfectants as the autopsy gels. The gels have a much greater penetrating ability.

Embalming Powder

As the name indicates, embalming powder is designed to preserve tissue. The fumes this powder generates help to preserve and disinfect tissues. Many contain *para*-dichlorobenzene crystals, which arrest mildew and mold. Paraformaldehyde is the chief ingredient of these powdered preservatives. Some embalming powders also serve as deodorants and disinfectants. They do not have the absorbent and drying qualities of a hardening compound. The embalming powder can assist in preservation of the walls and organs of autopsied bodies if placed directly on burned or decomposing tissue. These powders can also be used for preservation of stillborn infants, and can be applied to cancerous tissues, bed sores, and mutilated body parts. They help to preserve the tissues and control odors that may be present.

Embalming powder can also be put into the plastic garments placed on limbs with edema. When bodies are to be shipped to a distant point for interment, embalming powder can be placed in the casket to help control mildews or molds. These powders also help to control maggots and vermin.

Be certain to check the labels of embalming powders; some are preservatives, whereas others are merely disinfectants and deodorants. It would be helpful to purchase an embalming powder that serves all three purposes.

Sealing Agents

Sealing agents are used to prevent leakage from sutured incisions. The agent is placed in the incised area during suturing. If any moisture develops within the incision these agents absorb that moisture and are converted into a gelatinous material that helps to prevent leakage from the sutures. Two types of powder have been used for many years; more recently, a cream or "puttylike" material has been used.

The "putty" sealing agent can be used in various restorative procedures such as restoration of enucleated eyes, as a base for deep wound restorations, as a substitute for tissue builder, and to fill in sunken temple areas in autopsied bodies. It can be applied with a spatula or a specially designed injector.

Sealing agents are also surface glues. These help to ensure against any leakage from sutured tissues. Surface glues can be applied with a brush or can be purchased as a spray. Many of these agents can be directly covered with mortuary cosmetics when they are used in restorative work. Surface sealing agents work best on dry tissue surfaces.

SPECIAL-PURPOSE ARTERIAL FLUIDS

High-Index Fluids

The preservative arterial fluids have a formaldehyde index of 30 to 35 or slightly above. These fluids are designed for use in the preparation of difficult-to-embalm bodies. In addition to these difficult preparations, these fluids have two other uses. First, some embalmers use these fluids for routine preparations. Second, these fluids can be used to fortify or increase the firming and preservative qualities of regular arterial solutions.

> Example
>
> An embalmer mixes a solution of arterial fluid using a 22-index fluid and uses 8 ounces to the gallon for the solution. If firming of the body seems not to be happening in the second gallon and subsequent gallons, several ounces of the high-index fluid will be added to the solution to help boost the preservative strength of the solution.
>
> Keep in mind that solutions are always mixed from mild to strong—not the reverse. The embalmer never begins injecting a strong solution into the unautopsied body and then makes the solutions that follow milder. Embalming solutions are always increased in strength (if there is to be a change in solution strength).

The following statement from the Dodge Chemical Company regarding one of their special-purpose high-index fluids explains well the usage of this chemical:

The more severe the conditions of the body, the stronger the primary solution should be. When little drainage is anticipated, stronger concentrations and less total volume of solution should be used. When normal drainage is achieved, the volume of solution to be used will be governed by the size, weight and conditions of the body. In general, in treating bodies of "difficult" types, a good rule to follow is: more rather than less chemical—and less rather than more water. Water will not preserve nor will it arrest putrefaction—but it will create swelling and distension.

There are situations in which use of high-index fluid is advised:

- Bodies dead for extended periods (24 hours or longer)
- Bodies that have been refrigerated
- Bodies that have been frozen
- Bodies that have undergone extensive treatments with drugs
- Institutional bodies
- Bodies with traumatic injuries for which restorative treatments will be needed
- Bodies with evidence of decomposition
- Bodies with gangrenous limbs
- Bodies that are difficult to firm
- Bodies with skeletal edema
- Bodies dead from renal failure
- Bodies with bloodstream infections

Some companies produce two types of high-index fluids: **dehydrating** and **nondehydrating.** The nondehydrating fluid is designed to deliver a strong formaldehyde and preservative action with a minimum of dehydration. As with other arterial fluids, it is best to follow the dilutions recommended by the manufacturer. Most of the high-index fluids, when used as a "booster" fluid, work well with standard arterial fluids of other companies. Because of the problems encountered with delayed embalming and the wide use of drug therapy today, *this arterial fluid should always be kept on hand in the preparation room.*

Jaundice Fluids

A second special-purpose preservative arterial fluid is the jaundice fluid. Jaundice fluids are used not only to preserve the body but to hide or rid the body of mild yellow jaundice or to prevent yellow jaundice from converting to green jaundice. These fluids are most effective on the body that has only a mild jaundice discoloration as opposed to bodies with the deep jaundice discoloration. These fluids do little to remove this deep discoloration.

The conversion of yellow jaundice to green jaundice is an oxidation reaction; however, formaldehyde is a strong reducing agent. What appears to happen when excess formaldehyde is injected into jaundiced bodies is establishment of an acid condition. This condition now brings about the oxidation that converts the yellow to green. For this reason most jaundice fluids have a low index, and because of this low index it is important to follow the instructions of the manufacturer with respect to dilutions and quantity of fluid. Keep in mind that in treating the jaundiced body, preservation of the body must have precedence over the clearing of the jaundice discoloration. Never use a dilution *less* than that recommended by the particular jaundice fluid manufacturer.

There are four types of jaundice fluids.

Bleaching Fluids. Bleaching fluids bleach the discoloration. The chemicals employed in the formulations include peroxides, oxalic or critic acid, and phenols. These chemicals are usually employed in an alcohol medium.

Buffer System Fluids. Buffer systems are used to control the pH so that an acid condition does not develop in the tissues. According to Leandro Rendon of the Champion Company.

> When aldehydes react with proteins, one of the chemical reactions that occurs has been said to be that of a release of hydrogen ions which, of course, results in low pH which is acid in nature. A given amount of formaldehyde or aldehyde can unite with a given amount of protein to form a given aldehyde condensation resin. Once the proteins have received the necessary amount of aldehyde to form these condensation resins, any excess aldehyde tends to become more acid in character and, therefore, to cause oxidation changes.

The oxidation converts yellow jaundice to green jaundice. From another point of view, aldehydes, in combining with proteins or amino acids, increase the local acidity in the tissues by releasing proteins. The hydrogen ions that produce the acid condition result from the chemical reaction between the protein and the aldehyde. The yellow-orange pigment (bilirubin) is converted to the green pigment (biliverdin). It is *not* the formaldehyde that causes the oxidation (formaldehyde is a reducing agent). Rather, it is the chemical reaction (oxidation) that occurs as a result of acid present.

Coupling Compound System. The coupling compound system combines a chemical with the bile pigment to decolorize the pigment. A preinjection coupling compound, for example, a diazo agent in a nonacetic medium, is injected first. The aldehyde arterial injection follows. The system is complex, time consuming, and not always reliable.

Chemical Adduct System. In the chemical adduct system, a chemical is combined with formaldehyde; later, the formaldehyde is slowly released "on the spot," thus preventing an excessive buildup of hydrogen ions.

A final caution with regard to jaundice fluids: When using a jaundice fluid do NOT mix this fluid with other arterial fluids or preinjection fluids, unless the directions accompanying the jaundice fluid call for the use of a preinjection fluid. If a preinjection fluid is recommended, it would, no doubt, be best to use the preinjection fluid manufactured by the same company that made the jaundice fluid.

Tissue Gas Fluid

A variety of fluids have been manufactured by chemical companies to treat the condition known as tissue gas. This condition is caused by *Clostridium perfringens*. It is important that the directions for these fluids be carefully followed.

Infants and Children

Some chemical companies have produced fluids specifically for the embalming of infants and children. These arterial fluids generally have a low index and are very viscous. Care should be taken to follow the directions on the label.

KEY TERMS AND CONCEPTS FOR STUDY AND DISCUSSION

1. Define the following terms:
   Arterial fluid
   Coinjection fluid
   Hypertonic solution
   Hypotonic solution
   Osmosis
   Preinjection fluid
   Primary dilution
   Secondary dilution
2. List and define four special-purpose arterial fluids.
3. List and define four types of coinjection fluid.
4. Give five uses for a preinjection fluid.
5. List eight criteria that help the embalmer to determine the type, strength, and volume of arterial fluid.
6. List several purposes for addition of an active dye to arterial fluid.
7. Give several uses for autopsy gels.
8. List body conditions for which a special-purpose high-index arterial fluid would be best to use.
9. Give several uses for cavity fluid.

10. How many ounces of a 25-index arterial fluid must be used to prepare a 1-gallon 2.0% strength arterial solution? To prepare a 1.5% strength solution? To prepare a 3.0% strength solution?

11. If 8 ounces of a 20-index arterial fluid is used to prepare a 1-gallon solution of arterial fluid, what will be the strength of this solution? If 12 ounces of arterial fluid was used? If 6 ounces of arterial fluid was used?

12. How much water must be added to make a 2.0% arterial solution if 6 ounces of a 20-index fluid is used? If you desire to make a 1.5% solution? If you desire to make a 3.0% solution?

BIBLIOGRAPHY

Dhonau CO. *Defining Embalming Fluid*. File 100. Cincinnati, OH: Cincinnati College of Mortuary Science; 1928.

Dorn J, Hopkins B. *Thanatochemistry*. Reston, VA: Reston, 1985.

General chemical principles of embalming fluids. In: *The Champion Expanding Encyclopedia*, Nos. 365–371; Springfield, OH: Champion Co.; March–October 1966.

Pervier NC. *Textbook of Chemistry for Embalmers*. Minneapolis: University of Minnesota, 1961.

8

Anatomical Considerations

It is essential that the embalmer possess a sound understanding of and familiarity with the human form to efficiently approach and solve embalming problems. This chapter emphasizes those areas of anatomy most concerned with the embalming process. The orientation is strictly anatomical and space in the text is not consumed with considerations of the functional significance of any structure.

Before one can conceptualize the internal anatomy of the body, he or she must first be familiar with surface features and the manner in which they relate to underlying structures. A thorough knowledge of surface anatomy permits one not only to make appropriate skin incisions but also to anticipate which structures will appear when the incisions are made.

A portion of this chapter is devoted to the fundamentals of surface anatomy as it relates to underlying musculoskeletal and visceral structures. As a complete treatment of these topics is well beyond the scope of this text, this discussion is limited to those aspects of greatest importance to the embalmer.

All descriptions used throughout the text assume that the body is in the *anatomical position:* the subject is standing erect, the arms of the subject are at the sides with the palms of the hands facing the observer, the feet are together, and the subject is facing the observer.

The embalmer should have a detailed understanding of the blood vascular system. For each of the major vessels used in embalming, the anatomical guide, the linear guide, and the anatomical extent (limit) of each artery are given.

An **anatomical guide** is a method of locating a structure, such as an artery or vein, by reference to an adjacent known or prominent structure. A **linear guide** is a line drawn or visualized on the surface of the skin to represent the approximate location of some deeper-lying structure. The **anatomical extent (limit)** is the point of origin and point of termination of a structure in relation to adjacent structures.

As the blood in the veins flows in the *direction opposite* that of blood in the arteries, the anatomical extent and the linear guide for the veins would be the *opposite* of those of the respective artery. The anatomical guides for the arteries and the veins would be the same.

COMMON CAROTID ARTERY AND INTERNAL JUGULAR VEIN

Surface Features and Landmarks

Surface features of the neck that the embalmer should be able to locate and describe are the clavicle, mandible, angle of the jaw, mastoid process of the temporal bone, hyoid bone, sternum, sternoclavicular articulation, suprasternal notch, and thyroid cartilage of the larynx. The embalmer should also be familiar with one muscle, the **sternocleidomastoid (SCM)**. In addition, the location of the external jugular vein should be recognized. Underlying the skin in this area is a thin, delicate cutaneous muscle (a muscle of facial expression) called the **platysma,** the presence of which is indicated by the shallow, transverse wrinkles of the neck.

Consider first the anterior triangle of the neck. Draw an imaginary line along the midline of the neck between the tip of the mandible and the sternum. Extend this line superiorly along the anterior border of the SCM and then anteriorly along the lower margin of the body of the mandible. These three lines and their anatomical parallels describe the **anterior triangle.** In the midline, one can palpate (feel), from above downward, the hyoid bone and the thyroid and cricoid cartilages. The external carotid artery and several of its branches are located in the anterior triangle. Here, these vessels are relatively superficial, being covered only by skin and subcutaneous tissue.

Anterior Triangle of the Neck

The skin over the anterior triangle is thin and underlain by the thin, cutaneous platysma muscle. This muscle acts to alter the contour of the skin of the neck in much the same manner that the muscles of facial expression modify the appearance of the face. The significance of the muscle to the embalmer is that most structures of importance in the embalming process lie beneath the plane of this muscle. With the skin and platysma incised and reflected, the contents of the anterior triangle and the surrounding area are brought into view.

The SCM muscle is a useful guide to the anterior triangle. Attached to the mastoid process of the temporal bone and the manubrium of the sternum, the muscle courses obliquely along the side of the neck. On the muscle surface, one can identify the external jugular vein together with some of its tributaries. The external jugular and the internal jugular veins cannot be confused because of the relationship of the former to the outer surface of the SCM muscle.

Lying posterior and roughly parallel with the SCM muscle are the carotid sheath and its contents. The sheath is an investment of fascia that extends up into the neck and contains within it the common carotid (medial) artery, the internal jugular vein (lateral), and the vagus nerve (between the artery and vein). The lower portion of the sheath is crossed anteriorly by the central tendon of the omohyoid muscle. Identification of this muscle can guide the embalmer to the underlying carotid sheath and provide confidence that the operation has not progressed too deep.

If the sheath is incised, the upper portion of the internal jugular vein and the common carotid artery become visible. The vein lies lateral to and partially over-laps the artery. A few variable tributaries of the internal jugular vein may be seen crossing the carotid artery in this area. The vagus nerve (cranial nerve X) can be identified between and posterior to the two vessels within the sheath.

In the upper portion of the anterior triangle, the common carotid artery divides into internal and external carotid arteries and several branches of the latter may be identified here. The internal carotid, of course, has no branches until it enters the cranium.

Common Carotid Artery

Linear Guide. Draw or visualize a line on the surface of the skin from a point over the respective sternoclavicular articulation to a point over the anterior surface of the base of the respective ear lobes.

Anatomical Guide. The right and the left common carotid arteries are located posterior to the medial border of the sternocleidomastoid muscle, on their respective sides of the neck (Fig. 8–1).

Anatomical Extent. The right common carotid begins at the level of the right sternoclavicular articulation and extends to the superior border of the thyroid cartilage. The left common carotid begins at the level of the second costal cartilage and extends to the superior border of the thyroid cartilage.

Origins. The right common carotid is a terminal branch of the brachiocephalic artery. The left common carotid is a branch off the arch of the aorta.

Branches. There are no branches of the right common carotid, except the terminal bifurcation into the right internal and external carotid arteries. The left common carotid also has no branches, except the terminal bifurcation into the left internal and external carotid arteries.

Branches of the Right and Left External Carotid Arteries. Ascending pharyngeal, superior thyroid, lingual, facial,* occipital, posterior auricular, maxillary, superficial temporal (Fig. 8–2; also see Fig. 9–4).

Branches of the Right and Left Internal Carotid Arteries. Branches arising within the carotid canal, ophthalmic, anterior cerebral, middle cerebral, posterior communicating, choroidal.

Relationship of the Common Carotid to the Internal Jugular Vein. The internal jugular vein lies lateral and superficial to the common carotid artery.

---

*To raise the facial artery for injection, the incision is made along the inferior border of the mandible just anterior to the angle of the jaw.

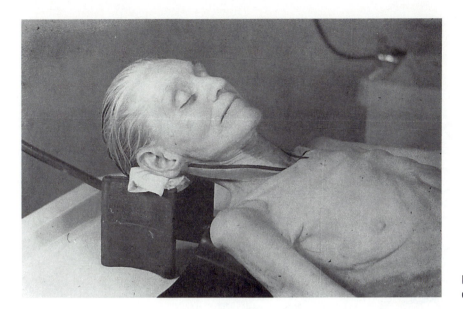

Figure 8—1. Linear and anatomical guides for the common carotid artery.

Contents of the Carotid Sheath. Internal jugular vein (lateral to artery), vagus nerve (between and posterior to artery and vein), common carotid artery (medial to vein) (Fig. 8–3).

THE AXILLA—SURFACE ANATOMY

When the arm is extended (or abducted) conceptualization of the axilla is easy. Think of a truncated pyramid: four walls, a base, and an apex that has been made flat and parallel with the base. Surface landmarks of the axillary region are the ribs and intercostal muscles and the anterior and posterior axillary folds. The most obvious boundaries of the axilla are its anterior and posterior walls, which comprise the anterior and posterior axillary folds. The anterior fold can be identified by grasping (with one hand) the mass of tissue on the anterior surface of the axilla on the contralateral side of the body. Most of the substance of this fold consists of the pectoralis major muscle with contributions from the pectoralis minor and the subclavius muscles.

The posterior axillary fold can be identified by grasping (with one hand) the tissue mass on the posterior side of the axilla on the contralateral side of the body. This fold consists of the latissimus dorsi, subscapularis, and teres major muscles. The medial axillary wall consists of ribs 2 through 6, which can usually be palpated even if they are not visible on the chest surface.

The serratus anterior muscle also contributes to the medial wall but is visible as a surface feature only in lean, muscular subjects. The shaft of the humerus makes up a portion of the lateral wall, and although it cannot be seen, it is easily palpated.

The biceps brachii and coracobrachialis muscles also contribute to the lateral wall. The former is discernible in virtually all subjects, whereas the latter is clearly de-

fined only in lean, muscular subjects. The apex of the axilla is an opening called the **cervicoaxillary canal,** which transmits structures from the neck into the arm and is bounded by three bony points of interest: the clavicle, the scapula, and the first rib. The cervicoaxillary canal is an important point of interest to the embalmer, particularly in autopsied bodies. Of the three landmarks that bound this canal, only the first rib is difficult to palpate. The base of the axilla is closed with dome-shaped fascia and skin on which the axillary hair is found.

Familiarity with the surface features of the axilla guides one to the important axillary contents, which include the axillary artery and its six branches, the axillary vein, and the many elements of the brachial plexus. The axillary sheath invests the major structures that leave the neck and pass through the cervicoaxillary canal to enter the axilla. On opening the axillary sheath, the first structure encountered is the axillary vein. If the extremity is abducted, the vein comes to lie over the axillary artery and partially obscures it.

The six typical branches of the axillary artery are fairly consistent and the axillary artery is relatively large. Identification of the artery within the sheath may prove difficult because of the many nerves of the brachial plexus which surround and partially obscure the artery. There are three large nerve cords of the brachial plexus: medial, lateral and posterior cords. They are grouped around the middle portion of the axillary artery in positions corresponding to their names.

Within the axilla, the nerve cords and some of the terminal branches form specific anatomical relationships with the axillary artery, making access to the artery sometimes awkward. These are large nerves in some cases, and care must be taken to avoid confusing elements of the plexus with the axillary artery. Careful inspection and the knowledge that the nerves surround the artery will

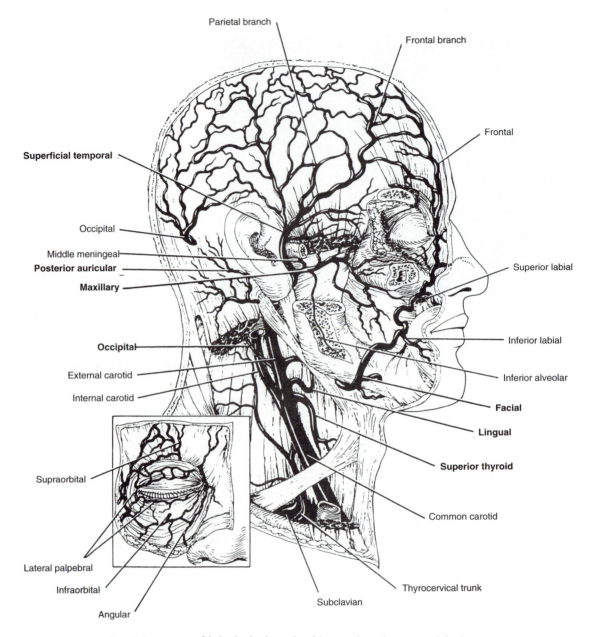

Parietal branch

Frontal branch

Frontal

Superficial temporal

Occipital

Middle meningeal

Posterior auricular

Maxillary

Superior labial

Inferior labial

Inferior alveolar

Facial

Lingual

Superior thyroid

Occipital

External carotid

Internal carotid

Supraorbital

Lateral palpebral

Infraorbital

Angular

Subclavian

Thyrocervical trunk

Common carotid

Figure 8–2. Cross section of the head and neck. Branches of the external carotid artery are underlined.

remove any confusion. *Approach to the axilla is made through an incision along the midaxillary line.*

AXILLARY ARTERY

Linear Guide. Draw or visualize a line on the surface of the skin from a point over or through the center of the base of the axillary space to a point over or through the center of the lateral border of the base of the axillary space. This line is parallel to the long axis of the abducted arm.

Anatomical Guide. The axillary artery is located just behind the medial border of the coracobrachialis muscle.

Anatomical Extent. The axillary artery extends from a point beginning at the lateral border of the first rib and extends to the inferior border of the tendon of the teres major muscle (Fig. 8–4).

Origin. The axillary artery is a continuation of the sub-clavian artery.

Branches. Highest (supreme) thoracic artery, thoracoacromial artery, lateral thoracic artery, subscapular artery, anterior humeral circumflex artery, posterior humeral circumflex artery.

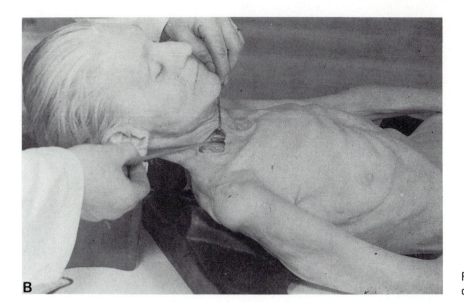

Figure 8–3. Raising the carotid artery. Note the suggested position of the embalmer. This is a posterior parallel incision.

Relationship of the Axillary Artery to the Axillary Vein. The axillary artery is located lateral and deep to the axillary vein.

Incision for Raising the Axillary Vessels. The incision is made along the anterior margin of the hairline of the axilla with the arm abducted.

BRACHIAL ARTERY

Linear Guide. Draw or visualize a line on the surface of the skin from a point over the center of the lateral border of the base of the axillary space to a point approximately 1 inch below and in front of the elbow joint.

Anatomical Guide. The brachial artery lies in the bicipital groove at the posterior margin of the medial border of the belly of the biceps brachii muscle.

Anatomical Extent. The brachial artery extends from a point beginning at the inferior border of the tendon of the teres major muscle and extends to a point inferior to the antecubital fossa (Fig. 8–5).

Origin. The brachial artery is a continuation of the axillary artery.

Relationship of the Brachial Artery and the Basilic Vein. The accompanying basilic vein is located medial and superficial to the brachial artery.

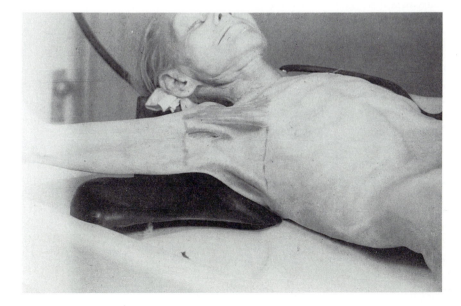

Figure 8–4. The axillary space is outlined and the location of the coracobrachialis muscle illustrated.

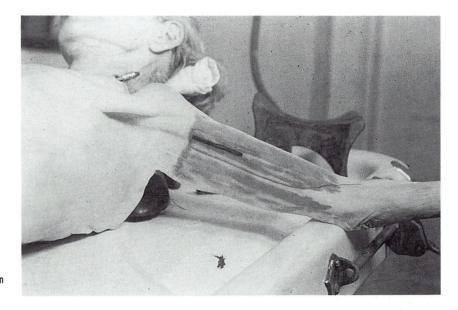

Figure 8–5. Linear guide, anatomical guide, and suggested incision location for the brachial artery.

Location of the Incision. The brachial artery is usually raised by an incision made along the upper one third of the linear guide.

DISTAL FOREARM

The distal forearm is the area in which the radial and ulnar arteries can be approached should they need to be raised for injection (Fig. 8–6). The radial artery lies on the lateral side of the forearm and the ulnar artery on the medial side. The distal forearm permits easy access to the radial artery. Surface features of importance here are the styloid process of the radius and the tendon of the flexor carpi radialis muscle. In the interval between these two structures lies the radial artery on the anterior surface of the styloid.

A pulse may be obtained here easily in the living subject. The styloid is the most distal and lateral bony structure in the forearm, and just medial to this, one can palpate the tendon of flexor carpi radialis. In the distal region, the fleshy bellies of the muscles tend to yield to long, usually well-defined tendons. Here, a layering of the musculature is evident. In the most superficial layer are four muscles including the pronator teres, flexor carpi radialis, flexor carpi ulnaris, and palmaris longus. Only the tendon of the pronator teres does not reach the distal forearm.

The second layer consists of one muscle with four tendons, one each leading to digits 2–5. This muscle is the flexor digitorum superficialis. The three muscles in the deep group are the flexor digitorum profundus, the flexor pollicis longus, and the pronator quadratus. Of these three, only the pronator has no long tendon. Some of these tendons are useful guides to the radial and ulnar arteries.

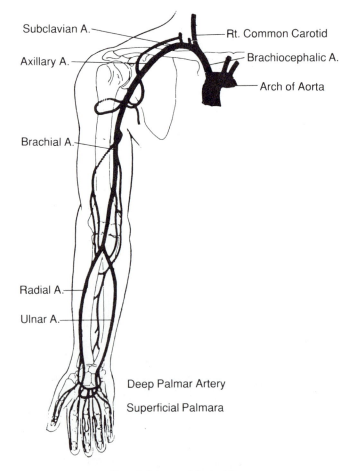

Figure 8–6. Arteries of the distal forearm.

Consider first the identification of the radial artery. An additional muscle, the brachioradialis, must be introduced here. This muscle is seen partially in the flexor compartment of the forearm. It is, nevertheless, an extensor muscle. In the proximal forearm, the radial artery is overlain by the brachioradialis muscle but at no point is the artery crossed by this or any other muscle. This situation keeps the radial artery superficial and permits easy access to it at any point along its course in the forearm. In the middle and distal forearms, the radial artery lies medial to the brachioradialis and lateral to the flexor carpi radialis. Its course is described by a line drawn from the middle of the cubital fossa to the medial side of the radial styloid process. It is easiest to approach the artery with an incision in the distal two thirds of the forearm along this line.

The ulnar artery is located on the medial side of the distal forearm. It lies between the tendon of the flexor carpi ulnaris muscle and the tendons of the flexor digitorum superficialis muscle. Here it will always be found traveling with the ulnar nerve, with which it should not be confused. Together with the venae comitantes, the nerve and artery will be found in a connective tissue sheath from which the vessels must be freed before beginning injection.

The course of the ulnar artery is indicated by a line curving medially from the midpoint of the cubital fossa to the pisiform bone in the wrist. An incision along the distal one third of this line permits access to the flexor carpi ulnaris muscle, which is then reflected medially to expose the ulnar artery.

RADIAL ARTERY

Linear Guide. Draw or visualize a line on the surface of the skin of the forearm from the center of the antecubital fossa to the center of the base of the index finger.

Anatomical Guide. The radial artery lies just lateral to the tendon of the flexor carpiradialis muscle and just medial to the tendon of the brachioradialis muscle.

Anatomical Extent. The radial artery extends from a point approximately 1 inch below and in front of the bend of the elbow to a point over the base of the thumb (thenar eminence).

Origin. The radial artery originates at the bifurcation of the brachial artery.

Relationship of the Radial Artery and the Vena Comites. Two small veins (venae comitantes) lie on either side of the artery. They may be helpful in locating the artery, for they generally contain some blood.

ULNAR ARTERY

Linear Guide. Draw or visualize a line on the surface of the skin from the center of the antecubital fossa on the forearm to a point between the fourth and fifth fingers.

Anatomical Guide. The ulnar artery lies just lateral to the tendon of the flexor carpi ulnaris muscle. (It lies between the tendons of the flexor carpi ulnaris and flexor digitorum superficialis).

Anatomical Extent. The ulnar artery extends from a point approximately 1 inch below and in front of the bend of the elbow to a point over the pisiform bone (hypothenar eminence).

Origin. The ulnar artery originates at the bifurcation of the brachial artery.

Relationship of the Ulnar Artery to the Venae Comitantes. Two small veins (venae comitantes) lie on either side of the artery. They can be useful in locating the artery for they generally contain some blood.

ARTERIES OF THE BODY TRUNK

Table 8–1 outlines the arteries of the body trunk and their branches (Fig. 8–7).

In embalming infants the ascending aorta (as it leaves the heart) or abdominal aorta can be used for injection points. A midsternal incision is used for the ascending aorta. An incision from the xiphoid process directed downward and to the left of the midline is used to raise the abdominal aorta.

In the adult, where partial autopsies have been performed or visceral organs are donated without autopsy, the abdominal or thoracic aorta can be used as a point of arterial injection.

EXTERNAL ILIAC ARTERY AND VEIN

Mention should be made of the use of the external iliac artery and vein as a site for arterial injection and blood drainage (Fig. 8–8). The external iliac artery is a continuation of the common iliac artery (the common iliac is one of the terminal branches of the abdominal aorta). The external iliac artery extends to a point under the center of the inguinal ligament. The artery lies exactly at this ligament lateral to the external iliac vein.

In the autopsied body this artery is used for the injection of the lower extremities. Injecting the external iliac artery rather than the common iliac in the autopsied body eliminates the need to clamp off the internal iliac artery (which usually has been cut during the removal of the pelvic organs). In the unautopsied body, when the

TABLE 8–1. ARTERIES OF THE BODY TRUNK

Artery	Description	Branches
Ascending aorta	Originates at the left ventricle; at its beginning the aortic semilunar valve should close, thus creating the pathway for arterial solution distribution	Right coronary artery Left coronary artery
Arch of the aorta	Center of arterial solution distribution	Brachiocephalic artery Left common carotid artery Left subclavian artery
Right subclavian	Begins at the right sternoclavicular articulation and extends to the lateral border of the first rib; in the complete autopsy (with neck organs removed), the branches need to be clamped	Vertebral artery Internal thoracic artery Inferior thyroid
Left subclavian	Begins at the level of the left second costal cartilage and extends to the lateral border of the first rib	
Descending thoracic aorta		Its branches include nine pairs of thoracic intercostal arteries

Descending abdominal aorta	Extends from the diaphragm to the lower border of the fourth lumbar vertebra	Parietal
		    Inferior phrenic
		    Superior suprarenals
		    Lumbar
		    Middle sacral
		Visceral (unpaired)
		    Celiac axis
		    Superior mesenteric
		    Inferior mesenteric
		Visceral (paired)
		    Middle suprarenals
		    Renals
		    Internal spermatic (male), ovarian (female)
		    Common iliacs (terminal)

body is very obese, the femoral vessels are located very deep and are hard to work with; however, the external iliac artery where it passes under the inguinal ligament is quite superficial, and this can be a good location if there is a need to use this vessel in the unautopsied obese body.

As insertion of an artery tube into the femoral artery (directed toward the upper area of the body) actually places the tip of the tube into the external iliac artery, the term *iliofemoral* is used by many embalmers to indicate use of the vessels at a site near the inguinal ligament.

INGUINAL REGION

The inguinal region is an area below the inguinal ligament in which the femoral vessels may be approached for injection and drainage. As a rule, the subcutaneous tissue in the thigh masks underlying soft tissue structures, so the embalmer must rely on bony landmarks in this area. Fortunately, the anterior superior spine of the ilium and pubic tubercle are easily identified. These two bony processes serve as attachments for the inguinal ligament. The positions of the underlying femoral vessels can be identified if the operator begins by placing the thumb of the left hand on the subject's right anterior superior iliac spine and the left middle finger on the subject's right pubic tubercle. If the operator's left index finger is now allowed to bisect the interval between his thumb and middle finger (i.e., bisect the inguinal ligament), the tip of the

index finger will indicate the approximate position of the femoral vessels in the thigh. The procedure can be repeated on the subject's left side using the operator's right hand. The incision to raise the vessel can be made on the linear guide.

FEMORAL TRIANGLE

The inguinal ligament serves as the base for this triangle whose two sides consist of the medial border of the sartorius and the lateral border of the adductor longus muscles (Fig. 8–9). In addition to skin and subcutaneous tissue covering the triangle, the roof consists of a dense sheet of fascia, the fascia lata, which attaches firmly to the inguinal ligament and encircles the thigh. This roof must be incised to expose the boundaries and contents of the triangle.

Lying on the surface of the fascia lata is the great saphenous vein which has coursed up the medial aspect of the thigh all the way from the foot. The operator should not mistake the great saphenous for the femoral vein. This potential mistake can be avoided simply by remembering anatomic relationships. **If the vein in question is lying on the surface of the dense, white fascia lata and if the fascia lata has not yet been incised, then the vein must be the great saphenous or one of its tributaries.**

If the great saphenous is followed, it disappears through an opening in the fascia lata called the fossa ovalis. This opening is not so glamorous as some text-

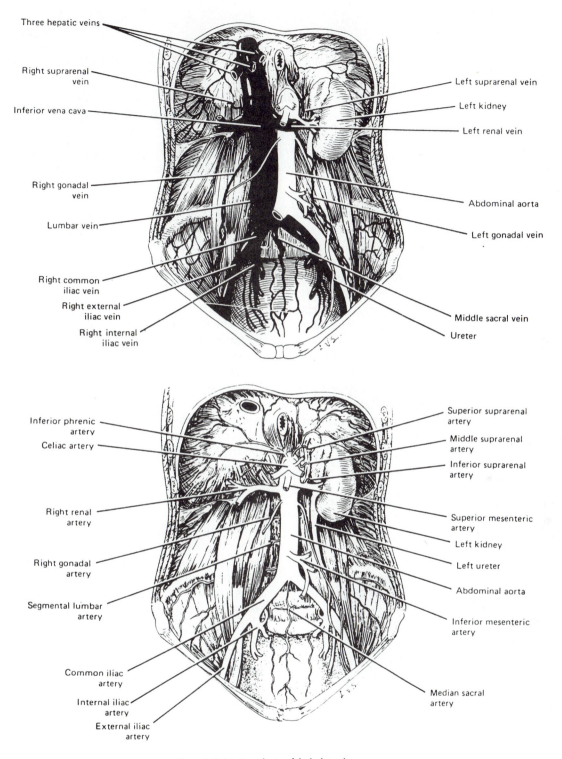

Figure 8–7. Arteries and veins of the body trunk.

books would have one believe. Rather, there is a hiatus in the fascia lata and the great saphenous insinuates itself through the fascia and empties directly into the femoral vein. So it is clear that identification of the great saphenous will lead directly to the femoral vein near the base of the femoral triangle. Around the hiatus one is likely to encounter inguinal lymph nodes, which may have to be resected.

When the roof of the triangle is incised and reflected, the contents and borders come into view. The femoral vessels are contained within the femoral sheath, which is a continuation into the thigh of abdominal wall and pelvic

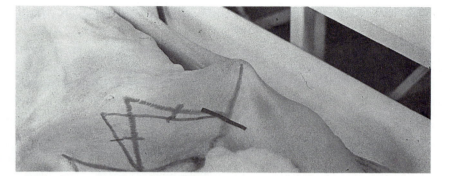

Figure 8–8. Incision location for left external iliac vessels. The linear guides are also shown.

fascias. The sheath is subdivided into three compartments which, from lateral to medial, contain the femoral artery, femoral vein, and lymphatic vessels and nodes. The most medial compartment is designated the femoral canal and is the site of femoral hernias. Therefore, a femoral hernia is always situated medial to the femoral vein. This relationship is an important one to remember if preparing a subject whose inguinal region is distorted (such as with a hernia).

To gain access to the femoral vessels, open each of the other two compartments separately. An incision in the sheath over each vessel will cause the artery and vein to be delivered easily. At the base of the triangle, the artery lies slightly anterior and lateral to the femoral vein and its position may be identified at the midpoint of the inguinal ligament. The vessels are best approached 1 to 2 inches from the base of the triangle, where they lie side by side and are easily accessible.

As the vessels approach the apex of the triangle, their relationship shifts to an anteroposterior one so that the femoral artery, femoral vein, deep femoral vein, and deep femoral artery lie one in front of the other, making accessibility to most of them somewhat difficult.

The most lateral structure at the base of the femoral triangle is the femoral nerve, which lies outside the femoral sheath. This very substantial nerve and its many branches should not be confused with the adjacent femoral artery because the nerve lies without the sheath.

The floor of the triangle is entirely muscular and different authors consider that either two or three muscles constitute the floor. Laterally, the iliopsoas muscle emerges beneath the inguinal ligament. Just medial to this lies the pectineus muscle. Certainly these two muscles contribute to the floor of the triangle. The disagreement comes about as a result of whether the medial or lateral border of the adductor longus muscle is considered to be the medial boundary of the triangle. The distinction is academic but in this text the adductor longus is treated as part of the floor for the following reason. The triangle is easily visualized in terms of the number 3. There are three borders: the inguinal ligament, the sartorius muscle, and the adductor longus muscle. Basically, three structures are contained within the triangle: the femoral nerve, the femoral artery, and the femoral vein. Each of these has branches or tributaries, but three major structures are present. Finally, if the adductor longus is considered to be a part of the floor, there are three muscles in the floor: the iliopsoas, the pectineus, and the adductor longus.

At the apex of the femoral triangle the femoral vessels, but not the femoral nerve, enter the subsartorial or adductor canal. Recognizing the relationships of the femoral artery and vein at the triangle apex facilitates the understanding of the anatomical relationships of these vessels after they emerge from the adductor canal and enter the popliteal fossa or space.

FEMORAL ARTERY

Linear Guide. Draw or visualize a line on the surface of the skin of the thigh from the center of the inguinal ligament to the center of the medial prominence of the knee (medial condyle of the femur).

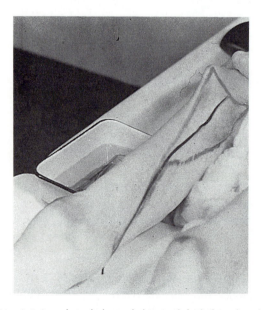

Figure 8–9. Femoral triangle showing the linear guide for the femoral vessels.

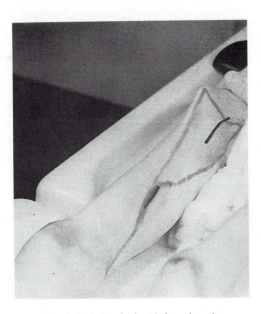

Figure 8–10. Incision for the right femoral vessels.

Anatomical Guide. The femoral artery passes through the center of the femoral triangle and is bounded laterally by the medial border of the sartorius muscle and medially by the adductor longus muscle.

Anatomical Extent. The femoral artery extends from a point behind the center of the inguinal ligament to the opening in the adductor magnus muscle (Fig. 8–10).

Origin. The femoral artery is continuation of the external iliac artery.

Branches. Superficial epigastric, superficial circumflex iliac, external pudendal, profunda femoris.

Relationship of the Femoral Artery and Vein. The femoral artery lies lateral and superficial to the femoral vein.

POPLITEAL FOSSA

On the posterior aspect of the knee two sets of tendons and two fleshy muscle heads can be identified. This describes the popliteal fossa as a trapezoid and can be subdivided into an upper femoral and lower tibial triangle.

The femoral triangle (not to be confused with the femoral triangle in the inguinal region) is bounded laterally by the long and short heads of the biceps femoris and medially by the tendons of the semimembranosus and semitendinosus muscles. The tibial triangle is limited medially and laterally by the diverging medial and lateral fleshy heads of the gastrocnemius muscle and, to a lesser extent, by the plantaris muscle laterally. The base of each triangle is an imaginary line drawn through the middle

of the joint. These surface landmarks serve as guides to the underlying popliteal vessels within the boundaries of the space.

The muscular boards of this fossa are overlain by a roof of deep fascia, subcutaneous tissue, and skin. Intrusion into this space provides access to the popliteal vessels for injection and drainage. After recognizing and dispatching minor vascular and nervous branches external to the deep fascia, the fascia is incised to gain access to the vessels. The major contents of the space include the tibial and peroneal nerves (from the sciatic) and their branches, the popliteal vein and its tributaries, the popliteal artery and its branches, and a good deal of fat and lymphatic tissue.

As the space is approached posteriorly, the first structures to be encountered are the tibial and peroneal nerves. The tibial nerve is the larger of the two and is located directly in the midline. The common peroneal nerve, on the other hand, leaves the sciatic nerve at about midthigh and courses down the lateral aspect of the popliteal space.

With the tibial nerve retracted, the popliteal vein comes into veiw, lying superficial (posterior) to the *popliteal artery, which is the deepest (most anterior) structure in the fossa.* Remember that this relationship was established as these vessels entered the adductor canal. The vessels are bound together by connective tissue, which must be loosened and reflected to gain access to the vessels. Several branches and tributaries of the vessels are also found in the fossa, but these need not be identified by name here.

Deep (anterior) to the popliteal artery, the floor of the fossa is formed by the lower end of the femur and a portion of the capsule surrounding the knee joint.

Linear Guide. Draw or visualize a line on the surface of the skin from the center of the superior border of the popliteal space parallel to the long axis of the lower extremity to the center of the inferior border of the popliteal space.

Anatomical Guide. The popliteal vessels are located between the popliteal surface of the femur and the oblique popliteal ligament.

Anatomical Extent. The popliteal artery extends from a point beginning at the opening of the adductor magnus muscle to the lower border of the popliteus muscle.

Origin. The popliteal artery is a continuation of the femoral artery.

Branches. Five pairs of genicular arteries, muscular branches.

Relationship of the Popliteal Artery and Vein. The vein lies posterior and medial to the artery. Because of the location of these vessels the vein can also be described as lying superficial to the artery.

DISTAL LEG

In the distal leg the superficiality of the anterior tibial artery makes it easily accessible as an injection site. The popliteal artery ends by dividing into two terminal branches: the anterior tibial artery and the posterior tibial artery. The branches begin at the lower border of the popliteus muscle. In the distal portion of the leg the arteries become superficial and can be used as points of injection for the foot. Injection could also be made toward the head to embalm the distal leg and thigh (Fig. 8–11).

The anterior tibial artery is the smaller of the terminal branches of the popliteal artery. As it approaches the distal portion of the leg it becomes very superficial.

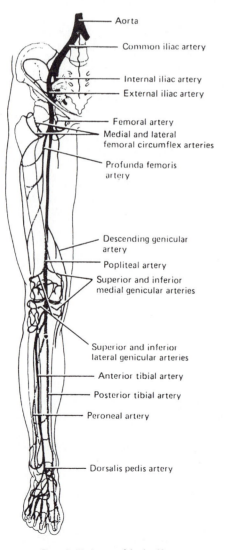

Aorta

Common iliac artery

Internal iliac artery

External iliac artery

Femoral artery

Medial and lateral femoral circumflex arteries

Profunda femoris artery

Descending genicular artery

Popliteal artery

Superior and inferior medial genicular arteries

Superior and inferior lateral genicular arteries

Anterior tibial artery

Posterior tibial artery

Peroneal artery

Dorsalis pedis artery

Figure 8–11. Arteries of the distal leg.

It can be raised by making an incision just above the ankle, just lateral to the crest of the tibia. In front of the ankle joint the anterior tibial artery now becomes the dorsalis pedis artery.

The posterior tibial artery is also one of the terminal branches of the popliteal artery and passes posteriorly and medially down the leg. In the area between the medial malleolus and the calcaneus bone, the artery can be raised by the embalmer for injection of the foot. The artery terminates by dividing into the medial and lateral plantar arteries.

ANTERIOR AND POSTERIOR TIBIAL ARTERIES

Linear Guide. *Anterior Tibial Artery:* Draw or visualize a line from the lateral border of the patella to the anterior surface of the ankle joint. *Posterior Tibial Artery:* Draw or visualize a line on the surface of the skin from the center of the popliteal space to a point midway between the medial malleolus and the calcaneus bone.

Anatomical Guide. *Anterior Tibial Artery:* The anterior tibial vessels are located in a groove between the tibialis anterior muscle and the tendon of the extensor hallucis longus muscle. *Posterior Tibial Artery:* The posterior tibia vessels are located between the posterior border of the tibia and the calcaneus tendon.

Anatomical Extent. *Anterior Tibial Artery:* The anterior tibial artery extends from a point beginning at the inferior border of the popliteus muscle to a point in front of the middle of the ankle joint on the respective sides. *Posterior Tibial Artery:* The posterior tibial artery extends from a point beginning at the inferior border of the popliteus muscle to a point over and between the medial malleolus and the calcaneus of the respective foot.

Branches and Tributaries of the Vessels. *Anterior Tibial Vessels, Posterior Tibial Vessels:* right and left peroneal branches, right and left dorsalis pedis arteries.

FOOT

Tendons passing onto the dorsum of the foot from the leg pass posterior to and are restrained by two thickenings of fascia, the superior and inferior extensor retinacula, which lie anterior to the ankle. Additionally, the anterior tibial artery and the deep peroneal nerve also pass deep to these retinacula. Only inconsequential superficial nerves and veins lie superficial to these retinacula.

Skin on the dorsum of the foot is thin and loosely applied. The subcutaneous tissue permits easy visualization of the venous network, which is so prominent here.

Tendons of two extrinsic muscles of the foot, the extensor hallucis longus and the extensor digitorum longus, are easily identified as they pass to the great toe and digits 2–5, respectively. The dorsalis pedis artery is situated in the interosseous spaces between the tendon of extensor hallucis longus and the first tendon of extensor digitorum longus as it passes to the second digit. An incision made from a point midway between the medial and lateral malleoli to the interosseous space will provide access to the dorsalis pedis artery.

Linear Guide (Dorsalis Pedis Artery). Draw or visualize a line from the center of the anterior surface of the ankle joint to a point between the first and second toes.

CONCLUSIONS

The anatomy of several potential injection sites has been considered. More than just vascular anatomy has been presented with the hope that complete familiarity with the anatomy of these regions will facilitate the work of the practitioner. Being aware of the anatomy peripheral to the blood vessels at an injection site and having a solid command of anatomical relationships in these areas should make the embalmer more comfortable with and more confident in his or her operations.

KEY TERMS AND CONCEPTS FOR STUDY AND DISCUSSION

1. Describe the anatomical position.
2. Define anatomical guide, linear guide, and anatomical extent.
3. Identify the surface landmarks and anatomical points of interest for the common carotid artery.
4. Give the linear guide and the anatomical guide for the common carotid artery.
5. List the eight branches of the external carotid artery and the areas they supply.
6. Give the bony boundaries of the cervicoaxillary canal.
7. Give the linear and anatomical guides for the axillary and brachial arteries.
8. Describe the relationship of the internal jugular vein to the common carotid artery, axillary vein, and axillary artery.
9. Give the extent of the axillary artery.
10. Give the linear guide for the radial and ulnar arteries.
11. List the branches, from right to left, of the arch of the aorta and the visceral and parietal branches of the abdominal aorta.
12. Give the anatomical guide and the linear guide for the femoral artery.
13. Describe the relationship of the femoral artery to the femoral vein.
14. Give the linear guides for the anterior tibial artery and the posterior tibial artery.

9

Embalming Vessel Sites and Selections

There are several anatomical locations on the dead human body at which arteries and veins may be elevated for the injection of chemical preservatives and subsequent drainage. One of the major objectives of making a pre-embalming analysis of the body is selection of the most logical and satisfactory vessels to employ for injection and drainage.

The proper selection of vessels should produce the most satisfactory results. This selection is based on a variety of intrinsic and extrinsic factors. Embalming analysis is not simply preembalming evaluation. During injection of the body, it may become necessary to select other vessels for injection and drainage. Therefore, an analysis of the progress of the embalming becomes necessary. These supplementary vessels needed to complete the injection of the body are called **secondary injection sites.**

TERMINOLOGY

Primary Injection Site(s)

In the unautopsied body the primary injection site selected at the start of the embalming process is the vessel(s) from which an attempt will be made to embalm the entire body. Primary injection may involve one of five techniques.

Single-Point Injection. An artery and vein at one location are used for injection and drainage (e.g., injection from the right common carotid artery and drainage from the right internal jugular vein).

Split Injection. The injection is made in an artery at one location and the drainage occurs from a vein at another location (e.g., injection of the right common carotid artery and drainage from the right femoral vein).

Restricted Cervical Injection. Both right and left common carotid arteries are raised; tubes are placed into them directed toward the head on both the right and the left side. One tube is directed toward the trunk into the right artery; the inferior portion of the left artery is ligated. Drainage is generally taken from the right internal jugular vein. During downward injection (toward the trunk), the arterial tubes directed toward the head remain open.

Multisite Injection or Sectional Injection. More than one artery is used for injection of the body (e.g., injection is begun from the right femoral artery but the embalming solution does not distribute to the left leg or the left arm; subsequently, the left femoral and the left brachial arteries are raised and injected).

Six-Point Injection. Six arteries are raised that will separately inject the head and the limbs: right and left common carotid arteries, right and left axillary (or brachial) arteries, and right and left femoral (or external iliac) arteries. Drainage can be taken from each location or from one location such as the right internal jugular vein.

There are also primary injection sites in the autopsied body. Generally, this would involve injection of the right and left external (or common) iliac arteries, the right and left subclavian arteries, and the right and left common carotid arteries; however, this selection depends on the extent of the autopsy. In partial autopsies, the aorta may often provide the primary injection location.

Secondary Injection Site(s)

A secondary point of injection is an artery (or more than one) other than those raised and injected in the primary injection procedure that is used to complete the arterial embalming of the body. Examples follow.

Unautopsied Body. In a one-point injection using the right common carotid artery, if arterial solution does not reach the left leg, the left femoral artery is raised and the leg injected. The left femoral artery would be the secondary injection point.

In a restricted cervical injection, the right common carotid is injected downward, but arterial solution does not enter the left arm. The left brachial artery is raised and the arm injected. The left brachial is the secondary injection point.

In another restricted cervical injection, the left arm does not receive arterial solution. The left brachial artery is injected, but the solution does not enter the left hand, so the left radial artery is raised and the hand injected. The left brachial artery and the left radial artery are both secondary injection points.

Autopsied Body. The right subclavian artery is selected to embalm the right arm. Arterial solution does not enter the arm, so the right axillary artery is raised and the arm injected. The axillary artery is considered the secondary injection point.

In a partial autopsy only the thoracic viscera have been removed. The abdominal aorta is injected downward. Arterial solution does not enter the right leg, so the right femoral artery is raised and injected. The femoral artery is the secondary injection point.

VESSEL SELECTION

Two of the most important objectives in making an embalming analysis of the body prior to the start of the embalming process is the selection of a vessel (or vessels) for injection of arterial solution and the selection of a vein for drainage.

In the unautopsied body, the vessel selected for beginning the arterial embalming can be called the **primary**
injection point. Most often this vessel is the common carotid, the femoral, or the axillary artery. From this vessel the embalmer will attempt to embalm the entire body. Sometimes two vessels can be selected as a primary injection point. The best example would be the decision to use the **restricted cervical method,** in which both right and the left common carotid arteries are raised at the start of the embalming process.

Autopsied Body

In the autopsied body, there are six primary injection points for each of the extremities: right and left common carotid, right and left femoral (external or common iliac), and right and left axillary (brachial or subclavian) arteries. The head must be injected separately. Embalming analysis does not stop once the injection of arterial solution has begun. During arterial embalming, the embalmer must ascertain which areas of the body are not receiving adequate arterial solution or no arterial solution at all. During arterial injection, a series of techniques can be used to stimulate a sufficient flow of arterial solution into these areas.

If these methods do not produce adequate results the embalmer must evaluate the situation and select additional vessels for injection or employ other embalming techniques, such as surface embalming or hypodermic embalming. Secondary injection points are those vessels that must be raised and injected to adequately arterially embalm body areas not reached by the arterial solution injected from the primary injection site.

Example 1. The embalmer selects the right common carotid as the primary injection point. During injection, the left leg receives little or no arterial solution. Attempts are made to stimulate the flow of arterial solution into the leg by elevating the pressure of the solution being injected; increasing the rate of flow of the injected solution and massaging the leg at the inguinal region do not provide satisfactory results. The embalmer, after injecting all other areas of the body, raises and injects the left femoral artery. This is the *secondary injection point.*

Example 2. In an autopsied body the right axillary artery is injected to embalm the right arm. Solution flows only as far as the elbow. Attempts to stimulate flow into the hand are not successful. The right radial artery is raised and injected. The right radial artery is the *secondary injection point.* Likewise, if the brachial or the ulnar artery is injected, it would be the secondary point of injection.

Unautopsied Body

In the unautopsied body there are four primary injection sites: the right common carotid artery, the right femoral artery (or external iliac artery), *both* the right and the left common carotid arteries (restricted cervical injection), and the right axillary artery (or brachial artery).

> With the problems encountered in embalming today, the three best choices for a primary injection point are the right (or left) common carotid artery, the right and left common carotid arteries (restricted cervical injection), and the right or left femoral artery.

The right side of the body is used for several reasons. Most embalmers are right-handed and find working on the right side of the body much easier. In addition, if the internal jugular vein is to be used for drainage, the right internal jugular leads directly into the right atrium of the heart and drainage instruments are much easier and more effective when inserted into the right internal jugular vein. It should be pointed out that selecting the left common carotid or left femoral vessels for injection points would afford the same advantages. There are a number of arguments against the use of axillary or brachial vessels as primary points of injection.

In selecting a primary point of injection, two criteria must be considered: factors concerning the artery or vein itself and general body conditions.

The embalmer should be able to locate and raise all the major vessels of the body without any difficulty. The routes of the vessels can be determined by the surface linear guides, and the embalmer should be thoroughly acquainted with the deeper anatomical relationships so the vessels can be located. *It is of primary importance that the embalmer be able to locate arteries of the body.* Drainage can always be taken from a separate vein or directly from the heart, but arterial solution supply into a particular body region must be by way of the arterial system.

Situations in which it may be necessary to isolate severed or cut portions of arteries to inject arterial embalming fluid for preservation include bodies on which extensive autopsies have been performed, bodies on which partial autopsies have been performed or from which only one or more organs and/or tissues for transplantation have been removed, and bodies resulting from traumatic accidents.

Arteries, veins, and nerves tend to be grouped together in their routes through the body. It is essential that the embalmer be able to distinguish between these structures (Table 9–1).

Nerves have a silvery appearance and, when examined with the naked eye, show striations along their surface. When cut, they have no lumen or opening and their cut edges take on a frayed appearance similar to the cut ends of a rope.

Veins are thinner than arteries. They contain valves, which arteries do not, but like arteries, when cut they do have an opening or lumen. When their sides are cut, veins collapse, creating a funnel effect.

TABLE 9–1. COMPARISON OF ARTERIES, VEINS, AND NERVES

Artery	Vein	Nerve
Lumen	Lumen	Solid structure
Creamy white	Bluish when filled with blood	Silvery white
Thick walls are demonstrated when artery is rolled between two fingers; edges of the artery easily felt	When vein is rolled between two fingers, walls collapse and edges are not felt	Solid structure is demonstrated when nerve is rolled between two fingers
Vasa vasorum may be seen on surface	Vasa vasorum not visible	Vasa vasorum not visible
Remain open when cut	Collapse when cut	Solid when cut; ends tend to fray
Generally empty of blood	Generally some blood or clotted material present	No blood present

Arteries have very thick walls as compared with healthy veins. Arteries are creamy white in appearance, and often, small vessels called the **vasa vasorum** can be seen over the artery surface (especially in arteries exhibiting arteriosclerosis). The most distinguishing feature of an artery is that if it is cut, the lumen remains open and very pronounced. The walls of the artery, unlike those of the vein, do not collapse. In addition, arteries are quite elastic and can easily be stretched after dissection and cleaning. It is most important that the embalmer be familiar with the relationship of arteries to veins where vessels are raised.

SELECTING AN ARTERY AS A PRIMARY INJECTION POINT

With respect to size (diameter) of artery, of the four choices for a primary injection point, the common carotid artery is the largest, for it is nearest to the heart. The femoral (or external iliac) is the second in size, and the axillary artery is the smallest in diameter. Actually, any artery could be used to inject the entire body, but the use of a vessel such as the radial or ulnar to embalm the entire body allows for a very slow rate of flow of arterial solution. In addition, it is difficult to build sufficient pressure in the arterial system to properly distribute and diffuse the arterial solution. The larger, more elastic arteries such as the common carotid and the femoral allow for use of the higher pressures and faster rates of flow that are often necessary to achieve uniform distribution of the arterial solution.

As for the accessibility of the artery, deep-seated vessels within the thorax or the abdomen are very difficult to use for injection of the adult body. In infants and children these vessels can be considered, for they are easier to reach. In the unautopsied adult body, vessels near the surface of the skin and with few branches can easily be raised to the surface of the incision. The common carotid arteries do not have branches (except their terminals) and, thus, can easily be raised to the skin surface. Likewise, the femoral arteries and the external iliac arteries (at the inguinal ligament) are not held tightly in position by large numbers of branches.

Presence of an accompanying vein is one of the most important factors in selecting an artery for injection of arterial solution. This accompanying vein is also a potential point of drainage. The common carotid artery is accompanied by the large internal jugular vein. On the right side of the neck this vein leads directly into the right atrium of the heart, and the right atrium is the center of drainage.

The size of the artery, its accessibility, and, finally, the possibility of draining from the accompanying vein must be considered in selecting an artery for injection. As previously stated, in the unautopsied adult body, this choice is among four vessels: (1) the common carotid artery, (2) the right and left common carotid arteries, (3) the femoral artery (or external iliac if raised at the inguinal ligament), and (4) the axillary artery (or brachial artery).

The second group of factors that must be considered (and the most important and variable factors in selection of a vessel for injection) is the conditions of the body or the external conditions that influence the choice of a vessel.

1. Age of the Body
   A. In the infant, additional vessels may be considered such as the ascending aorta or the abdominal aorta for injection.
   B. With respect to infants, the size of the artery may be the factor that determines which vessel can be used. The common carotid is the largest. A set of small infant arterial tubes should always be available.
   C. In the elderly, many times the femoral vessel is found to be sclerotic; the common carotid artery is rarely found to exhibit the condition of arteriosclerosis.
2. Weight of the Body
   A. In obese bodies the femoral artery is found quite deep in the upper thigh. Its depth should not preclude its possible use. If the vessel must be raised it should be raised at the inguinal ligament, or the external iliac artery can be used. At this location the vessel is the most superficial.
   B. Drainage is also a factor to consider with obese bodies. The internal jugular vein affords the best clearing of the body, especially the tissues of the face. Keep in mind that the weight of the viscera in heavy bodies provides a resistance to the flow of arterial solution as well as resistance to drainage.

C. In obese bodies large quantities of arterial solution are needed to adequately preserve the body. To avoid distension of facial tissues, it is best to select the right and the left common carotid arteries, which would be raised at the start of embalming.

A summary of the preceding statements points to the fact that the best approach to embalming obese bodies is to raise both right and left common carotid arteries (restricted cervical injection) and use the right internal jugular vein for drainage. In this manner large volumes (often of a strong solution) can be injected. This allows the use of higher injection pressures and faster rates of flow. It minimizes the necessity of raising other vessels, and in the obese body, especially if edema is also present in the tissues, the raising of secondary vessels can be very difficult.

   D. With very thin bodies care should be taken to minimize any destruction of the sternocleidomastoid muscle of the neck. It generally is very pronounced. All other factors taken into consideration, use of the femoral vessels, if possible, might prove advantageous in the preparation of these bodies.
3. Disease Conditions
   A. A condition such as arthritis may necessitate the avoidance of certain body areas; legs can be in the fetal position in the elderly or in bodies that have suffered from certain brain tumors, making use of the femoral vessel quite difficult (see Fig. 11–7).
   B. A goiter condition in the neck may make use of the carotid artery and the jugular vein difficult, because the vessels will be pushed out of their normal location.
   C. Malignancies or tumors or swollen lymph nodes in the neck, groin, or axillary area should be avoided for injection.
   D. Burned tissues should be avoided if possible; leakage will be a problem and suturing will be difficult.
   E. When edema is present in an area such as the upper thigh, raising a vessel should be avoided in this area; closure (suturing) may be difficult and leakage a problem. When edema is generalized (anasarca), large quantities of arterial solution must be injected. Here it would be best to use restricted cervical injection, raising both the right and left common carotid arteries. This allows the embalmer to inject large quantities of arterial solution. Many times, these arterial solutions are very strong. The

restricted cervical injection allows the use of large amounts of fluid to saturate other body areas without overinjecting the face. A separate, milder solution can then be used for injection of the head.

F. A *ruptured aortic aneurysm* dictates what additional (or secondary) arteries must be injected. Because, many times, arteriosclerosis is responsible for a ruptured aortic aneurysm, the common carotid would be the most logical vessel to use as a starting point for injection. Often, some circulation can be established in these conditions. In the majority, there is direct loss of all arterial fluid to the abdominal cavity, necessitating six-point injection of the body and treatment of the trunk walls, buttocks, and shoulders by hypodermic embalming.

G. When *scar tissue* is seen in a location where a vessel is to be raised (such as the upper inguinal area), no doubt surgery has been performed. Scar tissue beneath the skin can be very difficult to work with in raising vessels, and it may be wise, if possible, to use another vessel. If desiring to inject on the right side of the body it is suggested the left side be used.

H. *Gangrene,* particularly in the lower extremities, indicates the possibility that the deceased suffered from diabetes and that there is poor blood supply into the affected limb(s). Most often that poor blood supply is the result of arteriosclerosis. For example, if the foot or lower leg evidences gangrene, or a recent amputation is evident, the femoral vessel should be avoided as the primary injection point. Use of the carotid arteries is advised, as, generally, little arteriosclerosis is associated with these vessels.

4. Interruption of the Vascular System
   A. Mutilation or trauma: Automobile fatalities or accidental death can result in severed arteries. These conditions must be individually evaluated by the embalmer; arteries exposed as a result of the trauma may be considered as sites for injection. Likewise, standard points of injection such as the common carotid can be used and the severed arteries clamped during arterial injection. Secondary points of injection will, no doubt, be required.
   B. Ulcerations: Ruptured vessels can be the result of ulcerations. If this occurs in the stomach, there will be a great loss of blood during the agonal period. If sufficient arterial solution is lost during injection, the embalmer must select secondary points of injection to treat those areas of the body not reached by arterial solution.

> When arterial solution is evidenced in purge from the mouth or nose during arterial injection and there is still blood drainage, continue to inject arterial solution and evaluate the distribution of the solution.
>
> When arterial solution is evidenced in purge from the nose or mouth during arterial injection and there is no blood drainage, it would be wise to discontinue injection, evaluate the distribution of solution, and sectionally treat, by arterial injection, those areas not reached by sufficient arterial solution.

C. Autopsies: Partial autopsies must be evaluated by the embalmer as to the selection of arteries for injection. For example, if the viscera were removed only from the *abdominal cavity,* the portions of the body above the diaphragm could be embalmed by (1) injecting from the thoracic aorta upward and (2) injecting from the right common carotid and ligating the thoracic aorta. Even after a complete autopsy, there can be a choice of vessels depending on the lengths of vessels left by the dissecting pathologist. For example, the subclavian artery or perhaps the axillary artery can be used to inject the arm. If the external iliac arteries have been cut under the inguinal ligament, the femoral vessels may have to be injected. In some autopsies, the entire arch of the aorta may be present and most of the upper areas of the body can be injected from this point. Keep in mind that even in the autopsied body there can be a choice of vessels for injection.

5. Clotting
   Anytime an embalmer feels that clots may be present in the arterial system, particularly in the aorta, the femoral artery should *not* be used as the primary point of injection. The best choice, in this situation, is to begin the injection of the arterial solution from the common carotid, because if any coagula do break loose, it is better that this material be directed toward the legs. If instead the femoral artery is used, the coagula would be pushed up into the common carotid arteries and the axillary vessels. These arteries supply body areas that will be viewed. Clotting may be suspected in bodies that have been dead for long periods, in deaths from systemic infections and febrile disease, and in bodies of persons who were bedfast for long periods.

> When an embalmer suspects that the blood vascular system is heavily clotted or that distribution of arterial solution will be difficult, the best vessel to use in beginning the arterial injection is the common carotid artery, and drainage should be taken from the right internal

jugular vein. An even better method is to raise both common carotid arteries at the beginning of the embalming (restricted cervical injection). As the head is thus separately embalmed, the embalmer maintains control over solution distribution into the facial tissues.

6. Facial Tissue Distension

The possibility of distension of the facial tissues exists in bodies dead for long periods. Also, the facial tissues can easily distend during arterial injection in bodies that have suffered facial trauma or extended refrigeration or have been frozen. To maintain the most control over arterial solution entering the facial tissues, both common carotid arteries should be raised at the beginning of the embalming (restricted cervical injection).

7. Facial Discolorations

Quite often, after congestive heart failure or pneumonia, bodies show considerable blood congestion of the facial tissues, and the external jugular veins are often distended. If the head has been allowed to remain on a flat surface, it will, many times, exhibit intense livor mortis of the facial and neck tissues, especially if the deceased had been using medication that tended to thin the blood. In the preparation of these bodies, this intense discoloration necessitates the best possible drainage of the facial tissues. The right internal jugular vein is the best choice. It may be necessary to open and drain both internal jugular veins. Clearing of these tissues is also assisted by direct injection of arterial solution into the head, which is best achieved by raising and injecting the right and left common carotid arteries.

8. Volume and Strength of Arterial Solution

If a long delay has occurred between death and embalming, if the body shows evidence of decomposition, if death was due to uremic poisoning or burns, or if skeletal edema is present, the volume of strong arterial solution needed is large. To avoid running unneeded amounts of solution through the facial tissues, which can result in dehydration, and to avoid distension and possibly discoloration of the facial tissues, control must be maintained over the amount of arterial solution entering the head and the facial tissues. The best means of controlling solution entering the head and facial tissues is to begin the embalming of the body by raising both right and left common carotid arteries (restricted cervical injection).

9. Specific Requirements

These two examples illustrate specific requirements in selection of a primary or secondary injection site:

A. An embalmer preparing a body under orders from the military services must follow minimum standards, which may include the choice of vessels for injection.

B. Some hospitals allow arterial embalming prior to autopsy; in such situations the hospital may have preference as to the vessels to use for injection of the body.

To summarize, the major factors to consider in selecting a primary injection site are the age of the body, weight of the body, effects of disease, vascular system interruptions, clotting, facial tissue distension, facial discolorations, volume and strength of arterial solution, and legal considerations.

SELECTION OF SECONDARY INJECTION SITES

When arterial embalming solution has failed to distribute to a particular area, or if the embalmer feels an insufficient amount of arterial solution is present in a body area, the first consideration should be the direct arterial injection of that area. The artery chosen for injection of the body part needing arterial solution is called the *secondary injection site*. These secondary points of injection all involve treatment of the head or appendages. If there is insufficient arterial solution in any area of the trunk portion of the body, these areas are best treated by hypodermic injection of the area rather than by arterial treatment.

Three methods of embalming can be used to treat body areas that have not received enough arterial solution: (1) sectional arterial embalming, (2) hypodermic embalming, and (3) surface embalming.

Secondary points of injection could include injection of one or more of the following arteries in the *head*, the right and left common carotid and the right and left facial arteries; in the *arms*, the left or right axillary, brachial, radial, or ulnar artery; and in the *legs*, the left or right external iliac, femoral, popliteal, anterior tibial, or posterior tibial artery. As part of the ongoing embalming analysis the embalmer must make at conclusion of the injection of the body, he or she must determine what secondary injections are necessary to properly arterially embalm the areas where solution is needed.

Example 1. Suppose the primary injection site was the right femoral artery. Assume that there is no arterial solution in the entire left arm. It must be assumed that during arterial injection, attempts were made to stimulate the flow of fluid into the left arm, by massaging the arterial pathway, lowering the arm over the side of the table, using intermittent drainage, and increasing rate of flow and injection pressure. Assume there is a blockage before the left axillary artery. A clot or coagulum that was present in the abdominal aorta has been freed and has floated into the left subclavian artery. Now the embalmer must select a secondary injection site. It is almost certain that the left axillary or brachial artery may be used. Injection from this point should establish distribution of solution down the arm and into the hand.

Example 2. Using the same set of circumstances as in Example 1, assume that arterial solution reaches only as far down the left arm as the elbow. Now the embalmer must decide if injection of the left axillary or radial artery will establish distribution of the arterial solution down the remainder of the arm and into the hand *or* if the radial or ulnar artery (or both) should be raised, the hand injected, and then the arterial tube reversed and some solution injected back toward the elbow. Some embalmers would try first to inject the axillary or the brachial artery, hoping that a collateral route may still be open to distribute solution into the hand. If the clotted material is tightly lodged in the area where the brachial artery divides into the radial and ulnar arteries, then one or both of these arteries may have to be raised and injected to properly embalm the hand.

When secondary injection sites are injected, drainage can continue to be taken from the primary point of drainage. Some embalmers do, however, prefer to drain from accompanying veins. Exceptions would be the radial and ulnar arteries, where the veins are just too small for practical use.

Example 3. Assume a body has been embalmed using the right common carotid artery as the primary injection site. Drainage was taken from the right internal jugular vein. After embalming it is felt that the right leg does not have enough arterial solution. The embalmer raises the right femoral artery for a secondary injection site. She or he may inject the right femoral and drain from (1) the right internal jugular vein, (2) the right femoral vein, or (3) the heart (after beginning aspiration).

ELEVATION AND LIGATION OF VESSELS

After selecting the primary injection site, the embalmer elevates the vessels to the skin surface, ligates the vessels, and inserts the arterial tubes for arterial solution injection as well as a drainage device into a selected vein for drainage.

After injection of the arterial solution, the embalmer evaluates the body to determine if any further injection is necessary for regions that may have received an inad-

equate amount of preservative. If such areas are found, secondary injection sites are selected and an artery or arteries raised for direct injection into the areas needing additional solution.

This section of the chapter involves the general protocol for raising and ligating vessels. Later, the specific locations for incisions and the protocol for raising vessels with respect to the individual artery selected are examined.

1. Select instruments and prepare ligatures for the vessels to be used. Be certain arterial tubes, especially very small tubes, are clear and working before inserting them into an artery.
2. Locate vessels and their respective sites for skin incision by the linear guide on the surface of the skin.
3. Generally, make incisions where the vessels are nearest the skin surface.
4. In the dissection for the vessels, remember that muscles do *not* have to be cut to locate vessels, arteries, veins, and nerves. These run in groups *between* the muscles. The only muscle that may have to be divided for locating vessels is the sternocleidomastoid muscle.
5. After making the incision in the skin surface, use blunt dissection to find the vessels based on their anatomical guides and the location of surface vessels. A superficial vessel can be used to locate a deeper vessel by their anatomical relationship.

Example. When the internal jugular vein and the common carotid artery are raised, the vein is the superficial vessel. After a string is placed around the vein, it is pulled laterally, and the artery can easily be located on the medial side of the vein, a little deeper than the vein. The common carotid artery is described as being *medial* and *deep* in its relationship to the internal jugular vein.

6. The order in which vessels are raised varies, depending on the relationship of the artery to the vein. Two general rules should be remembered:
A. **When both the artery and the vein are to be used** (as in a one-point injection), **always raise the superficial vessel first.**
B. **When both the artery and vein are to be used at the same location** (as in a one-point injection), **always insert instruments** (arterial tube or drainage instrument) **into the deepest vessel first.**

Example. When raising the right internal jugular vein and the right common carotid artery, raise the vein *first*, for it is the more superficial. Pull the vein laterally, raise the *deeper* common carotid artery to the surface, open the artery, insert the arterial tubes, return to the vein, open the vein, and insert the drainage instrument.

7. Always use arterial tubes slightly smaller than the lumen of the artery into which they are to be inserted. *Do not* force arterial tubes into arteries.
8. If clotted material is present in an *artery,* especially in the common carotid artery, attempt to gently remove this material.
9. Arteriosclerosis does *not* always preclude use of an artery for injection. Starting from the incision, find the "softest" portion of the exposed artery. Some forms of arteriosclerosis actually form a "wall" around the lumen.
10. If an artery is accidently broken (arteries remain open and do not collapse) merely locate the two open ends and attach a hemostat to each. Carefully apply new ligatures and insert arterial tubes.

INSTRUMENTS AND LIGATURES

To raise an artery for injection and a vein for drainage, the following instruments may be used:

Instrument	Use
Scalpel	Making the incision; opening the artery or vein
Double-point scissors	Making the incision; preparing ligatures; opening the artery or vein
Aneurysm needle	Dissecting fat and fascia; elevating vessels at surface
Bone separator	Elevating vessels at skin surface
Arterial tubes	For insertion into the artery for injection of fluid
Drainage tube	For insertion into the vein for drainage control
Angular spring forceps	For insertion into the vein for drainage control (in lieu of a drainage tube)
Straight spring forceps	Passing ligatures around the vessels
Grooved director	Assisting in expansion of the vein for insertion of the drainage device

This list represents the minimum number of instruments. A variety of other instruments can also be used. These include arterial hemostats (for holding the arterial tubes in place within the artery; this is of great help in autopsy preparation), ligature passers, arterial scissors, and retractors. This list can also be reduced.

Ligatures for securing the arterial and drain tubes are generally linen or cotton thread. The cotton is somewhat thicker and softer, and many embalmers prefer it. Remember to cut these ligatures long enough so that you can get a good grip on the string to make a very secure tie. A length of 8 to 12 inches is comfortable to work with.

VESSELS USED FOR ARTERIAL EMBALMING

The arteries discussed in this chapter from the standpoint of injection site are the common carotid artery, femoral artery, external iliac artery, axillary artery, brachial artery, popliteal artery, radial artery, ulnar artery, facial artery, abdominal aorta, thoracic aorta, anterior tibial artery, and posterior tibial artery. With respect to these arteries, the area supplied, the considerations for their use, precautions, locations for incisions for raising the vessels, and the protocol for raising the vessels and inserting instruments when both the artery and vein are being used for an injection and drainage site are discussed.

Also discussed (along with the accompanying artery) is the use for drainage of the internal jugular vein, femoral vein, external iliac vein, axillary vein, and inferior vena cava. The location and use of the right atrium of the heart as a drainage point are included in the discussion. As the incisions for the veins are the same as those for the arteries, the student is asked to refer to the artery incisions.

Common Carotid Artery

To be accurate in the discussion of this vessel, consideration is given to the use of a single-point injection, but there follows a discussion of *restricted cervical injection,* which employs both right and left common carotid arteries.

The common carotid artery is the largest vessel the embalmer can raise from a superficial point in a body region outside the trunk area. The incision is made in the inferior portion of the neck. This large artery is closely situated near the *arch of the aorta,* which is the central distribution point for arterial fluid. The common carotid artery can well be described as the "best choice" for injection of the body, especially if there has been any time delay between death and preparation or if vascular difficulties are anticipated.

I. Regions Supplied
1. If the injection is directed superiorly, the head and face are embalmed.

2. If the injection is directed inferiorly, the opposite side of the face and head are embalmed as are the trunk and appendages.

II. Considerations
1. It is very large in diameter.
2. It has no branches except the terminal branches, so it is easily raised to the skin surface.
3. It is very elastic.
4. It is rarely found to be sclerotic.
5. It supplies fluid directly to the head.
6. It is situated close to the arch of the aorta.
7. It is accompanied by a very large vein that can be used for drainage.
8. Arterial coagula are pushed away from the head.

III. Precautions
1. The head may be overinjected.
2. If leakage occurs, it may be seen.
3. Some types of instruments, if improperly used, may mark the side of the face or jaw line.
4. The incisions may be visible with some types of clothing.

IV. Incisions for the Common Carotid and the Internal Jugular Vein
1. **Anterior lateral** (supraclavicular): The incision is made on the clavicle (collar bone) from a point near the sternoclavicular articulation and is directed laterally.
2. **Anterior vertical** (parallel): The incision is made from a point near the sternoclavicular articulation and is directed upward on the sternocleidomastoid muscle.
3. **Posterior vertical** (parallel): The incision is made posterior to the sternocleidomastoid muscle, 2 inches below the lobe of the ear, and is directed downward toward the base of the neck.
4. **Anterior horizontal:** The incision is made at the base of the neck from a point on the sternocleidomastoid muscle and is directed posteriorly.
5. **Flap incision (semilunar):** This incision is used by the operator when it is necessary to raise the vessels on both the right and left sides for injection or drainage. The incision extends from a point lateral and slightly superior to the sternoclavicular articulation and is directed downward on the upper chest wall, across and upward to a similar location on the opposite side. The pattern may be either a U or an inverted C in shape.
6. **Strap line:** This incision is adaptable to the embalming of females. The incision is made about 2 inches lateral to the base of the neck on the

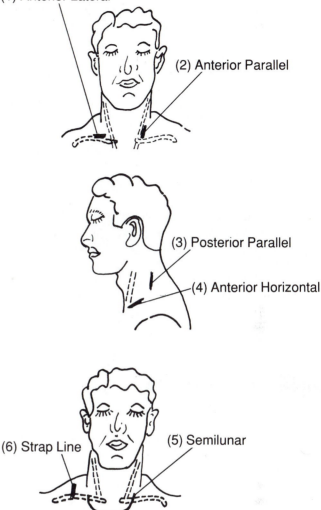

(1) Anterior Lateral
(2) Anterior Parallel
(3) Posterior Parallel
(4) Anterior Horizontal
(6) Strap Line   (5) Semilunar

line where the strap of the undergarments crosses the shoulder (Fig. 9–1).

V. Suggested Protocol for Raising the Common Carotid Artery and the Accompanying Internal Jugular Vein
1. Take a position *at the head of the embalming table.*
2. Turn the head of the body in the *direction opposite* that of the vessels being raised (i.e., if the right common carotid is being raised, turn the head to the left).
3. Place a shoulder block under the shoulders and lower the head of the body on the head block.
4. Make the incision. Dissect through (or cut through) the platysma muscle and the superficial fat and fascia.
5. The sternocleidomastoid muscle will exhibit an area where its fibers part at the clavicle (it looks like a triangle).

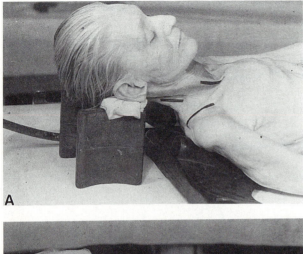

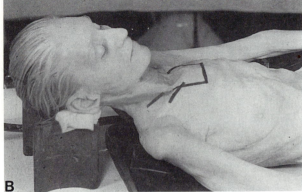

Figure 9–1. **A.** Anterior vertical, posterior vertical, and strap line incisions. **B.** Supraclavicular, semilunar, and anterior horizontal incisions.

6. Raise the *internal jugular vein*; put a ligature around the vein and pull it laterally.
7. Go *medial and deep* and locate the common carotid and bring it to the surface; put two strings around the artery; open the artery; insert arterial tubes superiorly and inferiorly; secure them with a tight ligature.
8. Return to the vein; open the vein and insert a drainage instrument (Fig. 9–2).

VI. Protocol if the Internal Jugular Vein Is Collapsed (and Cannot Be Easily Identified)
1. Make the proper incision.
2. Take a position at the *head of the table*.
3. Elevate the shoulders and lower the head.
4. Turn the head in the direction opposite that of the vessels being raised.
5. Palpate the common carotid artery after dissection.
6. Bring the artery to the surface and insert arterial tubes into the artery.
7. Begin arterial injection.
8. When vein becomes dilated, elevate it to the surface and ligate.

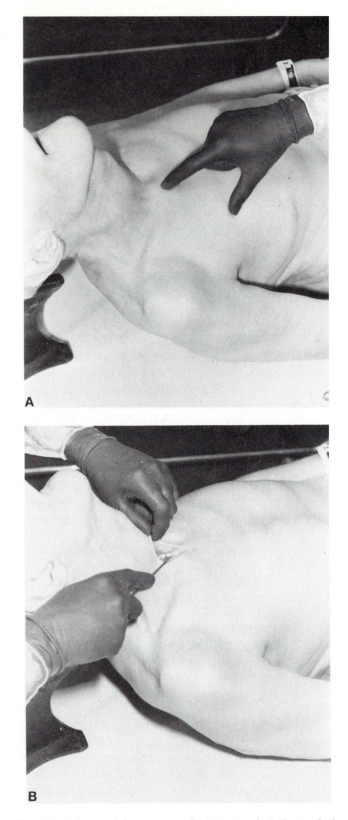

Figure 9–2. **A.** Point at which an anterior parallel incision is made. **B.** The (superficial) internal jugular vein is raised first.

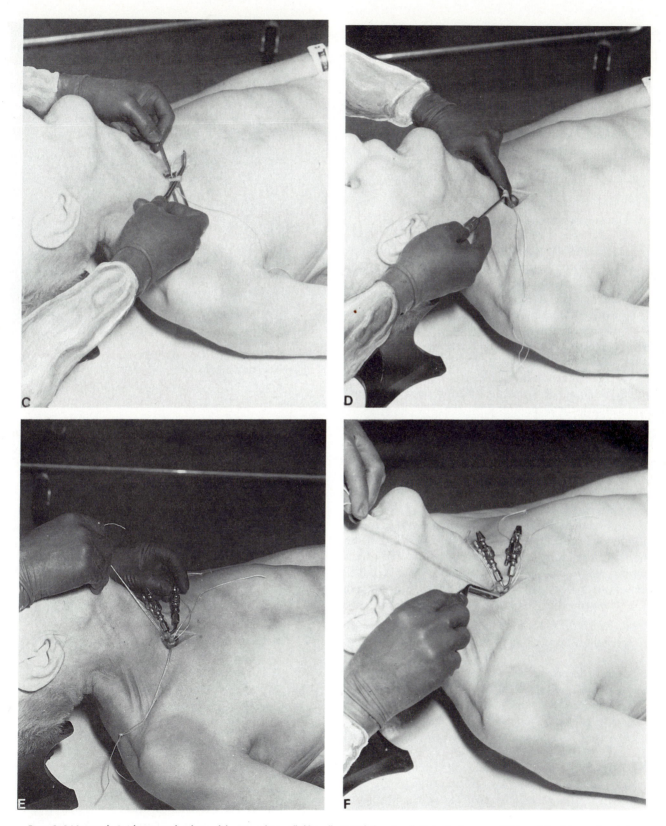

Figure 9–2 (*Continued*). **C.** A ligature is placed around the vein and it is pulled laterally. **D.** With the vein pulled laterally, the artery, which is medial and deep to the vein, is raised. **E.** Arterial tubes are placed into the common carotid and secured with ligatures. **F.** The operator elevates the vein and inserts a drainage instrument toward the heart. Note the suggested position of the operator throughout this procedure.

Internal Jugular Vein

The right internal jugular vein is in direct line with the right atrium of the heart. The right atrium is the central point of blood drainage in the dead human body. The left internal jugular, although a very large vein, does not lead directly into the right atrium. Instead, it joins with the left subclavian vein to form the left brachiocephalic vein, which crosses to the right side of the chest, joins with the opposite brachiocephalic vein, and forms the superior vena cava. For this reason, the right internal jugular vein is preferred as a drainage site.

I. Considerations
1. The vein is very large.
2. There is direct drainage from the face and head.
3. It is accompanied by the common carotid artery, which can be used for injection.
4. The right internal jugular vein leads directly through the right brachiocephalic and superior vena cava into the right atrium, allowing easy removal of clotted material that may be present.

II. Precautions
1. Leakage may be visible.
2. Drainage instruments, if improperly used, may mark the face.
3. The incision may be visible with some clothing.

Because of its size, its location with respect to the right atrium of the heart and its ability to directly drain the head, the right internal jugular vein certainly must be considered as one of the best possible sites for drainage during arterial injection.

An excellent method of embalming involves raising *both* the right and left common carotid arteries at the beginning of the embalming process. This method of embalming, ***restricted cervical injection,*** most effectively controls arterial solution entering the head and face (Fig. 9–3). The procedure follows:

1. Raise the right common carotid artery and the right internal jugular vein.
2. Insert an arterial tube into the right common carotid artery directed toward the head. Insert a second tube into the artery directed toward the trunk. *Be certain to keep the stopcock open* on the tube directed toward the head.
3. Insert a drainage device into the right internal jugular vein.
4. Raise the left common carotid artery only. Insert a tube into the artery directed toward the head. *Leave the stopcock open.* Tie off the lower portion of the artery.

The following are some advantages to use of the restricted cervical injection:

- The arteries are large.
- Carotids are very elastic and have no branches, so they are easy to elevate.

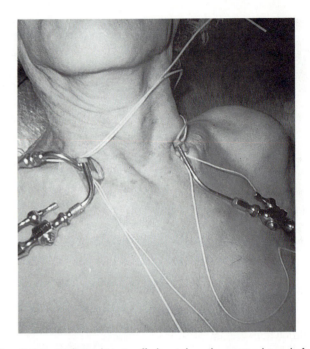

Figure 9–3. Restricted cervical injection affords control over the amount and strength of solution entering the facial tissues.

- The arteries are accompanied by the largest veins.
- The arteries are rarely sclerotic.
- Clots or coagula present in the arterial system will be pushed away from the head area.
- Solution is supplied directly to the head.
- This injection allows the best control over the amount of arterial solution entering the head.
- Two strengths of arterial solution can be used: one for the trunk and another for the head.
- Two rates of flow can be used: one for the trunk and a second for the head.
- Two pressures can be used: one for the head and another for the trunk.
- Large volumes of solution can be run through the trunk without overinjecting the head.
- Features may be set after the trunk is embalmed and aspirated if purging took place during injection.

Facial Artery

The facial artery can be used in two situations: in bodies that have been autopsied and the common carotid and portions of the external carotid removed; in bodies with clotting or sclerosis of the carotid artery, most frequently persons who have suffered from an extracerebral stroke.

The facial artery supplies arterial solution to the soft tissues of the face, the upper and lower lips, the mouth area, the side of the nose, and the medial tissues of the face and some portions of the lower eyelid. The artery is

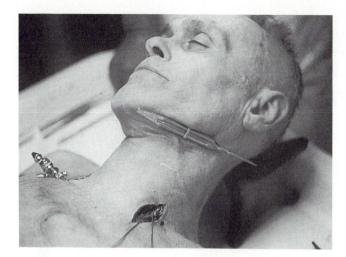

Figure 9–4. Right facial artery.

smaller than the carotid or femoral, and requires a very small arterial tube (see Fig. 8–2).

In life, the facial artery can be felt pulsating by touching the inferior margin of the mandible just in front of the angle of the jaw. It is in this same location that a small incision is made to raise the artery. Fibers of the platysma muscle have to be opened, and by moving the aneurysm needle along the inferior margin of the mandible, the embalmer can find the artery. This incision is best closed with super glue. If suturing is preferred, the use of dental floss for the stitching will be most beneficial (Fig. 9–4).

Axillary Artery

The axillary artery is a continuation of the subclavian artery. It begins at the lateral border of the first rib and passes through the cervicoaxillary canal (this canal is bounded by the first rib, clavicle, and scapula). This vessel can be used to embalm the entire body.

During the early years of embalming, when much work was done at the residence of the deceased, this vessel was preferred. The head received a large amount of solution, and the incision itself was easily hidden from view. It was a very "clean" artery to employ for injection, and drainage was generally taken directly from the right side of the heart by use of a trocar. Keep in mind that early arterial solutions were quite strong, so large volumes were not injected. The small volume would quickly clear the head when injection was from the axillary.

Today, the axillary is used principally as a secondary point of injection where there is insufficient arterial solution in the arm or hand. Also today, long delays result when hospitals have to request autopsies. Permission must be sought for organ donation, and frequently there are pathological problems such as generalized edema, in which cases the axillary artery is less frequently em-

ployed. In addition, the vein that accompanies the artery may not allow easy access for the passage of clotted materials.

I. Regions Supplied
1. If the arterial tube is directed toward the hand, the axillary supplies fluid directly to the arm and hand.
2. If the tube is directed toward the body, the entire body can be embalmed from this location.
II. Considerations
1. Arterial solution flows directly into the arm and hand.
2. The artery is close to the face.
3. The vessels are superficial.
4. The artery is close to the center of arterial solution distribution.
III. Precautions
1. The arm must be extended, especially if the vein is to be used for drainage.
2. The artery is small for injection of the whole body.
3. The artery is accompanied by a vein that is small for drainage.
4. There exists the danger of overinjecting the facial tissues.
5. There are numerous branches and, often, anomalies.
IV. Incision for the Axillary Artery and Vein
The arm should be extended (abducted) a little less than 90° from the body. The incision is made parallel to the linear guide. Many embalmers make this incision along the anterior margin of the hairline of the axilla.
V. Suggested Protocol for Raising the Axillary Artery and Vein
When the arm is abducted the artery will be found slightly anterior and deep to the axillary vein and the brachial plexus. The vein can be described as being located medial and superficial to the axillary artery (Fig. 9–5).
1. Abduct (extend) the arm and rest the distal portion of the arm on the hip of the embalmer. Try not to abduct the arm beyond 90°, as this tends to compress the structures in the arm.
2. Make the incision along the anterior margin of the hairline.
3. Begin the dissection and first locate the axillary vein. This will be a superficial vessel.
4. Place a ligature around the vein and pull the vein away from the incision and downward.
5. Go "above" and "behind" the vein to locate the artery.
6. Pass two ligatures around the artery.
7. Incise the artery and place arterial tubes into the vessel.

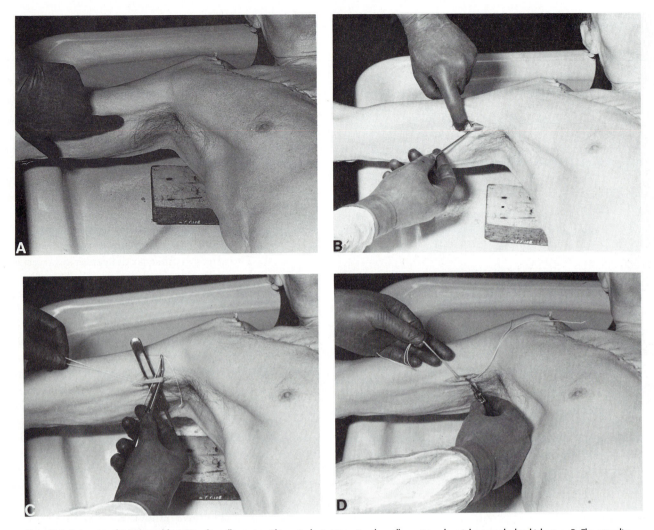

Figure 9–5. **A.** Location of incision used for raising the axillary artery. This particular incision raises the axillary artery where it becomes the brachial artery. **B.** The artery lies deep (behind) to the vein. **C.** Ligatures are passed around the artery. **D.** An arterial tube is inserted to demonstrate how the arm would be injected.

8. Return to the vein; pass a second ligature around the vein; open the vein and insert a drainage tube or forceps toward the heart.

Brachial Artery

The brachial artery supplies fluid directly to the arm and the hand. If the tube is directed toward the body the artery is large enough that the entire body can be embalmed from this point, but because of the small size of the brachial artery, injection would be quite slow and it would be very difficult to build effective arterial pressure. Drainage from the accompanying basilic vein is difficult, as this vein is quite small.

The incision for the brachial artery may be made anywhere along the upper half of the linear guide. The proximal third is preferred. Many embalmers make this incision about 1 inch above and parallel to the linear guide. To raise the artery the arm should be abducted.

Radial Artery

The radial artery supplies solution directly to the thumb side of the hand. It is quite superficial and may easily be palpated through the skin in the area of the wrist. The incision is made parallel to the artery directly on the linear guide, about 1 inch above the base of the thumb (Fig. 9–6).

Ulnar Artery

The ulnar artery supplies arterial solution directly to the medial side of the hand. The incision is made parallel to the vessel directly over the linear guide. Generally, the incision should terminate about 1 inch above the pisiform bone (Fig. 9–7).

There are times when injection of the axillary or brachial artery alone will establish adequate flow of solution into the arm and the hand. With heavy clotting, however, it is necessary to raise and inject both the ra-

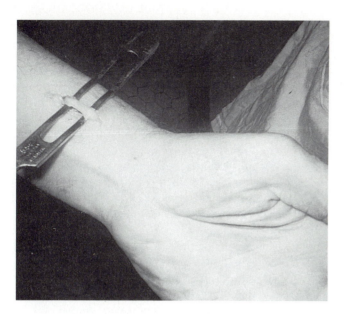

Figure 9–6. Left radial artery.

dial and the ulnar arteries to adequately embalm the hand. Also, a tube may be directed toward the arm from the radial or ulnar artery in an attempt to inject more solution into the arm area.

If there is difficulty clearing the hand, the embalmer may try injecting only the radial artery. When this is done digital pressure should be placed on the ulnar artery. By application of such pressure, short-circuiting of the solution will not occur and more solution will flow into both sides of the hand.

Some embalmers also raise the brachial artery in the area of the antecubital fossa, where the artery divides into the radial and ulnar arteries. The arterial tube can be directed into each of these arteries from this point, avoiding an incision in the wrist area, which may be a difficult area to tightly suture, especially if edema is present.

Femoral Artery

The second most frequently used set of vessels for arterial embalming comprises the femoral artery and femoral vein. The artery is located superficial and lateral to the femoral vein. Because it is a continuation of the external iliac artery and vein, this set of vessels is often referred to as the iliofemoral vessels. A tube placed into the femoral artery and directed toward the trunk of the body is actually placed into the external iliac artery. Likewise, a drainage tube inserted into the femoral vein and directed toward the heart is entered into the external iliac vein.

I. Regions Supplied
   1. When the injection is directed toward the foot, the artery directly supplies the leg and the foot.
   2. When a tube is directed toward the head, the artery supplies arterial solution to the opposite leg as well as the remainder of the body.
II. Considerations
   1. The artery is large.
   2. The incision is not visible.
   3. Both sides of the head may receive an even distribution of solution (especially important if dyes are used with the arterial solution).
   4. The artery is accompanied by a large vein, which can be used for drainage.
   5. With the proper instruments, it can be a "clean" method of embalming; no solution or blood will pass under the body.
   6. The head and arms can be posed without having to be further manipulated after embalming.
III. Precautions
   1. The most frequent reason for inability to use the femoral artery as an injection point is the presence of arteriosclerosis in the artery.
   2. In obese bodies, the vessels may be very deep.

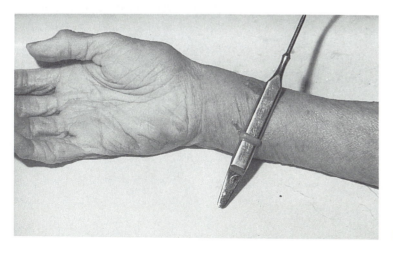

Figure 9–7. Right ulnar artery.

3. There is no control over the solution entering the head, especially when large volumes of solution must be injected or when strong solutions may be injected.
4. Coagula in the arterial system can be pushed into the vessels that supply the arms or the head, areas that will be viewed.
5. Large branches might be mistaken for the femoral artery.

IV. Incision for the Femoral Artery and Vein

This incision is made over the linear guide for the artery beginning at a point slightly medial to the center of a line drawn between the anterior superior iliac spine and the pubic symphysis. Some embalmers prefer to make the incision directly over the inguinal ligament; others prefer to make the incision an inch or more inferior to the inguinal ligament. The external iliac vessels at the inguinal ligament become the femoral vessels. The external iliac artery lies lateral and slightly superficial to the external iliac vein at the inguinal ligament. The code VAN can be used: the Vein is the most medial structure, then comes the Artery, and the most lateral structure is the Nerve.

V. Suggested Protocol for Raising the Femoral Artery and Vein
1. Stand at the right or the left side of the table.
2. Make the incision parallel to the vessels, on the linear guide through the skin and superficial fascia.
3. Dissect superficial fat and fascia bluntly. Observe the great saphenous vein, which is quite superficial.
4. Locate the sartorius muscle. The vessels are found along the medial side of this muscle.
5. Locate the femoral artery and dissect the artery free. Place a ligature around the superior and the inferior portions of the dissected artery.
6. Pull the artery laterally (toward the embalmer) and dissect medially and deeper to free the femoral vein.
7. Clean off the vein, being careful not to rupture it. Also, be careful around the tributaries, which may be full of blood. Bring the vein to the surface and pass one ligature around each end of the dissected portions of the vein.
8. Make an incision into the vein and insert the drainage device, tube, or forceps toward the heart. Tie the tube into the vein. (Keep the vein ligatures on the medial of the thigh and the artery ligatures on the lateral of the thigh.)
9. Bring the artery to the surface of the incision. Incise the artery and insert one arterial tube directed toward the head and a second tube directed down the leg. Secure both with the ligatures (Fig. 9–8).

Femoral Vein

The femoral vein may be used as a drainage point. The vein is large, and because of its location the incision will not be seen. Because of its location, the femoral vein is assisted by gravity in draining blood from the body.

I. Considerations
1. The vein is large.
2. With tubing attached to a drain tube, it can be a very clean method of drainage; water and blood need not come down over the table and under the body.

II. Precautions
1. The weight of the viscera can restrict drainage from the upper portions of the body.
2. Abdominal pressure from gases or ascites can exert pressure on the vein and restrict drainage.
3. In obese bodies, the vein is very deep.
4. Many tributaries flow into the femoral vein, and care must be taken not to rupture any of them.
5. Clots in the right atrium and upper areas of the vascular system may be difficult to remove.
6. Pressure on the heart from hydrothorax (as frequently seen in deaths from pneumonia) may make it difficult to establish good drainage from the right atrium and large veins of the head and arms.

Popliteal Artery

The popliteal artery is used as a secondary injection site when solution has not reached the area of the leg below the knee. Because of the inconvenient location of this artery, it is generally used only in special circumstances. Two examples are bodies resulting from mutilation and accidental deaths and arthritic bodies.

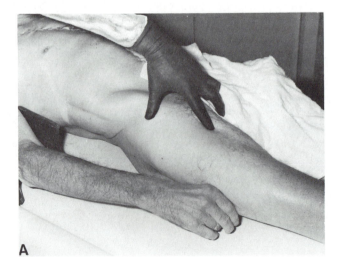

A

Figure 9–8. A. The femoral artery and veins are raised.

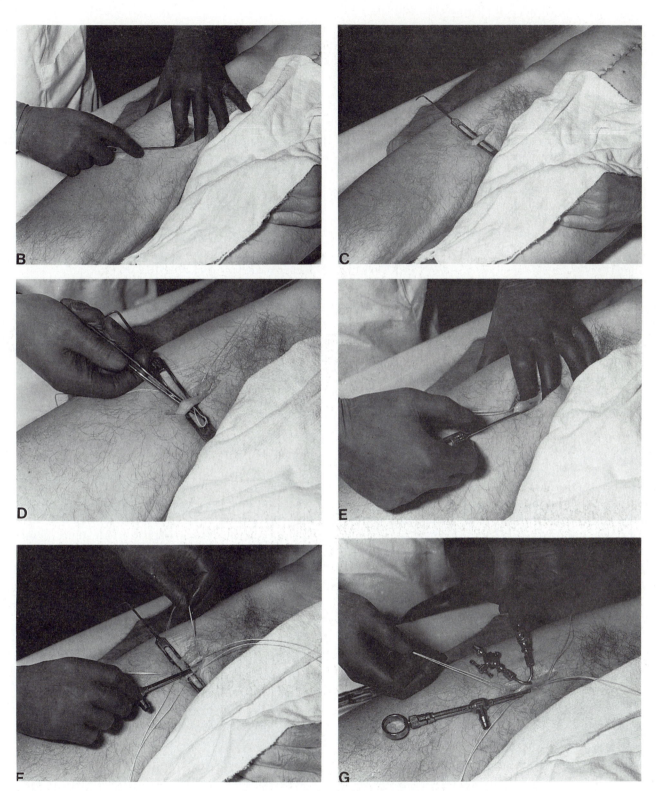

Figure 9–8. (*Continued*). **B.** The artery lies just lateral to the sartorius muscle. **C.** The femoral artery is superficial and slightly lateral to the vein. **D.** Ligatures are passed beneath the artery and it is pulled laterally, toward the embalmer. **E.** The femoral vein is raised; it is medial and deep to the artery. **F.** Ligatures are passed around the vein and a drain tube is inserted toward the heart. **G.** Arterial tubes are placed in the artery.

Most tissues of the body are best preserved and more uniformly preserved by arterial injection. As the legs will not be viewed, other methods of embalming can be used, including surface and hypodermic embalming. An attempt should be made, however, to inject the legs. The first choice would be the external iliac or the femoral artery. If these vessels are found to be sclerotic there will, no doubt, also be pathological problems with the other arteries of the leg, especially if gangrene or necrosis is present.

As previously stated, the popliteal is generally used when there has been an interruption of the arterial pathway, as in accidents or mutilations. The limbs of the arthritic body may be in such a position that the femoral vessels cannot be used, and, because of the "swayed" position of the legs, the popliteal artery may be easy to work with.

Two incisions can be used: (1) The body may be turned and the incision made down the center of the popliteal space, parallel to the artery. (2) If the body is not turned the knee can be slightly flexed and a longitudinal incision made along the posterior–medial aspect of the lower third of the thigh, actually just superior to the popliteal space (Fig. 9–9). Because of the location of the artery and the size of the vessels, the accompanying vein is not used as a drainage site.

Anterior and Posterior Tibial Arteries

The anterior and tibial arteries supply arterial solution directly to the portion of the leg below the knee and on into the foot. Unlike the superficial radial and ulnar arteries, which supply the distal portion of the arm and the hand, these arteries are deeper, making them more difficult to locate and to bring to the surface of the incisions. In addition, the skin covering the distal portion of the leg is very tight, making suture of the incisions very difficult. When suturing is difficult, leakage can become a problem.

With regard to arteriosclerosis, it would be most impractical to attempt to raise and inject the tibial arteries when the femoral artery is affected by arteriosclerosis, especially if gangrene or necrosis is present in the foot or in the distal portion of the leg. Treatment when the latter conditions are present is best accomplished by hypodermic treatment of the leg with cavity fluid; the leg should be painted with preservative autopsy gel and a plastic stocking containing embalming powder placed on the limb.

The incision for raising the anterior tibial artery is made along the lateral margin of the inferior third of the crest of the tibia. In the distal portion of the leg it lies at the superficial margin of the tibia. By using the aneurysm needle to dissect down along the tibia, the embalmer can locate the artery (Fig. 9–10).

The incision for the posterior tibial artery is made midway between the medial malleolus and the large calcaneous tendon.

Abdominal Aorta and Thoracic Aorta

The abdominal aorta and thoracic aorta are large vessels very deeply seated in the abdominal and thoracic cavities. They lie in the center of the body and can be found on the anterior surface of the spinal column. The thoracic or abdominal aorta may be used for injection after complete or partial autopsy or organ donation and in infants.

The thoracic or abdominal aorta may become a vessel for injection in certain bodies where an incision has been made from which the vessels can be dissected and identified. Such bodies might include those dying following recent surgery; bodies where partial autopsies have been performed or the bodies of organ donors.

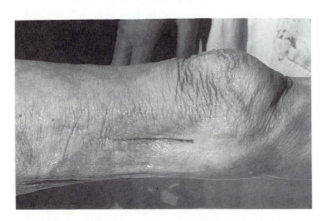

Figure 9–9. Incision location (optional) for the left popliteal artery.

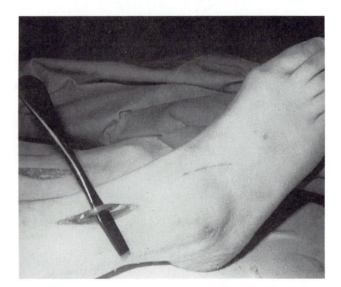

Figure 9–10. Right anterior tibial artery, lateral to the crest of the tibia.

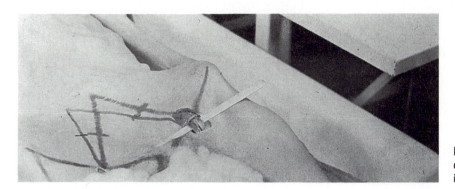

Figure 9–11. Linear guides and incision location for raising the left external iliac artery and vein. The artery is lateral to the vein at the inguinal ligament.

Drainage may be taken from a vein that the embalmer raises such as the femoral or internal jugular vein. Drainage may also be taken directly from the inferior or superior vena cava. Use of the aorta for injection and the vena cava for drainage is determined by the amount of exposure of these vessels created by the partial autopsy or organ removal.

In the unautopsied infant, the abdominal aorta can be exposed by making an incision to the left of the midline, beginning a few inches below the xiphoid process of the sternum and extending over the abdominal wall about 4 inches in length. The greater omentum is thus exposed. It can be reflected upward, and the small intestines can be pushed aside or lifted out of the abdominal cavity to expose the abdominal aorta and the inferior vena cava resting on the spinal column in the midline of the abdomen.*

The thoracic aorta in the infant can be exposed by making a midline incision down the center of the sternum. As the sternum is quite soft, a sharp scalpel can be used to divide it. The sternum is retracted and held in this opened position. The pericardium of the heart is now exposed and can be cut open with a pair of surgical scissors. After the pericardium is opened, the right auricle, the little earlike appendage at the top right side of the heart, can be cut open and used as a site for drainage. If the heart is moved to the right the descending thoracic aorta can be exposed as well as the arch of the aorta above it. The aorta can be opened and a tube inserted for injection. (See Chapter 16).

External Iliac Artery

For considerations on the use of the external iliac artery, see Femoral Artery. The incision is made over the inguinal ligament (Fig. 9–11). As the external iliac artery passes beneath the inguinal ligament it lies on the lateral side of the external iliac vein. If the leg is injected from this point, in the autopsied body, the artery supplies solution to the lower extremity and the anterior abdominal wall.

---

* These procedures should only be used when absolutely no other methods would produce satisfactory results; and when used be certain proper permission has been secured.

Internal Iliac Artery

The internal iliac artery is a branch of the common iliac artery that runs medially into the pelvic cavity. In the autopsied body, injection of this artery supplies embalming solution to the gluteal muscles and the peroneal regions.

Inferior Vena Cava

For completeness, at this point the inferior vena cava is discussed as a drainage point. This site can be used for drainage when a partial autopsy has been performed. If the contents of the thorax have been removed, the abdominal viscera and lower extremities can be injected (1) through the abdominal aorta or (2) by clamping off the aorta and injecting the femoral artery. With either point of injection, drainage can be taken directly from the remnants of the inferior vena cava. The inferior vena cava is located to the right of the abdominal aorta at the posterior portion of the diaphragm.

If the contents of the abdominal cavity have been removed in a partial autopsy, the thoracic viscera, head, and arms can be injected from the descending thoracic aorta. Or, the aorta can be clamped closed and the upper portions of the body injected from the carotid or axillary vessels. Drainage can easily be taken directly from the remnants of the inferior vena cava.

When drainage is taken from the inferior vena cava it is not necessary to place a drainage device in the vein. To create intermittent drainage the inferior vena cava can be closed shut with a hemostat. A large piece of cotton can also be held over the vena cava with a gloved hand.

Right Atrium of the Heart

When drainage is difficult to establish, the right side of the heart may be pierced with a trocar for drainage. The trocar is inserted into the right side of the heart and should be placed in the right atrium. Piercing of the heart should not begin until one-half to one full gallon of arterial solution has been injected.

To drain from the right side of the heart, the trocar is inserted through the abdominal wall at the standard point of entry (2 inches to the left and 2 inches above the umbilicus). The trocar is directed into the mediastinum area and intersects a line extending from the lobe of the *right* ear to the *left* anterior superior iliac spine. Actually, if the trocar is simply directed toward the right ear lobe, the point should pass into the right side of the heart. The aspirator can be stopped at this point and the drainage established by a gravity system.

It is wise to attach clear plastic tubing to the trocar so further movement of the trocar can be *stopped* immediately after it enters the heart. This very old method for removing blood during arterial injection was used when bodies were embalmed at the residence of the deceased.

MAKING THE INCISION INTO THE ARTERY AND VEIN

To open the artery or vein a scissors or scalpel may be used, depending on the preference of the embalmer. In the method most commonly employed to open the artery or vein, the embalmer simply makes a **transverse** cut into the vessel from the edge of the vessel to the center or just slightly beyond the center. Cutting too far may weaken the vessel enough that it will break into two pieces.

Very elastic arteries such as the carotid and the axillary arteries can easily be stretched to the surface of the incision. With arteries such as the femoral, when some sclerosis is present, raising the vessel to the skin surface can create great tension on the artery. Care should be taken in opening sclerotic vessels to avoid breaking the vessel. As soon as you observe the lumen in this type of vessel, cut no further.

A longitudinal incision may also be used to open vessels. Most embalmers prefer to elevate these vessels on a bone separator. Using a scalpel, cut a longitudinal incision in the center of the vessel running parallel to the vessel. Most embalmers prefer to use a scalpel: however, double-point scissors can also be used. The longitudinal incision is not recommended for opening sclerotic arteries. Many embalmers use this incision for veins, for it provides a large opening for drainage instruments. Two arterial tubes may be placed into position using this incision for the artery.

A combination transverse and longitudinal incision is preferred by many embalmers, especially for opening veins. It is also most helpful when a drainage tube is to be inserted, because it permits drainage from the opposite end of the vein. A wedge can also be cut into an artery or vein with double-point scissors or a scalpel. This method is not recommended for sclerotic arteries (Fig. 9–12).

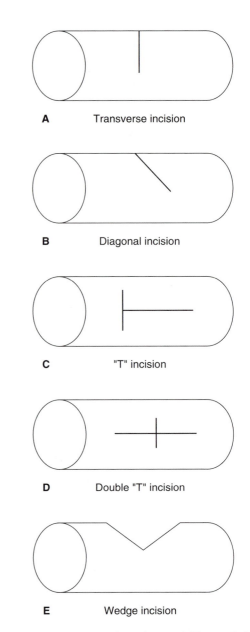

Figure 9–12. A. Transverse incision. **B.** Diagonal incision. **C.** "T" incision. **D.** Double "T" incision. **E.** Wedge incision.

KEY TERMS AND CONCEPTS FOR STUDY AND DISCUSSION

1. Define the following terms:
   multisite (sectional) injection
   primary injection site
   restricted cervical injection
   secondary injection site
   single-point injection
   six-point injection
   split injection
2. Differentiate between arteries, veins, and nerves.

3. List the nine major factors to consider in choosing an artery for injection and a vein for drainage.

4. List several advantages to use of the common carotid artery as a vessel for injection.

5. List the steps for raising and inserting instruments into the common carotid artery and the internal jugular vein.

6. List six incisions that can be used to raise the common carotid artery.

7. List the advantages to use of the restricted cervical method of injection.

8. Describe the relationship of the common carotid artery to the internal jugular vein.

9. Describe the relationship of the femoral artery to the femoral vein.

10. Describe the relationship of the axillary artery to the axillary vein.

11. Give the steps for raising and inserting instruments into the femoral artery and vein.

12. Describe where the incisions are made for raising the radial and ulnar arteries.

13. Describe several incisions that can be used to open an artery for insertion of the arterial tube.

14. List the incisions that can be used to raise and inject the popliteal artery.

10

Embalming Analysis

No one chapter in any embalming text can really cover embalming analysis. Likewise, one classroom lecture or even a series of lectures cannot possibly cover the entire scope of this subject. Embalming analysis is a summary of the entire embalming process that includes those relevant factors from the disciplines of anatomy, pathology, microbiology, and chemistry. Many think of embalming analysis only as a preembalming "diagnosis" of the body to determine the embalming treatments needed. An embalming analysis is not only a preembalming analysis; it is analysis of the body before, during, and after arterial and cavity embalming. In addition to recognizing the conditions of the body, the embalmer must have a complete knowledge of embalming methodology to make the analysis. The entire analysis should be documented in report form. If the body is being shipped to another funeral home, a copy of this document should also be sent.

The factors examined in making an analysis can be classified as intrinsic or extrinsic. Intrinsic factors are those conditions present within the body, for example, cause of death; manner of death; pathological conditions; bacterial influence; moisture level; age, weight, and body build; protein level; febrile conditions and effects; presence or absence of discolorations; postmortem changes (decomposition changes, pH of the body, presence or absence of rigor mortis); effects of drugs or medications; trauma; and surgery.

The extrinsic factors of embalming analysis are those conditions outside the body that have had a direct influence on the condition of the body. These include environmental factors (temperature, presence or absence of bacteria, humidity, vermin); length of time between death and preparation; and length of time expected between preparation and disposition.

The aim of this chapter is to approach embalming analysis not as treatment of a specific disease but as treatment of groups of conditions found in the dead human body. A recent death certification listed the following causes of death:

Cause	Duration
Respiratory failure	Hours
Chronic renal failure	1 year
Congestive heart failure	Years

EMBALMING ANALYSIS TIME PERIODS

1. Preembalming analysis — Treatments
2. Analysis during arterial embalming — Treatments
3. Analysis after arterial embalming — Treatments

A contributory cause listed *on the same certificate* was arteriosclerosis.

In addition to these disease processes, any one of which could eventually lead to death, this person had received medications for years. It would be impossible for the embalmer to evaluate each disease process and its effects and each drug administered and its effects. The embalmer must consider the effects these diseases and drugs had on the body and the *conditions* they produced.

In the preceding analysis, the embalmer would be most concerned with renal failure, for this disease process can leave nitrogenous wastes in the tissues. These nitrogenous wastes increase the preservative demand. Arteriosclerosis may make use of the femoral artery impossible as an injection site. The best vessels would be the common carotids. The best drainage point to relieve the engorgement of blood in the right side of the heart resulting from congestive heart failure would be the right internal jugular vein. In addition to these factors, the intrinsic general body conditions must be considered—age, weight, and senile changes. Finally, the embalmer must also consider the postmortem changes, the time between death and preparation, degree of rigor mortis, decomposition progress, and refrigeration of the body.

Very few causes of death determine the embalming technique. Three examples are death from a contagious or infectious disease, death from a ruptured aortic aneurysm, and death from renal failure. These causes of death (when known before embalming) can be very important to the embalmer. Some conditions take precedence over others, such as a body dead from renal failure but jaundiced. Preservation of the body must be the first concern of the embalmer. The body dead from renal failure must be treated with strong arterial solutions, and the jaundice condition must be a secondary consideration. The jaundice, no doubt, will worsen from the strong arterial solutions, but the face and hands can be treated later with opaque cosmetics. By using restricted cervical injection, the embalmer is able to inject large quantities of a very strong arterial solution into the edematous areas of the body which will help to overcome edema and the nitrogenous wastes in the tissues, both of which dilute and neutralize formaldehyde. The head could then be injected with a jaundice fluid to modify the effects of the jaundice condition in the facial tissues.

> The correct embalming treatment is dictated by the conditions of the body and not solely by the cause of death.

Suppose an apparently healthy man in his midfifties is traveling to work and suddenly dies from a massive coronary thrombosis. It is likely in such cases that the coronary arteries are the only vessels occluded by arteriosclerosis. His blood would be of normal viscosity and the tissues in general would not be debilitated. This presents a textbook picture of an "average" or "normal" case. The man would be brought to a medical examiner's office and placed in refrigeration where he would remain until he was identified and a medical examiner had signed a death certificate. This may take as long as 24 hours. The diagnosis on the death certificate might read "coronary thrombosis due to arteriosclerosis."

The embalming treatment required is that for a refrigerated body. Instead of larger volumes of a mild solution as indicated by the facts on the "certificate," proper treatment dictates that smaller volumes of stronger solution be used.

To achieve good results the embalmer must learn to observe. When raising the arteries note the condition of the vessels and the blood. When posing the features note the condition of the eyes, the eyelids, and the lips. An eye that is flattened and sunken in its socket indicates that the interval between death and embalming has been prolonged—the blood has thickened, separated, and settled to the dependent parts. In such cases, regardless of the cause of death, it is wise to raise both common carotid arteries, tie off the superior side, and inject toward the body only. In this manner the body can be injected with large volumes of strong solution under pressure. The head will receive sufficient solution via the vertebrals which are small enough to reduce the volume of solution per minute passing into the head, thereby making it possible to control distension.

While posing the body on the table, the embalmer notes the presence of edema in the lower extremities. This condition can prevail in heart disease or cancer deaths. It is more important for the embalmer to be aware of its presence than its cause. Whether or not edema is noted on the death certificate, it does *dictate* the type of embalming treatment.

Examine the abdomen for masses and the lower quadrant for the telltale green spot of decomposition. At the same time, observe for the presence of ascites. Regardless of the cause of the excess fluid in the abdominal cavity, its presence indicates the need to reduce this abdominal pressure prior to arterial injection. By doing so, pressure on the lower portion of the aorta and the inferior vena cava is eliminated, permitting better distribution of embalming solution and drainage of blood.

Another factor that can influence the embalming treatment is the presence of lesions. For example, decubitus ulcers may be present on the body even though they were not noted on the death certificate. In such cases the subject may have had an old nontraumatic cerebral hemorrhage or a bullet wound in the spine. Either condition would result in long confinement to bed and the resultant ulcerations. Again, regardless of the cause, the ulcers must be treated the same way.

Whatever the cause of death, the condition of the body is affected by the temperature of the environment, environmental moisture, the postmortem interval, the nature and amount of clothing, and airborne bacteria. There have been cases of postmortem contamination of the body with *Clostridium perfringens*. This negates all other pathological considerations for the embalmer. It is, of course, an example of an extreme case, but certainly does not detract from the view that embalming treatment, in general, should be based on the postmortem condition of the body rather than the medical causes of death.

Analysis is not only recognition of the conditions of the body and the effects of disease processes on the body; it is also selection of proper embalming techniques to deal with these conditions.

PURPOSE OF THE ANALYSIS

The purpose of an embalming analysis is to select those embalming procedures that provide a thoroughly sanitized and preserved body that closely resembles the lifelike appearance of the deceased.

Older embalming textbooks describe hundreds of diseases, poisons, and traumatic modes of death and the embalming treatment for each. Many of these treatments are still applicable today. Years later, several authors approached the subject by categorizing bodies by general conditions. From this approach came the "typing" of bodies. If embalming treatments are thought of in terms of the effect each disease has on the deceased, it is noted that the number of "types" of cases presented to the embalmer is fewer than the number of diseases. This gives the practicing embalmer a more practical approach to selection of the proper embalming technique. One of the best and most complete approaches to the "typing" of bodies is that of the late Professor Ray E. Slocum of the Dodge Chemical Company. In his approach to preembalming case analysis he established six categories or "types" of bodies. For each type he then prescribed a general embalming approach that included arterial fluids and their dilutions, recommended pressure for injection and rate of flow, primary injection and drainage points, and time period for cavity embalming.

The six body types are now described. Note that under Type II, there is mention of treating Type I bodies as if they were Type II if problems develop *during* injection of the body, indicating that this system included analysis *during* the embalming process.

CLASSIFICATION OF BODIES

Type I

Note: All bodies in this classification (the "average body") still retain some body heat.

1. Bodies dead of heart disease that have not undergone a lingering illness preceding death
2. Bodies dead of vascular diseases that have not been bedridden prior to death
3. Stout (obese) bodies in which there is no bloodstream or coccal infection
4. All bodies that have suddenly expired, not dead over 12 hours, except those requiring restorative treatments
5. Bodies dead of childbirth
6. Bodies not later specified that appear to have a normal or abnormally large protein content (as usually exists in fleshy bodies or where skin is dry)

Type II

1. Bodies not dead more than 24 hours that have low albumin content as indicated by moist or clammy tissue, usually with angular faces and still retaining body heat
2. Bodies not dead more than 12 hours from coccal infections
3. Bodies not dead more than 12 hours from uremic poisoning (uremia), diabetes, nephritis, dropsy, or any disease wherein the organs of elimination have not functioned properly for some time prior to death
4. Bodies not dead more than 12 hours where death occurred in a public institution
5. Bodies not dead more than 24 hours from wasting diseases such as tuberculosis and cancer
6. Bodies not dead more than 12 hours that require major restorative treatments
7. Bodies not dead more than 12 hours that may have been administered large quantities of drugs preceding death
8. Bodies that might have been classified as Type I but that have been dead long enough (but not over 24 hours) to have lost body heat
9. Bodies not dead over 12 hours that show evidence of considerable senile changes, such as extreme flabbiness of tissue
10. Bodies drowned but not in the water more than 24 hours in cold weather or 12 hours in warm weather
11. Bodies originally classified as Type I, in which the treatment recommended for that type was begun but difficulty is encountered in securing desired circulation, drainage, or tissue firming
12. Autopsied bodies not subjected to refrigeration that have not been dead more than 24 hours

Bodies placed in this classification are undoubtedly those that most frequently could cause embalming difficulties unless some consideration is given to the individual conditions present and plans are made to circumvent these conditions with specific treatments.

Type III

1. All bodies dead more than 24 hours that do not show evidence of advanced putrefaction
2. Bodies that have been frozen improperly and do not show advanced stages of putrefaction
3. Bodies that fail to respond to Type II treatment
4. Bodies in which the initial arterial injection was insufficient to the extent that reinjection became necessary for proper preservation, but wherein the advanced stages of putrefaction have not occurred
5. Autopsied bodies dead more than 24 hours

Bodies in this classification undoubtedly present a more serious problem to the embalmer than do Type I and II bodies. It is likely that the number of bodies in this classification will continually increase because of the ever-growing demands of medical science for more autopsies. In many instances, even though permission for autopsy is not secured from nearest kin, the bodies are held at hospitals pending attempts to secure such permission.

Type IV

1. Bodies dead of diseases affecting the biliary tract as evidenced by a jaundice discoloration, but still retaining body heat or dead not more than 12 hours prior to embalming
2. Bodies dead of asphyxiation or from any cause for which methylene blue* had been used intravenously as a resuscitory measure, but which have not been dead more than 12 hours
3. Bodies not dead more than 12 hours from Addison's disease

Type V

1. All bodies showing advanced stages of putrefaction
2. Bodies wherein "tissue gas" (*Clostridium perfringens*) or gas gangrene is present
3. Bodies that develop putrefaction after arterial injection
4. Bodies that require distal injection of gangrenous limbs
5. Bodies that require treatment for advanced stages of ascites wherein the limbs have become ulcerated

---

*This classification was written in the late 1950s.

Type VI*

1. Infants not dead more than 12 hours
2. Children under 12 years of age still retaining body heat (children over 12 years of age may be treated as recommended for adults)

As can be seen from the Slocum method of body typing, it is not the specific disease that concerns the embalmer but the condition that the disease produces in the body. This method of analysis, or *preembalming observations*, is the approach most embalmers take in determining what embalming techniques to employ. It would be too difficult to approach each body by the specific disease or effects produced by a specific drug.

Slocum lists the specific arterial chemicals and coinjection chemicals in his treatments for the different body classes. It would be impossible to list the specific treatments because the fluid dilutions vary depending on the product the embalmer selects. Nevertheless, it can easily be seen that Type I bodies require a mild arterial solution and equal amounts of coinjection chemicals. Type II bodies need stronger arterial solutions. The strongest solutions are needed for Types III and V. Special arterial solutions are needed for treatment of jaundiced Type IV bodies, and a mild solution is used for injection of Type VI bodies (infants).*

EMBALMING ANALYSIS, PART I: PREEMBALMING ANALYSIS

Embalmers consider four major factors in making a preembalming analysis, (factors also used in Slocum's method of analysis*): general conditions of the body, effects produced by disease processes, effects produced by drugs or surgical procedures, and effects of the postmortem period between death and embalming.

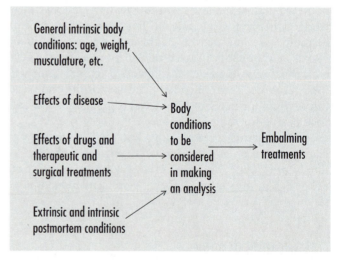

---

*Unlike the Slocum recommendations, this text takes the position that strength of all fluid solutions should be based on the preservative demands of the body.

The embalmer must be concerned with the *conditions* of the body he or she can touch or even smell. Most often, the embalmer does not know the cause of death at the time of embalming. The embalmer is also unaware of the medically prescribed drugs that the deceased may have been administered for long-term therapy. If the *conditions* of the body are treated, the exact cause of death or the chemotherapy used need not be known.

General Intrinsic Body Conditions

The general intrinsic conditions of the body include age, body weight and build, musculature, protein level, and general skin condition.

Age. *Child or infant:* Arteries and veins will be much smaller than in the adult; special sized instruments are needed for injection and drainage. Milder solutions may be needed (but preservative demands must determine solution strengths). A needle injector may not be usable for mouth closure. Positioning will vary from that for an adult.

Elderly: Arteriosclerosis may eliminate the use of the femoral artery as an injection point. Absence of teeth and dentures may create problems in setting features. Suturing may be needed for mouth closure if the jaw bone has atrophied.

Weight. *Emaciated:* Solution strengths may need to be reduced. Dehydration may create problems with eye closure and mouth closure.

Obese: Femoral vessels may be too deep to use for injection. Very large quantities of arterial solution will be needed. The internal jugular vein will afford the best drainage site. Restricted cervical injection will best control arterial solution entering facial tissues. There will be positioning problems.

Musculature: In the healthy adult with firm skin and well-developed musculature the embalmer can expect the embalming solution to result in very good firming of the body tissues. If there is a delay between death and preparation, this body can be expected to display intense rigor mortis, making it difficult to establish good distribution of the solution. Where bodies are wasted from disease and the musculature is not well developed and the skin is loose, the embalmer can expect little or no firming of the limbs from the embalming solution; swelling is expected if large volumes of mild solutions are injected. Senile, loose flabby tissue does not assimilate the arterial solution as well as healthy, firm tissues.

Disease Processes and the Cause of Death

The cause of death may not be known at the time of embalming; however, the embalmer can observe the effects that diseases have had on the body. For example, *jaundice* may be caused by the effect of drugs on the liver, the effect of drugs on red blood cells, obstruction of the bile duct, hepatitis, cancer of the liver, and hemolysis of red blood cells. It is the condition of jaundice that concerns the embalmer, not the disease that caused this condition.

The following excerpts, from an article written by Shor (1972) of the American Academy of Funeral Service, illustrate how the same disease can produce different conditions in different persons. (Remember that it is not the cause of death or the disease but the effects and conditions produced by the disease in the body that should concern the embalmer).

Let us begin by examining a very common disease and cause of death today—cancer. This pathological condition may attack and be confined to the stomach. In such an event the patient would not be able to retain foods, either liquid or solid, for weeks just prior to death. He actually might die of starvation although the primary cause of death would be cancer of the stomach.

Primary Condition Unimportant

The embalmer now is presented with a thin, emaciated, dehydrated subject. The primary condition in the stomach is of little significance to him.

Consider next another patient with the same basic disease—cancer. In this subject the malignancy is of the liver or the right suprarenal gland. The attendant enlargement of these structures bears down upon and obstructs the cisterna chyli, the lymph collecting station of the abdomen and lower extremities. This prevents the lymph from returning to the venous system from these areas. All of the parts drained by this system will become edematous and ascites will develop.

The primary cause of death in both examples is cancer. In one case we have a subject with edema, ascites and anasarca; in the other an emaciated, dehydrated subject. We should also note here that many other diseases can cause the above described conditions. (If we learn to treat the conditions, we will treat them successfully—regardless of the cause of death).

Let me illustrate this further. In incompetence of the right atrioventricular valve of the heart, the valve fails to close efficiently. During the diastole blood will regurgitate from the right ventricle to the right atrium. This, of course, reduces the amount of blood the right atrium can receive from the inferior vena cava. In turn, the amount of blood the vena cava receives from its tributaries is minimized. The resulting venous congestion in the lower venous system increases transudation of plasma and results again in edema and ascites. Whether the excess fluid is a result of cancer of the viscera or damage to the heart valves, the embalming treatment is the same.

Same Basic Treatment

By the same token, emaciation, whether caused by cancer of the stomach, actual starvation or pulmonary tuberculosis, requires the same basic embalming treatment.

Further inquiry into cancer shows that obstruction to the passage of bile into the intestinal tract can lead to the very common embalming problem, jaundice. This condition also can be caused by obstruction of the common bile duct—a disease not usually related to cancer. Here again, it is the symptoms and not the disease that pose an embalming problem.

A disease that is as common as cancer and can produce as varied a group of postmortem conditions is arteriosclerosis. Depending on the vessel or vessels involved, we can get a wide range of different embalming problems.

For example, let us consider renal arteriosclerosis. Here, the blood vessels carrying blood to the kidneys are impaired. As a result, the kidneys diminish in size and efficiency. Nitrogenous wastes and urea instead of passing out of the body via kidney and other excretory organs will remain in the bloodstream and tissue spaces. The result will be uremia, cachexia and possibly edema and ascites, as in some cancers. Arteriosclerosis can affect the vessels of the brain, causing a **stroke** which, in turn, can lead to other abnormalities. One of these is long-term **paralysis** of the extremities with the attendant atrophy and vasoconstriction. Another is long periods of confinement to bed, with the often attendant **decubitus ulcers.** A third is **immediate death** with *no special embalming problems.*

Again, the decubitus ulcers and the atrophied parts can stem from any other disease which confines the patient to bed for extended periods of time. In all these situations the resulting conditions cause much greater embalming problems than the disease that led to them. The embalmer must not overlook the fact that any two or three of the diseases discussed here can and do coexist. So can each disease exist in two or more forms. Therefore, a patient can die with cancer of the stomach and liver. A patient can have cancer of the liver and renal or cerebral arteriosclerosis. In reality, then, **an embalmer should ask, "What conditions exist?" rather than "Of what did the subject die?"**

The reader should not construe this article to mean that the author discourages the study of pathology. It is intended, rather, to encourage the student to correlate his studies of pathology with embalming. It is incumbent upon him to learn the embalming treatments for the basic postmortem conditions that create problems. If the conditions are identified and properly treated, the embalming procedure will succeed regardless of the disease that caused the condition.

Drug Treatments and Surgical Procedures

In the 1960s embalmers became increasingly aware that medications used for the treatment of disease were having a significant impact on embalming results. It was becoming increasingly difficult to establish firmness in the bodies, edema was becoming a frequent problem, and extravascular discolorations in the form of purpura and ecchymosis were more frequently seen along with jaundice and the loss of hair.

During the past 30 years, many articles have been written about the effects of specific drugs on the embalming process (see Chapter 23). Like the hundreds of diseases and their effects on the body, it would be impossible for the embalmer to attempt to embalm a body using chemical formulations designed to combat the effects of a specific drug. Most often a patient is given combinations of drugs, often over a long period. A drug does not always produce the same effects in each person. Here again, it is important that the embalmer have an understanding of the possible effects of drugs and of the fact that embalming problems often stem from the long usage of drug therapy. The embalmer must treat the conditions that can be observed in the dead human body and *not* the effects of a specific medication.

Some of the more common postmortem conditions that concern the embalmer in deciding what embalming treatments to use are those that have been brought about by the long-term usage of drugs. Remember that in addition to the conditions produced by the drugs, the embalmer must observe and consider the conditions produced in the body by disease, general body build, and postmortem changes.

Chemotherapeutic agents are toxic. The one axiom that can be universally applied to ALL chemotherapeutic agents is that they are *toxic.* Cellular changes occur when they are used, no matter which drug is administered. Even the relatively innocuous aspirin pill has its effects. Drugs have an effect on the skin, circulatory system, liver, and kidneys. Such changes may be comparatively minor in nature, limited to slight discolorations that respond readily to cosmetic treatment. But when they assume major proportions such as acute jaundice or saturate the body tissues with uremic poisons, the fixative action of the preservative chemicals contained in the arterial solutions used is seriously impaired (Table 10–1, Fig. 10–1).

In making a preembalming analysis, choice of embalming technique may be greatly influenced by whether death occurred during or immediately after surgery. Surgery could be the primary factor in an analysis, as illustrated in the following examples.

Heart Surgery or Aortic Repair. During these procedures the heart may be stopped for a period during which an artificial means of life support is used. Frequently, if death occurs during or shortly after this type of surgery, the face and neck are grossly distended with edema. Repair of an abdominal aneurysm may not always be successful, and the interruption in circulation will necessitate sectional arterial injection.

TABLE 10-1. EMBALMING COMPLICATIONS CREATED BY EXTENSIVE DRUG THERAPIES

Complication	Result
Immediate allergic reaction to the drug	Tissues appear swollen
	Discolored skin surface
	Possible skin eruptions
Liver failure	Edema (ascites); edema of lower extremities
	Increase in ammonia in the tissues (neutralizes formaldehyde)
	Purged caused by rupture of esophageal veins
	Gastrointestinal bleeding; fluid loss; possible purge
	Hair loss
	Jaundice
Renal failure	Increase in ammonia in the tissues
	Edema of tissues
	Gastrointestinal bleeding
	Pulmonary edema
	Congestive heart failure
	Discoloration of the skin (sallow color)
	Uremic pruritis of the skin
Damage to blood vessels	Skin hemorrhage (ecchymosis, purpural hemorrhage)
Damage to the walls	Breakdown of the skin; skin-slip often present
Clot formation (poor circulation of embalming fluids)	Breakage during arterial injection (causes discolorations)
Loss of cranial hair	
Growth of facial hair and hair on the forehead on women and children	
Creation of resistant strains of microbes	Disinfection treatment more difficult
	Exposure of embalmer to drug-resistant microbes
Cell membranes become less permeable	Creates "solid" edema that cannot be removed
	Makes passage of arterial solution into cell very difficult
Killing one type of microbe can stimulate growth of other types	Antibiotics used to kill bacteria give fungal organisms a chance to multiply
Jaundice	Breakdown of the red blood cell
	Liver failure
Congestive heart failure	Edema
	Drainage difficulties
	Facial discolorations
Scaling of skin (seen on facial tissues and between fingers	Death of the superficial cells
Difficult tissue firming	Protein degeneration
	Ammonia buildup in the tissues which neutralizes formaldehyde
	Presence of edema

Abdominal Surgery. Abdominal surgery on the bowel can result in peritonitis. There can be intense distension of the abdomen and bloodstream infection. These conditions require the use of a strong, well coordinated arterial solution.

Whenever death follows surgery, there exists the potential for leakage from arteries and veins involved in the surgical procedure. The embalmer should use dyes to indicate the distribution of arterial solution. It may be necessary to inject a greater volume of arterial solution to compensate for solution that may be lost to the abdominal or thoracic cavities.

All surgical bodies should undergo thorough cavity treatment. Be certain a liberal amount of undiluted cavity fluid is injected into the area where the surgery was performed. It is also a good precaution to inject some undiluted cavity fluid into the tissues surrounding the surgical incision. This decreases the formation of tissue gas in these tissues. Recent surgical incisions should be sutured before cavity aspiration and injection. It is most important in surgical deaths to reaspirate and possibly reinject the cavities.

Postmortem Interval Between Death and Embalming

The fourth component considered in the preembalming analysis comprises those events that can occur during the postmortem interval between death and embalming. Quite often the conditions that evolve during this period take precedence over the conditions created by disease or drugs or the general conditions of the body.

For example, a person dies of cancer and is very emaciated and jaundiced because of the effects of drugs on the liver, and the body is not discovered in its residence for 2 days. If the weather is warm or a furnace is running, the postmortem changes, such as rigor mortis, stain, and decomposition, will determine the treatments that the embalmer must employ to preserve, sanitize, and restore the body. The embalmer is not concerned with the jaundice (a condition that is also treated with mild arterial solutions).

The overriding factor to be considered is the degree of decomposition present. Bodies that have been dead for long periods and have begun to decompose demand the

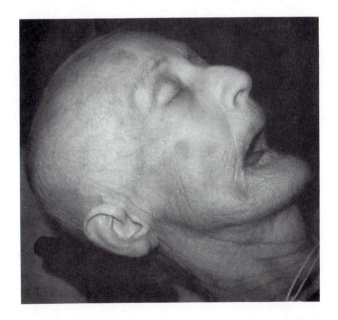

Figure 10–1. Loss of cranial hair but growth of facial hair, and emaciation in this female is the result of extensive chemotherapy.

use of very strong arterial solutions injected in such a manner and quantity as to limit the amount of swelling that easily occurs during injection of such bodies.

There are two aspects to the postmortem interval portion of embalming analysis: an **intrinsic consideration** and an **extrinsic consideration.**

The extrinsic consideration is the period between death and preparation. It also includes the environment surrounding the body during this period. It is always best to embalm as soon after death as possible. Embalming generally proceeds with fewer complications in bodies that still retain some heat than when there has been a protracted delay. The distribution and diffusion of embalming solution generally are much easier to establish when there is little time delay between death and embalming.

Two major postmortem factors that interfere most with good distribution of the arterial solution are rigor mortis and decomposition. Embalming the body before these changes are firmly established in the body helps to produce better results.

If there is to be a delay between death and preparation, refrigeration will help to slow the onset of many postmortem changes. Refrigeration, however, can create its own problems depending on how long it is used. Bodies in a warm environment rapidly undergo early postmortem changes that can create a number of problems for the embalmer. The embalmer must also keep in mind that many bodies released from a coroner or medical examiner's office were kept first in a warm environment—possibly for a long period—then placed under refrigeration. Frequently, these bodies will also be autopsied. Again, at this point, it is the postmortem conditions that have more influence on the selection of embalming technique than the cause of death or medication.

The intrinsic factors of the postmortem interval include those changes that occur within the body during the delay. Table 10–2 summarizes these changes and lists some of the embalming concerns they can create.

EMBALMING ANALYSIS, PART II: INJECTION OF THE BODY

The analysis is a continuous evaluation of the embalming procedure from the start of the embalming procedure until its conclusion. The second part of the analysis is an evaluation of the treatments begun in the preparation of the body. When a problem is encountered the embalmer must decide what new approach to take to solve the problem. The following are some of the concerns of the embalmer:

1. What areas of the body are receiving arterial solution? This can be noted by the presence of fluid dyes in the tissues and the clearing of discolorations such as livor mortis.
2. What areas are not receiving arterial solution?

TABLE 10-2. POSTMORTEM PHYSICAL AND CHEMICAL CHANGES

Change	Embalming Significance
Physical	
Algor mortis	Slows onset of rigor and decomposition
	Keeps blood in a liquid state; aids drainage
Dehydration	Increases the viscosity of the blood; sludge forms
	Partly responsible for postmortem edema; increasing preservative demands
	Darkens surface areas; cannot be bleached
	Eyelids and lids will separate; lips wrinkle; fingers wrinkle
	Could retard decomposition if severe enough
Hypostasis	Responsible for livor mortis and eventual postmortem stain
	Increases tissue moisture in dependent tissue areas
Livor mortis	Varies in intensity from slight redness to black depending on volume and viscosity of the blood
	Intravascular discoloration; can be cleared
	Can be set as a stain if too strong an uncoordinated arterial solution is used
	Keeps capillaries expanded; can work as an aid to distribution
	If it clears *by itself* it could serve as a sign of arterial solution distribution
Increase in blood viscosity	Sludge is created; intravascular resistance
	Postmortem edema can accompany problem
	Blood removal becomes difficult; distribution can be poor
Chemical	
Rigor mortis	Extravascular resistance
	Positioning difficult; features may be hard to pose
	pH not conducive for good fluid reactions
	Tissues swell easily
	False sign of preservation (fixation)
	After passage, firming is difficult
	Decomposition is usually minimal when present
	Increases preservative demand
Decomposition	Color changes; odor present; purges; skin-slip; gases
	Poor distribution of solutions
	Increased preservative demand
	Rapid swelling in affected tissue areas
Postmortem stain	Extravascular; cannot be removed; may be bleached
	Generally seen after the sixth hour; delayed problems
	Increased preservative demand
	False indication of fluid dyes
	Will turn gray after embalming; cosmetic problem
Postmortem caloricity	Sets off the rigor and decomposition cycles
Shift in the body pH	Interferes with fluid reactions
	Dyes can splotch
Hydrolysis	Speeded by heat; sets off rigor and decomposition cycles

Dyes will not be present and livor mortis, if present, will not be cleared; no firmness will be present.

3. What can be done to stimulate the flow of arterial solution into areas not receiving solution?
   A. Massage along the arterial route that supplies fluid to the area.
   B. Increase the pressure of the solution being injected.
   C. Increase the rate of flow of the solution being injected.

D. Lower, raise, or manipulate the body area.
E. Close off the drainage to increase the intravascular pressure.

4. What areas must receive sectional arterial injection? Areas that did not receive solution even after massage and changes in injection protocol must be injected separately.

5. Has the body as a whole received sufficient arterial solution and has the solution been of sufficient strength?
   A. A high-index arterial fluid can be injected or added to the remaining arterial solution to boost the preservative qualities of the solution.
   B. If there is doubt as to the amount of solution, inject additional amounts as long as there is no distension of the neck or facial tissues; inject until preservation is well established.

6. Has sufficient arterial solution been retained by the body? The most important portion of the solution being injected is that which **remains** in the body to preserve the tissues after blood and surface discolorations clear; intermittent drainage can be used to help the tissues retain more embalming solution. It has been estimated that more than 50% of the drainage is arterial solution.

7. Is the arterial solution having too much of a dehydrating effect on the tissues? A humectant coinjection fluid can be added.

8. Should additional fluid dye be added for internal coloring of the tissues? Additional dyes may be added throughout the embalming procedure.

9. If purge begins from the mouth or nose, what is its origin and cause? Let the purge continue during the arterial injection **unless** the purge is arterial solution. If the purge is arterial solution and drainage *continues, inject* additional arterial solution to make up for the preservative lost in the purge. If the purge is arterial solution and there is *no* drainage, it can be assumed there is a major rupture in the vascular system. Evaluate the amount of tissues embalmed and consider multipoint injections.

10. Are the tissues firming? This will depend on several factors; in conditions such as *renal failure, emaciation, edema,* and *wasting degenerative diseases,* firming may be very difficult to establish; poor firming can also be a result of the type of arterial fluid being used (some fluids have a slow firming action and others produce less firming of body tissues). If there is doubt as to the preservative needs of the tissues the arterial solution can be increased in strength either by preparing a new solution using a higher-index fluid or by using more concentrated fluid per gallon. A high-index fluid can be added to boost the strength of the solution being injected.

TO INCREASE ARTERIAL SOLUTION STRENGTH

1. Prepare a solution using a higher-index arterial fluid.
2. Add a higher-index arterial fluid to the present solution.
3. Add more concentrated arterial fluid to the present solution.

These are some of the items the embalmer evaluates during arterial injection and drainage of the body in this second phase of an analysis.

EMBALMING ANALYSIS, PART III: EVALUATION OF THE BODY AFTER ARTERIAL EMBALMING

The third phase of the analysis comprises evaluation of the body after the arterial solution and multipoint injections have been completed. Areas that are still lacking solution must now be treated by hypodermic injection or by surface embalming. Some of the following considerations are evaluated during this third phase of the analysis:

1. What body areas have not received arterial solution after primary and multipoint injections are completed?
   A. Look for the absence of fluid dyes, little or no firming of the tissues, and the presence of intravascular discolorations.
   B. Treatment now must be hypodermic injection of the area or surface embalming or a combination of both.

2. Should cavity embalming be done immediately after arterial injection or delayed several hours?
   A. This may depend on the time at which the body must be ready for viewing.
   B. In thin, emaciated bodies, an attempt may have been made to fill out the tissues with a humectant–restorative coinjection; this chemical should be given time to ensure the tissues are firmed before aspiration is done.
   C. If a body is dead from an infectious or contagious disease the embalmer may wish to delay aspiration to help ensure that any blood removed in the aspirated material will have time to mix with the arterial solution injected. With these bodies some embalmers inject a bottle of cavity fluid and wait several hours *before* aspirating; this helps to ensure disinfection of the aspirated materials.

3. Are the features set properly?
   A. Be certain that the mouth is dry. Remove moist cotton and replace it with dry cotton if purge developed during embalming or if moisture

leaked from the method of mouth closure where the skin was broken.

B. Lips and eyelids must not be moist if they are to be glued.

C. If the eyelids seem soft, cotton can be used for eye closure, and a drop of cavity fluid can be placed on the cotton to make an internal compress before adhesive is applied to the eyelids.

D. If residual air is present in the mouth after gluing, the lips can be cracked open or limited aspiration of the thorax can be done to remove the air.

4. What if purge developed during embalming?

A. Be certain the nose is tightly repacked and the mouth has been dried of any purge material.

B. Purge may be aspirated from the throat and nasal passages using a nasal tube aspirator.

C. Anal purge can be corrected after cavity embalming; force as much of the fecal material from the orifice; pack the anal orifice with cotton saturated with cavity fluid, phenol cautery fluid, or a chemical solution used for treatment of skin lesions. It may be necessary to use a pursestring suture around the anal orifice to ensure no further purge. Pants and coveralls or a diaper can be used to protect clothing from any further purge.

5. Is the body well groomed? Nails and hands should be cleaned, hands cupped, and fingers together.

6. Are the body and hair clean and dried? The body must be turned on its side to check for clots or debris that were not cleaned away. Turning the body allows it to be dried on all sides.

7. Have decubitus ulcerations been treated? Compresses should be removed from decubitus ulcerations or skin lesions and replaced with clean compresses and fresh chemical or embalming powder. Plastic stockings, pants, or coveralls can be placed on the body to hold the compresses in position.

8. Is there any leakage? Intravenous line punctures leak after arterial injection and even after cavity embalming. They should be properly sealed with a trocar button or super adhesive.

9. Are tracheotomy and colostomy openings closed? A pursestring suture can be used to close these openings. They should be packed with a cautery chemical and cotton. The tracheotomy can also be filled with some incision seal powder. These openings should be covered with glue and cotton after the suturing is completed.

10. Are incisions sutured? Sutures should be tight and not leaking. If leakage is present the sutures should be removed and the incision resutured.

These 10 items represent the type of evaluation necessary during the third and final stage of embalming analysis.

TREATMENTS

Embalming analysis ⟶ Treatments

The purpose of the analysis is to gather the information necessary to make the correct choices in treating

TABLE 10–3. EMBALMING TECHNIQUE VARIABLES

Description	Variation
Setting of features	Before embalming, during embalming, after embalming
Method of mouth closure	Needle injector, muscular suture, mandibular suture, dental tie
Method of denture replacement	Cotton, mouth former, kapoc, "pose" material
Method of eye closure	Cotton, eyecaps
Time for raising vessels	Before setting features, after setting features
Artery for primary injection	Right common carotid, right femoral, right axillary
Vein for drainage	Right internal jugular, right femoral, right axillary, heart
Method of injection/drainage	Single point, split injection, restricted cervical, six-point
Method of drainage	Continuous, intermittent, alternate
Drainage instrument	Drainage tube, angular spring forceps, trocar for heart drainage
Body treated with preinjection	Used, not used
Arterial fluid strength	Low index, medium index, high index
Arterial solution injected	Mild fluid solution, moderate fluid solution, strong solution
Coinjection fluid	Used, not used
Fluid dye	Used, not used
Fluid dye color	Pink, tan
Use of fluid dye	Mixed with all solution used, used only in last gallon of solution
Humectant coinjection	Used, not used
Time usage of humectant	Used in all solutions, used in final gallon only
Arterial solution strength	Same used for all solutions injected, mild followed by stronger
Pressure for injection	Low (2–10 pounds), medium (10–20 pounds), high (20 or more pounds)
Rate of flow	Very slow (5–10 ounces), medium (10–15 ounces), fast (more than 15 ounces)
Change of pressure	Not changed during injection, begin low then increase
Change of rate of flow	Not changed during injection, begin slow then increase
Volume of solution injected	Based on weight, edema, time dead, firming of tissues, other
Method of aspiration	Hydroaspirator, electric aspirator, air pressure
Time of aspiration	Immediately after arterial injection, delayed
Reaspiration	Performed, not performed
Method of trocar closure	Trocar button, sutured
Method of cavity fluid injection	Gravity injector, via embalming machine
Cavity fluid reinjected	Done, not done, done only if gases are present
Signs of fluid distribution	Fluid dye, clearing of livor, firming, combinations
Features glued after embalming	Performed, not performed
Type of glue used for features	Rubber-based glue, super glue
Treatment for lack of fluid	Local arterial injection, surface compress, hypodermic injection

the conditions observed. Through analysis of the body during and after arterial injection, the progress of the treatments is evaluated. If the treatments are not working, then new decisions and plans must be made.

Table 10–3 is by no means complete, but serves to illustrate some of the variables considered by the embalmer in choosing treatments to achieve good sanitation, preservation, and restoration of the body.

COMBINING BODY CONDITIONS AND EMBALMING TREATMENTS

Table 10–4 combines the embalming conditions often observed and of utmost concern to the embalmer. Again, as specific chemicals cannot be listed, a "general" treatment is described. This list combines the two major parts of an analysis: (1) observation of body conditions and (2) planning of treatment.

TABLE 10–4. BODY CONDITIONS AND EMBALMING TREATMENTS

Condition	Treatment
Normal body; some livor; dead less than 6 hours; no edema; no chemotherapy	Any vessel for injection and drainage, preinjection; mild to moderate solutions (3–5 gallons, will vary with body size); set tissue to desired firmness
Extensive livor of facial areas; dead less than 6 hours; no extreme pathology	Clear discolorations with a mild to moderate solution; jugular and common carotid recommended; step-up strength to set to desired firmness
Postmortem stain present; body in or out of rigor; dead more than 6 hours	Begin with strong coordinated arterial solutions; continue to increase after circulation is established; restricted cervical injection; slow injection; dye for tracer; section injection where needed; hypodermic and surface treatments where needed
Decomposition evident	Restricted cervical injection; strong coordinated solutions; dye for tracer; sectional/hypodermic and surface treatments where needed
Bodies refrigerated more than 12 hours; some rigor; livor	Solution stronger than average; avoid preinjection; dye tracer; circulation problems expected; restricted cervical injection
Jaundice; no edema; yellow	Jaundice fluid; mild solutions (however, must meet preservative demands); femoral vessels if possible, may respond to preinjection; dye for counterstain
Jaundice green	Cannot be cleared; solution strength based on preservative demands; plenty of dye to counterstain
Generalized edema of body	Start with solution a little above normal strength; continue to increase; if circulation should be poor increase to very strong solutions
Localized edema	Treat general embalming based on condition of the tissues; separate sectional embalming of area with edema; hypodermic and surface treatments
Extravascular discolorations from chemotherapy or pathology	Use solutions based on size of body, length of time dead, etc.; treat the discoloration when on hands and face with hypodermic and surface treatments
Autopsied; dead less than 12 hours	Moderate solutions; increase if needed to achieve desired firmness
Autopsied; dead more than 12 hours; refrigerated	Solutions stronger than normal; dyes for tracing; restricted drainage to help achieve circulation; higher pressure may be needed
Death from second-degree burns	Begin with strong solutions; use dye for tracer; death will be related to uremia; may need 100% fluid; do same if autopsied
Localized gangrene/ischemia/possible diabetic	Strong solutions when circulation problems are anticipated; bacterial complications can exist in these bodies; hypodermic/sectional and surface treatments to areas affected; dye for arterial tracing
Frozen bodies	Strong solutions; dye for tracer; restricted cervical
Emaciated with edema	Mild to strong solutions depending on circulation (it should be good); again if edema is localized, sectional embalming
Emaciated	Mild solutions in large volume; add humectants to last injection; restricted drainage
Generalized edema with jaundice	Always treat for preservation first; moderate to strong solutions; dye for tracer; inject until edema is treated
Trauma of face/black eyes/ lacerations/restorative work needed	Restricted cervical injection if not autopsied; strong solutions; dye for tracer
Infants/children with no pathological complications	Vessels (iliac/carotid/aorta) if not autopsied; standard arterial fluid; inject strength and volume as needed; based on weight and body conditions; dye for tracing
Dehydrated bodies not dead very long	Mild solutions; restricted drainage; humectants in last injection
Bodies with chemotherapy, some edema; skin hemorrhage; expect fixation problems	Use restricted cervical injection; strong solutions into trunk areas; dye for tracing; may help force fluid into tissue spaces
Eye enucleation/no other remarks	To control solution entering head use restricted cervical injection when body not autopsied; use a stronger than normal solution; do not preinject
Contagious disease	Use solutions a little stronger than normal (2–3%); run plenty of volume; avoid personal contact with "first" drainage; run volume and increased strengths depending on other body conditions, i.e., weight/edema
Obese	Begin with a slightly stronger than normal solution; after blood discolorations clear, strength may continue to be increased; first vessel choice common carotid/jugular; second choice external iliac
Arteriosclerosis noticed when raising a common carotid	Stronger than normal solutions; high pulsating pressure; dye for tracer; sectional; hypodermic and surface treatments
Arteriosclerosis seen when raising femoral as first vessel	Go to common carotid and jugular; use a solution a little stronger than normal; inject based on other body conditions

SOME GENERALIZATIONS

Whenver it is felt that circulation is going to be a problem because of pathology (arteriosclerosis), time delay since death, and other factors, the first choice should be the common carotid artery and internal jugular vein.

If the preceding conditions exist and it is necessary to run large volumes of solution or very strong solutions into the trunk regions, use the restricted cervical injection.

Whenever facial or neck swelling is anticipated or observed, use the restricted cervical injection.

After injecting a strong solution never inject weaker solutions into the same area; always inject *mild solutions* first, after which *stronger solutions* can be injected.

After livor and other intravascular discolorations are cleared, the best response is obtained with average or mild solution. After intravascular discolorations are cleared, solution strengths can be increased. At this time, some form of restricted drainage can be safely used (e.g., intermittent or alternate drainage).

KEY TERMS AND CONCEPTS FOR STUDY AND DISCUSSION

1. Define embalming analysis, intrinsic factors, and extrinsic factors.
2. List the three time periods of embalming analysis.
3. Explain the purpose of embalming analysis.
4. Describe the four categories of information used in embalming analysis.
5. Give a brief description of Slocum's six body classifications used in a preembalming analysis.
6. Discuss why the conditions present in the body are more important in an embalming analysis than the actual cause of death.
7. List several effects brought about by long-term drug therapy.
8. List postmortem physical changes and chemical changes.

BIBLIOGRAPHY

Chemotherapy and embalming results. In: *Champion Expanding Encyclopedia*. Springfield, OH: Champion Chemical; 1986:No. 570.

Frederick JF. *Effects of Chemotherapeutic Agents.* Boston: Dodge Chemical; 1968.

Shor M. Knowledge of effect of disease simplifies embalming. *Casket and Sunnyside,* September 1960.

Shor M. Conditions of the body dictate the proper embalming treatment. *Casket and Sunnyside,* November 1972.

Slocum RE. *Pre-embalming Considerations.* Boston: MA: Dodge Chemical, 1958.

11

Preparation of the Body Prior to Arterial Injection

The process of embalming the dead human body can be divided into three time periods, each containing procedures that are best performed within the specified period. The primary reason is that the preservative fluid used for embalming contains formaldehyde, and formaldehyde coagulates the proteins of the body. This coagulation (or preservation) of body protein brings about a firming and drying of the body tissues. Once set in a particular position the tissues are difficult to change.

Three time periods are described:

Preembalming   Period prior to injection of the arterial solution

Embalming   Period during which arterial solution is injected into the body

Postembalming   Period after arterial injection

In each period specific procedures are carried out. They all culminate in the complete embalmed body. In Chapter 1, complete chronologies for embalming autopsied and unautopsied bodies are detailed.

Analysis of the body is performed during each period. The treatments discussed in this chapter are based on the analysis made by the embalmer from his or her first observations of the body (pp. 23–25).

It is important that the student be aware that many procedures carried out in the preembalming period can be performed during the embalming or postembalming period. Because of the fixative and hardening action of the preservative solution, preembalming procedures such as shaving the body, setting the features, and aligning broken skin areas and bones can be done with greater ease prior to injection of the fixative arterial solution.

Body conditions and the skill of the operator may influence the period during which certain procedures are performed. For example, decomposition and the presence of stomach or lung purge may dictate that the mouth be closed after arterial embalming, once the cavity aspiration has been completed. Likewise, the mouth is usually sealed with an adhesive in the postembalming period but, if there is a problem of "buck" teeth, it may be necessary to glue the lips prior to injection of the arterial solution to achieve good mouth closure. The embalmer must learn to be flexible in technique, relying on the conditions of the body to dictate the order of embalming procedures.

An important reason for minimizing the procedures carried out during the period of arterial injection is that the embalmer should devote full attention to observation of solution distribution and drainage during injection of the embalming solution. Attention should be given to drainage problems and techniques to improve arterial solution circulation to all body areas. During the injection phase of embalming it is very important for the embalmer to employ as many techniques as possible to ensure **retention** of the arterial solution (Fig. 11–1).

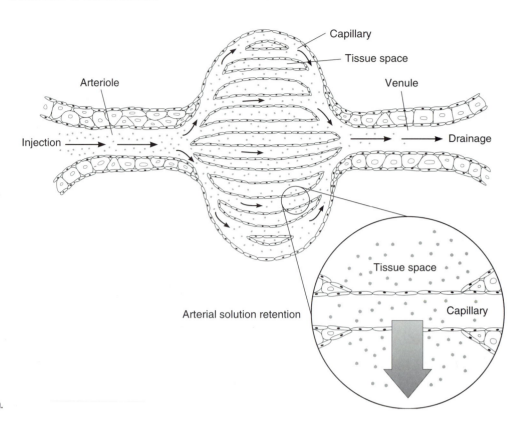

Figure 11–1. Arterial solution retention.

LEGAL REQUIREMENTS

Before the embalming process begins, it is important that the embalmer verifies with the funeral director to make certain that permission has been given for embalming the body. Many states require that permission be given in writing or by verbal order by the person in charge of final disposition. In addition, the Federal Trade Commission requires specific disclosures to the person arranging the funeral as to the price for embalming services and statements as to when embalming is not necessary for final disposition. Before any embalming is begun, it is imperative that the embalmer be certain permission has been given for preparation of the deceased.

PRELIMINARY PREPARATION

The embalming process begins when the deceased is placed on the middle of the embalming table. The body should be temporarily centered on the table with the head as near as possible to the upper end of the table.

Any clothing, sheeting, or body bag should be sprayed with a disinfectant. This helps to control vermin and odors. Standing at the side of the embalming table, the embalmer can gently roll the body toward him* by placing his hands on the shoulder and the hip of the deceased (Fig. 11–2A). After the body is slightly turned, the sheets may be pushed beneath the center of the body. (This is also a way to remove clothing.) Next, the embalmer rolls the body back to the supine position. He moves to the opposite side of the body, repeats the rolling process, and, thus, removes the sheeting that enveloped the body (see Chapter 2).

In moving a wrapped body the embalmer should always *pull* the body and not *push* it. For example, transfer of the body from the removal cot to the embalming table can be accomplished in three steps: (1) Place the removal cot next to the embalming table. (2) Stand on the opposite side of the embalming table and reach across the table to the deceased on the removal cot. (3) Pull the legs of the deceased onto the table first; then pull the portions of the sheet that envelop the trunk and shoulders (Fig. 11–2B).

It is easier to position the body on the embalming table while the deceased is wrapped or partially clothed. After clothes have been removed, the deceased can be

---

*As the traditional use of the pronoun *he* has not yet been superseded by a convenient, generally accepted pronoun that means either "he" or "she," the author will continue to use he while acknowledging the inherent inequity of the traditional preference for the masculine pronoun.

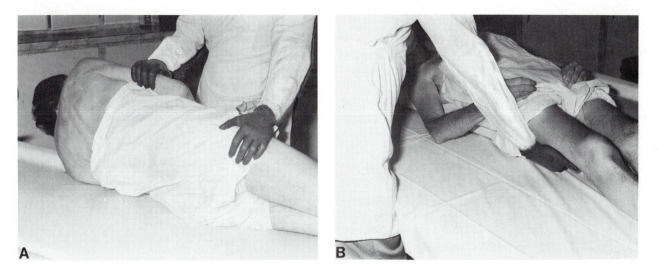

Figure 11–2. **A.** Turn the body by gripping the shoulder (upper arm) and the hip. **B.** The embalmer can easily move a body by placing one hand under the neck and one under the thigh and pulling the body toward him or her.

moved more easily if the embalming table is moistened with water. Clothing should be removed without cutting whenever possible, labeled and properly stored for dry cleaning, and returned to the family. Very soiled clothing and underclothing should be disposed of in a sanitary manner. All clothing should be checked for valuables. Rings, jewelry, and other valuables should be inventoried and securely stored until they can be returned to the family. Some embalmers protect rings on the deceased by placing adhesive tape around the ring finger. Others prefer to place a piece of string or gauze around the ring if it is to be left on the body during embalming. Glasses, jewelry, watches, and religious articles should be removed during embalming.

TOPICAL DISINFECTION OF THE BODY

After the sheeting or clothing has been removed and the body is placed in the center of the table, the surface and orifices of the body are treated with a topical disinfectant.[†] A good surface disinfectant should be used and should be either washed or sprayed onto the body. A droplet-type spray is preferred over pressurized sprays, which lose too much of the disinfectant to the surrounding air and can then be inhaled by the embalmer. Pressurized sprays also have the tendency to convert surface microbes on the body into airborne microbes. The surface disinfectant should be allowed to remain on the body several minutes. After topical disinfection, the body should be thoroughly washed with lukewarm water and

a good germicidal soap. The orifices should be cleaned and packed with cotton and the body dried.

QUALITIES OF A GOOD TOPICAL DISINFECTANT

1. It is active, not outdated.
2. It is effective against a wide range of microbes including viruses and fungi.
3. It destroys microbes and their products quickly.
4. It is a good deodorant for the body.
5. It does not bleach or stain the skin.
6. It is not irritating to the embalmer's skin or respiratory tract.

When sodium hypochlorite is used, it is important that the chemical be washed away with water before any contact is made with formaldehyde. Sodium hypochlorite and formaldehyde can combine to produce a carcinogenic product.

Disinfection of the body should also include the destruction of body lice or mites (scabies). If scabies is suspected, a commercial pediculicide should be applied to the skin and hair of the deceased. The embalmer should carefully handle these bodies so that the insects do not infest his skin. The embalmer should also carefully check for fly eggs or maggots, especially in the summer months or in warm climates. Fly eggs appear as yellowish clusters in the corners of the eyes, nostrils, or ears or within the mouth. If present, these eggs can develop into the eating larval stage known as maggots in 24 hours. Great

---

[†]Disinfectants are discussed in detail in Chapter 3.

care should be taken to remove all eggs. If the larval stage has begun, a larvicide can be used. Some success is achieved by flushing the affected area with kerosene, concentrated salt water, or a commercial mortuary product.

Maggots eat even embalmed tissue, so it is very important to remove and destroy them. To prevent flies from depositing eggs, keep the body covered. Nostrils can be packed in the summer months and small pieces of cotton can be placed in the nostrils (extending outside the nostril) when the body is left in the preparation room or is shipped. In the summer months, some funeral homes make a habit of covering the face of the body at night. Outside windows and doors of the preparation room should be screened. In addition, insecticides should be used if flies are present in the preparation room. Once fly eggs develop into the larval stage, the problem becomes very difficult, if not impossible, to control.

WASHING THE BODY

The body should be thoroughly washed with warm water and a germicidal soap. Special attention should be given to the areas to be viewed—the face and hands. These areas must be free of all debris for good cosmetic application after the embalming. If the skin of the hands, particularly between the fingers, is scaly, a solvent such as a dry hair shampoo or trichloroethylene can be used to remove the scaling skin. This condition can also be found on the forehead and parts of the face. This scale must be removed if cosmetics are to be applied. It is also useful to apply massage cream to these areas and wipe the cream away with a cloth after it has been worked into the pores of the skin. After thorough washing and rinsing, the body should be dried with toweling. Use disposable items in these procedures, for they can be destroyed and will not have to be laundered. Manipulation during washing and drying the body also helps to relieve rigor mortis.

The fingernails should be cleaned using soap, water, and a nail brush in the preembalming period. It is much easier to remove debris from under the nails at this time (use great care if an instrument is used to clean the nails). Any stains on the fingers or the nails can be removed with a solvent. Nail polish can be removed with a commercial remover or acetone. Trimming and brushing the nails greatly help to clean the fingers and nails.

CARING FOR THE HAIR

The hair can be washed at the beginning and at the end of embalming. Note the following points:

1. Wash the hair with warm water and a good germicidal soap; a commercial shampoo may also be used.
2. Washing the hair should deodorize the hair.
3. Hair rinses may be used to help untangle long hair. These products usually assist in deodorizing and styling the hair.
4. Blow-drying the hair helps to style the hair, for both men and women.
5. When in doubt as to styling the hair, comb or brush it straight back.
6. When hair is very thin and has a tendency to fall out, dry it before combing or brushing and avoid as much brushing or combing as possible.
7. Use cool water to remove blood from the hair.
8. If lice or mites are suspected, apply a commercial pediculicide before washing. Follow instructions for the use of this chemical.
9. When dandruff or scaling of the skin is present (often seen when therapeutic drugs have been used for longer periods), several washings may be necessary. The hair can also be washed with the "dry wash" solvent shampoos.
10. Do not comb curly hair when wet; knead the hair with a towel while blow-drying. This helps to retain the curl.
11. Plats should be combed out prior to shampooing.

SHAVING THE BODY

After topically disinfecting the body, washing and drying the hair and body surfaces, packing the mouth and nasal orifices, and temporarily positioning the body, the embalmer can shave the body. Facial hair should be removed from all bodies (men, women, and children). The nostrils should also be trimmed at this time. Shaving the body not only improves the appearance of the deceased but greatly assists in the application of cosmetics to facial tissues. If hair were to remain on the face, cosmetics (whether creams, liquids, or powders) would stick to the hair, making the appearance of the deceased quite unnatural.

The embalmer should check with the family with respect to a mustache or beard on a deceased male. It is much easier to remove a mustache or beard before arterial injection. Their removal when the family did not want them removed could create a legal problem for the funeral home. If there is doubt about shaving and the family cannot be consulted, embalm the body and shave later. This process is more difficult, but it is much easier to shave the body after embalming than restore a beard or mustache.

The administration of therapeutic drugs often induces growth of facial hair on females and children. Drug

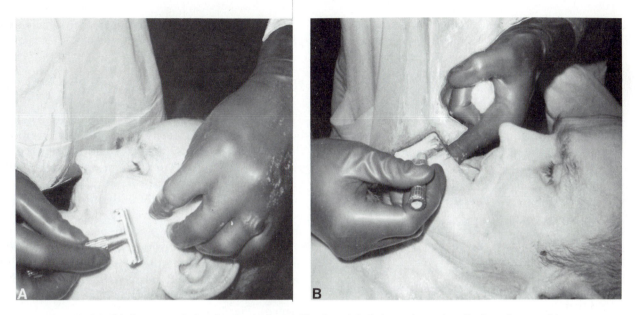

Figure 11–3. **A.** Slide the razor over the face, shaving in the direction of beard growth. **B.** The best results are achieved by shaving from several directions.

therapy can also induce hair growth on the forehead. In women and children, this facial hair is easily removed by lightly passing a safety razor over the facial tissues. Lather is not always necessary to remove this light growth. Shaving the forehead can be very difficult. Shaving lather should be applied and great care taken not to nick the skin. After shaving the forehead areas apply massage cream.

Note the following points in shaving the face:

1. Use a good, sharp blade; more than one blade may be needed to shave some bodies.
2. Use a double-edged safety razor, single stainless razor or straight edge.
3. Apply warm water to the face with a washcloth first.
4. Use shaving cream to lather the face.
5. When there is doubt about the length of side-burns, mustache, or beard, consult the family. If they cannot be reached, these areas can always be shaved after arterial embalming.
6. When using a new blade, it is wise to begin shaving on the left side of the face or in the neck area to slightly dull the blade.
7. Shave in the direction of hair growth; bodies vary, and sometimes shaving must be directed against or perpendicular to the growth.
8. Use small, short, repeated strokes over an area to achieve the closest shave; an area can be shaved repeatedly or (as stated in item 7) from one or several different directions (Fig. 11–3).
9. Clean the razor frequently with warm water.
10. Try to shave an area without lifting the razor off the face; apply pressure on the razor and "slide" the razor over the area being shaved.

11. Use a small piece of cotton or washcloth (gauze or cheesecloth) to pull the skin taut and make an even area for shaving; this is helpful in shaving the area immediately under the mandible and the upper neck area.
12. After shaving, wash the face with a washcloth and warm water; a thin layer of massage cream may be applied.

Razor abrasions are areas of the face where small pieces of flesh have been removed. Application of massage cream helps to prevent the area from dehydrating and turning brown. During arterial injection, arterial solution may leak through these nicked areas. It is important that a very small piece of wax be placed over these areas after cosmetics have been applied. This prevents the areas from further drying and showing through the cosmetic, especially when alcohol-type transparent cosmetics are used. If the area of the face that has been nicked is discolored and the face is to be treated with opaque cosmetics, use either cream or liquid opaque cover cosmetics. The massage cream can be omitted, for the opaque cosmetic needs dry skin free of any grease products for application.

If a beard or mustache or the face in general must be shaved after arterial injection, lather the face with a very moist, warm lather. Use a sharp, new blade in the razor. To avoid nicking the tissue, shave in small areas and keep applying lather to the area being shaved. When completed, apply a thin film of massage cream.*

---

*Shaving with an electric razor after vascular embalming and over a dry face is effectively used by some embalmers.

In shaving a beard, many embalmers first trim off the longer hair of the beard with shears or hair clippers. This process is not necessary; the beard can be shaved without the preliminary clipping. Shaving should be directed from the cheek areas downward over the face. Heavy growth may necessitate the use of several blades.

After the body has been shaved, massage cream may be applied. Some embalmers prefer that a light application of this cream be made after the features are set; others prefer to apply massage cream after embalming; some do not apply cream at all because of the type of cosmetic they will use. Massage cream has several uses:

1. It protects the face and hands from surface dehydration.
2. It prevents broken skin areas such as razor abrasions from dehydrating and turning dark brown.
3. It acts as a lubricant when the face is massaged to break up rigor mortis.
4. It is an excellent skin cleanser.
5. It provides a lubricating base that can be used for massaging the facial tissues, neck, and hands during arterial injection.
6. It protects areas of the face from damage if stomach purge from the mouth or nose occurs.
7. It provides a base for cream cosmetics.

There are two types of massage creams. One, the type generally sold by mortuary companies, has a greasy feel. The second is a face or hand cream that has a water base. After application, the cream can hardly be felt. The grease type may be more useful if the embalmer requires massage cream for use with mortuary cosmetics. In addition to creams that can be applied by hand, several spray antidehydrants are available; these are basically silicone or lanolin sprays. Whether a cream or spray, it need not be applied heavily. A very small amount adequately serves to protect the skin areas to which it is applied.

POSITIONING THE BODY

The objective of preembalming positioning is to make the body appear comfortable and restful in later repose in the casket. Preservative arterial solution firms the body proteins of the muscles in the position in which the embalmer places the body prior to arterial embalming. It is very difficult to reposition the body after embalming. The position of the body as it rests on the embalming table should approximate the desired position of the body when casketed. Three position levels are desired: (1) the highest level should be the head, (2) the middle level should be the ventral thoracic wall (chest), and (3) the lowest level should be the ventral abdominal wall (abdomen) (Fig. 11–4).

In addition to positioning the trunk of the body, the embalmer needs to properly position the arms, hands, legs, and feet (Fig. 11–5). The feet should be placed as close together as possible. During the embalming process, some embalmers prefer not only to place the feet together but also to elevate them. At this time, note should be made of any unusual size problems. If the body is quite obese the straight distance between the elbows should be measured. It is important with overweight bodies to position the arms so that the elbows are as close as possible to the upper area of the abdominal wall. This can save inches in the casket. Using an urn-shaped or oversized casket or turning the body slightly when it is placed into the casket will help to position these heavy bodies in the casket.

If length is a problem, an oversized casket should be ordered. Keeping the feet together and flexing the toes

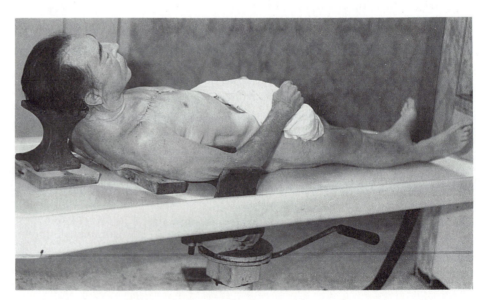

Figure 11–4. The three levels of position: head, chest, and abdomen.

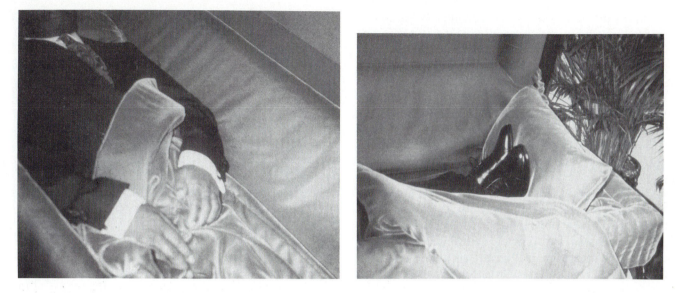

Figure 11–5. **A.** One pose in which hands, arms, and the blanket may be positioned. **B.** Straight legs and feet allow shoes to be shown, resting on the casket foot pillow.

save a little space. Flexing the legs as well as omitting shoes may also help. Oversized caskets may mean that an oversized vault is needed or that the casket cannot be placed in a crypt or a shipping container. In positioning the body, every effort should be made to use a standard-sized casket.

Caskets are available in the following dimensions:

METAL	Standard	6 ft 7 in. × 24 in.
	Oversized	6 ft 9 in. × 26 in.
		× 28 in.
		× 31 in.
WOOD	Standard	6 ft 3 in. × 22 in.
	Oversized	6 ft 6 in. × 24 in.
		× 26 in.
		× 28 in.

The body should be undressed, treated with a topical disinfectant, then washed and dried. The embalmer manipulates the limbs while undressing, washing, and drying the body to relieve rigor mortis if present. Rigor mortis may be responsible for the body being in a very undesirable position. It is necessary to remove the rigor by firmly manipulating the muscles.

When limbs are *flexed, rotated, bent,* and *massaged* to relieve rigor, capillaries are torn. This can lead to swelling during arterial injection and is one reason many embalmers do not attempt to relieve rigor. Avoid excessive exercise of the muscles in relieving rigor mortis. Breaking the rigor helps not only in positioning the body but also in removing extravascular resistance in the circulatory system. Relief of the rigor may result in better arterial solution distribution and also better drainage. A routine proposed for relieving rigor mortis follows:

1. Firmly rotate the neck from side to side.
2. Flex the head.
3. Push the lower jaw up to begin to relieve the rigor in the muscles of the jaw. Repeat this several times. If the mouth is firmly closed begin by pushing the mandible upward; then firmly push on the chin to attempt to open the mouth. Massage the temporalis and the masseter muscles on the side of the face. This may help open the mouth.
4. Flex the arm several times, then extend it. Finally, rotate the arm at the shoulder.
5. Grasp the fingers as a group on the palm side of the hand and attempt to extend all the fingers at the same time.
6. Grasp the foot and rotate it inward. Repeat several times. Attempt to flex the legs at the knee. Raise and lower the legs several times.

The body should be placed in a supine position in the center of the embalming table with the head located near the top of the table. This position allows adequate room for positioning devices for the head and arms. The carotid vessels can then be raised by the embalmer standing at the head of the table, the hair can be treated by the embalmer or hairdresser, and, if the table is "ribbed," water run on the table is kept off the body.

Establish the levels of positioning. Rest the buttocks on the table to establish the abdominal level. Next, place supports under the shoulders. Supports promote drainage from the head and neck areas and help relieve pressure on the internal jugular veins should the head be elevated too much. A variety of positioning devices can be used for shoulder supports. Some embalmers prefer that the support elevate the shoulders as much as 4 inches off the table. Additional head support would then be needed for the head rest. The chest and head are so elevated to prevent blood that remains in the heart after embalming from gravitating into the neck and facial tissues and graying these tissues. This discoloration is often referred to as **formaldehyde gray.**

Elevating the shoulders also helps to dry the body, for air can easily pass under a large area of the back. This elevation helps to keep any water on the table from contacting the skin of the back and the neck. It is easier to clean under the body. If the body is obese, a higher shoulder elevation will be needed to establish the three levels of positioning by raising the head and chest above the abdomen. In positioning the obese body, the higher shoulder support allows the embalmer to slightly lower the height of the head. By doing so, the chin can be pushed forward and thus elevated, creating some visible neck area. The neck will appear a little thinner when the chin is pushed upward.

Good elevation of the head and shoulders can also be very important in draining edema from the tissues of the face and neck. At the conclusion of the aspiration phase of cavity embalming as an **operative aid,** a trocar can be passed under the clavicles channeling the neck tissues; this establishes routes for the drainage of edema into the thoracic cavity. As a **manual aid,** a pneumatic cuff or elastic bandage can be applied to the external tissues of the neck to assist in the removal of edema (or swollen tissues).

Shoulders are elevated to (1) assist drainage, (2) keep water off larger areas of the back and shoulders, (3) prevent gravitation of blood into facial tissues after embalming, (4) assist in drying the body by allowing air to pass beneath the body, (5) assist in draining edema from the facial and neck tissues, and (6) position the head and chest higher than the abdomen.

If a problem should arise because of crippling of the limbs (the body cannot lie in an even supine position), a head block can be placed under one of the upper thighs (Fig. 11–6). This block prevents the body from turning from side to side. If placed under the left thigh, the block assists in turning the entire body slightly to the right.

POSITIONING THE HEAD

The head is adjusted on the headrest *after* the shoulders have been elevated. If the shoulders had to be elevated greatly, the headrest will need additional elevation. Placing a folded towel between the head and the headrest may be sufficient to elevate the head to the desired position. The head should be slightly tilted to the right about 15°. In some localities, the head is positioned straight without any turn. Custom, of course, dictates such protocol.

With obese persons the chin should be slightly elevated. This makes the neck look a little thinner and some-

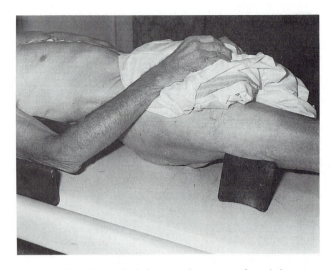

Figure 11–6. Blocking the thigh assists in the positioning of some bodies.

what visible. In positioning obese persons it may be helpful to leave the head straight. Turning the head can make the neck and jowl area look swollen and distended. Elevating the left shoulder in the casket turns the entire body slightly to the right. Should there be disfiguration on the left side of the face or if some of the hair has had to be shaved for surgical purposes, leaving the head straight can help to keep these problems from being seen.

If a kneeler is to be used during viewing of the body it should be placed in line with the shoulders. Viewers thus will see the profile of the body and, in particular, only the right side of the face. If the kneeler is placed at the center of the casket, both sides of the face can be seen (bilateral view). Any disfigurement on the left side of the face or any swelling of the face is more easily observed. In some areas of the country a "full-couch" casket is used. Should there be a disfigurement on the right side of the face, the "full-couch" casket allows the body to be turned so the left side of the face is viewed. A reverse-cap or special ordering makes it also possible to reverse the body in the half-couch casket.

POSITIONING THE HANDS AND ARMS

Prior to the start of the injection of arterial solution, the hands should be placed on the embalming table or even lowered over the table. This forces the blood in the veins of the arms to gravitate into the capillaries of the hands and may expand these tiny vessels. Once the embalmer sees that fluid is being distributed into the arms and hands, he can elevate the hands and place them on the abdominal wall. The elbows should be elevated off the embalming table with either a head block or an arm positioning device. Raising the elbows prevents them from interfering with drainage of blood or water that may be passing along the drains on either side of the table. The

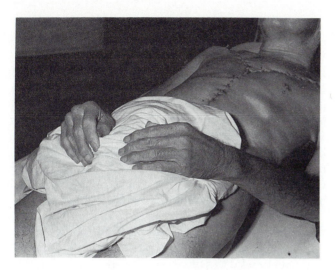

Figure 11–7. A sheet or towel can help in positioning hands and fingers.

elbows should be kept close to the sides of the body. This is very important in obese bodies. It may mean that an oversized casket will not have to be used.

Custom again dictates the position in which the hands should be placed. To help hold the hands in a cupped position and in proper place during embalming, a sheet or large towel can be mounded and the hands placed on top (Fig. 11–7).

Care should be taken to ensure that the fingers remain together (do not separate) and are slightly cupped. A large ball of cotton can be placed in the palm to cup the fingers, and masking tape or gauze can be used to keep fingers together during embalming. A drop of super adhesive between the fingers may be valuable in keeping fingers together.

POSITIONING PROBLEMS

A stroke, paralytic condition, or arthritis may contribute to distorted positions of the extremities (Fig. 11–8). Often the arms are drawn up on the chest and the hands are tightly clenched. In addition, there may be severe spinal curvature. When the spine is curved extra elevation of the head is necessary. A head block placed under a thigh helps to keep the body level. It may even be necessary to place straps around the body and table to hold the body in the correct position. Limbs can be gently forced, but if it appears that ligaments or skin wil be torn, leave the limbs in their position.

A **manual aid,** such as splinting and wrapping a limb, can be used to position a limb. The **operative aid** of cutting tendons should only be used when absolutely necessary. When the legs are drawn up, as in the fetal position, injection and drainage may be accomplished from the carotid location. Every attempt should be made to obtain good solution distribution, so the iliac or femoral vessels do not have to be raised and injected. After casketing, disfigured arthritic hands can be partly hidden from view by placing the casket blanket around the hands. This procedure and how they will be handled should be explained to the family prior to viewing.

Autopsied bodies present several positioning problems. If the spine is removed, it is very difficult, but very necessary, to place a shoulder block beneath the shoulders. The neck and shoulder have to be lifted to place the support under the shoulders. Some embalmers force a pointed wooden dowel into the foramen magnum at the base of the skull. This dowel extends down into the spinal

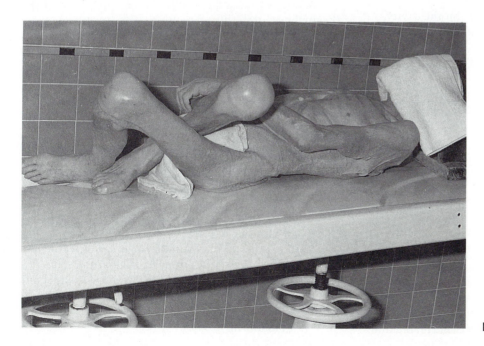

Figure 11–8. Severe arthritis of the lower limbs.

area of the neck and prevents the head from easily turning from side to side. Once the body is casketed, a wedge of cotton can be placed under the ear to help hold the head in proper position. Rigor mortis may or may not be present in autopsied bodies. If present in the arms, it should be relieved as much as possible. Attempt to keep the arms in the proper position during and immediately after injection.

After autopsy, sutures are completed and the body is washed and dried. It may be necessary to use strips of sheets to tie the arms into proper position. This is very important when the body is to be shipped to another funeral director. Do not let the arms lie at the sides of the body. Be certain they are properly positioned and, if necessary, tie them into position. These ties will later be removed when the body is dressed.

SETTING THE FEATURES

Generally, the features are set in the preembalming period. After the tissues are embalmed it may be difficult to align the tissues to obtain the desired expression. Features can be temporarily set when purge is expected. In this manner the mouth can be dried and the throat packed after the body has been aspirated. Features can be set during embalming, but manipulation of tissues during injection has a tendency to draw arterial solution into the area. This can result in swelling or overembalming of the facial tissues. By doing the steps involved in embalming separately, the embalmer can concentrate fully on each task.

Mouth Closure Sequence

1. Relieve the rigor mortis present.
2. Disinfect the oral cavity and clean the cavity.
3. Remove and clean dentures (if present).
4. Pack the throat area; if natural teeth and dentures are absent, also fill the entire oral cavity.
5. Replace dentures.
6. Close the mouth to observe the natural bite.
7. Secure the mandible by one of the methods of mouth closure.
8. Place the lips in a desired position, attempting to make the line of mouth closure at the level of the inferior margin of the upper teeth.
9. Embalm the body.
10. Check the mouth for moisture or purge material.
11. Seal the mouth.

One of four conditions exists when the mouth is set: (1) natural teeth are present; (2) natural teeth are present but several are missing; (3) dentures are present (complete set—well fitting, lower denture only—no upper denture, upper denture only—no lower denture, old and very loose fitting dentures, new ill-fitting dentures, partial plates); (4) neither dentures or natural teeth are present.

Dentures are personal property and many hospitals and nursing homes return them to the family with the belongings. Funeral directors should make every effort to instruct institutions to keep the dentures with the body. When death occurs at home, the persons removing the body should ask for the dentures. It is possible to open the mouth after embalming and insert dentures, but this task can be very time consuming and often difficult if a hard-firming arterial solution has been used.

The embalmer should relieve the rigor mortis before disinfecting the mouth. The mouth can be cleaned and dried with cotton. If purge is present, a nasal tube aspirator can be used to aspirate purge material. Disinfectant is poured into the mouth. The throat can be packed with cotton to help control purge and odor arising from the stomach or lungs. Some embalmers prefer to cover the cotton with massage cream so that the cotton does not draw purge material from the stomach or lungs, as a wick would do. If the body is to be shipped out of the country or is dead from a contagious disease, it may be mandatory that the throat and nose be packed with cotton saturated with a disinfectant.

The lips should be examined and loose skin removed. Massage cream or a solvent helps to remove any loose skin. A washrag moistened with cool water can be used to remove loose skin off the lips. Fever blisters should be opened and drained, and loose skin removed from the lip. A small cotton pack of a phenol cautery chemical can be placed over the area once the blister is removed to help seal the tissues. If the scab is hard to loosen, massage cream may be helpful. A scab can also be removed by loosening with a sharp scalpel.

Observe the "weather line." This helps to determine the thickness of the lips. A picture of the deceased, if available, is helpful in determining the correct expression. Remember, the upper mucous membrane is generally longer and thinner than the lower mucous membrane. (The mucous membranes are the "red" portions of the lips.)

Many problems may be encountered in setting the mouth. The expression of the deceased can be one of the most criticized areas of the embalming. A rare problem today, but one that is easy to solve, is buck teeth. Protruding upper teeth constitute the most problems. A simple method can be used to correct this condition:

1. Secure the jaw closed using one of the methods of mouth closure.
2. Place a strip of cotton over the lower teeth. This helps to push the lower lip forward.
3. Using rubber-based lip glue, secure the upper and lower lips together (super adhesive may also be used).
4. Embalm the body.

5. Reopen the mouth to be certain there is no purge or air in the mouth; then reglue the lips (Fig. 11–9).

Over the years, a variety of methods have been proposed for correcting the problem of protruding upper teeth. The preceding method works very well and is quite simple. The use of a super adhesive greatly facilitates the procedure. If there is a condition that warrants removal of the teeth or showing the teeth, the family should be consulted.

Securing the Mandible for Mouth Closure

Method 1: Needle Injector. A widely used method of mouth closure today involves the needle injector. A pin with an attached wire is driven by a hand-operated device into the center of the maxilla, and a similar pin with a wire attached is driven into the mandible in an opposing position (Fig. 11–10). The two wires are then twisted together to hold the mandible in position. The pin inserted into the maxilla should be placed at the center where the two maxillae fuse. This is called the *nasal spine.* Here, the bone is generally quite strong.

If dentures are to be used it may be wise to insert the teeth before the wire pins are driven into the maxilla and mandible. Most upper dentures at their center have a small notch, and the pin can be driven into the bone at the location of this notch. Some denture wearers exhibit an atrophy of the maxilla and mandible; other bodies exhibit a condition where these bones have become diseased

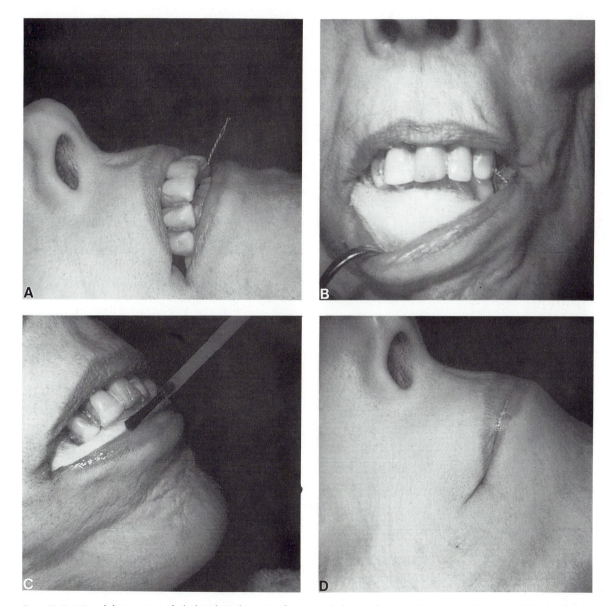

Figure 11–9. **A.** Preembalming treatment for buck teeth. **B.** Place a strip of cotton over the lower teeth to project the lower lip. **C.** Application of glue. **D.** End result.

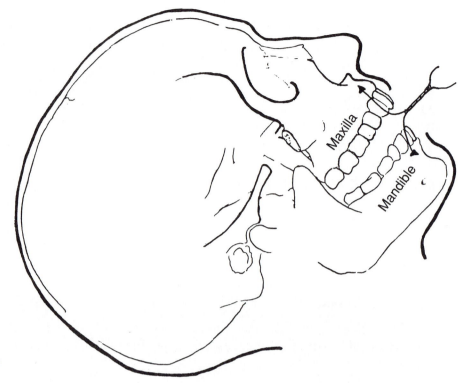

Figure 11–10. Needle barbs are inserted into the mandible and maxilla.

and are very porous. In both instances, it may be difficult, if not impossible, to use the needle injector to close the mouth. Suturing is then necessary. The embalmer can try various points along these bones to locate a solid point for the pins to be placed. The needle injector should be held at a right angle to the bone.

If the bones have been fractured, as often occurs in automobile accidents, four needle injector wires can be used. Place one on either side of the fracture so that two pins are inserted into the mandible. Then, insert two pins into the maxillae. The wires can then be *crossed*, making an ✕, and thus the fractured bones can be aligned.

It is important when inserting the pins into the bones that near the point where the skin from the mouth attaches to the gums, the skin be "torn" or pulled over the heads of the pins. This gives the fleshy portion of the lips better contact. Often, when bodies are shipped from another location and the lips are parted, all that needs to be done is to open the mouth and lift the skin over the pin heads to obtain good contact of the mucous membranes.

Method 2: Muscular Suture. In a muscular suture, a variety of needles and suture threads may be used:

*1. Open the mouth and raise the upper lip. Insert the threaded needle at a point where the upper lip joins the maxilla under the left nostril. The needle should slide along the bone and enter the

left nostril. Draw the threaded needle out of the left nostril. (By keeping the needle against the maxilla, a "pull" will not be noticed.)

2. Pass the needle through the septum of the nose. Keep the needle as close to the bone as possible. Direct the needle into the right nostril and pull the needle and thread from the right nostril.

3. Insert the needle into the base of the right nostril, keeping the needle against the maxilla. Push the needle into the area where the skin of the upper lip joins the maxilla.

4. Place the lower denture into the mouth first, then place the upper denture. If the denture is not available, fill the mouth with cotton or use a denture replacement.

5. Pull the lower lip out and insert the needle on the right side of the mandible at a point where the lower lip joins the gum. Be certain to keep the needle against the bone. Make a very wide stitch exiting the needle on the left side of the mandible in the same position where the lower lip joins the gum.

6. Tying the two free ends of the string together pulls the jaw up into position where the two mucous membranes will come into contact (Fig. 11–11).

The primary disadvantage of this method of mouth closure is that a pucker might result at the top of the chin that can easily be seen. Keeping all sutures close to the bones helps to relieve this problem.

_____

*Order is optional; suturing may begin with the mandible or maxilla.

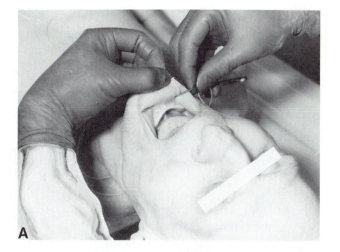

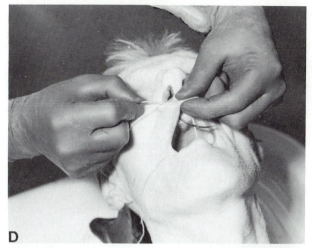

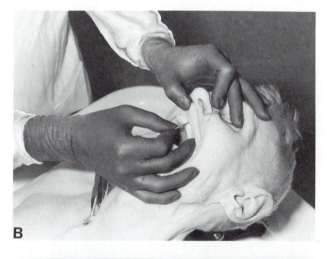

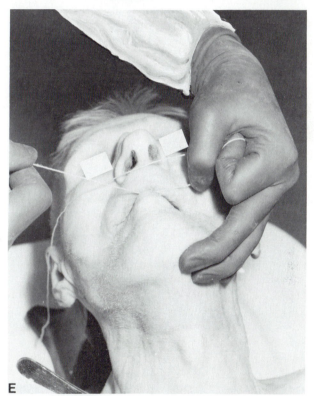

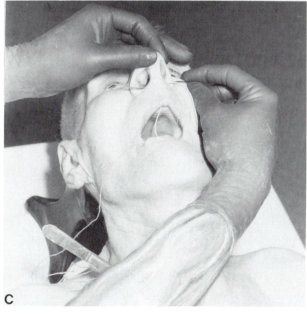

Figure 11–11. Muscular suture for mouth closure.

Method 3: Mandibular Suture. Mandibular suture is identical to muscular suture except that instead of placing the suture in the musculature of the chin, it is passed around the mandible.

1. Open the mouth and insert the needle at the center of the mouth at the base of the tongue behind the lower teeth at a point where the floor of the mouth joins the gum. Push the needle downward, exiting the point where the base of the chin joins the submandibular area.

2. Reinsert the needle into the same small hole at the base of the chin and pass the needle upward just in front of the center of the mandible, where the lip attaches to the gum. Now, the suture has passed completely *around* the mandible. By pulling on both ends of the suture the string will "saw" itself through the soft tissues until it reaches the mandible. The small hole can be cov-

ered with a small piece of wax after cosmetics are applied. It should not prove to be a leakage problem. If it does, place a drop of super adhesive on the area.

3. If dentures are used, insert the lower dentures at this point and tie the two ends of the suture together. In this manner, the lower dentures are tied into position. This is an excellent manner for securing loose-fitting dentures.
4. Insert the upper dentures if they are being used.
5. Pass the threaded needle into the left nostril as in the muscular method of mouth closure.
6. Complete the suture by tying both free ends of the suture together (Fig. 11–12). A bow may be tied in case an adjustment needs to be made.

This method of mouth closure is excellent to use when the body is to be shipped to another funeral home. It ensures that the mouth will not open during transport.

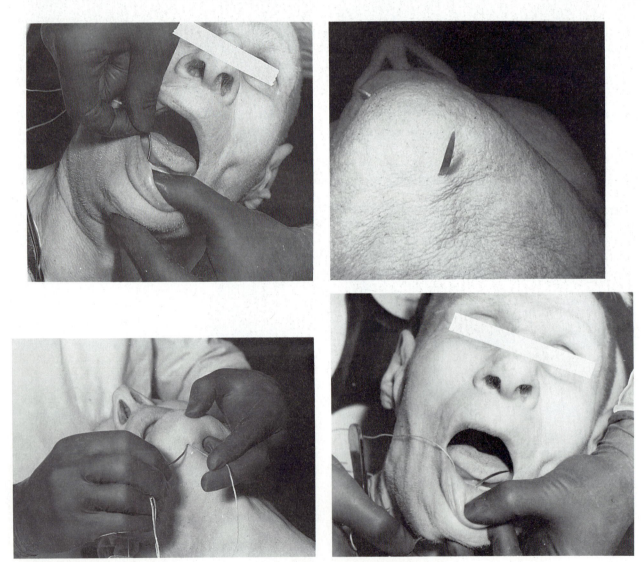

Figure 11–12. Mandibular suture for mouth closure.

Method 4: Dental Tie. To use the dental tie of mouth closure the deceased must have natural teeth on both the mandible and the maxilla. A thin thread or dental floss is tied around the base of one tooth in the upper jaw and one tooth in the lower jaw. The two strings are then tied together to hold the jaw in position. Opposing incisor teeth are generally used, but any of the front teeth can be used. It would be too difficult to use the molars. In addition to securing normal mouth closure the dental tie helps to align a fractured jaw. Several dental ties can be used to align a jaw (Fig. 11–13).

The following methods of mouth closure are included for completeness. Most are outdated or are specific, but are not used routinely.

Method 5: Drill and Wire. A small hole is drilled through the mandible and a similar hole is drilled through an opposing point on the maxilla. A small wire is passed through the holes and the wire is secured to hold the jaw in position. In lieu of a wire, thread can be passed through the holes with a suture needle. This method has been used over the years to align jaws that have been fractured. Be certain that the drill being used is properly grounded and that care is taken not to cut the fleshy portion of the lips.

Method 6: Chin Rest. The chin rest consists of two small prongs that are inserted into the nostrils. Attached to the two prongs is a sliding support, which can be placed under the chin to hold the chin in the desired position. This method of mouth closure is very old and depended on the harsh, very firm reaction obtained with early embalming fluids. These fluids rapidly and rigidly firmed the tissues. After the tissues of the face and jaw firmed, the device was removed.

Method 7: Gluing the Lips. Gluing the lips has little value as a method of mouth closure. Its use as a method of mouth closure is limited to infants and children. The lips are sealed prior to arterial injection. After the fluid has firmed the body, the lips can be reopened and the mouth dried and checked for air or purge material and then resealed. This method is not recommended for adults.

Modeling the Mouth

Raising the mandible and securing it in position are only parts of the process of mouth closure. Once the lips have been brought into contact the embalmer must create a pleasing and acceptable form.

Natural teeth, when present, create the foundation. It is helpful to place some cotton over the molar teeth to slightly fill out the posterior area of the cheek. This is necessary when the body is emaciated. Keep in mind that with all bodies, gravity tends to result in some sagging of the cheek area. Placing cotton or mortuary putty over the area of the molar teeth helps fill out the area and to slightly lift the tissues into their normal position. After embalming, tissue builder can be injected to elevate these tissues.

When natural teeth are present but several are missing, cotton, mortuary putty, kapoc, or nonabsorbent cotton is used to fill in the missing teeth after the mouth closure is secured. This helps to give an even curvature to the mouth.

When all natural teeth are missing and no dentures are present, the throat can be packed with cotton and the oral cavity with cotton, nonabsorbent cotton, kapoc, or mortuary putty. Secure the jaws into position using one of the methods of mouth closure. A mouth former can be placed over the jaw bones, but if a mouth former is used, it should be placed over the jaws prior to securing mouth closure. The needle injector wires or the suture thread helps to hold the mouth former in position. These formers come in a variety of materials such as plastic, cardboard, or metal, and can be trimmed to fit securely. A substitute can be made with cotton or mortuary putty.

If cotton is used to replace missing dentures, use long strips. **Remember the horseshoe curvature of the mandible and the maxillae.** The cotton should be placed in such a manner that a small portion covers the mandible and the maxillae, the same way a denture does. Always model the upper teeth first. Some embalmers prefer to wet the cotton strips they use to model the mouth. Squeeze out the excess water and place the cotton strips. This prevents the cotton from sinking. If mortuary putty is used as a dental replacement, inject it using a long nozzle injector. The mouth can easily be molded to obtain the horseshoe curvature (Fig. 11–14).

When there are dentures but no natural teeth, insert the dentures prior to using the needle injector or suturing the mouth closed. The dentures should be cleaned and disinfected. Cotton placed on the tongue can help to hold the dentures in position. The mandibular suture method of mouth closure can be used to tie the lower denture into position. If dentures do not fit well attempt to use the upper denture. The upper denture gives the best foundation for the curvature of the mouth. It can be held in position by placing cotton or mortuary putty in the area normally occupied by the lower denture. If the denture is new and does not appear to fit, do not use it. When placing dentures in the mouth, **always insert the lower denture first. After it is in position insert the upper denture.** In most people, the line of mouth closure (where the two mucous membranes meet) is located at the inferior margin of the upper teeth. So, establishing the curvature of the upper teeth is the key to a natural appearance.

There are occasions when rigor is so intense the jaws cannot be opened. It is still wise to use some form of mouth closure. In these instances, if dentures are in the mouth, it is impossible to remove them for cleaning. Spray a disinfectant into the mouth and dry and clean the buccal cavity with cotton swabs.

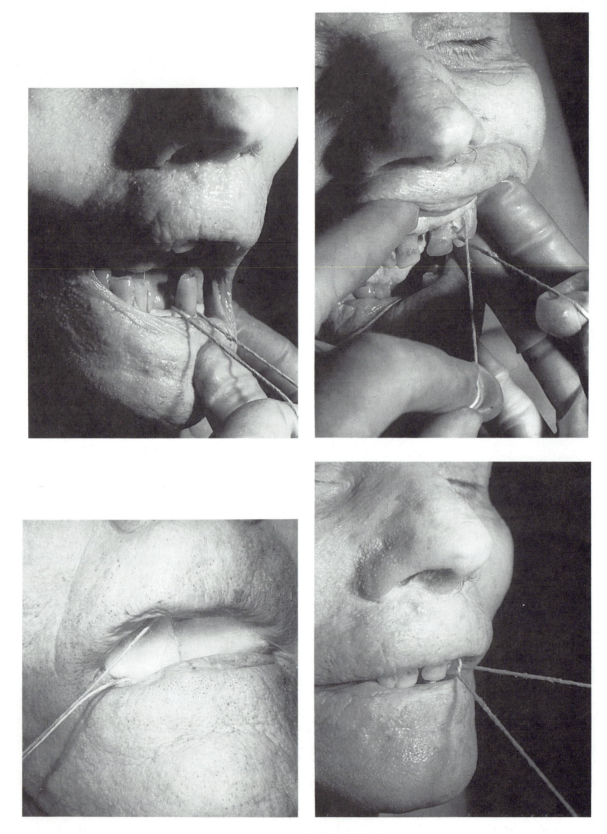

Figure 11–13. Dental tie.

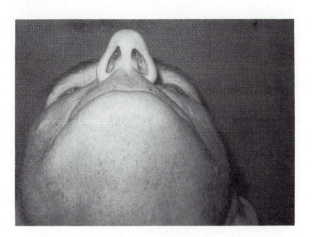

Figure 11–14. Bilateral view of face. Note the curvature of the mouth.

Positioning the Lips

After the mouth has been closed and the cheeks padded, the line of closure should be established. Always keep in mind the curvature of the mouth. In the bilateral view of the mouth (looking from the chin upward) the horseshoe curvature of the mouth is easily observed. By keeping this curvature in mind, the embalmer avoids making the mouth look flat and straight. The center of the mouth should give the most projection. Try to obtain some depth at the corners. **The mouth is convex in curvature from corner to corner.** The line of closure is along the inferior margin of the upper teeth. Inserting a small amount of cotton high on the maxillae, on a line from the corner of the mouth to the center of the closed eye, helps to raise the area surrounding the corner (angulus oris eminence) (Fig. 11–15).

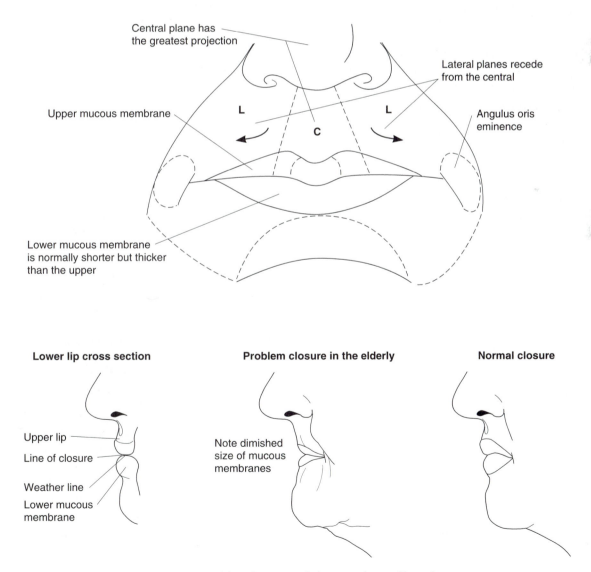

Figure 11–15. Lines of closure for positioning the lips. Various closure profiles are shown.

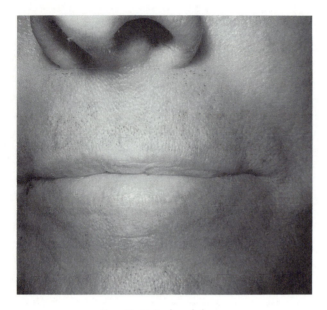

Figure 11–16. Good mouth closure.

This angulus oris eminence [the area surrounding the corner of the mouth (angulus oris sulcus)] can be reinstated with tissue builder after arterial embalming. The upper lip (mucous membrane) is usually thinner and longer than the lower lip. This appearance can be reproduced when cosmetics are applied. The weather line (the line between the moist and dry portions of the lips) helps to determine the thickness of the lips. As already mentioned, any scabs or loose skin should be removed from the lips as soon as possible, prior to embalming. To hold the lips in position during embalming the following products can be used (Fig. 11–15): lip seal creams (very thick massage creams), petroleum jelly, rubber-based eye and lip glue (for gluing the lips), and super adhesive (for very difficult problems).

Application of a thick cream to the lips during embalming to hold them in position also helps to smooth wrinkles on the lips. Natural wrinkles or lines in the mucous membranes are vertical, but lines from dehydration are horizontal. Place a very thin film of lip cream on each lip, and then bring the lips into contact. They tend to slightly pull away from each other. In doing so, the horizontal wrinkles will be removed. After embalming, wrinkled lips can be corrected by gluing, tissue building, or waxing. These same three methods can be used if the lips are slightly separated after embalming (Fig. 11–16). Some embalmers find it helpful to keep the lips *slightly separated* during arterial injection. This allows the mucous membranes to round out and prevents the lip closure from presenting a tight or pursed look.

If the lips are glued *prior* to embalming, they should be opened *after* embalming to be certain there has been no solution leakage into the mouth during injection or that there is no purge material. In addition, air from the lungs can be forced into the mouth and should be released. The lips can then be reglued if desired.

CLOSURE OF THE EYES

In establishing the line of eye closure, keep the following items in mind. The upper eyelid (superior palpebra) forms two thirds of the closed eye; the lower eyelid (inferior palpebra) forms one third of the closed eye. The line of closure is located in the lower one third of the eye orbit. The line of closure is not level and the inner corner of the line of closure (inner canthus) is slightly above the outer corner of the eye (outer canthus).

The general procedure for eye closure can be summarized:

1. Closure of the eyelids is generally done prior to arterial injection. It is easier to close the eye than the mouth after the body has been embalmed, but establishing a good line of closure may be difficult.
2. The eyes can be cleaned with moist cotton. Like all areas of the body, the eyes should be disinfected with a topical disinfectant spray. Conjunctivitis and herpes infections of the eye could be communicable to the embalmer. In addition to cleaning the surface and corners of the eyes, clean the lashes.
3. Cleaning the eyes also helps to relieve rigor mortis in the muscles of the eyelids. If the face is emaciated or dehydrated, the eyelids may have to be stretched slightly to establish closure. This can be done by placing the smooth handle of an instrument such as a pair of forceps or an aneurysm needle, under the eyelid and gently stretching the lids.
4. To help establish the anterior projection of the closed eye and to keep the lids closed, use an eyecap or cotton. These are inserted under the lids.
   A. Eyecap: These plastic or metal disks are approximately the size of the anterior portion of the eyeball. They are generally perforated, and the small perforated projections help to hold the lids closed. The convex shape of the cap helps to maintain the convex curvature of the closed eye. The cap itself prevents the eye and lids from sinking into the orbit should the body begin to dehydrate. Should the eyes be sunken, use several caps or two caps with mortuary putty or a piece of cotton sandwiched between to elevate the closed eyelids.
   B. Cotton: Cotton may be placed under the closed eyelids to keep the lids closed, elevate the lids, and establish the convexity of the closed eye. A piece of cotton about the size of a nickel can be used. Lift the upper lid and insert the cotton under the upper eyelid with an aneurysm handle or forceps. Lift the upper eyelid over the cotton and place it in its proper position. Evert the

lower eyelids and insert the cotton into the area covered by the lower eyelid. Lift the lower eyelid into position. If the eyelids do not seem to contain enough arterial solution after embalming, a drop or two of cavity fluid can be placed on the cotton. The lids should then be glued. This will make a preservative pack *under* the eyelids. If preservation is needed, dehydration from the cavity fluid should not be a concern (Fig. 11–17).

In cases of extreme emaciation or dehydration, the eyes can be sunken and the eyeball itself can be dehydrated. The eyelids have to be exercised and stretched to secure closure. Preembalming gluing of the lids may be helpful. The lids should abut but not overlap. In these difficult closures, however, overlapping may be necessary, and if the lids must be overlapped an attempt should be made to show some of the lower eyelid.

Some embalmers place massage cream under the lids. This is easily done by coating the eyecap or the cotton used for closure with a small amount of cream. The difficulty in using massage cream under the eyelids is that a solvent has to be used to clean the cream from the line of closure if the lids have been glued. **Difficult closures can easily be corrected today by using super adhesive to hold the lids together.** Super glue is helpful when during transport from another funeral home, the eyelids have separated. Simply exercise the lids and use super glue to hold them closed. Care should be taken at the start of the embalming to be certain the small inner corner of the eye (the inner canthus) is closed. If this area dehydrates, the brown discoloration can be quite noticeable.

PACKING THE ORIFICES

A topical disinfectant should be sprayed over the outer surfaces of the anal and vaginal orifices. Cotton packing saturated with phenol solution, undiluted cavity fluid, or autopy gel should be placed into the vaginal and the anal orifices. Some embalmers prefer to do this after embalming, because they prefer that any discharges from these orifices be allowed to exit the body during embalming. After arterial and cavity embalming, the orifices are tightly packed and the body washed.

The nasal cavity as well as the throat and ears should be packed with cotton prior to embalming. The throat must be packed before the features are set. If purge develops, however, all soiled packing should be removed and replaced with dry packing after the body has been thoroughly aspirated.

TREATMENT OF INVASIVE PROCEDURES

The following effects of invasive procedures may be treated by the embalmer before, during, or after em-

balming. They are listed here because the analysis of the body is made in the preembalming period. Also, several of these conditions should be treated during the preembalming period.

Surgical Incisions. Check the suture to see if the healing process has begun. If the sutures are recent, the area can be disinfected at this time and cauterized with a surface pack or hypodermic injection of a phenol cautery. Temporary metal sutures can be removed with a hemostat after arterial injection, and the surgical incision tightly sutured using a baseball suture. Incision seal powder can be placed within the incision to ensure against leakage. Glue can later be placed over the surface of the suture after the body has been washed and dried. If the incision is in a visible area, super adhesive or a restorative suture may be necessary. The small metal "staples" can be removed by grasping them in their center with a hemostat; then move the hemostat from side to side to allow the small, bent metal edge embedded in the skin surface to be freed.

Feeding Tubes. Tubes that enter the mouth or the nostrils should be removed in the preembalming period. These tubes, if left in place for any time, can mark the corners of the mouth or nose. When the tubes have been in the patient's mouth or nose for several weeks, the surrounding skin may be destroyed. Massage of these areas during arterial injection helps to restore them to their normal contour. After embalming, it may be necessary to use restorative wax, tissue builder, or super adhesive to restore these areas.

Abdominal Feeding Tubes. A feeding tube may also be inserted into the stomach through a small incision in the abdominal wall and a second incision in the stomach wall. These tubes can be removed after arterial embalming. The area of the abdomen should be disinfected. A small piece of cotton saturated with phenol, autopsy gel, or undiluted cavity fluid can be inserted into the abdominal opening after the tube is withdrawn or cut. A small pursestring suture can be used to close the abdominal opening. A trocar button can also be used if the opening is small enough.

Surgical Drains. Surgical drains can be removed after arterial embalming. Drain openings should be packed with cotton saturated with phenol, autopsy gel, or undiluted cavity fluid. A small pursestring suture is used to close the opening. This should be done prior to cavity embalming.

Intravenous Tubes. Any tubing placed into the circulatory system, whether an artery or a vein, should remain in place until the arterial embalming is completed. These invasive devices did not hamper circulation during life, and leaving them in place will not interfere with arterial in-

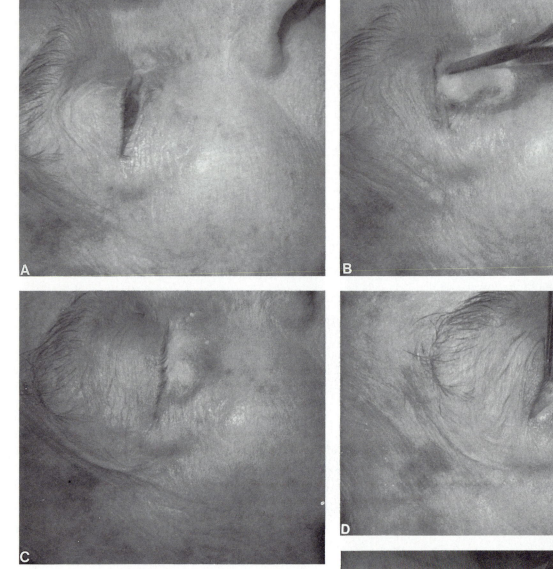

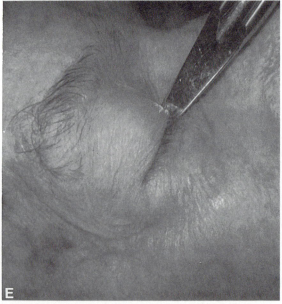

Figure 11–17. Eye closure with cotton.

jection or blood drainage. They can be removed after arterial and cavity embalming is completed. When these tubes are removed from areas that will not be seen after the body is dressed, their openings can be enlarged with a scalpel and a trocar button can be inserted to prevent leakage. Super adhesive can also be applied to these openings, especially in visible areas such as the back of the hands or the neck.*

Tracheotomy Tubes. Tracheotomy tubes should be removed in the preembalming period and the area disinfected. Some cotton saturated with a disinfectant or cautery agent can be placed in the opening to disinfect the respiratory passages. It is best not to seal these passages until after arterial embalming. Should any purge develop in the lungs or stomach, this opening in the base of the neck provides an outlet for the purge material. The embalmer may encounter two types of tracheotomies: With the older tracheotomy the skin around the opening contains a great amount of scar tissue. It is not possible to close the opening with a pursestring suture. Pack this type of tracheotomy with cotton and incision seal powder (or mortuary putty) to the surface level of the skin; then place glue over the opening. With the recent tracheotomy there is little or no scar tissue around the opening. After packing with cotton and incision seal powder, a small pursestring suture can be made to close the opening. Dental floss can be used for the suture to hide the opening.

Colostomy. The colostomy bag and the surrounding abdominal wall area should be disinfected. Some embalmers remove the bag, empty its contents, disinfect and deodorize the inside of the bag, then reattach it. Most embalmers prefer to remove the bag after arterial embalming. Insert a piece of cotton saturated with phenol solution, undiluted cavity fluid, or autopsy gel into the abdominal opening. Sometimes a portion of the bowel is exposed. Apply the cotton to this portion of the bowel and use the cotton to gently push the bowel into the abdominal cavity. Close the opening with a pursestring suture. Surface glue and cotton can be applied to prevent any leakage. The bag and its contents (which were removed) should be deodorized and disinfected by pouring some undiluted cavity fluid into the bag. The bag and its contents can then be destroyed.

Urinary Catheter. A catheter can be inserted into the urinary tract through the urethra or the abdominal wall. It can be removed prior to arterial embalming. Cut the small side vent with scissors to allow the dilated balloon located within the bladder to collapse. Then pull the catheter from the body. If the catheter was inserted through the abdominal wall, a small pursestring suture can be used to close the opening. In females, the urethra

*Disposal of any invasive device into the blood vascular system may be regulated by OSHA standards if an infectious disease is present.

can be packed with cotton saturated with cavity fluid, autopsy gel, or a phenol cautery chemical after the catheter is removed.

REMOVING CASTS

Sometimes, casts are not removed by the hospital, or death may occur at home where it would be impossible to remove the cast. Most embalmers remove the cast if possible. If the entire leg is in a cast it may be very difficult to remove it and, of course, the cast would not be visible after the body is dressed. The difficulty involved in leaving a cast in place is that the embalmer cannot ensure that embalming solution was distributed to the area covered by the cast. The cast must also be protected from drainage during the embalming; it can, of course, be elevated and covered with plastic.

There are two types of casts: the older plaster type and the new fiberglass type. Both must be sawed open. Sometimes the fiberglass, if thin enough, can be cut open. Some arm casts can be pulled off the body. Some embalmers own a vibrating cast cutting saw or borrow one from a hospital. These devices reduce the time needed to remove the cast. In some locations, the body can be taken to a local hospital, and the hospital personnel will remove the cast. Casts should be removed prior to arterial embalming.

PREEMBALMING TREATMENTS

Skin Lesions and Ulcerations

As the embalmer undresses, disinfects, washes, and dries the body, he should look for rashes, lesions, infected areas, decubitus ulcers, and skin cancers. After cleansing the body the embalmer should begin treatment of these areas immediately (1) to disinfect the affected area, (2) to preserve the tissues surrounding the lesion, (3) to dry the tissues, and (4) to deodorize the tissues. These areas should be of concern to the embalmer for the following reasons:

1. They can be a source of contamination to the embalmer, for example, staph infections and herpes infections.
2. The area is generally necrotic and decomposition of the superficial and deep tissues can already be in progress.
3. Blood supply to the actual necrotic and infected tissues is poor so there will be little or no contact between injected arterial solution and the diseased tissue.
4. Odors may be present that will easily be noticed even after embalming, dressing, and casketing.
5. Necrotic tissue can contain anaerobic gas bacillus microbes that can produce gas gangrene.

A common example of necrotic and infected tissue is the decubitus ulcer. These ulcerations, also known as bedsores, result from limited circulation into areas where there is pressure contact, usually with the bedding. Hospital staph infections result and the necrotic tissue can grow from a small red mark to involve the greater portion of the hip, buttocks, or shoulder. These areas and any area of infection (e.g., pustules) should be sprayed with a topical disinfectant. If one is not available, the area can be swabbed with undiluted chlorine bleach or undiluted cavity fluid. **Do not use the two together.**

If the ulcerated area is covered with a bandage, saturate the bandage with undiluted cavity fluid, undiluted phenol cautery solution, or undiluted autopsy gel. Later, remove the bandage and inject the necrotic tissue with the fluid and solution. If there are no bandages, place a compress of cotton saturated with undiluted cavity chemical, undiluted phenol cautery solution, or autopsy gel over the area during embalming.* This helps to control odors, to preserve the necrotic tissue, and to destroy any microbes and their products that may be present. Hypodermic treatment of the walls of these lesions after embalming is very important, as gas bacillus (*Clostridium perfringens*), a source of tissue gas, may be present.

After embalming and treatment by hypodermic injection and fresh surface preservatives, cotton compresses with embalming powder can be applied to the area. If the hip or buttocks is affected, a large diaper can be made with sheeting. The embalming will do some preserving but, more important, it will control odors. When handling these lesions, the embalmer should always wear gloves (double gloves preferred), gown, and mask. Plastic goods such as coveralls, pants, and plastic stockings can be placed on the treated area.

Lacerations and Fractures

A laceration is defined as a jagged tear in the skin. In the preembalming period, a laceration should be cleaned of any blood or dirt present. This is easily done with germicidal soap and cool water. After the edges of the laceration are cleaned, the torn skin should be aligned. Several small bridge sutures of dental floss can be placed along the laceration to hold the edges in position during embalming. If the laceration is in a body area that will not be viewed after arterial injection, the laceration can be sewn with a baseball suture, using incision seal powder within the laceration to prevent leakage. If the laceration is in an area of the body that will be seen, some massage cream can be placed around the area after the bridge sutures are in place. This protects the good skin.

During embalming, arterial solution escapes from the laceration. After embalming, dry the laceration, treat

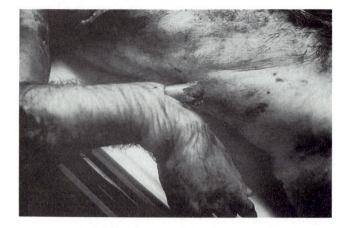

Figure 11–18. Compound fracture of the radius.

the edges with a hypodermic injection of phenol cautery solution, and then either suture or glue them closed. Some embalmers prefer to place a compress of undiluted cavity fluid or autopsy gel over the lacerated tissues during embalming to ensure good preservation of the torn tissues.†

When bones are fractured (Fig. 11–18), the embalmer is able to observe the distortion by touch or sight. He should make every attempt to align bones, especially facial bones, in the preembalming period. If skull bones or facial bones are fractured, small incisions may have to be made to realign them. Because so many situations can arise regarding fractures, the best advice is simply align all fractures *prior to embalming.*

Abrasions

An abrasion is defined as "skin rubbed off." The embalmer encounters two types of abrasions:

Dry Abrasion. Dry abrasions are abraded areas that have dehydrated. The area resembles a scab. The tissue is dark brown to black, very rough and firm to the touch. It may be the remains of an old abrasion. Or, if it occurred at the time of death, perhaps the body has been dead for a while or the body has been kept in a refrigeration unit, where air passed over the body and dehydrated the abraded tissues.

Moist Abrasions. Moist abrasions are abraded areas that are moist to the touch; some bruising may be present. A fall on a carpeted area can easily bring about an abrasion on that part of the face that came into contact with the carpet.

In the preembalming period, for abrasions located on visible body areas (face, head, neck, arms, or hands), clean the affected area as some blood may be present.

---

*Cover with plastic to control odor and fumes and to prevent the chemical from dehydrating.

†Cover with plastic to contain fumes.

Moist abrasions can be covered with a compress of undiluted cavity fluid, phenol cautery solution, or autopsy gel. During embalming, arterial solution passes through the abraded tissues. After embalming, the objective should be to dry these abrasions so the tissues *will turn brown*. A hair dryer can be used to dry moist abrasions. *Cosmetics can only be applied to dry tissues.*

Skin-Slip or Torn Skin

Skin-slip should be removed and the underlying tissues treated by immediately packing the denuded tissue with undiluted cavity fluid, phenol solution, or autopsy gel. When the embalmer is satisfied that adequate preservation has occurred and that the area is disinfected and deodorized, he can allow the area to air dry or dry it with a hair dryer. Blisters (Fig. 11–19), scabs, torn skin, and other conditions should always be treated in the preembalming period by removing the skin that will not be receiving arterial solution, preserving and cauterizing the denuded skin surface, and, finally, drying the skin. These areas discolor, but they can then be treated with an opaque cosmetic if they are in a visible location. During arterial injection, solution may seep from the affected skin areas. This helps to ensure good preservation.

Gases

During undressing, disinfecting, and cleaning of the body, the embalmer should determine if gas is present in the cavities or body tissues. There are three sources of gas in the dead human body.

Subcutaneous Emphysema: Gas or Air in the Tissues. Subcutaneous emphysema originates from invasions into pleural cavi-

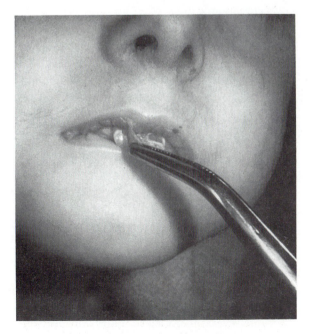

Figure 11–19. Fever blisters.

ties. When gas is detected in the tissues and neither odor nor skin-slip is present, examine the body for punctures that may have been made into the lungs, recent tracheotomy, or fracture of the clavicle, sternum, or ribs. Subcutaneous emphysema can be widespread from the scrotum of the male into the limbs and face.

Gas from Decomposition. If there has been a time delay, signs of decomposition may be present, as may discoloration, odor, purge, skin-slip, and gas. This gas can accumulate in the viscera, body cavities, or skeletal tissues.

True Tissue Gas. The source of this gas is Welch's bacillus (*Clostridium perfringens*). It is an anaerobic spore former and thrives on dead necrotic tissue. The microbe can be passed from body to body through contaminated cutting instruments. A very strong odor of decomposed tissue is present. The condition continues to increase and may begin in the agonal and postmortem periods. Because it spreads so rapidly and is so hard to control, viewing of the body may be impossible. Its presence should immediately be recognized and appropriate steps taken to control it. Use extreme care to disinfect all cutting instruments used in the embalming. Disposable scalpel blades should be removed and placed in an OSHA-approved sharps disposal unit and the trocar immersed in concentrated arterial solution using a coinjection chemical specifically designed for bodies with "true tissue gas."

When gases are present in the tissues, distension and swelling may also occur. The gas can be felt by moving the fingers over the tissues. It feels as if it were stuffed with cellophane tissue. This movement may also produce a crackling sound, called *crepitation*. There is only one way to remove gas from tissues. The tissues must be opened and the gas allowed to escape.

In the preembalming period, the greatest concern is distension of the abdomen. Severe distension may restrict the flow of arterial solution and blood drainage. The abdomen should be punctured and the gas allowed to escape.

1. Make a puncture with a scalpel approximately at the standard point of trocar entry—2 inches to the left and 2 inches above the umbilicus. This in itself may allow enough gas to escape that sufficient pressure will be relieved.
2. Insert a trocar at the standard point of entry and, keeping the point high over the viscera, attempt to relieve the gases.
3. Make a small 3- to 4-inch incision over the abdominal wall, possibly opening some of the intestinal viscera, to allow gas to escape.
4. Make an opening with a scalpel on the abdominal wall and insert a "pointless" trocar or large drain tube.

TABLE 11–1. GASES CAUSING DISTENSION

Type	Source	Characteristics	Treatments
Subcutaneous emphysema	Puncture of lung or plural sac; seen in cardiopulmonary resuscitation treatments; puncture wounds to thorax; rib fractures; tracheotomy	No odor; no skin-slip; no blebs; gas can be extreme, present even in toes; can create intense swelling; rises to highest body areas	Gas will escape through incisions; establish good arterial preservation; channel tissues after arterial injection to release gases
"True" tissue gas	Anaerobic bacteria; *Clostridium perfringens*	Very strong odor of decomposition; skin-slip; skin blebs; the condition and amount of gas increase; spore-forming bacterium may be passed by cutting instruments to other bodies	Use of special "tissue gas" arterial solutions; localized hypodermic injection of cavity fluid; channel tissues to release gases
Gas gangrene	Anaerobic bacteria; *C. perfringens*	Foul odor; infection	Strong arterial solutions; local hypodermic injection of cavity chemical
Decomposition	Bacterial breakdown of body tissues; autolytic breakdown of body tissues	Odor may be present; skin-slip in time; color changes; purging	Proper strong chemical in sufficient amounts by arterial injection; hypodermic and surface treatments; channel to release gases
Air from embalming apparatus	Air injected by embalming machine (air-pressure machines and hand pumps are in limited use today)	First evidence in eyelids; no odors; no skin-slip; amount would depend on injection time—most would be minimal	If distension is caused, channel after arterial injection to release gases

If the facial tissues and the upper chest areas evidence the presence of gas, it would be advantageous to raise both common carotid arteries for injection. The half-moon incision, running from the center of the right clavicle to the center of the left clavicle, is useful. This incision allows gases to escape. Gases already present in the face can be channeled, after embalming, and allowed to exit through these incisions.

It is important that the embalmer determine the type of gas present. True tissue is very rare, but most difficult to control. The gas most frequently seen is subcutaneous emphysema. This is generally found when a rib has been fractured during the administration of cardiopulmonary resuscitation (CPR). Table 11–1 outlines the characteristics of these gases.

Ascites

When the abdomen is tightly distended, the embalmer should determine if the distension is caused by gas or edema. Often, simply the insertion of the trocar into the upper areas of the abdomen can determine the difference. If there is generalized edema of the tissues and tortuous veins are visible over the abdominal wall, the presence of edema in the abdomen (ascites) can be expected. If the abdomen is very tense this fluid should be removed prior to arterial injection, for it will create a resistance to the flow of arterial solution and interfere with blood drainage.

Not all the ascites fluid need be removed, only enough to relieve the intense pressure in the abdomen. An easy method is to insert a trocar, not at the standard point of trocar entry but at a point a little lower on the abdominal wall in the area of the right or left inguinal area or in the hypogastric area (right and left lower quadrants). This lower point allows the ascites fluid to gravitate from the cavity. Insert the trocar, keeping the point directed under the anterior abdominal wall. This instrument can be left in this position during the entire embalming. Drain enough ascites fluid to relieve the intense pressure. Placing a hand on the abdominal wall and applying slight pressure can assist. Attaching tubing to the trocar can provide a direct drain of any ascites fluid directly into the sewer system or into a container where it can be disinfected.

KEY TERMS AND CONCEPTS FOR STUDY AND DISCUSSION

1. Define the following terms:
   abrasion
   ascites
   colostomy
   dental tie
   embalmer's gray
   eyecap
   laceration
   larvicide
   maggot
   mandibular suture
   mucous membranes
   muscular suture
   needle injector
   subcutaneous emphysema
   tissue gas
   tracheotomy
   weather line
2. List the qualities of a good topical disinfectant.
3. List several rules for shaving.
4. List several uses of massage cream.
5. Name the three levels of position.
6. List several reasons for placing a support beneath the shoulders.
7. List several methods of mouth closure.
8. Describe methods of eye closure.

12

Distribution and Diffusion of Arterial Solution

Arterial embalming could also be called "capillary embalming." The capillaries, the smallest blood vessels of the body, link the injected embalming solution with the cells of the body. The embalming solution that passes from the capillaries to the tissues effects the embalming. This chapter discusses the movement of arterial solution through the blood vascular (intravascular) and interstitial (extravascular) systems of the body. On reaching the capillaries, the embalming solution, by a series of passive physical transport systems, moves to the cells of the body.* The movement of embalming solution from the intravascular to the extravascular location is called *fluid diffusion*. The remainder of the embalming solution, which passes into the venous system of the body, helps to remove the blood and its discolorations, which exit the body in the form of drainage.

The ability of the embalmer to retain as much preservative within the body as possible without visible distension of the tissues is a key factor in thoroughly preserving and sanitizing the body.

Arterial embalming involves two distinct processes: *Distribution of arterial solution* is the movement of arterial solution from the point of injection throughout the arterial system and into the capillaries (perfusion). *Diffusion of arterial solution* is the movement of arterial solution from inside the vascular system (intravascular)

*Passive transport systems require no energy by the cell to operate.

through the walls of the capillaries to the tissue spaces (extravascular).

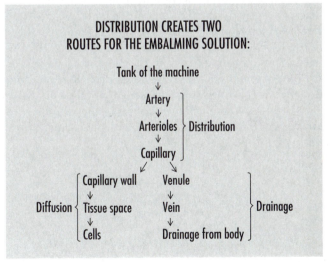

DISTRIBUTION CREATES TWO ROUTES FOR THE EMBALMING SOLUTION:

Tank of the machine
↓
Artery
↓
Arterioles } Distribution
↓
Capillary

Diffusion { Capillary wall   Venule
↓   ↓
Tissue space   Vein   } Drainage
↓   ↓
Cells   Drainage from body

From this simple diagram, it can be seen that fluid distribution and diffusion occur at the same time once the vascular system has been filled. These processes work similar to a lawn sprinkler or soaker hose. Arterial solution fills the vascular system, much like water fills the hose to reach the sprinkler. Some of the arterial solution flows through the walls and pores of the capillaries into the tissue spaces, as water passes through the holes in the sprinkler to reach the grass. The major difference is that all the water is sprayed out of the sprinkler. In embalming, a portion of the arterial solution stays inside the capillaries and flows into the veins to be removed as drainage.

CLINICAL OBSERVATION

In the embalming of a body that has been dead a long period and in which decomposition has begun, injection can result in the immediate swelling of tissues. This swelling occurs because the capillary walls (only one cell in thickness), after being decomposed, can no longer hold arterial solution. Arterial solution thus flows from the large arteries into the small arterioles and then directly into the interstitial spaces. As almost all the arterial solution enters the interstitial spaces, the tissues become distended. In embalming this type of body, it is important to inject a strong arterial solution, so that the maximum amount of preservation is achieved with minimum tissue distension. This is particularly important for the face and hands if the body is to be presentable for viewing.

The material drained during embalming of the body is a mixture of blood, arterial solution, and interstitial fluid. It has been demonstrated that as much as 50% of the drainage can be arterial solution. As the vascular system is basically a "closed" system, the arterial solution must pass through the walls and small pores of the capillaries to enter the interstitial spaces (Fig. 12–1). In these tissue spaces a fluid surrounds and bathes the cells of the body. In life, this tissue fluid serves to transport the nutrients and oxygen carried by the blood to the cells, as the blood remains in the blood vascular system and does not have direct contact with the cells. The tissue fluid also carries the wastes of cell metabolism to the blood vascular system, where they are carried to the organs of the body that dispose of these wastes.

A similar process occurs in arterial embalming. Arterial solution flows through the arteries into the capillaries. A portion of the solution leaves the capillaries and passes into the fluid in the tissue spaces. Eventually it moves to and enters the cells and makes contact with the cell proteins. In this manner, the cells of the body are preserved or embalmed. The embalming solution that leaves the capillaries and eventually embalms the cells is the **retained fluid.** It is the retained fluid that embalms.

The arterial solution that remains in the capillary and is pushed ahead into the venules and veins and is eventually drained from the body serves only to clear the vascular system of blood. This solution can embalm only the walls of the vascular system. The vascular system is extensive and the preservation of arteries, capillaries, and veins would, no doubt, diminish decomposition of the body. Nevertheless, muscle cells and connective tissue cells account for the bulk of the body, and their preservation is essential if decomposition is to be halted and a thorough and extended preservation of the body achieved.

Drainage is a combination of **blood, arterial solution,** and **interstitial fluid.** It is easy to see how blood and embalming solution are elements of the drainage, but interstitial fluid becomes part of the drainage through two routes. In living bodies, excess interstitial fluid is carried away from the spaces between the cells by the lymph system. This system empties into certain large veins of the body. In the embalming process, some embalming solution diffuses into the interstitial fluid and is removed by the lymph system. Even more importantly, embalming solution is present in the capillaries, and as it moves through the capillaries it draws some tissue fluid with it into the drainage. This explains why dehydration often occurs in areas such as the lips and the fingers during injection: more tissue fluid is being removed than is being replaced by embalming solution.

Arterial embalming involves both physical and chemical applications. Filling the arterial system by forced injection with some apparatus that pushes solu-

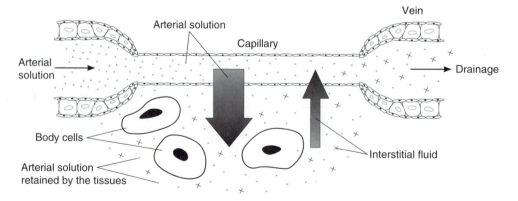

Figure 12–1. Drainage and retention of arterial solution.

tion into the body under pressure involves physical procedures. Control of the drainage is a physical process. Some of the injected solution is forced through the walls of the capillaries simply by the physical process of filtration.

The arterial fluid is chemical in nature. When properly diluted it makes a homogenous solution that is described as hypotonic. Through the physical processes of osmosis and dialysis, this hypotonic solution passes from the capillaries into the interstitial spaces. The preservatives in the solution chemically combine with the proteins in the body cells and the protein in microorganisms and their products to form new compounds and alter the proteins in such a manner that the tissues are preserved and sanitized.

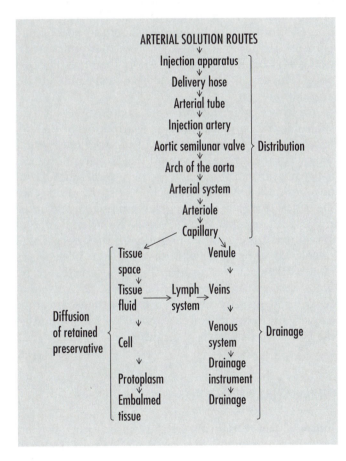

ARTERIAL SOLUTION INJECTION

Arterial embalming begins with the injection of a preservative solution, under pressure, into an artery of the body.* Arterial (vascular) embalming can be defined as the injection of a suitable arterial (embalming) solution,

*Some embalmers may prefer to begin the arterial embalming (of the unautopsied body) by injecting a preinjection arterial solution.

under pressure, into the blood vascular system to accomplish **temporary preservation, sanitation,** and **restoration** of the dead human body. The solution moves from the arteries to the capillaries and then passes through the capillaries to come into contact with the body cells. A portion of the embalming solution remains in the capillaries to remove the blood and its products from the vascular system in the form of drainage. This drainage is taken from a vein of the body.

It is necessary to inject an embalming solution under pressure. Even transfusions of blood into living persons are done under pressure, by elevating the container containing the blood. Some early embalming injection apparatus were just as simple. A solution of embalming chemical was elevated above the body to create the pressure needed to distribute the solution throughout the body. The body offers resistance to the injection of the solution. As the solution is injected into the vascular system by way of an artery, the resistances are described in relationship to the vascular system. Resistances within the blood vessels are called **intravascular resistances;** resistances outside the blood vessels are called **extravascular resistances** (Fig. 12–2).

Extravascular and intravascular resistances have their greatest effect on arterial solution distribution. Poor or good distribution of the arterial solution results in poor or good diffusion of the embalming solution, respectively. Pressurized injection is needed primarily to overcome these resistances that interfere with arterial solution distribution. As embalming solution travels from the large central trunk of the arterial system (the aorta) into the arterial branches (arterioles and capillaries), the diameter of the arterial system actually *expands* because of the innumerable branching of the vessels. The injection pressure needed to force the solution through the narrow arteries *decreases* by the time the solution reaches the capillaries.

The arterial solution at the microcirculation level can take three routes: (1) A portion flows through the capillaries, where some of the embalming solution passes through the walls of the capillaries to embalm the tissues. (2) The portion that remains in the capillaries flows on to the venules. This embalming solution helps to remove the blood from the capillaries and the veins and eventually exits as drainage. (3) The remaining embalming solution flows through direct connections that link arterioles and venules. It eventually exits as drainage.

Intravascular pressure (IVP), which brings about pressure filtration that moves the embalming solution from the capillaries into the interstitial spaces, is no doubt created by the pressure from the machine and the expansion of the elastic arteries. This pressure effects fluid filtration through the walls of the capillaries. Pressure filtration is one of the major processes by which embalming solution enters the tissue spaces. Intravascular pres-

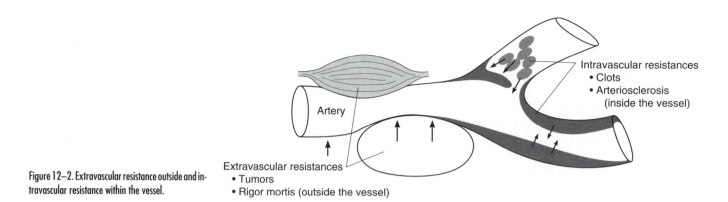

Figure 12–2. Extravascular resistance outside and intravascular resistance within the vessel.

sure also remains with the fluids that flow on into the venous system. This is what helps to create the small (approximately ½ pound) pressure that the drainage exhibits. No doubt a lot of the drainage pressure is brought about by arterial solution flowing directly through connecting routes—directly from arterioles to venules and not passing through the capillary routes.

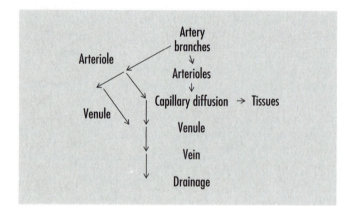

During life, some capillaries remain devoid of blood as a result of vasoconstriction. Also, some areas of the body are engorged with blood because of the activity of the body, which causes vasodilation. For example, in a person who is running, more blood is concentrated in the muscles being used rather than in those muscles not being used. At death, the vascular system relaxes and thus increases its capacity. As a result, the embalmer can inject a large volume of solution without causing immediate distension of the tissues or drainage.

The drainage from the average body generally amounts to one half or less of the total volume of arterial solution injected. It is the intent of the embalmer that 50% or more of the arterial solution injected be retained by the body for the embalming of cells and tissues. The embalmer must make every attempt to promote even distribution of the embalming solution throughout the body and to have the tissues retain as much embalming solution as possible. A general guide over the years has been

1 gallon of a properly mixed arterial solution for every 50 pounds of body weight. This should be sufficient to meet the preservation and sanitation demands of the body. Thus, for the average 165-pound body, the injection of 3 to 4 gallons of solution should be adequate to preserve and sanitize all tissues. To achieve this saturation it may be necessary to use more than one injection point. This depends on the evenness of distribution of the arterial solution.

Extravascular and intravascular resistances are responsible for nonuniformity in distribution of the embalming solution. The diameter of the artery, as well as the size of the arterial tube, and the diameter of the delivery hose from the machine to the arterial tube all produce resistance. As a point for injection, the artery with the largest diameter, generally the common carotid or the femoral artery, should be selected. An arterial tube of maximum size should be inserted into the artery. Small radial arterial tubes are of little or no value in vessels as large as the common carotid. Smaller arterial tubes are used for sectional or localized injections. The valve that controls the rate of flow of fluid and the diameters of the delivery hose and arterial tube constitute factors outside the body that determine resistance.

INTRAVASCULAR RESISTANCE

Intravascular resistances can be caused either by narrowing or obstruction of the lumen of a vessel. This narrowing or obstruction is brought about by conditions found either within the lumen of the vessel or within the walls of the vessel. The *lumen* can be *obstructed* by blood, antemortem emboli, antemortem thrombi, and postmortem coagula and thrombi.

As the embalming solution flows from the aorta into the narrowing branches of the arterial tree, the lumen of the arteries also narows. A coagulum that is loosened and moved along with the solution will eventually clog a small distributing artery. Arterial coagulum could never be reduced to a size where it could pass through arterioles and capillaries. When a coagulum reaches an arterial branch through which it can move no further, distribution of solution beyond this point is stopped. The only way tissues beyond this point can receive embalming solution is through the collateral circulation.

Intravascular resistance resulting from *narrowing of the lumen* can be caused by arteriosclerosis, most frequently seen in the arteries of the lower extremities; vasoconstriction, frequently seen on one side of the body as a result of a stroke; arteritis, brought about by inflammation of the artery; and intravascular rigor mortis, postmortem narrowing caused by rigor mortis of the smooth muscles in the arterial walls. Unlike extravascular resistance, the embalmer can do little to remove intravascular resistance.

EMBALMING PROCEDURES FOR INTRAVASCULAR PROBLEMS

The following embalming techniques can be used when intravascular problems are anticipated:

1. Use sufficient pressure and rate of flow to uniformly distribute the arterial solution. A slow rate of flow can help to prevent coagula in the arteries from floating free and clogging smaller branch arteries. Once circulation is established, a faster rate of flow can be used.
2. If arterial coagula are anticipated (i.e., bodies dead for long periods, gangrene evidenced in distal limbs, and death from infections) inject from the right common carotid artery (or restricted cervical injection). This pushes arterial coagula away from the arteries that supply the head and arms (the areas to be viewed). The legs can be injected separately, if necessary, or treated by hypodermic and/or surface embalming.
3. Avoid using a sclerotic artery for injection. The common carotid is rarely sclerotic, whereas the femoral and iliac arteries are frequently sclerotic.
4. Use the largest artery possible for the primary injection point. This is usually the common carotid, external iliac, or femoral artery.
5. Use an arterial tube of proper size so that it will not damage the walls of the artery.

EXTRAVASCULAR RESISTANCE

Extravascular resistance is pressure placed on the outside of a blood vessel. This pressure is sufficient to collapse or partially collapse the lumen of the vessel. The embalmer is better able to reduce or remove extravascular resistance than intravascular resistance. Therefore, the following discussion of extravascular resistances includes techniques that can be used to reduce or remove the pressures that these resistances place on blood vessels.

Rigor Mortis. The postmortem stiffening of the voluntary skeletal muscles is a strong extravascular resistance. Rigor mortis is not a uniform condition. It may be present in some muscles and absent in others. This can cause a very uneven distribution of arterial solution. Embalming prior to or during the onset of rigor is generally recommended. When rigor is present, gentle but very firm manipulation and massage of the muscles help to reduce the degree of stiffness. The massage and manipulation can be done prior to and during arterial injection.

Gas in the Cavities. Decomposition gases in the abdominal cavity can exert enough pressure to push the large abdominal aorta and inferior vena cava against the spinal column, thus causing these vessels to narrow or collapse. Most frequently this pressure can be removed at the beginning of the embalming by puncturing the abdominal wall with a trocar or scalpel. It may also be necessary to puncture some of the large and small intestines. This can easily be done without fear of interrupting the circulation.

Expansion of the Hollow Viscera During Injection. Too rapid an injection of arterial solution, especially in bodies dead for long periods, can result in expansion of the hollow visceral organs. This expansion causes the abdomen to swell and places sufficient pressure on the aorta and vena cava so as to collapse their lumens. Stomach purge often accompanies this abdominal distension. Insert a trocar into the abdominal cavity, keeping the point just beneath the anterior abdominal wall, and puncture some of the distended intestines.

Tumors and Swollen Lymph Nodes. These distended growths and organs can place pressure on the blood vascular system, creating distribution and drainage problems. Sectional injection may be necessary. A higher injection pressure and pulsation may help to obtain good distribution. Massage and manipulation may also help to encourage solution distribution and drainage.

Ascites and Hydrothorax. Enough fluid may accumulate in the thoracic and abdominal cavities to interfere with blood drainage and arterial solution distribution. Drainage from several sites may be necessary. The ascites can be removed or relieved by inserting a trocar into the abdominal cavity or inserting a drainage tube through a puncture made in the abdominal wall.

Contact Pressure. Portions of the body that push against the embalming table or against positioning devices (such as shoulder blocks) may not receive enough arterial solution. Contact pressure can restrict the flow of solution into the shoulders, buttocks, and backs of the legs. During embalming, these areas should be manipulated and massaged to relieve the pressure from the contact with the embalming table.

Visceral Weight. In all bodies, abdominal viscera create some resistance. In obese bodies, however, there can be sufficient visceral weight on the large vessels in the abdomen to restrict drainage and possibly solution distribution. Higher pressures, pulsation, and a more rapid rate of flow may help to overcome this resistance. Manipulation and massage of the abdominal area may also assist distribution and drainage.

Bandages. An Ace bandage or any bandage wound around an extremity should be removed prior to arterial injection. They can disrupt drainage from the hands and feet. During injection, even a patient identification band can be a source of vascular resistance.

Skeletal Edema. Skeletal edema can be intense enough that it exerts extravascular resistance to the distribution of embalming solution as well as a resistance to blood drainage. Numerous conditions, from pathological disorders to drug treatments, can bring this about (Fig. 12–3). These intense edemas are frequently seen postoperatively, particularly after open-heart or vascular surgery. Higher injection pressures, pulsation, manipulation, and massage assist in distribution and drainage. Sectional embalming may be necessary.

Inflammation. Inflamed tissue can swell to the extent that vascular constriction results. Higher injection pressures, pulsation, and massage may assist in distributing arterial solution into these body areas. Sectional and hypodermic embalming may be necessary.

COMBINED RESISTANCE

Extravascular and intravascular resistances rarely exist in and of themselves. In embalming the "average" body, a combination of resistances is found. For example, in embalming a 62-year-old man who died from a myocardial infarction, resistances might originate from rigor

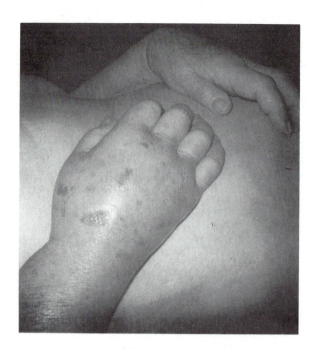

Figure 12–3. A right hand and arm distended with edma.

mortis (because of delay between death and preparation), arteriosclerosis (some degree of sclerosis can be found), contact pressure (possible in every body), and blood in the dependent portions of the vascular system.

These four sources of resistance demonstrate that even in a sudden death, vascular resistances are present that can restrict good arterial distribution and blood drainage. In the preceding example, the rigor may be intense enough that distribution is reduced to the point where sectional embalming is required. If the person had been taking an anticoagulant the blood may remain in a liquid form and postmortem clotting would be diminished. Thus, arterial distribution and blood drainage would be much better.

At the time of death invasive treatments and drugs administered could cause extensive ecchymoses on the backs of the hands or extreme antemortem subcutaneous emphysema, resulting in gross distension of the tissues of the neck and face. Delays between death and preparation greatly increase the amount of postmortem coagula in the vessels.

All these hypothetical factors demonstrate that the embalmer must prepare each body on the basis of the conditions exhibited by the individual body. The embalming analysis must be based upon the individual body conditions. As the embalming progresses, further analysis must be made as to the extent of arterial distribution, volume of drainage, clearing of discolorations, amount of tissue distension, degree of firming, and any new conditions that arise.

NEED FOR RESISTANCE

Resistance is not a totally negative factor in arterial embalming. If there were total resistance on the arteries no distribution could take place. If there was total resistance on the veins, drainage would not be possible and distension of the tissues would result. In embalming any body a certain amount of resistance is found throughout the vascular system. The injection pressure is greatest on the arterial side of the capillaries. This pressure overcomes arterial resistances and helps to distribute the embalming solution. The resistance in the capillaries and on the venous side of the capillaries slows the embalming solution and helps to hold it within the capillaries, giving the solution an opportunity to diffuse; brings about a more even distribution of the embalming solution, because it reduces short-circuiting of the embalming solution; and helps the tissues to retain more embalming solution, for it allows for better filtration of the embalming solution into the tissues.

If there were no resistance, the embalming solution would pass directly through the capillaries and into the drainage. To illustrate the problems that arise when there is little or no resistance, take the case of a person who dies from a ruptured aneurysm of the abdominal aorta. Some solution may be distributed, but most of the embalming solution will follow the path of least resistance through the torn artery and fill the abdominal cavity.

During injection and drainage of the body, most embalmers create resistance to effect better penetration of the embalming solution and reduction of the loss of solution. Intermittent or alternate methods of drainage are used. The solution is injected against a closed drainage system, which creates the resistance. In addition, some embalmers inject the last ¼ to ½ gallon of embalming solution with the vein used for drainage tied off. Aspiration can be delayed several hours. This technique helps the capillaries to hold the embalming solution and gives the solution time to diffuse.

Figure 12–4 illustrates the need for some degree of resistance. Figure 12–4A shows little or no resistance. The solution rushes through the tissues, resulting in tissue dehydration. Filtration is reduced, solution can easily short circuit, and the evenness of distribution is reduced.

Figure 12–4B demonstrates total resistance, perhaps a situation in which there is very extensive blood clotting. Once the system is filled, tissue distension becomes a major problem and uniformity of distribution is reduced.

Figure 12–4C represents a movable resistance, such as liquid blood in the venules and veins or the use of intermittent drainage. Blood removal is more complete, distribution is more uniform, and, most important, more

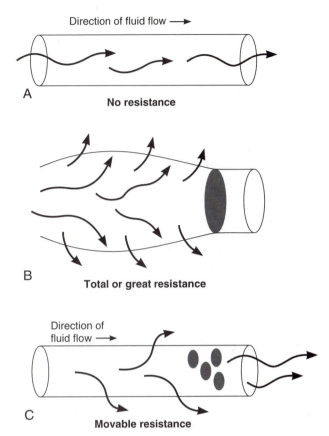

Figure 12–4. **A.** No resistance. **B.** Total or great resistance. **C.** Movable resistance.

embalming solution is retained by the body with a minimum of tissue distension.

PATHS OF LEAST RESISTANCE

When vascular resistances are present in a body, the arterial embalming solution always distributes to those areas where little or no resistance exists. As a result, certain body areas receive too much solution and others do not receive enough. Three questions must be asked: (1) Is the embalming solution flowing into the blood vascular system? (2) What body areas *are* and what areas *are not* receiving embalming solution? (3) Has a body area received *sufficient* arterial solution?

Three indicators can be used to tell if arterial solution is being distributed throughout the vascular system:

1. A drop in the fluid volume in the tank of the embalming machine.
2. When the rate-of-flow valve is opened on the centrifugal injection machine, there should be a drop on the pressure gauge. This drop is the **differential pressure.** The greater the drop, the greater the rate of flow. The differential reading of "10" in

Figure 12–5B indicates that the embalming solution is being injected twice as fast as it would if the differential reading is "5" (Fig. 12–5A). The fact that the dial dropped to 5 or 10 from the reading of 15 when the rate-of-flow valve was closed indicates that solution is entering the body. As the solution fills the vascular system, the dial may rise. This shows that more resistance is being encountered. To keep the rate of flow at the original speed, the pressure has to increase. Increasing the pressure increases the differential reading.

Example. The machine is turned on with the rate-of-flow valve (or the stopcock) turned off. (*No* solution is entering the body). The pressure is set at 20 pounds. The rate-of-flow valve is now opened and the dial drops to 15 pounds. The differential reading is 5. After a gallon and a half is injected, the needle on the dial rises to 18. This indicates the system has been filled and more resistance is being encountered. To establish the original rate of

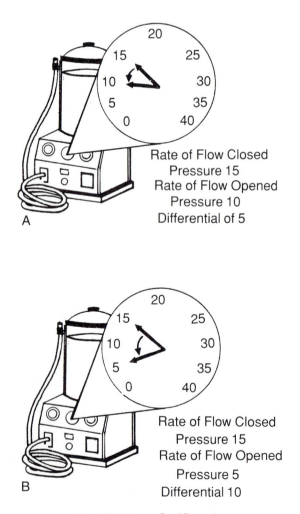

Rate of Flow Closed
Pressure 15
Rate of Flow Opened
Pressure 10
Differential of 5

A

Rate of Flow Closed
Pressure 15
Rate of Flow Opened
Pressure 5
Differential 10

B

Figure 12–5. Pressure–flow differentials.

flow, try to open the rate-of-flow valve so the needle drops to 15. If this does not happen, increase the pressure to 23 pounds. If the dial remains at 18 the differential is again 5, and this was the original rate of flow. Differential "pressure" is a good indicator of the resistance in the body. It may also indicate that an arterial tube is clogged. (The tube should always be checked prior to use to be certain it is clean).

3. There should be drainage if the solution is entering the body and making the proper circuit through the arteries, capillaries, and veins.

Once it has been determined that the arterial solution is entering the body at a rate of flow and pressure that do not cause distension, the embalmer must determine which body regions are receiving arterial solution and which areas are not. A group of indicators known as the *signs of arterial solution distribution and diffusion* help to make this determination. Most of these indicators, such as the presence of fluid dye in the tissues, demonstrate only the presence of embalming fluid in skin regions.

The dermis, the deep layer of the skin, is very vascular and offers little resistance to the flow of embalming solution, as the solution flows rapidly and easily into the surface areas of the body. The embalmer can easily detect the presence of embalming solution in the skin. Concern must be given to the deep tissues such as the muscles. It is very important that solution distribute to these body tissues, which offer more resistance. To achieve this deeper penetration of solution, the drainage can be restricted and massage must be very firm. Penetrating agents in the arterial solution also promote the passage of solution into the deeper tissues.

The skin areas offer little resistance to the flow of solution; also, some localized areas can receive large amounts of arterial solution. These areas are generally in the vicinity of the artery injected. Solutions will establish pathways where they quickly pass through a group of capillaries near the artery being injected. The fluid then passes rapidly into the drainage. This frequently happens when injection and drainage occur at the same location. This short-circuiting reduces the total volume of fluid available for saturation of other body areas.

In recent years, many direct connections between arterioles and venules have been discovered in the microcirculation of the blood. Here, again, is a route that offers little resistance to the flow of fluid. Embalming solution can rapidly pass from the arterial system to the veins without distributing to the tissues. Restricting the drainage can reduce the amount of arterial solution lost in these direct routes.

Once the embalmer determines that solution is entering the body and where it is within the body, it must be determined which body areas have received sufficient solution. There is no positive test for determining if a body area has sufficient solution. If there is any doubt, the embalmer should raise an artery that supplies the area and make a separate injection. If the area is very localized, hypodermic or surface embalming can be used. With local injections, it is wise to increase the strength of the injected chemical to help ensure good preservation. It is better to slightly overembalm an area than to risk the chance that an inadequate amount of preservative has reached the area.

INJECTION PRESSURE AND RATE OF FLOW

Injection pressure is needed to overcome intravascular and extravascular resistances. The pressure needed is created by the injection apparatus (embalming machine); it can be as simple as a gravity percolator or as complex as some of the centrifugal pumps.

Injection pressure is the amount of pressure produced by an injection device to overcome initial resistance within the vascular system.

Rate of flow is the amount of embalming solution injected in a given period, or the speed at which the embalming solution enters the body. The rate of flow is generally measured in ounces per minute.

Injection pressure and rate of flow are related, but not identical. Of the two, the rate of flow is the factor of most concern to the embalmer. The ideal rate of flow can be as much arterial solution as the body can accept as long as (1) the solution is evenly distributed throughout as much of the body as possible, and (2) there is little or no distension of the tissues. The ideal pressure is the amount needed to establish this rate of flow.

By use of a centrifugal pump or air pressure machine, it is possible to have a set pressure with the rate of flow valve closed. It is then possible to open the rate-of-flow valve to a certain point to establish the desired rate of flow and to open the rate-of-flow valve on a centrifugal pump and adjust the pressure to a point where the machine injects the desired number of ounces of solution. *In use of a centrifugal pump injector, it is recommended that the pressure be set with the rate-of-flow valve closed.* The pressure set with the rate-of-flow valve closed is called the *potential pressure.* When the rate-of-flow valve is opened the resultant pressure reading is called the *actual pressure.* The difference between actual pressure and potential pressure is the rate of flow or the *differential pressure.*

There are many theories as to the amount of pressure and rate of flow that should be used. Keep in mind that these factors vary in different ways:

1. From body to body: Bodies injected shortly after death when rigor is not present and some body heat is retained can be injected much faster than bodies that have been refrigerated many hours. A low pressure can be used to establish a high rate of flow in a recently deceased body.
2. In different body areas: Fluids always follow the path of least resistance. Areas such as the skin and vascular organs easily accept fluid. Resistance is greater in tissues where arteriosclerosis is present in the arteries or in body areas where blood has clotted or coagulated in the vessels.
3. As embalming proceeds: As embalming proceeds, resistance increases (a) when vessels are empty and fluid rapidly enters the body (after the vessels fill, more resistance is created), (b) when the preservative in the fluid acts on the capillaries, allowing less fluid to flow into the tissue spaces (more fluid will then be directed into the drainage), (c) when the tissue spaces become filled to capacity with arterial solution, and (d) when arterial clots move and block small arteries and venous coagula are hardened by the preservative solution, making them more difficult to remove.

It can easily be seen that pressure and rate of flow can vary from body to body, within the same body, or at different times in the embalming process.

Some claim that high pressures are required to force the preservative solution through the blood vascular system out to the tissues. Such advocates of high pressure also insist that the drainage be permitted to flow freely; that is, drainage should not be restricted. Naturally, at the high pressures with which the solution is injected in such cases, the drainage cannot be restricted without producing swelling. Consequently, the solution injected under such pressures tends to follow the path of least resistance. This means that if the vein is left open during the entire embalming operation, the injected solution is often forced rapidly through the circulatory channels (arteries, arterioles, capillaries, venules, veins), making very little contact with the tissue cells, which should be thoroughly saturated to be preserved. Under such conditions, much of the injected preservative solution is lost by way of the drain tube without having achieved its intended purpose—preservation of the soft tissues.

At times it may be necessary to increase, for short intervals, the pressure normally used to obtain distribution of the injected solution. After death, and depending on the cause of death, some blood vessels may collapse because the volume of circulating blood has decreased, the vessels contain no blood. Increase in the pressure or rate of flow may well promote filling of the vessels and start good distribution. When this has been accomplished, the amount of pressure can be reduced to somewhere between 2 and 10 pounds, depending on the case, that is, on the amount of drainage that is being taken. The pressure used at that time should be sufficient to maintain a rate of injection that is slightly greater than the amount of drainage. (On the average, the total drainage will equal approximately one half of the total volume of solution injected.)

Some embalmers are left with the impression that they can get by with a "one-point" injection on *every* case merely by using high pressure (20 pounds to as high as 100 pounds) as indicated on the embalming machine pressure gauge. They forget the pathology: sclerotic vessels may not permit enough fluid to reach remote body areas. Such a condition usually requires a "six-point" injection for complete and thorough embalming; the cause of death may have produced a condition in which the capillaries are easily ruptured by increased pressure, thereby permitting fluid loss. Rupture of the tiny superficial vessels as a result of injection pressures causes the injected solution to "hemorrhage" into the surrounding tissue areas and accumulate under the skin.

There exists much misunderstanding with respect to the pressure that may exist inside the body as a result of the injection of solution. The gauge on the device used for injection indicates the pressure at which the fluid is leaving the machine; this is not necessarily the pressure that exists within the body.

Ideal pressure is then defined as the pressure needed to overcome the vascular resistances of the body to distribute the embalming solution to all body areas. It can easily be seen that a one-point injection may require very little pressure; however, if the left leg does not receive arterial solution, a high pressure may be needed to inject solution down this leg using the left femoral artery if the vessels of the leg are sclerotic because of diabetes.

The *ideal rate of flow* is defined as the rate of flow needed to achieve uniform distribution of the embalming solution without distension of the tissues. In embalming a body dead from a sudden myocardial infarction, a faster rate of injection can be used if death occurred within 2 or 3 hours of embalming rather than if death occurred several days previously and there was some evidence of decomposition. In the latter situation, a rapid rate of flow would easily bring about distension of the tissues.

There are two strong schools of thought on injection rate. Some embalmers prefer a low pressure and a rapid rate of flow. (Note: Injection machines have been developed on this idea of low pressure but high rates of flow.) Other embalmers feel a high pressure but a very slow rate of flow is ideal. The following compromise might be acceptable. A moderate rate of injection for the *"average unautopsied"* body is 1 gallon over 10 to 15 minutes. The pressure needed to achieve this flow could range from 2 to 10 pounds (Fig. 12–6.) Postmortem coagula are found in the arteries as well as the veins. Using

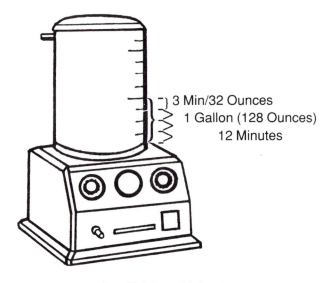

3 Min/32 Ounces
1 Gallon (128 Ounces)
12 Minutes

Figure 12–6. Average injection rates.

slower rates of injection may help to keep these coagula from moving to smaller distal arteries where the vessel would become blocked and diminish or completely stop the distribution of arterial solution from that point.

Not all bodies can be injected within the same set time at the same rate of flow and injection pressures. As soon as distension is evident, injection should be stopped. The injection pressure can be reduced, the rate of flow can be reduced, or sectional embalming can be done. Likewise, if arterial solution is not entering some areas of the body, the rate of flow can be increased, the pressure can be increased, or sectional embalming can be done.

High pressures are not always necessary. If pressures ranging from 2 to 10 pounds are used with intermittent or restricted drainage after surface discolorations have been cleared, the following effects are possible: removal of blood from the main as well as the collateral circulation; saturation of soft tissues by the injected solution; and buildup of intravascular pressure, restoring moisture and retaining a sufficient amount of solution to produce thorough preservation.

Remember that for the injected embalming solution to accomplish its function of preservation, it must reach and penetrate *all* tissue areas. Merely flushing the solution through the blood vascular system and out the drain tube does not achieve the intended purpose. It requires time for the preservative solution to diffuse out of the capillaries and penetrate, and saturate tissues. If high pressures and a fast rate of flow are employed in injecting the embalming solution, then the technique should also include some compensating factor, such as the use of large volumes of solution, the use of pulsation, and the tying off of the vein as the last half-gallon of solution is injected to retain a sufficient amount of the preservative material. The injection pressure must be adopted to suit the needs of the individual body. Studies have demonstrated best results can be obtained by injecting (the unautopsied body) at a *moderate* rate of flow, 12 to 15 minutes per gallon of arterial solution, accompanied by a sufficient arterial injection pressure to maintain the desired rate of flow; 2 to 10 psi is recommended to ensure distribution and diffusion of the chemicals. Higher pressures and faster rates of flow may be necessary when sectional embalming is used for problem areas that did not receive sufficient arterial solution.

> The foregoing would be under "ideal" conditions. The *ideal rate of flow* and the *ideal pressure* will vary from body to body. The "ideal" of these two factors is the pressure necessary and the rate of flow necessary to overcome the resistances and evenly distribute the preservative solution throughout the entire body, while at the same time the body retains as much of the preservative solution as possible without distension or dehydration of the body tissues.

CLINICAL DISCUSSION

To many embalmers the gauge on a pressurized fluid injection machine indicates the pressure that is being exerted within the body's blood vessels. Such a belief, however, is fallacious. The pressure gauge actually relates the resistance to the flow of the arterial solution. The pressure or force of the stream of embalming solution depends on a number of significant influences within the body and on the mechanical arrangement of the injector itself.

For example, if a centrifugal embalming machine is filled with fluid and the end of the rubber tubing is allowed to discharge the fluid back into the tank uninhibited, the volume of fluid pumped out would increase as the pressure is increased if the rate of flow remains unchanged. If the pressure is set at a constant rate, the volume pumped out would decrease as the rate of flow is reduced, and the pressure would tend to increase as the resistance to the flow increases. A simple illustration of the effect of end resistance on rate of flow and pressure is obtained by filling the tank of a centrifugal machine and setting the controls to deliver a moderate amount of pressure and rate of flow. After the machine is running, pinch off the rubber tubing so as not to totally occlude the fluid from flowing, and note the gauge readings. The restriction (resistance) causes the pressure to *increase* markedly and the rate of flow to *decrease* substantially.

The relationship between machine gauge pressure, rate of flow, and events within the blood vascular system is difficult to equate. There is a steady decline in pressure from the high point recorded on the embalming injector pressure gauge to the smallest arteries. Pressure is dissipated against the channel walls while moving through the rubber tubing (the size of arterial tube), through blood vessels, and against the blood (thick or thin) and clots within the blood vascular system.

In a living person, blood pressure falls from its exit at the left ventricle through the blood vascular system to its entrance into the right atrium. It is commonly acknowledged that within a normal healthy aorta, blood flows at about 15 inches per second. By the time the blood reaches the capillary bed, which has 700 to 800 times the volume capacity of the aorta, flow diminishes to about one-fiftieth of an inch per second. As the blood flow passes into the venous side, the vessels increase in size and diminish in volume capacity. Thus, blood pressure and flow slowly increase.

Many factors influence blood pressure and the blood vascular system in life. In younger people, free from vascular diseases, the arteries expand on systole and, thus, exert pressure to move the blood as their elastic walls contract and return to normal size in response to the pressure. In persons with arteriosclerosis the walls are no longer fully elastic; the arteries do not expand and, therefore, offer more resistance, which is reflected as an increase in blood pressure. Additional factors influence blood flow when arteriosclerosis is present. There is usually a reduction in the diameter of the lumen of the artery almost to the point of occlusion. The roughening of the intimal coat resulting from the calcium deposits interrupts the flow of blood.

Temperature plays a part in increasing or decreasing blood flow in the living. Cold tends to cause vasoconstriction, whereas heat tends to cause vasodilation. When considering possible postmortem influences on the rate of flow of embalming solution and pressure, remember that rigor mortis may restrict the flow of the solution if not relieved; warm fluid (at or near 100°F) may be more efficient than cold fluid; and various tumors, accumulations of ascites, and body position may exert profound alterations in rate of flow and/or embalming solution pressure by compressing blood vessels and increasing resistance to the flow of embalming solutions. Ruptured blood vessels further alter the "normal" postmortem pressure/resistance relationship by permitting the escape of embalming solution from blood vessels into surrounding tissues at low pressures. Increasing the injector pressure output rarely improves the situation.

CENTER OF ARTERIAL SOLUTION DISTRIBUTION

The ascending aorta and the **arch of the aorta** are the center of arterial distribution. The arch is a continuation of the ascending aorta and gives off three large branches from its superior surface. From right to left, these are the **brachiocephalic artery,** which supplies the right side of the head and right arm; the **left common carotid artery,** which supplies the left side of the head and face; and the **left subclavian artery,** which supplies the left arm. The *arch* continues as the *descending thoracic aorta* through which the embalming solution is distributed to all other parts of the body.

The arch of the aorta is a continuation of the *ascending aorta,* which begins at the left ventricle. The embalming solution is injected into the arteries of the body and not into the veins because of the valve at the beginning of the ascending aorta called the *aortic semilunar valve.* This valve is situated between the left ventricle of the heart and the ascending aorta. As embalming solution is injected, the ascending aorta fills and causes the aortic semilunar valve to close (Fig. 12–7). Once it is closed, the arteries of the body can begin to fill with the embalming solution. If the valve fails to close, or leaks, the left ventricle fills with embalming solution. If this happens, the cusps of the left atrioventricular (bicuspid valve) close, allowing the arteries of the body to fill.

If, for some reason, both the aortic semilunar valve and the bicuspid valve fail to close (solution injected under too much pressure), arterial solution will flow to the lungs through the pulmonary veins, which could create a purge. The solution might flow into the right ventricle through the pulmonary artery, and from the right ventricle to the right atrium, from which it would exit through the drainage.

SIGNS OF ARTERIAL SOLUTION DISTRIBUTION AND DIFFUSION

Each embalmer has a set of criteria that he or she uses to tell if arterial solution has reached an area of the body. It is best that more than one indicator be used. Remember that even if embalming solution is present in an area, sufficient solution of the proper strength must be present. Most of the signs of distribution and diffusion are surface indicators. Concern must always be given to the deeper tissues and organs that cannot be seen.

SIGNS OF ARTERIAL SOLUTION DISTRIBUTION AND DIFFUSION

- Dye in the tissues
- Fluorescent dye observed using black lights
- Distension of superficial blood vessels
- Leakage from intravenous punctures
- Blood drainage
- Clearing of intravascular blood discolorations
- Loss of skin elasticity (beginning firming)
- Drying of the tissues
- Rounding of fingers, lips, and toes
- Bleaching of the tissues
- Firming of the tissues

Dyes. The most reliable sign of arterial distribution and diffusion is the presence of an active fluid dye in the tissues of the skin. As active fluid dyes stain the tissues, they act not only as a sign of solution distribution, but clearly demonstrate solution diffusion. The dyes help to prevent formaldehyde gray and provide an excellent internal cosmetic. They are available in pink and suntan. Many arterial fluids contain active dye, but additional dyes may be added separately to the arterial solution.

Fluorescent Dye. A coinjection arterial chemical that contains a fluorescent dye that cannot be seen without the use of a "black light" is available for injection with the preservative arterial solution. When the lights of the embalming room are extinguished and a "black light" is held over the body, areas of the body in which the coinjection

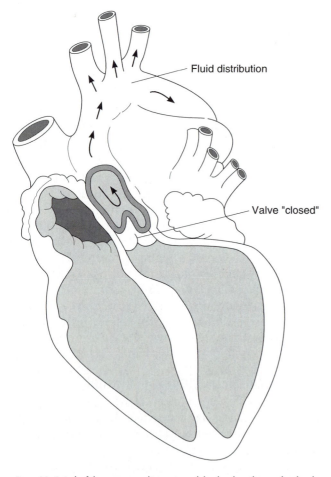

Fluid distribution

Valve "closed"

Figure 12–7. Arch of the aorta, ascending aorta, and the closed semilunar valve closed.

fluorescent dye is present glow a bluish white. This coinjection fluid is similar to active fluid dye, except that the coinjection dye cannot be seen on the body surface. It is important to remember that fluid dyes indicate only surface profusion of the embalming solution.

Clearing of Intravascular Blood Discoloration.

It is most important that the livor mortis be observed prior to the injection of arterial solution (Fig. 12–8). Livor is found in the dependent body areas. The fingertips and nail beds should be carefully inspected. Depending on the cause of death and the position of the body, livor may be present even in the face. If this blood discoloration is pushed on, it should lighten, indicating that the blood present is still in the vascular system. During injection, the livor mortis should be removed. Many times the "breaking up" of large areas of livor mortis can easily be observed. Once this breakup begins, the area can be massaged.

Distension of Small Surface Vessels.

When fluid reaches certain body areas such as the hands, feet, or temple of the face, small vessels can often be observed by their distension. It should be pointed out that gravitated blood can also cause the veins to rise when hands are placed on the embalming table. Gas in the cavities can cause small vessels to distend. Observe vessel areas (e.g., temples, backs of hands) prior to and during arterial injection to be certain any distension of the vessel(s) is brought about by arterial injection.

Loss of Skin Elasticity.

As the solution begins to firm the tissues, skin areas exhibit a loss of elasticity. When the skin is gathered and gently pulled upward, it slowly settles back into proper position.

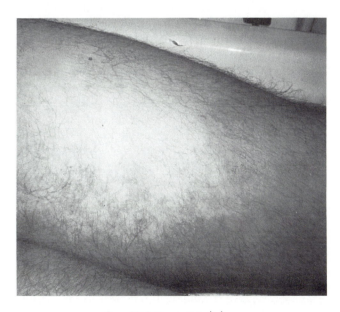

Figure 12–8. Livor mortis in the legs.

Firming (Fixation) of the Tissues.

Rigor mortis can easily be mistaken for firming of the tissues by the arterial solution. It is most important that in making the preembalming analysis of the body, the **presence of rigor** be noted. Some bodies exhibit little or no firming after good embalming. These are usually bodies that have been treated with large doses of drugs, that have small amounts of muscular protein, or that have been dead for long periods. Most bodies exhibit some degree of firming depending on the amount and strength of embalming chemical injected. Firming, although not a foolproof sign of embalmed tissue, is nevertheless an indicator that most embalmers rely on as a sign of arterial distribution. Some embalming chemicals are designed to produce tissues that are only slightly firm or that exhibit no firming. Different embalming chemicals affect the degree and speed of tissue firming.

Drying of the Tissues.

As arterial solution reacts with the tissues to the skin, the surface of the body dries slightly. Areas not reached by the embalming solution often appear shiny and somewhat moist to the touch. This is not a very reliable sign of distribution and should *not* be relied on as an accurate indicator. Bodies that are dehydrated prior to embalming exhibit dry skin tissues *before* arterial solution is injected.

Bleaching of the Tissues.

Some arterial fluids produce a mottled effect of the skin when the solution is present. This mottled coloring is caused by the bleaching quality of some arterial fluids. Dyes in the embalming solution, however, can mask this bleaching effect. Bleaching is not a reliable sign of arterial fluid distribution.

Blood Drainage.

The presence of blood drainage indicates that embalming solution is being distributed to the tissues and organs of the body. It does not, however, indicate what specific areas of the body are receiving arterial solution. As a sign of distribution, it does not account for short-circuiting of arterial solution. Some body areas might be receiving too much and other body areas might not be receiving any solution. Excellent preservation can be accomplished with little or no drainage. In embalming bodies for dissection, many medical schools take no drainage. The blood is used as a vehicle for the concentrated embalming solutions; however, distension is generally very evident. In "waterless embalming," very concentrated solutions but in much smaller volumes are used than in standard embalming (i.e., 1 to $1\frac{1}{2}$ gallons would be injected in waterless embalming; 2 to 4 gallons would be injected in standard embalming). Limiting drainage again helps to make the blood the vehicle for dilution and distribution of the concentrated chemical solution.

Leakage From Punctures. When intravenous needles are removed by the hospital after death, during the embalming process, fluid or blood drainage can be seen exiting from these intravenous sites. This is a good indication that arterial solution is reaching these body areas. Some embalmers puncture the skin with a large-gauge needle or the tip of a scalpel (in an area not to be viewed) to see if embalming solution seeps from the skin.

Rounding of Fingers, Lips, and Toes. With some embalming formulations the tips of the fingers, lips, and toes slightly plump when reached by the arterial solution. Depending on the method of drainage and the strength of the embalming solution, the reverse can happen; these areas can wrinkle when fluid reaches them as a result of dehydration. It is an unreliable test of distribution but may be very evident in some bodies.

> Most embalmers use several signs of distribution to ensure that a sufficient amount of arterial solution has reached a body area. The most reliable in the preceding list are dyes, clearing of intravascular blood discolorations, and firming of tissues.

OBSERVATIONS PRIOR TO INJECTION

Several signs of arterial solution distribution and diffusion can be confused with several postmortem changes. It is important that the embalmer note these changes prior to injection so they are not mistaken as a sign of arterial distribution.

Observe for the presence or absence of livor mortis in all body areas prior to the start of the arterial injection. Examine the nail beds. Some degree of livor is generally present. In some bodies, however, depending on the position of the hands, the livor may gravitate from the fingers and hands. If this were not noted at the start of the embalming, the *absence* of the livor could be mistaken for clearing of the livor by the arterial injection.

Note the degree of rigor mortis present in the tissues. An attempt should always be made to relieve the rigor prior to injection. This is not always possible in areas such as the legs or jaw. Rigor can easily be mistaken for firming of the tissues by the arterial solution.

Observe the distension of veins or small arteries. Veins on the backs of the hands can be distended before arterial solution injected as a result of gravitation of the blood. Gases in the cavities or conditions such as ascites or hydrothorax can put pressure on the diaphragm and heart and cause small vessels to fill with blood. This distension or its absence should be noted prior to arterial injection.

Note any discoloration of the skin. Skin of refrigerated or frozen bodies or bodies dead from carbon monoxide poisoning may have a pinkish hue. If fluid dyes are used, this color gives the appearance of embalmed tissue. It is important to note this discoloration (resulting from hemolysis) prior to arterial injection.

Check for firmness of the tissues. Tissues of bodies placed in refrigeration, as many are done today, not only appear to be embalmed (hemolysis) but also feel slightly firm, as embalmed tissue. This firming is due to the slight firming of subcutaneous fatty tissues as a result of the refrigeration. This condition should be noted with refrigerated bodies so it is not mistaken for distribution and firming by the arterial solution.

These factors should all be noted in making a pre-embalming analysis. Active dyes in the arterial fluid serve as the best indicator for the presence of arterial solution in a body region.

IMPROVING ARTERIAL SOLUTION DISTRIBUTION

Several mechanical (or physical) procedures improve the distribution of the arterial solution. The embalmer may also use a combination of these procedures.

1. Increase the rate of flow of the arterial solution being injected.
2. Increase the pressure of the arterial solution being injected.
3. Inject the arterial solution using pulsation.
4. Restrict the drainage; use intermittent drainage and the alternate method of drainage.
5. Massage the body. Massage should be firm, not merely rubbing the surface of the body. Massage should be directed along the arterial routes (e.g., if solution is not entering the legs, massage should first be concentrated on the inguinal areas; once solution enters the leg the remainder of the arterial route can be massaged and flexed).
6. Inject an adequate volume of embalming solution. Often, when large volumes of embalming solution are injected, body areas that received little or no arterial solution during the early part of the embalming receive solution after 2 or 3 gallons has been injected.

Treatments for specific areas may also be applied. For *facial tissues,* massage the neck where the common carotid arteries are located. For the *arms,* lower them to the sides or over the embalming table; massage should first be concentrated in the axilla (Fig. 12–9). For the *fingers,* massage the radial and ulnar artery areas of the fore-

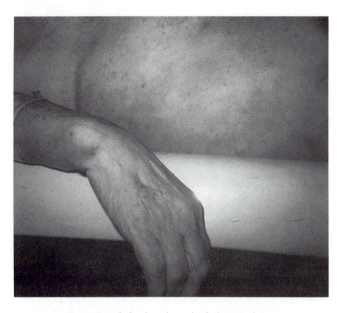

Figure 12–9. The hands are lowered to facilitate circulation.

arm and then massage the sides of the fingers (where the vessels are located); pressure can also be applied to the nailbeds. For the *legs,* massage the inguinal areas over the femoral arteries, flex the legs, and turn the foot inward; this helps to "squeeze" the muscles of the legs.

Massage can attract arterial solution to an area. Areas such as the lips and eyelids often respond well to massage (when it is needed). Squeezing the lips can attract solution into the labial tissues. Care should be taken that swelling or dehydration (wrinkles) do not result.

Body areas that receive no solution or inadequate amounts of arterial solution should be injected separately. If distribution is still a problem, restricting drainage from the limb, massaging, increasing the pressure or rate of flow of injection, or using pulsation with higher pressures may all help to distribute solution into a particular body area.

CLINICAL EXAMPLE: ONE-POINT INJECTION USING THE COMMON CAROTID ARTERY

The right arm does not appear to be receiving arterial solution. The axillary area is massaged and the arm lowered over the side of the table. There is still no solution in the arm. Raise and inject the axillary or brachial artery. Use a higher pressure if desired. Thoroughly massage along the arterial route. Assume that the hand does not receive solution. Raise the radial or ulnar artery and inject.

Remember that solution must enter a body region before it can reach a specific location. Arterial solution cannot enter the fingers if it is not entering the arm.

When doubt exists as to whether a body area has received any or an adequate amount of arterial solution, make every attempt to raise the artery that supplies the area and separately inject the area.

Stimulation of arterial solution distribution is a three-step procedure:

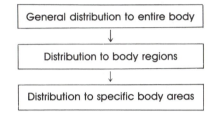

General distribution to entire body
↓
Distribution to body regions
↓
Distribution to specific body areas

DIFFUSION OF THE EMBALMING SOLUTION

The key to arterial embalming is arterial fluid *diffusion.* Fluid diffusion can be defined as the passage of some elements of the injected embalming solutions from within the capillary (intravascular) to the tissue spaces (extravascular). The capillary network of the blood vascular system is so vast that a pin can hardly be inserted into the living skin without rupturing a sufficient number of these smallest of blood vessels to cause bleeding (Fig. 12–10).

Capillaries are the smallest blood vessels. They link the smallest arteries (arterioles) to the smallest veins (venules). They are actually the extensions of the inner linings of these larger vessels. Their walls are composed of endothelium, which lines the entire vascular system and is made up of flat, single-layered cells called *squamous epithelium.* These very thin-walled cells form the semipermeable membranes through which substances in the blood must pass to reach the body cells.

Blood does not have direct contact with body cells. All of the cells (e.g., muscle cells, nerve cells) are surrounded by a liquid called interstitial (tissue) fluid. Blood nutrients and oxygen must pass through the walls of the capillaries and into the interstitial fluid. These products diffuse through the tissue fluid to reach the body cells. This same movement occurs in embalming. The arterial solution must pass from the capillary, through the walls of the capillary, into the interstitial fluid, and finally to the body cells. It must then enter the cells of the body and react with the protoplasm protein.

METHODS OF ARTERIAL SOLUTION DIFFUSION

The start of this chapter stated that "arterial embalming could actually be called capillary embalming." It is at the capillary level that most embalming begins. (Additionally, the contents of the blood vascular system,

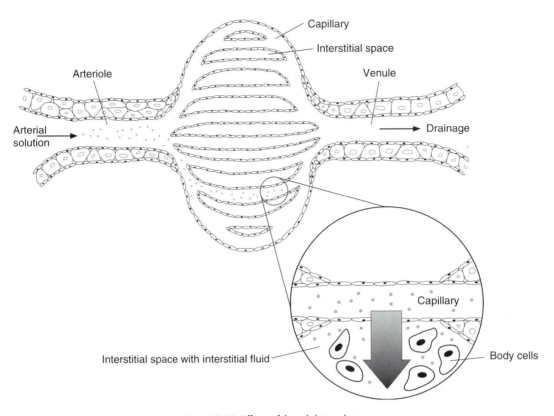

Figure 12–10. Diffusion of the embalming solution.

including any microbes or their agents in the blood, and the lining of the blood vascular system are disinfected and preserved as the embalming solution passes through the vessels.) From the capillaries, embalming solution moves to the interstitial fluid that surrounds each cell. The solution makes contact with proteins in the interstitial fluid, proteins in the cell membranes, and proteins in the cytoplasm of the cell.

Physical (or passive) transport mechanisms are responsible for the movement of embalming solution from within the capillaries to the tissue spaces. The energy needed to move the solution through the walls of the capillary originates from a nonliving mechanism. Passive mechanisms can move materials through dead cell membranes (capillaries). The major passive (or physical) transport processes for the movement of embalming solutions are pressure filtration, osmosis, and dialysis.

Pressure Filtration

Pressure filtration caused by intravascular pressure (IVP) is one of the most important passive transport systems for the passage of embalming solution from the capillary to tissue fluid. In this process both the solute and solvent portions of the embalming solution pass into the interstitial fluid. Penetrating agents (wetting agents, surface tension reducers, or surfactants) in the concentrated embalming fluid lower its surface tension. The reduction of

surface tension makes the embalming solution "wetter," and it can more easily pass through the minute pores and the cell membranes of the capillaries.

Intravascular pressure places enough pressure on the embalming solution to force it through the pores and cells of the capillary walls. This is similar to the effect of a lawn soaker hose. Some of the solution enters the tissue spaces to mix with the interstitial fluid. The embalming solution that remains in the capillary pushes on to remove the blood and exits as part of the drainage.

In the agonal period, respiration can become difficult and shallow. Sufficient oxygen is not delivered to the blood. As a defense mechanism, the pores between the cells of the capillaries expand in an attempt to get more oxygen. It is theorized that at death the capillaries are permeable, for their pores are still expanded. As a result, embalming solution can easily be filtered (or pushed) through these pores (caused by intravascular pressure). In some bodies, the capillaries may have begun to decompose. The injected solution can now easily flow through the broken capillaries into the tissue spaces. When this happens the body tissues easily distend. This is seen in bodies that have been dead for long periods. These bodies easily swell and there is little or no drainage.

Likewise, when the limbs are exercised to break up rigor mortis, many capillaries may be torn. The muscle tissues can rapidly swell on injection and, again, drainage is minimal. In bodies in which decomposition is evident or rigor is present, stronger solutions should be used so preservation can be achieved with a minimal amount of solution. This keeps swelling at a minimum. Pressure filtration is, no doubt, one of the primary mechanisms by which embalming solution comes into contact with the interstitial spaces and fluids (Fig. 12–11).

Osmosis

Osmosis is a passive transport mechanism involved with liquid (or solvent) movement. It is the passage of a solvent (such as water) through a semipermeable membrane from a dilute to a concentrated solution. Embalming solutions are more dilute (or less dense) than the interstitial fluids that surround the body cells. The interstitial fluids and the embalming solution are separated by the walls of the capillaries, which are semipermeable. Some of the chemical compounds found in the interstitial fluid cannot move through the capillary walls into the blood vascular system. The more dilute solution, in this case the embalming solution, is described as hypotonic, meaning it is more dilute or less dense than the interstitial fluid. For example, in mixing a 1-gallon solution of embalming solution, assume that 8 ounces of concentrated fluid is added to 120 ounces of water; for every ounce of embalming fluid, 15 ounces of water is used as a dilutant.

Some of the hypotonic embalming solution will easily pass through the walls and minute pores of the capillary to enter the interstitial spaces and mix with the interstitial fluid. It will then travel through the interstitial fluid and come into contact with the cells. Again, the process of osmosis will occur. This time the mixture of interstitial fluid and embalming solution will pass through the cell membrane and the preservatives will enter the cytoplasm of the cell. All along this route, contact of the preservative solution is made with proteins whether they are in the walls of the capillaries, in the interstitial fluid, in the membranes of the cells, or in the cytoplasm of the cell. New substances are being made between the protein and the preservative. In this manner, the process of preservation occurs.

When the directions are not followed and embalming solutions are made too weak (too dilute), these solutions will rapidly pass through the capillaries into the tissue fluids. Not only can swelling occur, but inadequate preservation results. These tissues become "waterlogged" with the weak solution, and the process of decomposition can actually be speeded. A reverse condition can be created by mixing solutions that are too concentrated. These concentrated solutions can cause the moisture in the interstitial fluid to move into the capillaries, bringing about dehydration. In conditions such as edema, a more concentrated (or dense) embalming solution can be used.

When the embalmer dilutes the concentrated arterial fluid with water, this dilution is called **primary dilution**. In addition to water, coinjection fluid may also be used as a diluent in addition to such chemicals as humectant and water softener. These solutions are described as being hypotonic for embalming the average body under normal moisture conditions. They allow some moisture to be added to the tissues and assist in retaining tissue moisture.

Within the tissue spaces, where the interstitial fluid is present, dilution of the arterial fluid continues. This dilution of the embalming solution that occurs in the tissues of the body is called the **secondary dilution**. The moisture found in the tissues dilutes the fluid. In addition, the fluid that remains in the capillaries and exits with the drainage is also diluted by the liquid portion of the blood. The secondary dilution of the fluid can be very great in bodies with skeletal edema.

In making an embalming analysis the embalmer must evaluate the moisture conditions of the body. Are the tissues dehydrated? Are the tissues moist as a result of edema? Or are the tissues normal? On the basis of these observations the primary dilution is prepared. On the labels of embalming fluid most chemical manufacturers indicate the number of ounces of concentrated fluid to use per gallon based on the moisture content of the body.

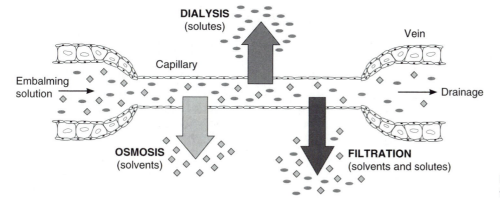

Figure 12–11. Summary of "fluid diffusion": pressure filtration, osmosis, and dialysis.

Dialysis

The third method of passive transport by which the embalming solution passes from the capillaries to the cells is dialysis. Dialysis is the diffusion of the dissolved crystalloid solutes of a solution through a semipermeable membrane. Interstitial fluid, cytoplasm of the body cells, and embalming solutions are composed primarily of the solvent water. Dissolved in these solutions are very small solutes called **crystalloids** and very large solutes called **colloids.**

The embalming solution in the capillary is separated from the interstitial fluid by the semipermeable membrane of the capillary wall. The cytoplasm within the cell is separated from the interstitial fluid by the semipermeable **cell membrane.** In dialysis, small crystalloids can diffuse through the semipermeable membranes, but large colloids in the solutions cannot. Water is the primary solvent in embalming solutions; alcohols and glycerine are other examples. The solutes in embalming fluids are various crystalloids such as salts, preservatives, and germicides and colloids (humectants). Interstitial fluid comprises the solvent water and various crystalloid salts and colloids (proteins, enzymes, etc.). Crystalloids in the embalming solution can diffuse through the capillary semipermeable membrane into the interstitial fluid. These preservatives, germicides, dyes, and so on then spread through the interstitial fluid and again pass through the cell membrane to enter the cytoplasm of the cell.

To repeat, dialysis is the diffusion of crystalloids across a semipermeable membrane that is impermeable to colloids. It is the process of separating crystalloids (smaller particles) from colloids (larger particles) by the difference in their rates of diffusion through a semipermeable membrane.

MOVEMENT OF EMBALMING SOLUTIONS FROM OUTSIDE THE CAPILLARIES TO INSIDE THE CELLS

Fluid diffusion was defined as the movement of embalming solution from within the capillary (intravascular) to the interstitial fluid (extravascular). Embalming solution does not stop moving once it leaves the capillary and enters the interstitial space to mix with the interstitial fluid. The interstitial fluid (intercellular or tissue fluid) is a viscous solution similar to the cytoplasm found inside the cells of the body. It contains inorganic chemicals, proteins, carbohydrates, and lipids dissolved in water. This fluid surrounds the cells of the body and is the connection between the blood vascular system (capillaries) and the body cells. Embalming solution must pass from the capillaries into the interstitial fluid, spread through the interstitial fluid, and finally enter the cells of the body (Fig. 12–12). Once inside the body cells, the

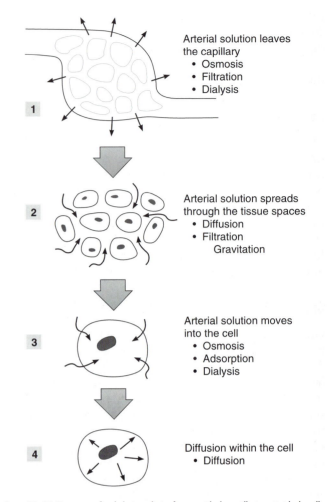

Figure 12–12. Movement of embalming solution from outside the capillaries to inside the cells.

embalming solution again diffuses to come into contact with all portions of the cell.

The concentrated embalming elements are spread through the interstitial fluid by the passive transport systems called *diffusion* and *filtration gravitation*. Passage of embalming solution into the body cells is brought about by the passive transport systems of **adsorption, osmosis,** and **dialysis.**

Diffusion

Diffusion means scattering or spreading. Small particles such as molecules are always moving in all directions. For example, place a drop of fluid dye into a gallon of water and let the solution of dye and water set without stirring. In a short period, the entire gallon of water is slightly and evenly colored by the dye. The concentrated drop of dye has spread through the water. Diffusion occurs from a region of high concentration to a region of lower concentration. In a similar manner, once the embalming solution passes into the interstitial fluid it spreads (or diffuses) through the interstitial fluid to come into contact with the cells of the body. By the processes of dialysis, adsorption, and osmosis it passes into the cell and, once in the cell, spreads through the cytoplasm by diffusion.

Adsorption

The cytoplasm of the body cells is composed of a continuous aqueous solution (cytosol) and all the organelles (except nucleus) suspended in it. The fluid inside the cells of the body is called a **colloidal dispersion.** The large colloid molecules, because of their large surface area, tend to *adsorb* molecules. Colloidal dispersions in cells adsorb molecules from the surrounding interstitial tissue fluids. In this manner, some of the embalming solution present in the interstitial fluid is adsorbed into the body cells.

Gravity Filtration

Gravity filtration is the extravascular settling of embalming solution by gravitational force into the dependent areas of the body. This passive transport system helps to move embalming solution throughout the interstitial fluid. In the embalmed body gravity filtration is responsible for the movement of embalming solution into the dependent tissues—lower back, buttocks, and backs of arms, legs, and shoulders. It may be of some value in moving embalming solution into those areas that are in contact with the embalming table. This slow movement continues for some time after the injection of solution. This is *not* a gravitation of fluids through the vascular system. It is extravascular movement of the solution through the interstitial fluid.

Summary

Passive transport systems require some amount of time to work. Pressurized injection, the penetrating agents found in the arterial fluids, and pressure filtration constitute the primary transport system for the movement of arterial solution from the capillaries to the tissue spaces. Osmosis, dialysis, gravitation filtration, and diffusion all take longer. Many embalmers prefer a delay between injection and cavity aspiration. In addition to a delay, many embalmers prefer to inject the last half-gallon of arterial solution with the drainage closed. This method allows a maximum filtration pressure to be established. The delay between injection can be 1 or 2 hours. Some embalmers feel several hours is needed. There should be some interval between injection and aspiration, even if it is only the time in which incisions are sewn and the body washed and dried. This interval gives the solutions an opportunity to fully penetrate the capillaries.

KEYS TERMS AND CONCEPTS FOR STUDY AND DISCUSSION

1. Define the following terms:
   Actual pressure
   Adsorption
   Arterial fluid
   Arterial solution
   Arterial solution diffusion
   Arterial solution distribution
   Arterial solution perfusion
   Arteriole
   Capillary
   Center of arterial solution distribution
   Contact pressure
   Crystalloid
   Dialysis
   Differential pressure
   Diffusion
   Drainage
   Extravascular resistance
   Gravity filtration
   Hypertonic solution
   Hypotonic solution
   Ideal pressure
   Ideal rate of flow
   Injection pressure
   Interstitial
   Interstitial fluid
   Intravascular resistance
   Lumen
   Osmosis
   Passive transport system
   Potential pressure
   Pressure filtration
   Primary dilution
   Rate of flow
   Retained embalming solution
   Secondary dilution
   Semipermeable membrane
   Signs of distribution
   Solute
   Solvent
   Venule
2. Discuss the movement of arterial solution from the machine to an individual body cell.
3. Why would the ascending aorta and the arch of the aorta be considered the "center of arterial solution distribution"?
4. Why is some resistance valuable to drainage?
5. Discuss fluid dilutions for the normal (moisture content) body; emaciated and dehydrated body; body with skeletal edema; and body with ascites and/or hydrothorax but no skeletal edema.

BIBLIOGRAPHY

Anthony CP. *Textbook of Anatomy and Physiology.* St. Louis, MO: CV Mosby; 1979:40–53.

Arnow LE. *Introduction to Physiological and Pathological Chemistry.* St. Louis, MO: CV Mosby; 1976:66–73.

Dhonau CO. *The ABCs of Pressure and Distribution,* File 86. Cincinnati, OH: Cincinnati College of Embalming.

Dhonau CO. *Manual of Case Analysis.* 2nd ed. Cincinnati, OH: The Embalming Book Co.; 1928.

Frederick JF. The mathematics of embalming chemistry, Parts I and II. *Dodge Mag,* October–November 1968.

Johnson EC. A study of arterial pressure during embalming. In: *Champion Expanding Encyclopedia.* Springfield, OH: Champion Chemical; 1981:2081–2084.

Zweifach BW. The microcirculation of the blood. *Sci Am,* January 1959.

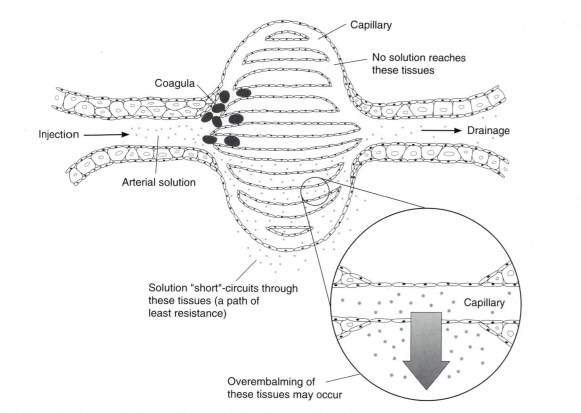

Figure 13–2. *Continued.* **B.** The greatest disadvantage of the one-point method of injection and drainage is the short-circuiting of arterial solution. Solution has a tendency to find direct routes from the arterioles to the venules in the region around the injection site. This can account for overembalming of the area near the injection site and loss of a large amount of arterial solution through the drainage.

RIGHT FEMORAL ARTERY, RIGHT INTERNAL JUGULAR VEIN

Insert a drainage instrument into the right internal jugular vein directed toward the heart.

Insert an arterial tube into the right femoral artery directed toward the right foot.

Insert an arterial tube into the right femoral artery directed toward the trunk and head of the body.

Inject the right leg and foot first; drainage is taken from the jugular.

Inject the trunk and head of the body; drainage is taken from the jugular.

RIGHT COMMON CAROTID ARTERY, RIGHT FEMORAL VEIN

Insert a drainage instrument into the right femoral vein directed toward the heart.

2. Insert an arterial tube into the right common carotid artery directed toward the right side of the head.

3. Insert an arterial tube into the right common carotid artery directed toward the trunk of the body.

4. Inject down the right common carotid first to embalm the trunk of the body and left side of the face; drainage is taken from the femoral vein.

5. Inject the right side of the head; drainage is taken from the femoral vein.

A similar process is used to inject from the axillary artery and to drain from either the internal jugular vein or the right femoral vein. If pathological or physical problems exist in the body, the veins and arteries on the left side can be used. Most operators, being right-handed, find working on the right side of the body more convenient. Split injection does require two incisions and, therefore, requires more time for suturing and for the preparation of vessels.

13

Injection and Drainage Techniques

During arterial embalming of the body, four processes take place *at the same time:* (1) *injection* of the arterial solution at a set rate of flow and pressure from the machine, (2) *distribution* of the embalming solution through the blood vascular system, (3) *diffusion* of the embalming solution from the blood vascular system (capillaries) to the cells and tissues, and (4) *drainage* of the contents of the blood vascular system, some of these tissue fluids, and a portion of the embalming solution.

When all four of these processes are successful, a sufficient amount of embalming solution is delivered to the tissues to achieve a uniform preservation and sanitation of the body tissues without distension. These processes remove intravascular discolorations, color the tissues, and establish the proper moisture balance in the tissues so that dehydration or overly moist tissue is not a problem.

In Chapter 12, discussion centered on the distribution of arterial solution and the mechanisms by which arterial solution is retained by the body. Injection involves not only pressurized injecting apparatus but the equally important artery (or arteries) used for injection and the vein (or veins) used for drainage. In the unautopsied body, the ideal artery for injection is the largest artery, the aorta. Its location, however, makes the aorta an impractical choice. The best location for drainage is the right atrium of the heart, but again, its location within the thoracic cavity makes it an impractical choice. Therefore, the ves-

sels used for injection and drainage should be as close as possible to both the aorta and the right atrium.

ARTERIES FOR INJECTION/VEINS FOR DRAINAGE

Arteries are used for injection of arterial solution, because, unlike some of the long veins of the body, they *do not* have valves. When arterial solution is injected "down" the leg, the drainage is returned "up" the leg through the veins. In life, blood flows back to the heart. In embalming, drainage flows in a similar direction, toward the heart.

INJECTION TECHNIQUES

Embalming of the unautopsied body begins when the embalmer selects a suitable artery or combination of arteries (as in restricted cervical injection) from which the arterial solution can be distributed throughout the *entire body.* This first choice of a vessel is called the **primary injection site.** Should injection of the embalming solution from the primary injection point fail to distribute the fluid to all body areas, other arteries must be raised and injected. These additional arteries are referred to as **secondary injection sites.**

Embalming analysis continues throughout the embalming process. In the preembalming period, an artery and vein are selected for the primary injection and drainage sites on the basis of the following criteria:

One-point injection — Injection and drainage from one location

Split injection — Injection and drainage from separate locations

Multipoint or sectional injection — Injection at two or more sites

Restricted cervical injection — Raising of both common carotid arteries at the start of injection

One-Point Injection

In single-point injection, one location is used for both injection and drainage. The most frequently used one-point injection sites are the right common carotid artery and the right internal jugular vein, the right femoral artery and the right femoral vein, the right external iliac artery and the right external iliac vein, and the right axillary artery and the right axillary vein.* The common carotid and the femoral arteries are the most frequently used one-point injection sites today. The axillary artery is least used. Years ago, when most embalming was performed at the residence of the deceased and a minimum amount of very concentrated fluid was injected, the axillary, no doubt, was the most frequently used artery because the head could easily be cleared of discoloration, and drainage could easily be collected from this site or by drainage from the right atrium of the heart. Also, the incision would not be seen by the family after the preparation.

CRITERIA FOR SELECTION OF AN ARTERY
AS AN INJECTION SITE

1. Size (diameter) of the artery
2. Effect on posing the body
3. Incision location if leakage is a possibility (if edema is in the area of the artery)
4. Practicality of drainage from the accompanying vein
5. Depth of the location of the artery
6. Flexibility of the artery because of its branches
7. Proximity of the vessel to the arch of the aorta

---

*Reference is made to Chapters 8 and 9 concerning the advantages and disadvantages of each artery and vein as a point for injection or drainage. The left vessels could also be used.

CRITERIA FOR SELECTION OF A VEIN FOR DRAINAGE

1. Size (diameter) of the vein
2. Proximity to the right atrium of the heart
3. Discolorations of the face and neck (blood)
4. Ease with which vein can be brought to the surface because of tributaries
5. Depth of vein

Today, embalming necessitates the use of large volumes of embalming solution. The internal jugular or femoral vein allows for better drainage than the small axillary or basilic veins. Many embalmers prefer the one-point injection when possible because only one incision is required. Many bodies can be embalmed using a one-point injection. Studies have demonstrated that better distribution of the arterial solution is accomplished when multisite injection is used. Procedures for such an injection from the three major sites are as follows:

RIGHT COMMON CAROTID, INTERNAL JUGULAR VEIN

1. Insert an arterial tube into the right common carotid artery directed downward toward the trunk of the body.
2. Insert an arterial tube into the right common carotid artery directed upward toward the right side of the face, leaving the stopcock *open*.
3. Insert a drainage instrument into the right internal jugular vein *directed toward the heart*.
4. *Inject* the trunk of the body; several gallons of solution are required for the adult body.
5. Inject sufficient solution up the right side of the head.

RIGHT FEMORAL ARTERY AND VEIN

1. Insert a drainage tube *directed toward the heart* into the femoral vein.
2. Insert an arterial tube directed toward the right foot into the femoral artery.
3. Insert an arterial tube directed toward the trunk (head) of the body.
4. Inject the right leg first.
5. Inject the trunk, arms, and head.

See Figure 13–1.

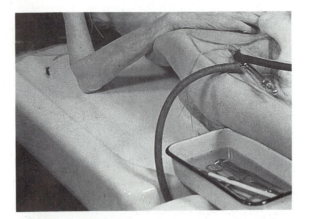

Figure 13–1. Single-point injection and drainage from the right femoral artery and vein. Note the concurrent disinfection of the instruments. A hose is attached to collect drainage from the drain tube.

RIGHT AXILLARY ARTERY AND VEIN

1. Insert an arterial tube into the axillary artery directed toward the right hand.
2. Insert an arterial tube into the right axillary artery directed toward the trunk and head of the body.
3. Insert a drainage instrument in the axillary vein directed toward the heart.
4. Inject the head and trunk first.
5. Inject the right arm.

See Figure 13–2A.

The greatest disadvantage of the one-point method of injection and drainage is the short-circuiting of arterial fluid. Fluid has a tendency to find direct routes from the arterioles to the venules or through only portions of the capillaries in the region around the injection site. This can account for overembalming of the area near the injection site and loss of a great amount of arterial solution through the drainage.

Short-Circuiting of Arterial Solution

Fluids follow the path of least resistance. Quite often the skin area is the path of least resistance, for the skin has a greater amount of capillaries than most deeper body tissues. The skin areas surrounding the injection and drainage points frequently receive a greater volume of solution (Fig. 13–2B). Embalming in which only the skin and superficial portions of the body and not the deeper tissues receive solution has been referred to as **shell embalming**. Massage, manipulation, and restriction of drainage all help to reduce shell embalming and to en-

courage movement of arterial so[lution] and deep tissues.

There are direct connections venules. In life, direct connections venules help to divert blood int[o] most nourishment. After one-poi[nt] circuiting pathways are quite fre[e] a result, the solution does not ente[r] instead, rapidly passes from the a[rte]nous side of the blood vascular syst[em] from the body. This is often seen in a one-point injection and drainage[.]

Coagula in the arterial system *into minute arterial tributaries*. So paths of least resistance and quickly venous system. Once there, it can the drainage site. The short-circuit[ing] caused not so much by the use of o[...] by the unrestricted drainage (Fig. 1[.]

Split Injection

Split injection is the injection of sol[ution] and the drainage from a separate lo[cation] reduces short-circuiting of the soluti[on] establish a more even distribution of t[...] The most frequently used combinati[on] split injection method is the right in[...] (drainage) and the right femoral artery the embalmer begins with a one-point femoral vessels, but soon finds dif[ficulty] drainage. Raising the internal jugul[ar] solves the drainage problem. Some em[balmers] use this type of injection and drainage of split injection include the following:

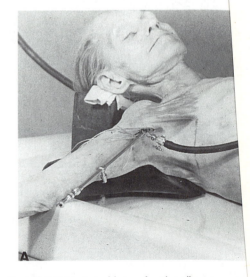

Figure 13–2. **A.** Injection and drainage from the axillary artery and ve[in] size of these veins, this method is not used often today. (*Continued*)

Multisite (Multipoint) Injection

Multisite injection is vascular injection from two or more arteries. Multisite injection can be used as the primary injection technique. If the embalmer is preparing a body dead for a long period and anticipates poor solution distribution and possibly tissue distension, he or she can *begin* the embalming using a multisite injection. The embalmer would raise several arteries for injection; drainage is taken from each injection location or from one drainage point. More often, multisite injection is used after a one-point injection has resulted in poor distribution. In this case several secondary arteries must be raised to embalm the various body areas receiving inadequate amounts of solution. Six-point injection involves three major pairs of vessels: common carotid, femoral (external iliac), and axillary (brachial).

The multisite procedure ensures thorough distribution throughout the body. Multisite injection may be required for bodies that are to be shipped to certain countries and for bodies of U.S. armed services personnel. This type of injection allows different solution strengths to be used in different body regions. Each area is directly injected, and the volume and strength of solution injected into an area depend on the preservative demands and amount of tissue distension of that area.

The procedure for the six-point injection follows:

1. Raise the right internal jugular vein and insert a drainage instrument directed toward the heart.
2. Raise the right common carotid artery and insert an arterial tube directed toward the trunk of the body. Also insert a tube directed toward the right side of the head.
3. Raise the left common carotid and insert a tube directed toward the left side of the head. Tie off the lower portion of the artery.
4. Raise the right axillary (or brachial) artery and insert an arterial tube directed toward the right hand. Tie off the upper part of the artery.
5. Raise the left axillary (or brachial) artery and insert a tube directed toward the left hand. Tie off the upper part of the artery.
6. Raise the right femoral artery and insert an arterial tube directed toward the right foot. Tie off the upper portion of the artery.
7. Raise the left femoral artery and insert an arterial tube directed toward the left foot. Tie off the upper portion of the artery.
8. Inject in the following order: right leg, left leg, right arm, left arm, trunk of the body (inject down the right common carotid), left side of the head, right side of the head.
9. Drainage can be taken from the right internal jugular vein for all body areas injected, or drainage may be taken from each accompanying vein.
10. The body may be aspirated before injecting the head, if purge has been a problem.

Note: The six-point injection technique is similar to embalming the autopsied body, with the exception of the visceral organs and the trunk.

Multisite injection may also involve injection of a distal body part. For example, a one-point injection is used but solution fails to reach the right hand. Here, perhaps, injection of the right radial or ulnar artery is necessary. Any combination of two or more arteries for injection constitutes a multisite injection.

SITUATIONS THAT MAY REQUIRE A MULTISITE INJECTION

1. When a body area does not receive arterial solution
2. Bodies dead for long time periods
3. Bodies that show evidence of decomposition
4. Death caused by a ruptured aortic aneurysm
5. Bodies dead of highly contagious diseases involving the blood vascular system (this method of injection maximizes tissue saturation with embalming chemicals).
6. When disposition of the body is delayed for some period
7. In following military regulations
8. When a one-point injection has been used but embalming solution purge develops and drainage stops (distribution cannot be observed)
9. Bodies with generalized edema
10. Bodies that are difficult to firm
11. Bodies that exhibit poor peripheral circulation
12. Bodies that exhibit poor distribution after a one-point injection is completed
13. Bodies with true tissue gas
14. Bodies that must be reinjected because of poor preservation *after* cavity embalming
15. Autopsied bodies

Restricted Cervical Injection*

In restricted cervical injection, both common carotid arteries are raised so that the head can be separately injected (Fig. 13–3). With many of the distribution and drainage problems encountered in embalming today, this

---

*Much of this information was supplied by David. G. Williams, Pittsburgh, Pennsylvania.

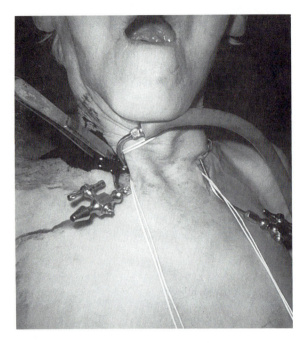

Figure 13–3. Restricted cervical injection.

method has become a standard practice in many funeral establishments.

1. Raise the right common carotid artery and insert an arterial tube directed toward the trunk of the body. Insert an arterial tube directed toward the right side of the head and leave the stopcock *open*.
2. Insert a drainage instrument into the right internal jugular vein directed toward the heart.
3. Raise the left common carotid artery and insert an arterial tube directed toward the left side of the head; *tie off the lower portion of the left common carotid artery and leave the stopcock open*.
4. Inject the trunk of the body *first;* drainage is taken from the right internal jugular vein. (Solution entering the head by collateral circulation exits through the two open stopcocks. Only the trunk of the body is embalmed.)
5. Inject the left side of the head.
6. Inject the right side of the head.

The restricted cervical injection is recommended in several situations.

Bodies with Facial Trauma. With restricted cervical injection a minimum volume of a very strong solution is injected to preserve and firm tissues with a minimum amount of tissue distension.

Bodies in Which Facial Distension Is Anticipated. When there has been a long delay between death and preparation, when bodies have been refrigerated, or when frozen bodies exhibit decomposition changes, restricted cervical injection allows the trunk to be saturated with large amounts of strong solution while the head and facial tissues are injected separately to control distension.

Bodies in Which Eye Enucleation Has Been Performed. Restricted cervical injection allows complete control over the strength and amount of solution entering the facial tissues and thus helps to control distension of the eyelids.

Bodies with Generalized Edema. A large volume of solution can be injected into the trunk areas. Frequently, if facial tissues are not edematous, a milder solution can be used for injection of the head to prevent distension and/or dehydration of the tissues.

Difficult-to-Firm Bodies. With many of the drugs used today protein levels in the body can be low. Restricted cervical injection allows the embalmer to inject large quantities of preservative solutions without overembalming the facial tissues.

Bodies with Distribution Problems. Restricted cervical injection allows the use of high pressures and high rates of flow without distending the facial tissues.

Bodies with a High Formaldehyde Demand. Burned bodies and bodies dead from renal failure require large amounts of preservative. Restricted cervical injection allows the embalmer to inject strong solutions of special-purpose high-index fluids without overembalming the facial tissues.

Bodies in Which Purge is Expected. In a body that purges prior to arterial injection, the purge often continues during the embalming process. Examples include bodies with esophageal varices (as in alcoholism); bodies that suffered pneumonia, tuberculosis of the lungs, and ulcerations of the upper digestive organs; and bodies that show decomposition changes. Restricted cervical injection allows the embalmer to embalm the limbs and trunk areas, then *aspirate the body,* set the features, and embalm the head. This eliminates the necessity to reset the features if purge occurs.

It can easily be seen that restricted cervical injection can be a routine embalming technique, similar to the one-point injection. With the difficulties encountered in embalming today (time delays, poor distribution as a result of vascular clotting, edema, and difficulty in firming as a result of drug therapy), more embalmers are using restricted cervical injection as their primary injection method.

The restricted cervical method of injection affords the *greatest control* over entry of arterial solution into the head. Because the tubes that are directed upward are left open while the trunk is injected, any solution that does reach the face and head via the collateral circulation *exits* the carotid arteries through the open arterial tubes.

cervical injection is used with both common carotid arteries and the right internal jugular vein.

Solution Strength. A very strong arterial solution is prepared, and in some cases, 100% arterial fluid is used. One solution suggested contains 16 ounces of a high-index arterial fluid (25-index or above), 16 ounces of a coinjection chemical, 16 ounces of water, and 1 to $1\frac{1}{2}$ ounces of arterial fluid dye. This solution is designed to immediately preserve, dry, and firm the tissues.

Pressure. The solution is mixed in the machine. When a centrifugal injection machine is used, the pressure with the rate of flow valve *off* should be set at 20 pounds or above.

Method of Injection. Connect the injection hose to the arterial tube in the left common carotid artery. Be certain that the arterial tubes used are as large as the arteries allow. Turn the machine *on* with the rate-of-flow valve closed. Set the pressure at 20 pounds. Once the hoses are connected, open the rate-of-flow valve a full turn and immediately turn it *off*. This creates a "pulse" type of fluid flow. The solution is injected in a strong spurt, under high pressure, for only a moment. Repeatedly turn the rate-of-flow valve on and off until sufficient solution has been injected. Only a minimum amount of solution is needed because of its strength. The excess dye indicates the presence of the solution in the tissues. In addition, the dye helps to prevent graying of the tissues. Next, the right side of the head is injected in the same manner. High pressure is used, but the rate-of-flow valve is turned on and off for only a moment each time. The purpose of this method of embalming is to inject a very strong solution throughout all the facial tissues but to use the minimum amount of solution. In this manner, maximum preservation is achieved with a minimum of tissue distension (Fig. 13–4).

ADVANTAGES TO THE USE OF RESTRICTED CERVICAL INJECTION

1. Amount of arterial solution entering the facial tissues can be controlled.
2. Large volumes of arterial solution can be injected into the trunk without overinjecting the head and face.
3. Two solution strengths can be used: one for the trunk and limbs and another for the head and face.
4. Arterial coagula, if present in the aorta, are pushed toward the lower extremities.
5. Different pressures can be used to inject the head and the trunk.
6. Different rates of flow can be used to inject the trunk and the head.
7. The trunk can be injected first and the body aspirated to stop purging; the features can be set *after aspirating,* and then the head injected last.
8. Arteriosclerosis is rarely seen in the carotid arteries; they are very large vessels and very elastic.
9. The common carotid arteries have no branches (except their terminal branches) and, thus, are easily raised to the surface.
10. Clots present in the right or left carotid artery can be identified and removed.
11. The carotid arteries allow direct injection of the head and facial tissues.
12. The carotid arteries are accompanied by the large internal jugular veins, which directly drain the head and face.
13. The *instant tissue fixation* technique can be employed.
14. For jaundiced bodies, only the head is treated with jaundice fluids.

INSTANT TISSUE FIXATION

A variation of the restricted cervical injection in which a very strong arterial solution is used is **instant tissue fixation.** This embalming technique is used for injection of the head (although other body areas can be similarly treated) when swelling of the face is anticipated (as in bodies that show evidence of decomposition) or when trauma has damaged facial tissues. This technique is used when the tissues must be dry and firm for restorative treatments, when pathological conditions such as tumors exist, or when cancerous tissue must be dry and very firm for its excision and facial reconstruction. In this method of injection very little drainage is taken as only a minimal amount of arterial solution is injected. The restricted

VARIATIONS OF INJECTION TECHNIQUES

The autopsied body presents its own injection problems. When the body has undergone a complete autopsy, generally a six-point injection is used; each body extremity is embalmed separately. After partial autopsies, or when organs have been removed for donation, the routine varies with the access to the abdominal or thoracic aorta.

After the partial autopsy and in bodies from which abdominal or thoracic organs have been removed, the aorta may be an injection point. Infants may also be embalmed from the ascending or abdominal aorta, for this vessel is much easier to raise in the unautopsied infant than it is in the adult body. Secondary injection sites may also be needed in autopsy preparations and would most

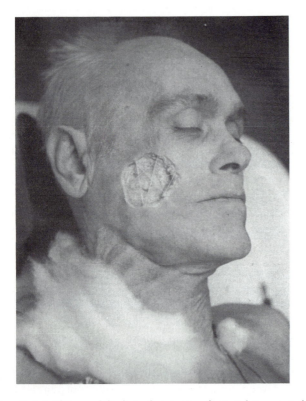

Figure 13–4. Facial tissues embalmed using the instant tissue fixation technique prior to the removal of a cancerous tumor of the right cheek.

likely involve the more distal arteries such as the radial, ulnar, popliteal, and facial.

DRAINAGE

As stated at the beginning of this chapter, four processes occur at the same time in the embalming of the average body: (1) injection of the solution, (2) distribution of the solution, (3) diffusion of the solution, and (4) drainage. Distribution and diffusion of arterial solution are discussed in Chapter 12.

Drainage is brought about by displacement. As the arterial solution fills the vascular system the contents of the vascular system are displaced. There are 5 to 6 quarts of blood in the vascular system of the average body. This accounts for approximately 8% of the body weight. At death, there is generally a wave contraction of the arterial system. This contraction forces the greatest volume of blood into the capillary and venous portions of the blood vascular system after death.

It has been estimated that after death, 85% of the blood is found in the capillaries, 10% in the veins, and 5% in the arteries. Amounts of blood in the vascular system vary depending on the cause and manner of death. In addition, the blood will gravitate into the dependent body regions over time. This engorges the dependent capillaries with blood (livor mortis) and leaves the less dependent tissues free of most blood.

Contents of Drainage

In addition to blood, the drainage also contains arterial solution and interstitial fluid. As arterial solution flows into the capillary, a portion of the solution passes through the walls of the capillary and is retained by the body. This retained preservative is the portion of the embalming solution that preserves, sanitizes, moisturizes, and colors the body tissues. Some of the embalming solution moves through the capillaries, into the venules and veins, and exits as part of the drainage. It has been estimated that 50% or more of the drainage taken during embalming is actually embalming solution.

The color and consistency of the drainage change during injection of the body. During injection of the first gallon of embalming solution, drainage contains more blood than in subsequent injections. As the blood in the vascular system is gradually displaced and replaced with embalming solution, the drainage lightens in color and becomes thinner. The initial drainage is the most dangerous; however, all drainage should be carefully controlled and splashing should be avoided. Collection and sanitation of drainage may be warranted with diseases such as hepatitis and AIDS.

As the embalming solution passes through the capillaries some of the interstitial fluid in the tissue spaces enters the capillaries by osmosis because of the high concentrate of the embalming solution, especially when strong arterial solutions are used. Some interstitial fluid may enter the drainage through the lymphatic system. Dehydration can result when too much interstitial fluid is removed. In bodies with edema, the edema is removed in much the same way that interstitial fluid is taken from the tissue spaces.

LYMPHATIC CIRCULATION

The lymphatic vessels originate as blind-end tubes called lymph capillaries (Fig. 13–5). These tubes are located in the spaces between the cells. The lymph capillaries are larger and more permeable than the blood capillaries. They converge to form lymph channels called the lymphatics. These lymphatics have valves similar to those of veins and contain lymph nodes along their routes. Their fluid eventually enters the blood vascular system by flowing into the thoracic and the right lymphatic ducts. The thoracic duct empties lymph into the junction of the left subclavian vein and the left internal jugular vein. The lymph from the right lymphatic channel empties into the junction of the right subclavian vein and the right internal jugular vein.

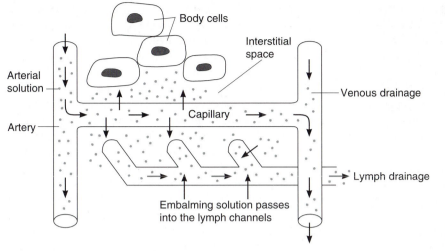

Figure 13–5. Drainage consists of blood, interstitial fluid, and embalming solution.

In life, the lymph is composed of the fluids that pass from the blood through the walls of the capillaries. Here it is called tissue or interstitial fluid. More fluid enters the interstitial spaces from the blood than is directly reabsorbed back into the bloodstream by the capillaries. This excess fluid is drained by the lymph system. Once the interstitial fluid enters the lymph capillaries it is called lymph. At the time of death these lymph channels can be the site of large numbers of microbes. The lymph system is part of the defense system for protecting the body from pathological microbes. Embalming solution will diffuse from the interstitial spaces into the lymph channels. Massage and manipulation of the body during injection combined with the use of restricted drainage help to move embalming fluid throughout the lymph system.

Embalming solution can be diffused through the lymphatics in the following order: lymphatic capillary → lymphatic vessel → lymph nodes → lymph vessels → lymphatic trunk → subclavian veins.

Drainage can then be said to consist of blood, interstitial fluid, and arterial solution (Fig. 13–6). Bacteria and microbial agents and their products that have entered the blood vascular system before or after death are also removed in the drainage. In bodies with skeletal edema, the edematous fluid may be part of the drainage. Coagula should also be included in the contents of drainage. Several types of clotted materials are present in drainage; however, all clotted material comes from the *veins* or from a heart chamber. It is impossible for any arterial coagula to pass through the capillary beds and enter the venous side of the circulatory system. The following coagula can be identified:

■ Postmortem coagula: These coagula are not actual clots, but simply blood inclusions that have congealed and stuck together; they can be large and dark.
■ Postmortem clots: These clots are multicolored. The bottom portion of the clot is dark, for it was formed by red blood cells that gravitated to the dependent part of a vessel. The clear layer on the top of the clot is a jellylike layer of fibrin.
■ Antemortem clots: Clots such as thrombosis form in layers—a layer of platelets, followed by a layer of fibrin, followed by another layer of platelets, and so on.

The viscosity of the blood can vary depending on the cause of death and the time between death and embalming. As the body gradually dehydrates after death,

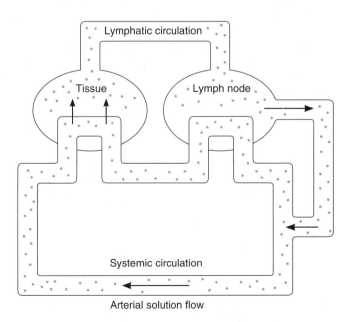

Figure 13–6. Lymphatic and systemic circulation.

the viscosity of the blood increases. Bodies that have been refrigerated for very short periods after death, have been administered drugs such as heparin or dicumarol, or have died from carbon monoxide poisoning exhibit low blood viscosity.

The volume of drainage is not equal to the volume of embalming solution injected. A large portion of the blood vascular system, particularly the arteries, is empty at death. This entire area must be filled, which accounts for the delay often noted between injection and the start of the drainage. At the conclusion of the embalming, the arterial system is filled; some of the injected solution is found in the capillaries and the veins, and some has passed through the capillaries to be retained by the tissues and cells.

In some bodies, there will be little or no drainage.

> As long as the solution is distributing and there is no swelling or discolorations in the tissues, drainage need not be a concern.

Sometimes, there is little to drain, as illustrated in these examples.

1. In cases of esophageal varices and ruptured ulcerations of the digestive tract (blood has been lost to the lumen of the esophagus, stomach, or intestines), drainage actually occurs within the intestinal tract.
2. Accidental death could cause the spleen or other internal organ to rupture; blood is lost from these sites and drainage also occurs at these ruptures.
3. Traumatic death may result in a large loss of blood outside the body. This hemorrhage decreases the volume of blood available for drainage.
4. Insertion of the drainage tube into the femoral or external iliac vein may tear the vein, allowing drainage to flow into the abdominal cavity.
5. When a preinjection embalming solution is used, a portion of the blood is removed. At the time of arterial solution injection, there is less blood to drain.
6. Pathological or tubercular lesions may account for a blood loss in life and an internal site of drainage at the time of solution injection.
7. Bloodstream infections frequently cause extensive clotting, and anemic diseases reduce blood volume; these factors contribute to poor distribution and low drainage volume.

Often in bodies in which hemorrhage into the digestive tract or abdominal cavity occurred prior to death, there may be a gradual swelling of the abdomen as the solution is injected and some of the drainage (and arterial solution) fills the digestive tract or abdominal cavity. This drainage can be removed with a trocar. Likewise, hemorrhage into the stomach, esophagus, or lung tissues can result in a purge during injection. The purge will take the form of drainage. It is possible to drain from the mouth if a stomach ulcer has ruptured large veins. Aspiration can later remove these fluids. Some medications cause gastrointestinal bleeding. If this bleeding was intense, a major portion of the drainage may flow into the intestinal tract during arterial injection.

The bodies just described may demonstrate two forms of drainage: internal, into a cavity or hollow organ, and external, through the drainage tube or exit as purge.

Good drainage can be expected under the following conditions:

1. The interval between death and preparation is short; the body retains some heat.
2. The body shows early evidence of livor mortis, indicating that the blood has a low viscosity and can easily be moved.
3. Death was not the result of a febrile disease or a bloodstream infection.
4. Skeletal edema is present.
5. The body is jaundiced.
6. The person had been treated with blood thinners (e.g., heparin and dicumarol), resulting in low blood viscosity.
7. The body was refrigerated shortly after death but not for a long period.
8. Death was due to carbon monoxide poisoning.

Purpose of Drainage

Bodies to be used for dissection are often embalmed but not drained. Bodies dead for long periods can be slowly embalmed without draining, and are suitable for viewing. Years ago, small volumes (1 to 1½ gallons) of arterial solutions were injected, drainage was limited, and the blood that remained in the vessels was expected to act as a vehicle to gradually spread the fluid through the body. Machine injection not only improved arterial solution distribution and diffusion but increased the volume of blood drainage. Fluid is drained for many reasons:

1. To make room for the arterial solution. Distension would result without removal of some of the blood (especially today, when 3 to 5 gallons of preservative solution is injected into the average body).
2. To reduce a secondary dilution of the arterial fluid. The blood in the capillaries can dilute the embalming solution. This dilution would be very

small if a major portion of the blood is drained as the result of injecting large volumes of arterial solution.

3. To remove intravascular blood discolorations. Livor mortis is a postmortem intravascular blood discoloration. Discolorations such as carbon monoxide and capillary congestion are antemortem blood discolorations. Injection of arterial solution accompanied by blood drainage should greatly reduce or remove these discolorations.

4. To remove a tissue that rapidly decomposes. Blood is a liquid tissue that rapidly decomposes after death, and decomposition of the blood can result in discolorations, odors, and formation of gas.

5. To remove an element that speeds decomposition. Blood, a portion of which is liquid, can hasten hydrolysis and the decomposition of the body tissues. Moisture is needed for decomposition and blood can provide that medium.

6. To remove bacteria present in the blood. With some diseases, microbes normally found in the intestine can translocate to the bloodstream. After death, this translocation greatly increases. Removal of blood as drainage helps to reduce microbial agents in the body.

7. To prevent discolorations. When the blood in the body (hemoglobin) mixes with the formaldehyde of the arterial solution methyl-hemoglobin can form, which produces a gray color in the tissues (formaldehyde gray).

8. To reduce swollen tissues. When pitting edema is present in the skeletal tissues, it is possible to remove some of the edematous fluid via the blood drainage from the body.

In some bodies drainage is most important in clearing very pronounced discolorations, especially when the face, neck, and hands are affected. In some very thin bodies, with little or no livor mortis, drainage is not as copious, nor as necessary. The importance of drainage varies from body to body. If a primary purpose for drainage must be stated, it would be that the drainage makes room for the arterial solution so it can be evenly distributed to all tissues of the body with a minimum of distension.

Center of Drainage

The center of drainage in the dead human body is the right atrium of the heart (Fig. 13–7). The superior vena cava returns blood to this chamber from the head and the upper extremities. The inferior vena cava returns blood from the visceral organs, trunk, and legs. If the internal jugular vein is used as a drainage point, all blood from the lower extremities and visceral organs must pass

through the right atrium to be drained. Likewise, if drainage is to be taken from the right femoral vein, blood from the arms and head must pass through the right atrium. After death, blood in the right atrium frequently congeals. This condition warrants drainage from the right internal jugular vein where an instrument, such as angular spring forceps, can be placed directly into the right atrium to fragment this coagulum.

Some embalmers also use two locations for drainage. An example of the two-point (above and below the heart) drainage technique would be when the primary drainage site is the femoral vein. When the face and upper extremities begin to flush and discolor, the internal jugular vein is opened as the "above heart" drainage site.

> Drainage instruments are inserted into the vein and directed toward the heart.

Drainage Sites

The primary drainage site is the location from which drainage is first taken. In the unautopsied body, the veins most commonly used for drainage are the right internal jugular vein, the right femoral vein, and the right external iliac vein.

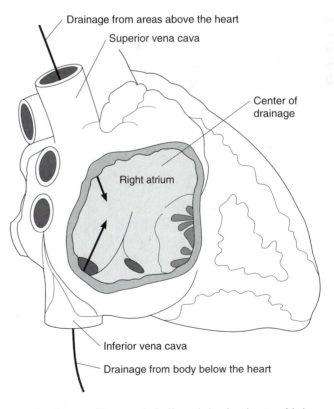

Figure 13–7. The center of drainage in the dead human body is the right atrium of the heart. The superior vena cava returns blood to this chamber from the head and the upper extremities. The inferior vena cava returns blood from the visceral organs, trunk, and legs.

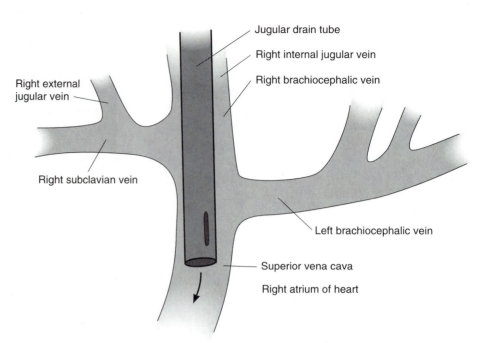

Figure 13–8. Drainage tube placed in the right internal jugular vein.

Axillary and basilic veins can be used, but their small size and the need to extend the arm make these veins an impractical choice. *Any vein can be used for drainage, whether it is large or small or on the right or left side of the body.* In unusual circumstances, even the external jugular vein can be used if the internal jugular vein is obstructed by a cancerous growth or a large attached thrombosis.

> A broken vein can still be used as a drainage site; if an instrument such as angular forceps cannot be inserted, a groove director may be used. Following injection the area can be dried and the ends of the broken vein ligated.

Should a vein tear while it is being raised, the following steps can be taken to attempt to place an instrument in the portion of the vein leading to the heart:

1. Force as much blood from the vein as possible.
2. Clean the area using a very large piece of absorbent cotton.
3. Observe where blood is seeping from the broken portion of the vein.
4. Clamp an edge of the wall of the broken vein with a small serrated or rat-toothed hemostat, or place the hemostat across the entire broken portion of the vein.
5. Gently insert a drainage device toward the heart; if the vein has been torn into two pieces do not remove the hemostat.
6. After embalming, pass a ligature around the distal portions of the vein (holding the torn vein with the hemostat).

In Chapter 9, the advantages and disadvantages of the various veins for drainage are discussed, as are the incision locations and the relationships of veins to arteries. The internal jugular vein is the most valuable drainage point. It is the largest systemic vein that can be raised in the unautopsied body. The right internal jugular vein leads directly into the right atrium of the heart. Figure 13–8 illustrates why the *right* and not the left internal jugular vein is most frequently used for drainage. Should there be a complication with the right internal jugular vein, the left can be used, but note that the vein turns to the right, often making insertion of a drainage instrument difficult. The angular spring forceps is the easiest drainage instrument for both right and left internal jugular veins.

A secondary drainage point is often used when the femoral vein is used as the primary injection and drainage point. If there is a blockage in the right atrium or the right internal jugular vein, the neck and face can begin to flush. The neck veins distend and the neck tissues may begin to distend. The right internal jugular vein should be raised and opened as a secondary drainage site. If it is impossible to use the jugular veins as drainage sites attempt to use the axillary or direct heart drainage.

Direct Heart Drainage*

The right atrium of the heart can be directly drained using a trocar (Fig. 13–9). This very old method of drainage was often used when embalming was performed at the residence of the deceased. The drainage could be conve-

---

*This method is not intended for use as a primary drainage technique but only in special situations where a vein cannot be used for drainage.

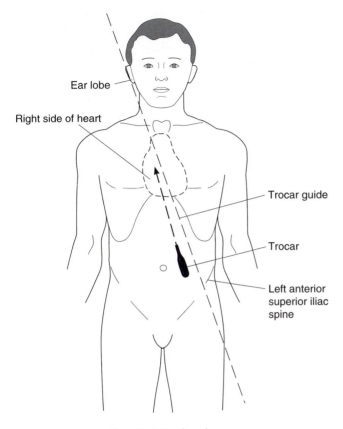

Figure 13–9. Direct heart drainage.

niently collected in bottles, which could be taken back to the funeral parlor to be emptied.

To drain directly from the right atrium of the heart, start by injecting approximately ½ to 1 gallon of embalming solution to fill the vascular system. To drain the heart, insert the trocar at approximately the standard point of entry, 2 inches to the left and 2 inches above the umbilicus. Drawn an imaginary line across the body connecting the *left* anterior superior iliac spine and the lobe of the *right* ear. Direct the trocar toward a point where this line crosses the right side of the sternum. This point is approximately at the level of the sternum where the fourth rib joins the sternum. Be certain to keep the trocar slightly to the right of the sternum. The trocar point should be kept in the anterior portion of the mediastinum. If there is sufficient pressure in the right atrium, simply placing the trocar in the heart chamber should be sufficient to start drainage. The trocar can be attached to the hydroaspirator.

Do not turn the hydroaspirator on to full suction; half is quite sufficient. Insert the trocar with the hydroaspirator running. As soon as the heart is pierced the hydroaspirator can be turned off. Most hydroaspirators are lower than the height of the embalming table, so a natural gravity system is established. It is important that a plastic hose be used on the trocar, for the embalmer

can then see immediately when the right side of the heart has been punctured.

If the embalmer is unfamiliar with this technique of drainage it can easily be practiced. Begin cavity aspiration by aspirating the right side of the heart first. The embalmer need not pierce only the right atrium with the trocar; the right ventricle can also be pierced. There should be sufficient pressure in the right side of the heart that the suction of the aspirator on the trocar can open the right atrioventricular valve and, in this manner, drain the right atrium. Should the trocar puncture the ascending aorta or the arch, sufficient embalming solution may be lost to necessitate a six-point injection. This method of drainage is efficient to use on the body of an infant, child, or adult.

Drainage Instrumentation

A large variety of drainage devices are available. The most standard drainage instruments are the drainage or drain tube and the angular spring forceps. Drainage tubes are made especially for use in the internal jugular vein (Fig. 13–10). These tubes are very large in diameter and short in length. Axillary drain tubes are long and slightly curved for insertion into the axillary vein.

Axillary drain tubes are not very large in diameter. A variety of drainage tubes are made for the femoral vein; they come in a wide range of diameters and lengths. One type of iliac drain tube is designed to be inserted into the external iliac vein, and the tip of the tube reaches into the right atrium of the heart; they are approximately 2 to 2½ feet long and can be made of plastic, metal, or rubber. **Drain tubes are inserted into veins and directed toward the heart.** Some embalmers prefer to lubricate these devices with massage cream to facilitate their entry into the vein. Drain tubes contain a plunger rod, which also can be lubricated with massage cream. After each use drain tubes should be disassembled and flushed with cool, soapy water.

Many times, a drainage tube cannot be fully inserted into the vein; it should not be forced. As long as a portion of the tube can be inserted, it will keep the vein expanded. Changing the position of the tube in the vein often assists with the drainage. Tubes should be tied into a vein, but loosely enough so that their position can be changed.

Advantages of the Drain Tube	Disadvantages of the Drain Tube
The tube keeps the vein expanded.	The size of the opening is limited to the diameter of the tube.

Advantages of the Drain Tube

The "stirring" rod helps to fragment coagula.

Drainage can be shut off to build intra-vascular pressure.

Disadvantages of the Drain Tube

The tube can block the opposite portion of the vein.

The tube can block other veins.

Coagula cannot be grasped.

The tube may mark the face or interfere with positioning of the head.

The tube can easily be pushed through the vein into a body cavity.

The head can be positioned to the right.

The forceps does not mark the face.

Coagula can be grasped.

It does not block other venous tributaries.

Drainage may splatter onto the table.

Embalmer's contact with the drainage is increased.

Angular spring forceps can be used to assist drainage from any vein; however, this drainage device is generally used with the right internal jugular vein. The 8-inch angular spring forcep fits conveniently into the superior vena cava and the upper portions of the right atrium.

Advantages of the Angular Spring Forceps for Jugular Drainage

It provides a very large opening for the the drainage

Disadvantages of the Angular Spring Forceps

It may have to be removed to close the vein for intermittent drainage.

The angular spring forceps is convenient to use for drainage from the right internal jugular vein. It *does not block* drainage from the left innominate vein, right subclavian vein, or upper portion of the right internal jugular vein. These tributaries can be blocked if the jugular drain tube is used. It provides a wide opening for the passage of coagula and it allows the right side of the head to drain. Large masses of coagula can be broken and easily removed from the superior vena cava and the right atrium. The head can easily be positioned without the forceps marking the side of the face.

The **groove director** is used to assist in the insertion of a drainage tube or forceps into the vein. The groove director is inserted into the vein first. Once it is in place, the drainage instrument is slid along the grooved portion of the instrument. The grooved portion should face the lumen of the vein.

Methods of Drainage

Most embalmers use a compromise of embalming techniques. For example, it is recommended that 1 gallon of

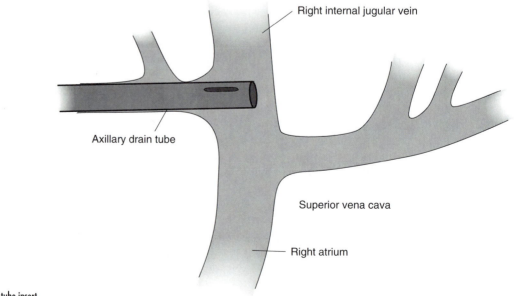

Figure 13–10. Drainage tube insert.

arterial solution be injected over 10 to 15 minutes. Embalmers can, however, inject this amount of solution in a shorter period if necessary. A 2% arterial solution is recommended as the standard solution. Many embalmers would be hesitant to begin injections with a solution of this strength so they begin with a milder solution and increase to the 2% level once circulation is established.

The same is true of the relationship between injection and drainage. Many embalmers use a combination of drainage methods. They begin the injection using continuous drainage and then restrict the drainage (using intermittent drainage) after the blood discolorations clear.

METHODS OF DRAINAGE IN RELATION TO INJECTION

Alternate
Concurrent
Intermittent

Alternate Drainage. In alternate drainage, the arterial solution is never injected while drainage is being taken. A quart or two of arterial solution is injected; then the arterial injection is stopped and venous drainage commences. This is allowed to continue until drainage subsides; then the drainage instrument is closed. The process is then repeated. Injection and drainage are alternated until the embalming is completed. Because 1 or 2 quarts of fluid is constantly injected into a confined system, it is believed that a more uniform pressure is developed in all parts of the body. More complete distribution of arterial solution is achieved and more complete drainage results. Fluid diffusion is enhanced, for pressure filtration is increased. This method increases preparation time and care must be taken to avoid distension.

Concurrent (Continuous) Drainage. In concurrent drainage, injection and drainage are allowed to proceed at the same time throughout the embalming. This method is less time consuming than the alternate method, and there is less chance of distension.

Distension is possible with any method of drainage or injection. As soon as distension is evident, stop injection.

Because of the open drainage, it may be difficult to attain a pressure sufficient to saturate tissues throughout the body. Clots (in the venous system) may not be dislodged when the concurrent method is used. Fluid will follow the path of least resistance and "short-circuit,"

and more embalming solution may be lost to the drainage. This method of drainage may dehydrate and wrinkle body tissues. It has value in the preparation of bodies with skeletal edema, for which dehydration is encouraged.

Intermittent Drainage. Another method of drainage involves continuous injection and intermittent drainage (Fig. 13–11). When drainage is difficult the vein is closed to build up pressure and encourage drainage. The intermittent method is considered a compromise between the alternate and the concurrent methods. In this process the injection continues throughout the embalming and the drainage is shut off for selected periods. Some embalmers stop drainage until a particular amount of solution is injected (1 or 2 quarts); others stop drainage until surface veins are raised. It is important that surface intravascular blood discolorations clear before intermittent drainage is begun. This method is less time consuming than the alternate method, encourages fluid distribution and pressure filtration, helps to prevent short-circuiting of the embalming solution and its loss to the drainage, and promotes retention of the embalming solution by the tissues. Intermittent drainage helps the body to retain tissue fluid (which provides a proper moisture balance) and is recommended when colloidal fluids such as humectants or restorative fluids are used to slightly distend emaciated tissues.

Techniques for Improving Drainage

The necessity for drainage has already been discussed. In summary, drainage (1) allows for a thorough distribution of the embalming solution, (2) prevents distension of the body tissues, and (3) prevents adverse discolorations. Creation of good drainage can be done in two periods, prior to injection of the preservative solution and during injection of the preservative solution. Preembalming techniques include the following:

- Selection of a large vein: Preference is generally the internal jugular or the femoral.
- Selection of a large drainage instrument: An angular spring forceps or drainage tube is used.
- Injection of a preinjection fluid: Follow the manufacturer's dilution of the chemical and volume of the chemical injected. If a preinjection chemical is not used, a mild arterial solution can be injected to clear blood discolorations and establish circulation.
- Removal of extravascular pressure such as gas and fluids in the abdomen.

During injection, techniques include the following:

- Use of drainage devices to fragment clots

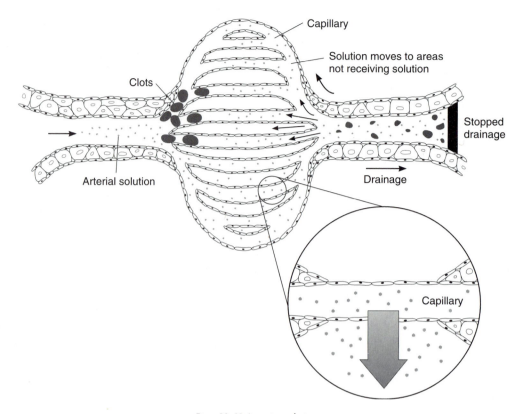

Figure 13–11. Intermittent drainage.

- Use of massage and pressure applied over the heart and/or liver to move venous clots
- Increase in the rate of solution injection or increase in the pressure of the solution being injected
- Intermittent and alternate forms of drainage techniques
- Selection of another drainage site if necessary

Disinfection of the Drainage

The initial drainage presents the greatest risk to the embalmer when the cause of death was bloodborne infection (AIDS, hepatitis, or bloodstream sepsis). At present, the Occupational Safety and Health Administration permits bulk blood, suction, and aspirated fluids to be carefully drained into a sanitary sewer system. To prevent a minimum of contact as blood is being drained, tubing may be attached to the drain tube. If a drainage forceps is used running water should direct blood drainage immediately into the sewer system.

As drainage and injection proceed, formaldehyde from the fluid becomes part of the drainage and disinfects the blood and its microbial contents. Some embalmers recommend injecting as much arterial solution as possible prior to draining into bodies dead from contagious disease and, several minutes later, beginning the drainage. This interval allows the blood and the embalming solution to mix.

KEY TERMS AND CONCEPTS FOR STUDY AND DISCUSSION

1. Define the following terms;
   alternate drainage
   concurrent drainage
   instant tissue fixation
   intermittent drainage
   multipoint injection
   one-point injection
   path of least resistance
   restricted cervical injection
   six-point injection
   split injection
2. List the advantages of using restricted cervical injection.
3. List the contents of drainage.
4. List the purposes for drainage.
5. List several techniques for stimulating drainage.
6. Complete the following distribution problems:

One-Point Injection and Drainage

Skeletal tissues   Trace arterial solution from the femoral artery (tube directed downward) to the right greater toe; drain from the right femoral vein.

Skeletal tissues	Trace arterial solution from the right femoral artery to the left side of the upper lip; drain from the right femoral vein.
Visceral tissues	Trace arterial solution from the right femoral artery to the fundus of the stomach; drain from the right femoral vein.

Split Injection and Drainage

Skeletal tissues	Trace arterial solution from the right femoral artery to the right greater toe; drain from the right internal jugular.
Skeletal tissues	Trace arterial solution from the right common carotid to the left upper lip; drain from the right femoral vein.
Visceral tissues	Trace arterial solution from the right common carotid to the appendix; drain from the right femoral vein.

Restricted Cervical Injection

Skeletal tissues	Inject the right common carotid down to reach the left lower lip; drain from the right internal jugular
Skeletal tissues	Inject the right common carotid down to reach the right upper lip

	(with the stopcock directed upward closed); drain from the right internal jugular.
Visceral tissues	Inject down the right common carotid to the tissues of the left lung; drain from the right internal jugular.

BIBLIOGRAPHY

Investigating factors relating to fluid retention during embalming, Parts I and II. In: *The Champion Expanding Encyclopedia.* Springfield, OH: Champion Chemical; August–September 1979:Nos. 499 and 500, 2013–2020.

Kroshus J, McConnell J, Bardole J. The measurement of formaldehyde retention in the tissues of embalmed bodies. *Director* 1983;March/April:10–12.

Mechanics of proper drainage. In: *Champion Expanding Encyclopedia.* Springfield, OH: Champion Chemical; November–December 1973:No. 442, 1785–1788.

Removal of blood via the heart. In: *Champion Expanding Encyclopedia.* Springfield, OH: Champion Chemical; May 1976:1885–1888.

Shor M. An examination into methods old and new of achieving greatest possible venous drainage. *Casket and Sunnyside* 1964;July:20.

14

Cavity Embalming

Cavity embalming, or cavity treatment, is the second major procedure in the preservation and sanitation of the dead human body.

The oldest methods of embalming, dating back to the Egyptians, included treatment of the viscera. Until the "modern era" of embalming, most embalming techniques involved not only removal of the viscera (evisceration) from the thoracic and abdominal cavities, but removal of the brain from the cranial cavity. Embalmers using these early embalming processes recognized the difficulty in preserving the body if some method of visceral treatment was not practiced. With the invention of the "trocar" toward the end of the 19th century, embalmers began to move away from a direct incision approach to preserve and sanitize the contents of the body cavities.

There is a need to continue the preservation and sanitation process after arterial embalming. Purulent materials, blood, and edematous fluids within the body cavities, along with possibly unembalmed tissues, continue to decompose and remain an excellent medium for bacterial growth. Untreated microbes can become a source of gases and possibly contagion.

Even preserved tissues are subject to reversal and breakdown as long as there are untreated or partially embalmed body areas. The aspiration procedure and subsequent profusion with cavity fluid are designed to reach the substances and microbes found in the spaces within the thoracic, abdominopelvic, and sometimes cranial cavity. In addition to these substances, those materials found within the hollow viscera and portions of the visceral organs themselves that are not reached by arterial injection are treated in the process of cavity embalming.

Cavity treatment is normally a two-step process: aspiration of the cavities and their contents and injection of a strong preservative/disinfectant chemical. This process takes place after the arterial embalming. Often, depending on the condition of the body, the process involves subsequent steps of reaspiration and reinjection of the cavities.

There may be occasions when cavity treatment is *not* employed in preparation of the body, for example, when the body is bequeathed to a medical school (where the school permits vascular preparation of the body for viewing by the family and public), and when a hospital allows the body to be arterially embalmed prior to a postmortem examination (autopsy).

There are also situations in which arterial embalming is not possible. Cavity embalming along with surface and hypodermic embalming woud be the principal means of preserving and sanitizing the remains. These cases include badly decomposed and badly burned bodies.

This is *not* a visible process. The work should proceed in an orderly fashion so that all areas of the cavities are treated. Large numbers of microbes may be found within these spaces, which are prefect media for postmortem microbial growth. Thorough cavity treatment prevents gas formation and subsequent purging of the body.

CHRONOLOGY OF CAVITY TREATMENT

1. Arterial embalming
   A. Limited treatment of the abdominal cavity prior to or during arterial injection if the abdominal wall is very tense
      a. Drainage of edema from the abdominal cavity if ascites exists
      b. Removal of gases if the abdomen is tightly distended with gas
   B. Limited treatment of the thoracic cavity
      a. Limited aspiration of the thorax if subcutaneous emphysema is present.
2. Aspiration of the cavities
   A. Time of treatment
      a. Immediately after arterial injection
      b. Several hours after arterial injection
3. Order of aspiration
   A. Thoracic cavity and its contents
   B. Abdominal cavity and its contents
   C. Pelvic cavity and its contents
4. Injection of the body cavities
5. Closure of the trocar point of entry
6. Washing and drying of the body
7. Possible reaspiration
8. Possible reinjection

> Direct treatment in cavity embalming, other than arterial injection of the contents of the body cavities and the lumina of the hollow viscera, is usually accomplished by aspiration and injection.

Cavity treatment after vascular injection accomplishes as complete a preservation and sanitation of the dead human body for funeralization as possible. Vascular injection alone does not reach all spaces of the body and may not treat all tissues of the body whether visceral organs or skeletal tissue.

Not all microorganisms die with the host. Many survive some time after somatic and cellular death. During the agonal period and then the postmortem period following somatic death, microbes from the hollow intestinal organs enter the bloodstream and lymph channels where they translocate to the skeletal tissues and interstitial fluids. In tissues not reached by arterial treatments, the decomposition cycle can occur and produce undesired effects. Cavity treatment attempts to treat visceral tissues that may not have been reached by arterial solution. It creates an unfavorable environment in the internal organs and destroys the media on which these microbes can grow and multiply.

TABLE 14–1. CONTENTS OF THE HOLLOW VISCERA THAT MUST BE TREATED

Organ	Contents to be Aspirated or Treated
Lungs, trachea, bronchi	Blood, edema, purulent material, gases
Stomach	Hydrochloric acid, undigested food, blood, gases
Small intestine	Gases, undigested foods, partially digested foods, blood
Large intestine	Gases, fecal material, blood
Urinary bladder	Urine, pustular material, blood
Gallbladder	Bile
Pelvis of the kidney	Urine, pustular material, blood
Heart	Blood
Inferior vena cava, portal veins	Blood

Cavity embalming treat the **contents** of the hollow viscera (Table 14–1), the **walls** of the visceral organs not embalmed by arterial injection, and the **contents** of the spaces between the visceral organs and the walls of the cavities.

The contents of the hollow portions of the viscera are not perfused during arterial injection. Materials within these spaces continue to decompose if untreated, and the resulting products of decomposition may cause **odors, gas formation, and purge.** The gases may move into the skeletal tissues and cause distension of viewable areas such as the face and hands.

It is impossible to determine which visceral organs did or did not receive arterial solution. The embalmer cannot look at these organs for "signs of arterial distribution," so cavity embalming serves to *ensure* that the walls and parenchyma of the hollow viscera and the stroma and parenchyma of the solid organs are embalmed.

The solid organs treated by cavity embalming are the pancreas, spleen, kidney, brain, liver and lungs.

Undigested or partially digested foodstuffs within the stomach and small intestines, as well as the gases and liquids resulting from the breakdown of these materials, are removed by the aspiration process. Those not removed are treated by the injection of cavity fluid (Table 14–2). If these materials are not removed or treated, gases could form, placing sufficient pressure on the stomach and diaphragm to create purge from the oral or nasal cavities.

TABLE 14–2. CAVITY CONTENTS THAT MUST BE TREATED

Cavity	Material to be Treated
Thoracic	Blood, edema, purulent material, gases
Pericardial	Blood, edema
Abdominal	Blood, edema, purulent material, gases
Pelvic	Blood, edema, purulent material, gases
Cranial	Blood, edema, gases

Note. The liquids in these cavities not only *decompose;* they serve as *media for bacteria* and as a *diluent* for cavity chemicals.

Purge from the *mouth* originates from either the contents of the *lungs,* the contents of the *stomach,* or the throat area (esophageal veins that hemorrhage) (Table 14–3). Purge from the *nose* can also originate from the lungs, stomach, or throat. If fecal material is not removed or treated by cavity chemicals, it can cause sufficient gases to form within the abdomen to cause a lung purge (by pressure on the diaphragm) or stomach purge. In addition, purge from the *anal orifice* is quite possible. Rectal hemorrhage can be a source of bloody purge from the anal orifice.

Cranial purge is very rare. Gases within the cranial cavity can spread into the facial tissues through the various foramina that lead from the cranial cavity to the soft facial tissues. Generally, a liquid or semisolid purge from the cranial cavity is the result of a fracture of the temporal bone. The point of exit of the purge is the ear. If gas is of sufficient pressure to exit the cranial cavity, the eyes and eyelids will be distended.

In some diseases, infections of the brain or meninges may lead to formation of gases or edema in the cranial cavity. Hemorrhages from a stroke can also cause blood and edema to accumulate in the cranial cavity. **It is rare for disease to cause cranial purge.** In bodies in which decomposition is advanced, sufficient pressure may be present to cause a purge from the cranial cavity.

Foramina in the area of the *eye* that serve as pathways for gas that affects the eye and surrounding tissues include the optic foramen, superior orbital fissure, inferior orbital fissure, infraorbital foramen, supraorbital foramen, anterior ethmoidal foramen, and posterior ethmoidal foramen.

In certain preparations such as after recent cranial surgery (gunshot or trauma to the head or advanced decomposition), aspiration and injection of a few ounces of cavity fluid into the cranial cavity may prevent the buildup of gas in the cranial cavity. The point at which the aspirating device is introduced into the cranium is discussed later in this chapter.

It should be mentioned here that it is not necessary to aspirate the brain of an adult who suffered from hydrocephalus. The bones at this time in life are ossified and the condition should present little problem in embalming.

TABLE 14–3. DESCRIPTION OF PURGE

Source	Orifice	Description
Stomach	Nose/mouth	Liquids, semisolids, dark brown "coffee ground" appearance; odor; acid pH
Lungs	Nose/mouth	Frothy; any blood present is red in color, little odor
Brain	Nose/ear/eyelids	Gases can move into tissues of the eye, fractures can cause blood to purge from the ears, creamy white semisolid brain matter may exit through a fracture or the nasal passage

Some embalmers routinely aspirate and inject the cranial cavity on every body. There is a very heavy arterial supply to the brain through both the internal carotid arteries and the vertebral arteries. In the majority of embalmings these routes should supply sufficient arterial solution to the brain and even to the cerebrospinal fluid.

In preparation of the unautopsied stillborn child or infant, the embalmer should consider the need for cranial treatment. The stillborn or infant brain can decompose very rapidly. Carefully evaluate for the presence of gases in the tissues around the eyes and give consideration to the time between death and preparation. It may be most advantageous in these preparations to at least inject some cavity fluid into the cranial cavity with a large hypodermic needle.

INSTRUMENTATION AND EQUIPMENT REQUIRED

A scalpel, pointed trocar, several feet of rubber or plastic hose, a device to create a suction or vacuum, and a receptacle (usually a sewer service, jar, or pail) are the items need to accomplish the process of aspiration. After aspiration, a gravity cavity injector or other injection device is connected with tubing to the trocar to apply the disinfectant/preservative chemicals. To close the opening in the body wall, a needle and ligature or trocar button and inserter are used. A disinfection tray or basin is needed for cleaning and disinfecting the scalpel, needle, trocar, and tubing.

Instruments Used to Create a Vacuum

Hydroaspirator. The hydroaspirator is installed on a cold water line, preferably over a flush sink; when the water is turned on, a vacuum is created. Proper operation of the equipment depends on the water pressure of the water line. A vacuum breaker is normally a part of the hydroaspirator and protects against a backflow into the water line. Local ordinance directives for proper installation of the aspirator may require other vacuum breakers at different heights above the water level of the receptable into which the aspirant flows.

The student unfamiliar with the hydroaspirator should "experiment" with this device. A few ounces of material such as blood passing through the water of the hydroaspirator can give the appearance of a very large quantity of material. Although it is helpful to observe the material passing through the hydroaspirator, it is more important to observe the material being withdrawn from the body at a position near the trocar. A piece of plastic or glass tubing can be inserted into a portion of the tubing used for aspiration. Clear tubing can be used so the aspirated material can be observed. Some trocars have a glass portion in the handle that allows the material flowing through the trocar to be observed.

Hydroaspirators can become clogged with small pieces of solid or semisolid material, for example, fatty tissue from the abdominal wall. There is a distinct sound change when this happens. Water then *reverses* and flows into the tubing, trocar, and body cavity. The hydroaspirator should be shut off immediately and the hose removed from the trocar. An attempt should be made to "flush" the material from the hydroaspirator. If this is unsuccessful, the hydroaspirator may be disassembled and the material removed from the inside of the device.

Electric Aspirator. An electric aspirator contains an electric motor with an encased impeller on the shaft. The impeller creates the suction. A small-diameter water line may be attached to the encasement for lubrication of the impeller. The electric aspirator is perhaps more expensive and requires more maintenance than the hydroaspirator. The electric aspirator may be the preferred device in funeral homes where there is low water pressure. An attachment to the electric aspirator allows the embalmer to add a disinfectant solution to the materials being aspirated.

Hand Pump. A dual-purpose piece of equipment, the hand pump, permits removal of air or forces air into an enclosed airtight container. Drawing the air out of the container creates suction and is used for aspiration. Forcing the air into the container of embalming solution forces the solution out and is used to generate flow for injection. In the past, a glass jar with a "gooseneck" and the hand pump were commonly used. The "gooseneck" is the rubber stopper that makes the jar airtight. The stopper has two openings for two hose attachments. One hose allows air movement out of the jar, and the second hose leads to a trocar. This method is little used today.

Air Pressure Machine. The air pressure machine operates on the same principle as the hand pump The machine has two outlets. One creates a vacuum; the other can be used to force air into a jar. Again, a "gooseneck" is employed. The concentrated aspirated material is collected in the jar. Care should be taken to use jars specially made for aspiration, as there is a danger of glass implosion. The contents of the jar can be poured into the sewer line, or, if the embalmer desires to disinfect the contents, they can be treated in the jar prior to being released into the sewer system.

Instruments Used in Aspiration

Trocar. A trocar is a long hollow needle (metal tube) with a removable sharp point that is available in varying lengths and bores. Whetstones or other sharpening devices can be used to keep the points honed, or the point can be replaced. The trocar is used to pierce the wall of the abdomen and the walls of the internal organs in the thoracic and abdominal cavities. The trocar, attached to the suction device, is used to withdraw the contents of the organs and residual fluid that has pooled in the cavities. The trocar is also used to introduce the disinfectant/preservative solution over and into the internal organs.

An 18-inch long, $\frac{5}{16}$-inch-bore trocar is used in aspiration of the abdominal and thoracic cavities of the adult body. Opening the cavities after the trocar has been used would reveal all of the organs in their *proper positions*. The embalmer would have to examine the viscera for the *pierce marks* made by the trocar, as these punctures close.

The *infant trocar* is approximately 12 inches in length and about $\frac{1}{4}$ inch in diameter. It is used in cavity treatment of infants and children. Many embalmers also use it for hypodermic injection of preservative chemicals into areas of the limbs or trunk not reached by arterial embalming.

Complete disinfection/sterilization of the trocar is important. Microorganisms have been carelessly transferred from one body to another via the trocar. Trays of sufficient size and length for the trocar are needed whether the chemical or autoclave method of sterilization is used. For example, after its use in a body with true tissue gas, an improperly cleaned trocar can harbor the spore-forming *Clostridium perfringens*.

Tubing. Clear plastic or rubber tubing 6 to 8 feet in length and $\frac{3}{8}$ to $\frac{1}{2}$ inch in diameter is needed to connect the trocar to aspiration devices. The wall of the tubing must be thick enough to preclude collapse as the suction is generated. Clear or semiclear tubing permits visual examination of the material being removed and aids in determining which organ or space is being aspirated.

Nasal Tube Aspirator. A 10-inch, 90° curved metal tube with a $\frac{3}{16}$-inch bore, the nasal tube aspirator is designed for aspiration of the nasal/oral cavity. It is placed through the nasal opening or between the lips. The primary problem in the use of this instrument is the diameter of its opening. Even a small semisolid particle can easily clog this instrument.

Autopsy Aspirator. The autopsy aspirator is an 8- to 10-inch long, $\frac{3}{8}$-inch-bore metal tube. A collector is attached to one end and a hose to the other. This equipment is used for aspiration of the cavities of the autopsied body, and has a number of openings to prevent clogging of the instrument. The aspirator can be set to operate while the body is being embalmed. The nonclogging feature is designed to free the embalmer's hands so constant attention is not needed.

VISCERAL ANATOMY

The embalmer should constantly be aware of the internal structures he or she is attempting to preserve. Although comprehensive treatment of the internal anatomy is beyond the scope of this textbook, it is appropriate to include here limited descriptions of internal soft tissue structures to provide the embalmer with a quick reference source should he or she encounter a simple anatomical question or problem. Resolution of more complex problems is, of course, deferred to complete textbooks of anatomy.

Head

The interior of the cranial vault comprises anterior, middle, and posterior cranial fossae in which portions of the brain and brain stem are located. The frontal lobes of the cerebrum rest on that portion of the skull floor created by the anterior cranial fossa. The temporal lobes, hypothalamus, and midbrain cover the floor of the middle fossa. The large, posterior fossa houses the medulla, pons, and entire cerebellum.

Neck

The thyroid gland is a bilobed endocrine gland that partially covers the thyroid cartilage of the larynx and extends inferiorly as the sixth tracheal ring. The two lobes are usually, but not always, connected by an isthmus, which crosses the midline at about the level of the second, third, and fourth tracheal rings. The common carotid and inferior thyroid arteries are found posterior to the two lobes. Lateral to the lobes are the internal jugular veins. Posteriorly, the trachea is related to the straight muscular tube of the esophagus.

Thorax

Although the lungs are properly described as contents of the thorax, remember that their apices extend above the level of the first rib into the neck under the cupola. The right lung comprises three lobes and the left lung two lobes, although this is subject to some variation. The left lung is further characterized by the presence of a cardiac notch or impression to accommodate the ventricles of the heart. Medially, both lung surfaces relate to the contents of the mediastinum and contain the hilar structures, that is, the pulmonary vessels and the main-stem bronchi.

Inferiorly, the lungs are related to the diaphragmatic pleura and the diaphragm.

The heart is positioned retrosternally in the middle mediastinum and extends from the second intercostal space inferiorly to the fifth. The lateral cardiac margins extend beyond the lateral margins of the body of the sternum. The great vessels arise from the base of the heart at the level of the second intercostal space, behind the upper portion of the body and the manubrium of the sternum.

Abdomen

The majority of abdominal viscera consist of some part of the digestive apparatus, which is mainly tubular with some modifications and specializations of this basic structure in various locations. As the straight-tubed esophagus passes through the diaphragm and enters the abdomen, it quickly gives rise to the stomach. The remainder of the alimentary or digestive tube, in order, consists of the duodenum, jejunum, ileum (small intestine), cecum, ascending colon, transverse colon, descending colon, sigmoid colon, rectum (large intestine), and anus. Organs that facilitate digestion include the gallbladder, liver, and pancreas.

A rather peripatetic organ, the stomach is one whose location varies with changes in the position and orientation of the body. It is, therefore, difficult to describe specific relationships of the stomach. Similarly, the shape of this organ is dependent on the amount and type of foodstuffs contained therein as well as the extent to which the digestive process has progressed. A "typical" stomach possess greater and lesser curvatures, a fundic region that extends above the level at which the esophagus enters, and a pyloric region at the junction of the stomach and the duodenum.

The C-shaped duodenum is the first part of the small intestine and consists of four parts, which are either numbered one, two, three, and four or named superior, descending, transverse, and ascending. The superior portion is only partially covered by peritoneum and is, therefore, the most mobile of the four parts, as the others are entirely retroperitoneal. The descending portion typically receives the common bile duct and the main pancreatic duct, the contents of which facilitate digestion. The transverse portion crosses the body from right to left at the level of the fourth lumbar vertebra and continues as the ascending portion, which emerges from the peritoneum and gives rise to the jejunum.

The first 40% of the remainder of the small intestine is the jejunum, which cannot be grossly distinguished from the other 60%, which is the ileum. Internal and microscopic structures, together with vascular patterns associated with each organ, allow discrimination between the two. The distinctions are most obvious at the extreme ends. These organs occupy much of the abdomen and both are suspended by a fan-shaped mesentery from the posterior body wall.

The large intestine can be distinguished grossly from the small bowel by the presence of three longitudinal strips of muscle, the taeniae coli, sacculations, and fatty appendages called epiploic appendices, none of which is found on the small intestine.

A diverticulum, the cecum, marks the beginning of the large intestine and extends inferiorly beyond the level at which the ileum joins the ascending colon. The cecum is situated in the right iliac and hypogastric regions. Opening from it is the vermiform appendix. Extending superiorly from the cecum is the retroperitoneal ascending colon, which continues to the right colic or hepatic flexure, inferior to the liver in the right lumbar region. Here, the colon turns sharply to the left in the umbilical region, as the transverse colon. This is a freely movable portion of the large bowel, suspended by the transverse mesocolon from the posterior body wall and extending to the left colic or splenic flexure in the left hypochondriac and lumbar regions. Here, the colon again becomes retroperitoneal and descends to the level of the iliac crest as the descending colon. In the left iliac region, the descending colon forms the sigmoid colon which is once again freely movable, being suspended by the sigmoid mesocolon. Anterior to the third sacral vertebra, the sigmoid colon gives way to the rectum which in humans is not really straight as its name implies but is curved, following the curvature of the sacrum and coccyx.

The largest gland in the body is the liver, which develops as an outgrowth of the digestive tract and retains a functional and anatomical relationship with it. It rests in the right hypochondriac and epigastric regions. The upper surface of the liver is higher on the right than on the left and lies in relationship with the inferior surface of the diaphragm from which it is suspended by the coronary ligaments. On the inferior surface of the liver is the gallbladder, whose cystic duct is joined by the common hepatic duct from the liver to form the common bile duct which empties into the second (descending) portion of the duodenum. The gallbladder and the lower portion of the right lobe of the liver lie anterior to the right hepatic flexure in the right lumbar region.

The pancreas lies cradled in the arms of the C-shaped duodenum and extends across the midline from the right to the left at about the level of the second lumbar vertebra. The major subdivisions of the pancreas include the head, neck, body, and tail. The main duct of the pancreas typically joins the common bile duct immediately as they both enter the second part of the duodenum, but the patterns of the ducts from the liver, gallbladder, and pancreas are subject to considerable variation.

The remaining unpaired organ in the abdomen is the spleen, which is located in the left hypochondriac region. Lying in the umbilical left and right lumbar regions are the usually paired kidneys. These lie along the posterior body wall, with the right slightly lower than the left because of encroachment by the large right lobe of the liver. Both kidneys lie at the level of the umbilicus and both are retroperitoneal. In its own separate capsule at the superior pole of each kidney is a suprarenal gland.

Pelvis

Internal pelvic viscera in the male include the prostate gland, seminal vesicles, urinary bladder, and rectum. The last structure was already discussed; the first three are considered here. The prostate gland is situated at the base of the urinary bladder, surrounding the prostatic or initial portion of the male urethra. The gland is difficult to visualize in the pelvis but can be palpated as a firm structure if fingers are introduced into the pelvis around the neck of the bladder immediately anterior to the rectum. In addition to its continuity with the urinary bladder, the prostate also receives secretions from the paired seminal vesicles, which lie posterior to the prostate and communicate with it by means of ejaculatory ducts. The latter structures form as a result of the union of the ducts of the seminal vesicles and the distal ends of the vasa deferentia.

The urinary bladder is situated behind the pubic symphysis in the midline and its shape and size are dependent on the volume of urine contained within it. This muscular, distensible structure receives urine from the kidneys via the paired ureters, which open posterolaterally into the bladder.

In the female, the urinary bladder occupies a position similar to that in the male but is separated from the rectum by the intervening uterus and its adnexa. In addition to the uterus and bladder, other visceral structures in the female pelvis include the ovaries, uterine tubes, and vagina. The muscular unpaired uterus is positioned in the midline and is supported by a double layer of peritoneum called broad ligament. The uterus is divided into several parts including the fundus, body, and cervix.

The fundus projects above the level at which the uterine tubes communicate with the uterine cavity. At the distal end of the body is a thick, muscular constriction known as the cervix. Through the cervix, the cavity of the uterus communicates with the vagina, which is a distensible tube, flattened anteroposteriorly. The uterine tubes communicate with the opening directly into the abdominal cavity and the uterine cavity. The abdominal cavity, therefore, opens to the external environment via the uterine tubes, the cavity of the uterus, the cavity of the cervix, and the vagina. The paired ovaries are located on the posterior aspect of the broad ligament on either side of the uterus. The uterus, tubes, and ovaries are supported by an elaborate system of "ligaments" derived from reflections of the peritoneum.

CONTENTS OF THE ABDOMEN: THE NINE-REGION METHOD

To establish the nine abdominal regions (Table 14–4), extend two *vertical* lines upward from a point midway between the anterior superior iliac spine and the symphysis pubis. Draw two *horizontal* lines. Join the upper line to the lowest point of the costal margin on each side, at the level of the inferior margin of the tenth costal cartilage. Join the lower horizontal line to the tubercles on the respective iliac crests (Fig. 14–1).

Quadrant Method

There is a second method of dividing the abdomen into regions and that is the **four region plan.** A *horizontal* line is drawn from left to right through the *umbilicus.* A *vertical* line is drawn down the midline of the body. This establishes upper right and left quadrants and lower right and left quadrants (Fig. 14–2).

These topographical systems of dividing the abdomen serve to give the practitioner an approximate location of the various abdominal organs. The embalmer should have a thorough knowledge of the location of the visceral organs. This understanding is important in the

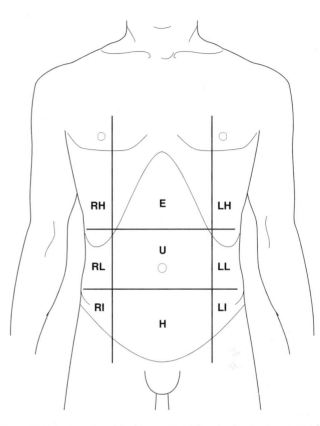

Figure 14–1. The nine regions of the abdomen. RH, right hypochondriac; E, epigastric; LH, left hypochondriac; RL, right lumbar; U, umbilical; LL, left lumbar; RI, right inguinal; H, hypogastric; LI, left inguinal.

process of cavity embalming. It is also valuable when one or more organs have been donated to an organ bank or when partial autopsies have been performed. In addition, the embalmer should have a complete understanding of the relationship of the vascular system to the visceral organs.

Trocar Guides

The efficiency of using the trocar to pierce the internal organs and aspirate their contents is enhanced by the use of trocar guides. **The main guides are to reach the stomach, cecum, urinary bladder, and the heart.** The guides all originate at the common insertion point—2 inches to the left and 2 inches superior to the navel. The point of the trocar is inserted into the abdomen and kept close to the anterior abdominal wall until the specific organ is reached.

Guide for the Right Side of the Heart. Move the trocar along a line from the left anterior–superior iliac spine and the right earlobe. After the trocar has passed through the diaphragm, depress the point and enter the heart (Fig. 14–2).

TABLE 14–4. THE NINE ABDOMINAL REGIONS

Right Hypochondriac	Epigastric	Left Hypochondriac
Part of the liver	Stomach including cardiac and pyloric openings	Part of liver
Part of right kidney	Portion of liver	Stomach, fundus and cardiac regions
Greater omentum	Duodenum, pancreas	Spleen
Coils of small intestine	Suprarenal glands and parts of kidneys	Tail of pancreas
Gallbladder	Greater omentum	Left colic splenic flexure
		Part of left kidney
		Greater omentum

Right Lumbar	Umbilical	Left Lumbar
Lower portion of liver	Transverse colon	Part of left kidney
Ascending colon	Part of body kidneys	Descending colon
Part of right kidney	Part of duodenum	Coils of small intestine
Coils of small intestine	Coils of small intestine	Greater omentum
Greater omentum	Greater omentum	
Right colic (hepatic) flexure	Bifurcation of the abdominal aorta and inferior vena cava	

Right Inguinal (iliac)	Hypogastric	Left Inguinal (iliac)
Cecum, appendix	Bladder in adults if distended	Part of descending colon
Part of ascending colon	Uterus during pregnancy	Sigmoid colon
Coils of small intestine	Coils of small intestine	Coils of small intestine
Greater omentum	Greater omentum	Greater omentum

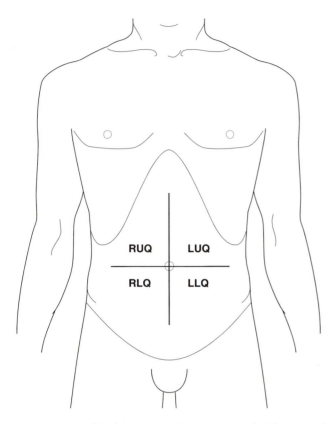

Figure 14–2. Division of the abdomen into quadrants. RUQ (LUG), right (left) upper quadrant; RLQ (LLQ), right (left) lower quadrant.

Guide for the Stomach. Direct the trocar point toward the intersection of the fifth intercostal space and the left mid-axillary line (established by extending a line from the center of the medial base of the axillary space inferiorly along the rib cage); continue until the trocar enters the stomach (Fig. 14–3).

Guide for the Cecum. The trocar is directed to a point three fourths of the distance on a line from the pubic symphysis to the right anterior superior iliac spine. When the point of the trocar is approximately 2 inches from the line, the point is depressed 2 inches and then thrust forward to pierce the cecum as it is trapped against the pelvis (Fig. 14–3).

Trocar Guide for the Urinary Bladder. Keep the point up near the abdominal wall directing the trocar to the median line of the pubic bone (symphysis pubis) until the point touches the bone. Retract the trocar slightly, depress the point slightly, and insert into the urinary bladder.

PARTIAL ASPIRATION PRIOR OR DURING ARTERIAL TREATMENT

Cavity embalming, complete aspiration and injection of cavity fluids, *follows* arterial injection and drainage.

There is one exception to this rule: When the abdomen is tightly distended with gas or edema this pressure should be relieved *prior to or during* arterial injection. The presence of fluid (as in ascites) or gas in the abdomen can be great enough to act as an *extravascular resistance*. This resistance may also interfere with drainage. Drainage may be difficult to establish until this extravascular pressure is relieved.

Two methods can be employed:

First, using a scalpel, puncture the abdomen at the standard point of trocar entry 2 inches left and 2 inches superior to the umbilicus. (Later, this point can be used for aspiration and injection.) Then insert a trocar or blunt instrument such as a large drain tube into the cavity and aspirate the gases or edema. It may be more useful to make this puncture in the lower area of the abdomen in the right or left inguinal area or the hypogastric region of the abdomen. From this point edema will be able to gravitate easier from the abdomen, and if gases are the trouble, it may be easier to pierce the *transverse colon* with a trocar from this more distant point (Fig. 14–4).

Second, using a scalpel, make a small incision in the abdominal wall. Dissect into the abdominal cavity. A portion of the large intestine can be incised if gas is the problem; edema drainage can be taken from the opening. Cover this opening with cotton or gauze saturated with a disinfectant so microbial agents are not released into the air.

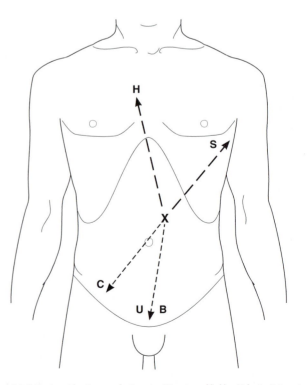

Figure 14–3. Trocar guides. S, stomach; C, cecum; UB, urinary bladder; H, heart; X, insertion point.

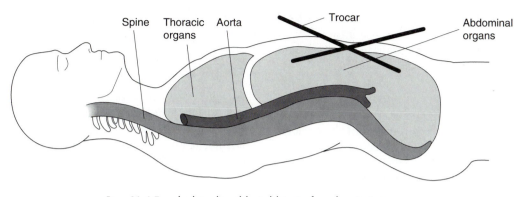

Figure 14–4. Trocar levels to relieve abdominal distension from edema (ascites) or gases.

The first method using the trocar is much cleaner and will be found to be generally more effective in relieving abdominal pressure (gas or edema) prior to or during arterial injection.

If the neck is distended and discolored prior to injection using the standard trocar point of entry, direct the trocar along the lateral abdominal wall through the diaphragm and into the thoracic cavity. The problem could be hydrothorax, and this can be removed to relieve pressure on the heart and neck veins. Care must be taken not to interrupt circulation.

ANTEMORTEM SUBCUTANEOUS EMPHYSEMA

A condition where there is an exceptional and noticeable amount of gas in the tissues *prior to embalming* is antemortem subcutaneous emphysema. Many times the facial tissues will be quite distended, the tongue will protrude, gases may be felt all along the thoracic walls, and, in the male, the scrotum may be distended with gas.

If there is no odor and if there are no signs of decomposition, palpate for a broken rib or examine the body for a puncture wound to the thorax or a very recent tracheotomy opening. Look for large needle punctures over the skin of the rib cage. This condition is brought about by a rupture or by the puncturing or tearing of the pleural sac of the lung. Air was forced into the tissues as the person struggled to breathe air. If the condition is severe enough, try and remove some of this gas *prior to arterial embalming.*

Insert the trocar into the abdomen at the standard point of entry, then direct the point through the diaphragm, keeping the point just under the rib cage so as not to damage any of the large vessels. This should help to relieve some of the gases. Likewise, using a carotid incision will help to relieve gases from the neck tissues. Removal of these gases can be better accomplished by channeling and/or lancing the tissues after the arterial injection is completed.

TIME PERIOD FOR CAVITY TREATMENT

There are two periods during which cavity aspiration and injection can take place: immediately following arterial injection and several hours following arterial injection. Most embalmers will certainly delay aspiration for a short period following arterial injection if it is only for a matter of a few minutes while the arteries and veins used for injection are being ligated and the embalming machine rinsed and cleaned. This time delay will allow the intravascular pressure to assist the diffusion of the arterial solution from the capillaries into the interstitial spaces. It is best to inject the last quarter to one-half gallon of arterial solution with the drainage closed, being careful to remove the arterial tubes and drainage devices quickly and to tie off the vessels so as much pressure as possible remains within the vascular system. A short delay of several minutes can then follow.

Now the aspirating begins. It is wise to do the aspirating PRIOR TO SUTURING. Aspiration takes the pressure off the vascular system and, thus, decreases the chances of leakage from the incision should some small vessels leak.

It should be stated that some funeral homes do not do the cavity embalming until the time of dressing and casketing. Many embalmers do the cavity embalming immediately at the conclusion of the arterial embalming. The theory of aspiration shortly after arterial injection has the following advantages:

1. Large numbers of microbes that can easily multiply and accelerate decomposition are removed as soon as possible.
2. Removal of the microbes prevents the possibility of translocation of the microbes to the skeletal tissues.
3. Removal of these microbes prevents or minimizes the production of gases that could cause purge.
4. Immediate aspiration removes materials that

could purge if sufficient gases were generated during the delay.

5. Removal of the contents of the hollow viscera and cavities eliminates a bacterial medium.

6. **Most important,** removal of blood from the heart, liver, and large veins helps to prevent blood discolorations.

7. If there has been some distension of the neck or facial tissues during arterial injection, immediate aspiration decreases the swelling. This is often seen in bodies dead from pneumonia when hydrothorax is present.

The second theory is to have a long delay prior to aspirating the body. Some embalmers delay aspirating for 8 to 12 hours. The theory is to allow a maximum time for the arterial solution to penetrate into the tissue spaces. Some embalmers feel the delay helps to preserve the walls of the visceral organs. This will then make the walls easier to pierce with the trocar when the aspirating is done. If a humectant coinjection or a humectant restorative "to fill out" emaciated tissue has been used, some chemical manufacturers suggest that the last half-gallon be injected with the vein ligated and a delay made between arterial injection and aspiration. This delay gives the tissues time to firm.

ASPIRATION TECHNIQUE

The standard point of trocar entry is located 2 inches to the left of and 2 inches superior to the umbilicus. This point is used for the standard trocar; from it the embalmer is able to reach all areas of the thoracic, abdominal, and pelvic cavities. The trocar should also be able to reach above the clavicle into the base of the neck. A second reason for using this point, especially with infants and children, is that the liver is on the right side of the body. At the location where the trocar is inserted, it is easier to move the instrument from point to point. If it were inserted on the right side, the trocar would be entangled in the solid tissues of the liver.

During the aspiration of the cavities, the trocar can be withdrawn enough to let some air pass through the instrument. This helps to "clean out" materials in the tubing and the instrument. Some embalmers withdraw the trocar several times during aspiration and plunge it into a container of water to flush out the tubing and trocar.

A moistened cloth saturated with a disinfectant solution can be used to clean the barrel of the trocar as well as any matter that may exist around the abdominal opening during the aspiration process.

An orderly method of aspiration should be employed. Remember that gases are usually found in the anterior portions of the abdominal and thoracic cavities.

Liquids gravitate to the posterior portions of the cavities. If each cavity is "fanned" from right to left, most of the viscera are pierced. This "fanning" can be done in about three levels of depth.

Begin by inserting the trocar and aspirating the most anterior portions of the cavity. Then progress from right to left within the middle portion of the cavity, and finally from right to left through the deepest portions of the cavity. Treat both abdominal and thoracic cavities in this manner. The "trocar guides" can be used to aspirate the hollow viscera such as the stomach, heart, urinary bladder, and cecum.

Let the trocar "sit" for a while until an area filled with liquid is thoroughly drained. This is necessary when treating bodies with ascites, hydrothorax, or ruptured vessels such as the aorta.

RECENT SURGERY OR ORGAN REMOVAL

If the deceased was an organ donor or died during the course of an operation and no autopsy was performed, the surgical incision or the incision used to remove the organ(s) may or may not have been loosely closed by the hospital. For such bodies, the following protocol simplifies treatment of the cavities:

1. Disinfect the surgical incision with a *phenol solution.*
2. Arterially embalm the body.
3. Remove loose sutures, surgical staples, and so on, and open the incision.
4. Swab the edges of the incision with a phenol solution.
5. Suture closed the incision using a tight baseball suture. If possible, use sufficient quantities of incision seal powder.
6. *Aspirate the cavities and inject cavity fluid.*

Any surgical drainage openings should be closed by suture or trocar button *prior* to aspiration of the cavities.

PARTIAL AUTOPSIES AND ORGAN DONATIONS

After a partial autopsy on an adult, the unautopsied cavity can be difficult to treat from the cavity that has been opened. It is much simpler to treat the walls of the autopsied cavity by hypodermic treatment and painting with autopsy gel. Fill the cavity with an absorbent material and saturate the material with a cavity fluid. Suture the cavity closed. *Now treat the unautopsied cavity* by aspirating the cavity and its visceral contents. Inject a sufficient quantity of cavity fluid.

DIRECT INCISION METHOD

In the treatment of bodies that have recent surgical incisions or from which organs were removed after death, resuturing followed by aspiration and injection with the trocar is recommended.

An alternate method can be used, a method that was employed as an alternative to cavity treatment via trocar many years ago. In this *direct incision method* of cavity treatment, the *embalmer* makes a midline incision over the abdominal wall and, from this point, treats the visceral organs and the cavities by lancing and draining the organs and sponging or aspirating their contents within the cavity. Either cavity fluid is poured over the various organs or the organs are directly injected with a parietal needle or large hypodermic needle.

This method of direct cavity treatment can be used when the cavity has been opened by recent surgery, an organ(s) has been removed for donation, or partial autopsy has been performed. The method is not only time consuming and unsanitary, but access to both thorax and abdomen is difficult.

ORDER OF TREATMENT

There is no specific order of treatment, but the embalmer should proceed in an orderly fashion in treating the cavities to ensure that no areas are missed. Years ago some instructors taught that each organ should be separately treated. That is, the stomach was aspirated (with one puncture) and then, without removing the trocar, the stomach was filled with cavity fluid. The embalmer then moved on to treat another organ until all hollow viscera and cavities had been embalmed.

A suggested order might be *thoracic* cavity, abdominal cavity, and pelvic cavity. Likewise, when injecting cavity fluid, inject the thoracic cavity first, then the abdominal and pelvic cavities.

ASPIRATION OF THE THORACIC CAVITY

At the standard point of entry, direct the trocar into the thoracic cavity. A good point at which to begin aspiration is the right side of the heart, using the trocar guide of an imaginary line running from the left anterior superior iliac spine to the lobe of the right ear. Intersect this line with the trocar in the mediastinal area. This technique also provides practice for those occasions on which the trocar may have to be used as a drainage instrument (which will have to be inserted into the right atrium of the heart). Next, aspirate the anterior chambers of the right and left pleural cavities. Direct the trocar a little lower and pierce the central portions of the lungs and the heart.

> Observe what is being aspirated. Clear tubing is a help. Remember, the hydroaspirator may be 10 feet away from the body. Look through clear tubing at what is being immediately removed from the body.

Finally, aspirate the deep areas of the pleural cavities. If hydrothorax is present, edematous liquids will be found, often in great quantities. Be certain that the trocar is directed to either side of the vertebral column where the great vessels enter and leave the lungs. This also aspirates the bronchial tubes leading to the trachea.

ASPIRATION OF THE ABDOMINAL CAVITY

After aspiration of the thorax, the trocar can be withdrawn and the stomach aspirated. Use the trocar guide. Move the trocar toward a point established along the *left* midaxillary line, at about the level of the fifth intercostal space. As the trocar moves toward this point it should pierce the stomach.

Several passages can be made through the stomach wall. Aspiration not only *removes* gases, liquids, and semisolids from the organs, but also *pierces* the viscera so that cavity fluid can better penetrate the visceral organs. Next, the cecum and bladder can be aspirated again using the trocar guides.

In similar "fanning" movements, aspirate the entire abdominal cavity again. Try to establish three levels. *Remember, gases, when they can move, will be in the anterior portions and liquids in the posterior portions of the cavities.*

In aspiration of the abdomen, the small intestines and the greater omentum have a tendency to cling tightly to the small holes located in the point and shaft of the trocar. For this reason, it is best to keep the instrument in constant motion, except when a large amount of liquid such as edema in bodies with ascites is being drained. Removing the trocar from time to time helps to prevent clogging of these small holes.

Pay special attention to the posterior of the liver. It is here that the great vessels enter and leave this organ. The liver is very difficult to preserve. Therefore, numerous passes with the trocar should be made through the solid portions of this organ. Also give special attention to the large intestine, especially the *transverse colon.* Check the previous* charts to observe the location of this intestinal organ. The large intestine, especialy the transverse portion, should be thoroughly pierced to allow the escape of gases and to assist later in penetration of the cavity fluid.

To assist the trocar in piercing the abdominal organs, place external pressure on the abdominal wall. Do this with a gloved hand. Hold the trocar with one hand

and apply the pressure with the other. Apply pressure gently on the abdominal wall. To facilitate passage of the trocar through the coils of the small intestine, in addition to applying pressure on the abdomen, pass the trocar to a bony part such as the ilium or pubic bone. In this way, the point of the trocar will pass through the intestine rather than push it aside or slip around it.

Another method that can be used in aspirating the *abdomen* and inferior portion of the thorax is to insert the trocar in the center of the right or left inguinal region of the abdomen. Long passes can be made with the trocar, which will pass through the lumen of the intestines as the point forges ahead through the diaphragm. Many embalmers feel they can better pierce the large and small intestine from this point of trocar entry.

TREATMENT OF THE MALE GENITALIA

After aspiration of the pelvic and abdominal cavities of the male, the trocar need *not* be inserted into the scrotum to aspirate this organ. Cavity fluid should, however, be injected into the shaft of the penis and the scrotum if these organs appear not to have received arterial solution.

To enter the scrotum direct the point of the trocar to the most anterior portion of the symphysis pubis. Draw back slightly on the trocar and direct the point over the top of the symphysis pubis into the scrotum. In cases of hydrocoele, edema of the scrotum, make several such passages into the scrotum. Be careful not to puncture the organ. Then, with a cloth placed around the scrotum, much of the water can be forced into the pelvic cavity. Later, undiluted cavity fluid can be injected into the scrotum.

Another condition less frequently encountered is a hernia involving the scrotum. A portion of the intestines moves into the scrotum. This condition can be severe enough to make dressing the body difficult. The trocar should be directed into the scrotum to pierce the loops of the intestine and remove as much of the content as possible. Later, this area should be injected with cavity fluid. The embalmer can also use the trocar to pull the intestine back into the abdominal cavity. This is slowly accomplished by pulling on the intestine with the point of the trocar. Gradually, the intestine can be manipulated into the abdominal cavity. This will make dressing of the body much easier.

CRANIAL ASPIRATION

The point of entry in cranial aspiration is the right or left nostril. A small trocar is introduced into the nostril and pushed through the *cribriform plate of the ethmoid bone.*

At this point the instrument enters the anterior portion of the cranial cavity (Fig. 14–5). It is not possible to move the trocar into the posterior portion of the cavity; therefore, any gases present must be removed from this anterior position.

Inject only a few ounces of concentrated cavity fluid. This is done by using a hypodermic syringe with a long needle. After injecton, tightly pack the nostril with cotton to prevent leakage.

INJECTION OF CAVITY CHEMICALS

After the complete aspiration of the thoracic and abdominal cavities, preservative/disinfectant cavity chemicals are placed within the cavities over the viscera. *Concentrated cavity fluid* is always used. In cases of hydrothorax or ascites or where blood has escaped during arterial injection or during aspiration of the organs, the fluids—blood and edema—dilute the cavity fluid.

The volume of chemical is determined by the mass of tissues to be treated, which is estimated on the basis of body size and weight. On the average, for a body weighing 150 pounds, 16 ounces of undiluted cavity chemical is used for each (thoracic, abdominal and pelvic) cavity. Larger bodies may require considerably more chemical. Smaller bodies, such as infants, require less.

Prior to cavity chemical injection, it is necessary to wash and flush the trocar thoroughly. All organic materials must be flushed from the trocar if concentrated cavity fluid is to pass through the instrument. The undiluted cavity chemical may be injected by two methods: gravity injector and machine injection. The gravity injector is attached directly to the 16-ounce bottle of cavity fluid. A hose connects the injector to the trocar. The higher the bottle is raised, the faster the fluid flows into the body. A small opening on the side of the gravity injector allows air to flow into the cavity fluid bottle. By placing a finger over this opening, the embalmer stops the flow of cavity fluid. This can be done when the trocar must be withdrawn to change its position within a body cavity. After use, the gravity injector, tubing, and trocar should be rinsed with cold water to disperse all the cavity fluid. The trocar can then be immersed in a cold liquid sterilant.

In machine injection, three bottles of cavity fluid are placed in the tank of the embalming machine. The delivery hose is then connected directly to the trocar. Pressure and rate of flow should both be set very low. The tubing alone can hold several ounces of cavity fluid. Following injection, make certain that the cavity chemical is thoroughly rinsed from the machine. Wash the machine with warm water and ammonia and then run fresh cold water through it.

The chemicals are sprayed or made to flow over the *anterior surface* of the viscera close to the anterior wall of the thoracic and abdominal cavities. The cavity chem-

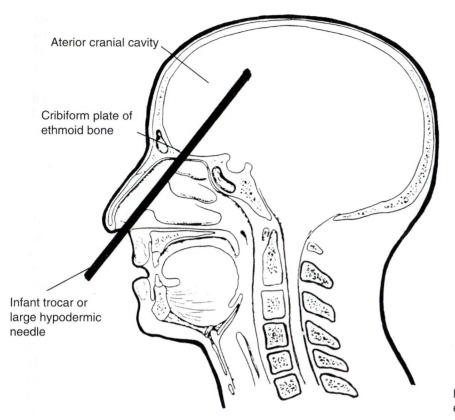

Aterior cranial cavity

Cribiform plate of
ethmoid bone

Infant trocar or
large hypodermic
needle

Figure 14–5. Anterior cranial cavity and cribriform plate of the ethmoid bone.

icals gravitate through the openings in the viscera made by the trocar and are absorbed by or rest on the posterior surface of the cavity walls.

After the cavity fluid is injected, some embalmers make several passes with the trocar through the abdomen and thorax to release gases that may have been displaced to the surface of the cavities. This movement of the trocar helps to distribute the cavity fluid. Cover the open end of the trocar with a cloth saturated with disinfectant so formaldehyde fumes and/or body gases are not released into the air.

After the trocar puncture has been closed and during the postembalming washing and drying of the body, *turn the body on its sides* not only to wash and dry the back and sides of the body, but also to distribute the cavity fluid and bring any trapped gases to the surface of the cavities.

The cavity chemicals should be kept in the body and not be allowed to spill or run onto the surface of the abdominal wall. Use a wet cloth to wrap the trocar and cover the opening in the body as the fluids are injected. If cavity chemicals accidentally flow onto the surface of the body, immediately flush with cold running water.

It is possible to inject cavity fluid into the trachea or esophagus. If the nasal passages or throat has not been tightly packed with cotton when the features were set, this fluid can exit when the body is turned to be dried after it is washed. Limited aspiration can be done with the

nasal tube aspirator after the body is placed into a supine position. The nasal passages can be tightly packed with cotton. Open the lips and, using dry cotton, make certain all the liquid is dried from the mouth. Likewise, clean and pack the nose again. If the embalmer feels that cavity fluid purge may be a problem during dressing and casketing, he should reaspirate the thoracic cavity at this time, giving special emphasis to the posterior of the neck, where the trachea and esophagus are located. Packing the throat and nasal passages with an abundant amount of cotton prior to embalming can help reduce the chance of cavity fluid purge.

CLOSURE OF THE ABDOMINAL OPENING

To complete the aspiration procedure, the opening in the body wall is closed. Several methods can be used. Each embalmer uses his or her own preferred method. The plastic, threaded trocar button provides complete closure and is easily removed if further aspiration and reinjection are necessary later.

Two sutures are commonly used to close the trocar opening: the **purse-string** (Fig. 14–6) and the **"N" or reverse stitch.** Sutures offer the advantage of a complete closure. A bow can be used to secure the suture. It can easily be opened if reaspiration is necessary. To minimize

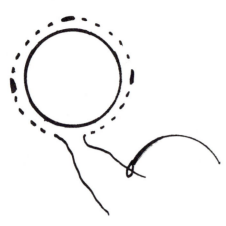

Figure 14–6. Purse-string suture.

exposure to any fluid that may leak from the abdominal opening, if the embalmer plans to suture the opening closed, place the stitch after aspiration, just before the cavity fluid is injected. After injection, pull the suture tight to close the opening.

The barrel of the trocar can enlarge the abdominal opening if there is poor integrity to the abdominal skin to a size where a trocar button would be impossible to use. This condition necessitates the use of sutures for closure.

Some embalmers do not close the trocar openings but allow them to remain open for the escape of any gases. If this is done the opening should be covered with cotton and the cotton covered with plastic to prevent any soilage of the clothing. This technique is not recommended when the body is being shipped.

REASPIRATION/REINJECTION

A body must be reaspirated and reinjected with cavity embalming chemicals whenever the possibility exists that tissues or cavity contents (liquids, gases, semisolids) have not been thoroughly saturated with disinfectant preservative chemicals. The procedures are the same as those used in the initial cavity embalming. The entire cavity is aspirated and cavity chemicals applied.

In some funeral homes, policy mandates that *every body* be reaspirated prior to dressing and casketing, whereas others reaspirate only when it is felt absolutely necessary. Some embalmers not only reaspirate but reinject at least one full bottle of cavity fluid after reaspiration.

The following situations require reaspiration and reinjection:

1. A noticeable amount of gas escapes when the trocar button is removed.
2. The body is to be transported to another funeral home.

3. Final disposition of the body is to be delayed.
4. Decomposition is evident prior to embalming.
5. Abdominal surgery has been performed recently.
6. The body is obese.
7. The body shows evidence of gas (distension of the veins of the neck or backs of the hands) or purge or distension of the abdomen is present.
8. Death was due to blood infections or infectious diseases of the abdomen, thorax, or visceral organs (e.g., bacteremia, peritonitis, pneumonia).
9. Death was due to drowning, or purge was evident prior to, during, or after arterial embalming.
10. Ascites is present.

KEY TERMS AND CONCEPTS FOR STUDY AND DISCUSSION

1. Define the following terms:
   aspiration
   cavity embalming
   electric aspirator
   hydroaspirator
   infant trocar
   purge
   reaspiration
   trocar
2. Give several reasons for aspiration.
3. Distinguish between stomach purge and lung purge.
4. Describe how the abdomen is divided into nine regions; name each region.
5. Describe how the abdomen is divided into quadrants.
6. List the major visceral contents of the nine abdominal regions.
7. Give the trocar guides for the following organs: (a) right side of the heart, (b) stomach, (c) cecum, and (d) urinary bladder.
8. Describe four means of creating a vacuum for aspiration.
9. Discuss the various means of closing the trocar opening in the abdominal wall.
10. Give the standard point of trocar entry into the abdomen and explain why this location is used.
11. List conditions that necessitate reaspiration of the body.
12. Explain why partial aspiration may be necessary prior to or during arterial injection.
13. Explain why cavity embalming is performed.
14. List the advantages and disadvantages of immediate cavity treatment and delayed cavity treatment.

BIBLIOGRAPHY

Burke PA, Sheffner AL. The antimicrobial activity of embalming chemicals and topical disinfectants on the microbial flora of human remains. *Health Lab Sci* 1976;13(4):267–270.

Cavity fluids. In: *Champion Encyclopedia*. Springfield, OH: Champion Chemical; 1975:No. 454, 1833–1836.

Dorn JM, Hopkins BM. *Thanatochemistry*. Reston, VA: Reston; 1985.

Grant ME. Cavity embalming. In: *Champion Encyclopedia*. Springfield, OH: Champion Chemical; 1987:2338–2341.

Proper cavity treatment. In: *Champion Encyclopedia.* Springfield, OH: Champion Chemical; 1974:No. 449, 1813–1816.

Rose GW, Hockett RN. The microbiological evaluation and enumeration of postmortem specimens from human remains. *Health Lab Sci* 1971;8(2):75–78.

Tortora GJ. *Principles of Human Anatomy*. 3rd ed. New York: Harper & Row; 1983.

Weed LA, Baggenstoss AH. The isolation of pathogens from tissues of embalmed human bodies. *Am J Clin Pathol* 1951;21:1114.

Weed LA, Baggenstoss AH. The isolation of pathogens from embalmed tissues. *Proc Soc Mayo Clin* 1952;27:124.

15

Preparation of the Body After Arterial Injection

POSTEMBALMING TREATMENTS

The process of embalming is divided into three periods: preembalming, embalming, and postembalming. Preembalming procedures are carried out before arterial injection of the body and include setting of the features, positioning of the body, selection and elevation of vessels for injection and drainage, and selection and preparation of the embalming fluid.

During embalming the arterial solution is injected. In this period, activities include the selection of proper pressures and rates of flow to distribute the arterial solution, massage and manipulation of the body to promote fluid distribution, control of drainage to help distribute the fluid, removal of surface blood discolorations and promotion of the retention of arterial fluid for preservation, use of humectants and dilute arterial solutions to moisturize dehydrated bodies, use of high-specific-gravity, concentrated arterial solutions to dry bodies with skeletal edema, and maintenance of a good moisture balance in the "normal body."

In the embalming period an embalming analysis is made to determine what body areas have not received arterial solution. Procedures to promote fluid solution distribution to these areas are instituted, and, if necessary, a secondary artery is raised to inject the area devoid of fluid. Most embalmers pause a short time between injec-tion and cavity embalming to flush and clean the embalming machine, remove drainage instruments and ligate veins, remove arterial tubes and ligate arteries, and clean blood and drainage materials from the embalming table. Cavity embalming is usually carried out during the embalming period; however, some embalmers prefer to wait several hours between injection and cavity embalming. When this is done, cavity embalming is considered to be carried out during the *postembalming* period.

The following treatments are generally carried out after the arterial and cavity embalming. **The order of treatment is optional.** Each is discussed in detail in this chapter.

1. Preservative treatments for areas that did not receive arterial solution or did not receive *sufficient* arterial solution
2. Closure of embalming incisions
3. Removal (and closure of the opening) of invasive devices, for example, pacemaker, intravenous needles, surgical drains, colostomy apparatus
4. Washing of the body, turning of the body to dry and inspect for posterior lesions
5. Final treatments for ulcerations and discolorations
6. Corrective treatments for purge and packing of all orifices

7. Removal of gases or edema from viewable facial areas
8. Inspection of mouth for purge or moisture; resetting of features if necessary, and insertion of false teeth if these were not available before embalming
9. Application of adhesives to eyes and mouth
10. Dressing with plastic garments
11. Repositioning, if necessary
12. Terminal disinfection of instruments and preparation room and personal hygiene
13. Preparation of documentation, shipping instructions, and so on

TREATMENT OF AREAS NEEDING ARTERIAL SOLUTION

The primary embalming point is the artery (or arteries) that the embalmer chose as a site from which to embalm the entire unautopsied body. If areas of the body have not received fluid or have not received sufficient arterial solution, the embalmer should inject the area through a secondary injection point.

Example. If the embalmer began by injecting and draining from the right femoral artery and vein, and solution did not reach the left forearm and hand, he or she should first inject the axillary, brachial, radial, or ulnar artery to secure preservation of the forearm and hand by arterial injection. If fluid is not distributed to these areas through the secondary injection sites, the embalmer must now use one or more other methods of embalming to preserve these tissues.

Appearance of Areas Not Receiving Arterial Solution. Areas that have not received arterial solution do not show evidence of fluid dye. Intravascular blood discolorations may still be present. The tissues exhibit no preservative fixation.

When doubt exists as to whether an area has received any or sufficient solution, the simplest corrective treatment is to inject the area arterially with a slightly stronger arterial solution.

Appearance of Areas Receiving Insufficient Arterial Solution. Determining if a body region contains arterial solution is not as easy as determining if a body area has received *NO FLUID*. Fixation is not as intense as normally would be expected. Dyes may be blotchy and not as intense. If there is doubt, follow the preceding rule and inject the area. Later, these areas can darken, gases may form, and skin-slip is a possibility.

SUPPLEMENTAL EMBALMING TREATMENTS

There are two supplemental methods of embalming: *surface embalming and hypodermic embalming*. These supplemental embalming methods are used to treat small areas, such as the eyelids, mouth, and fingers, or to treat large body areas that could not be injected because of arteriosclerosis, trunk walls that did not receive arterial fluid, or the side of the face when the common carotid is occluded.

Surface Embalming*

Surface embalming can be used to treat intact skin that has not received sufficient arterial fluid. It can also be used in "raw" skin areas, for example, broken skin, skin-slip, burned tissues, and surface lesions. Surface embalming may be applied to both *external* and *internal* body surfaces, for example, the buccal cavity of the mouth, underneath the eyelids, within the nasal cavity, underneath the scalp in autopsied bodies, and the inner trunk walls in autopsied bodies.

The chemicals used for surface embalming may be liquids, gels, or powders. The liquids most frequently used include accessory surface embalming chemicals and cavity fluid. Cotton compresses saturated with an accessory chemical specifically formulated for the treatment of intact skin are most frequently used both for viewable and for nonviewable body areas. Surface chemicals also include strong formulations of phenol. These chemicals are designed to bleach, dry, and cauterize tissue. Cavity fluid compresses may be used to treat intact and broken skin.

Cavity fluid and the accessory surface chemicals may be milder than phenol solutions and are designed to preserve, bleach, dry, and deodorize the tissues. The stronger phenol solutions bleach, preserve, dry, and cauterize tissues. Cotton should be soaked with the chemical and applied to the skin area needing fluid. The cotton should then be covered with plastic. The plastic reduces the fumes and keeps the compress from drying. The compress may need to be left on several hours.

Gels constitute a second surface embalming chemical. Years ago, formalin creams were used for surface embalming. In the early 1960s, surface preservative gels were introduced. These can be applied directly to the skin with a large brush or they can be poured onto cotton and applied as a pack. The gels are available in an almost-liquid form of very low viscosity or in a very heavy "jelly" of very high viscosity. When used on external surfaces, gels should also be covered with plastic to reduce fumes and to prevent evaporation. These chemicals are designed to penetrate the tissues. They should remain affixed to

---

*When any surface chemicals are used, the compress or gel should be covered with plastic so as to reduce fumes and to prevent the surface chemical from evaporating.

nonviewed body areas. Cotton compresses with the liquid surface preservatives should also remain on body areas that will not be viewed. In areas that will be cosmetically treated and viewed, the chemicals should be left on the skin several hours.

Arterial fluid is not recommended as a surface embalming chemical, for the dyes present in the fluid stain the skin surface. Their penetrating strength and preservative strength may be less than those of cavity fluid, accessory surface chemicals, or gels. When a surface compress (gel or liquid) is removed from an area to which cosmetics will be applied, the area should be cleaned with a solvent before cosmetic treatment begins.

Specific Treatments

Specific areas are discussed to show how surface embalming can establish good preservation.

Mouth, Lips, and Cheeks. Cotton can be placed over the dentures and saturated with cavity fluid, using a hypodermic needle and syringe to moisten the cotton. The lips can then be glued; the preservative works from the inside of the mouth to preserve the tissues. Cosmetic treatment can be immediately implemented using this method of preservation.

Eyelids. Cotton can be used for eye closure or a small piece of cotton can be inserted over the top of an eyecap. The cotton can be moistened with a few drops of cavity fluid and the eyelids sealed with an adhesive. Cosmetic treatment can begin immediately (Fig. 15–1).

Dehydration. If tissues need the preservative they will not dehydrate. Underembalmed tissue can dehydrate faster

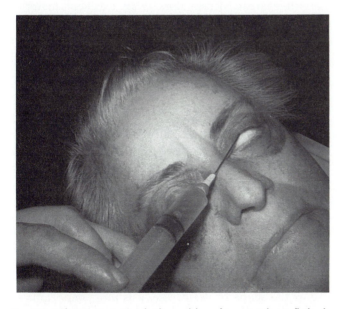

Figure 15–1. Placing cotton moistened with several drops of concentrated cavity fluid under the eyelids ensures good preservation of the lids. Cosmetic treatment can then begin.

than well-embalmed tissue. Gluing the eyes and mouth further reduces any dehydration problems. Visible areas treated by internal surface compresses or hypodermic preservative treatments can be cosmetized using a cream-based cosmetic to retard dehydration.

Nose. Cotton saturated with preservative fluid can be inserted into the nostrils. It can later be pushed back far enough that it will not be noticeable.

The preceding areas can also be treated with external surface packs; however, the application of cosmetics must be delayed.

For areas that will not be seen, such as the leg or foot, the gel can be applied to the skin surface or poured into a plastic stocking. The latter reduces fumes and makes application easier.

Surface embalming powders have been used for many years.* Diapers can be used to apply the powder or the powder can be placed in plastic garments such as stockings, coveralls, or pants after the garments are in position. Powders can also be used to treat the interior walls of the abdomen and thorax in the autopsied body. Powders are not as effective as gels or liquids. Read the label to be certain the powder is a preservative and not just a deodorant. (Note: *An excellent way to treat a gangrenous limb is to pour preservative gel into a plastic stocking along with some preservative powder. Place the stocking on the leg. The powder sticks to the sides of the stocking along with the gel. This combination helps to establish preservation and control odors.*)

Hypodermic Embalming

The second and most effective supplemental method of embalming is hypodermic embalming. This method is used to treat small localized body areas or large areas, such as the trunk walls of the autopsied body or a limb that did not receive sufficient arterial fluid and cannot be injected arterially.

Hypodermic injection involves the use of a hypodermic syringe and needles ranging from 6 to 19 gauge and of varying lengths. The larger needles (6 gauge) are useful for large areas. An infant trocar or specially designed hypovalve trocar can be connected to the centrifugal embalming machine for the injection of large body areas.

The arterial solution used for arterial injection can be used for hypodermic injection. It is recommended that it be strengthened with cavity fluid or a high-index arterial fluid. This type of solution should be used only on

---

*When embalming powders are being used, the embalmer must wear a protective particulate mask and the room should be properly ventilated to remove powder particulate and fumes.

body areas that will not be viewed, as the dye in the fluid can blotch the skin. Cavity fluid as well as specially designed accessory embalming chemicals may be used for hypodermic embalming. Phenol solutions should be reserved for localized treatments of discolored areas or tissues when bleaching of tissues is necessary. The phenol solutions would not be used for routine supplemental hypodermic embalming.

In nonviewable areas where the infant trocar or hypovalve trocar has been used, the punctures can be sealed with a trocar button. In facial areas, where hypodermic needles would be used, most of the injections can be made from inside the mouth. In this manner, leakage will not exit onto the face. Unlike tissue builder, these chemicals have a tendency to seep from the point of puncture. If the inside of the nose is to be used as an entry point for hypodermic embalming, use the nostril **opposite** the side of the face being treated. For example, if the right cheek needs arterial fluid, inject the right cheek for the left nostril. Pass the needle under the septum and enter the right cheek or upper right mouth. This reduces fluid leakage. In the autopsied body large portions of the face can be reached through scalp incisions.

The hands and fingers can be injected from the palmar surface of the hand or from between the fingers. Super adhesive can be applied to prevent leakage.

The nose can be treated hypodermically by inserting the needle inside the mouth. The ear can be reached by hypodermic injection from behind the ear. Application of super adhesive to the punctures prevents leakage.

For larger areas such as the arm and leg, the infant trocar can be inserted into the area of the cubital fossa of the arm to reach the arm and forearm. The leg can be treated by inserting the infant trocar on the medial side of the leg just inferior or superior to the knee. From this point, both the thigh and lower leg can be reached.

Combination Treatments for Large Areas

Certain conditions such as arteriosclerosis, gangrene, and edema require additional injection of the legs. If arterial treatment is unsuccessful the legs can be injected hypodermically. In addition, surface embalming can also be used. The legs can be painted with autopsy gels and embalming powder can be placed into the plastic stockings. A combination of supplemental embalming methods (hypodermic and surface) is used.

In the trunk area, hypodermic injection is used when edema is present. Coveralls can be applied and embalming powder or autopsy gel painted over the areas being treated. When edema is a problem in the elbow area, hypodermic treatment can be used and the area painted with autopsy gel and wrapped with gauze. A plastic sleeve can then be placed over the treated area.

CLOSURE OF INCISIONS

Today, two methods are used to close incision: sutures and super adhesive. Regardless of the method of closure, the embalmer must follow several steps to prepare all incisions for closure:

1. Be certain all vessels are securely tied. This prevents any further leakage.
2. Dry the incision with cotton.
3. If there is edema in the surrounding tissues, force as much liquid out of the incision as possible.
4. Do not suture until after cavity aspiration; aspiration relieves pressure on the vascular system and helps to prevent leakage.
5. Tightly close all sutures.
6. During suturing or prior to gluing, place an absorbent powder (or absorbent clay, "mortuary putty") in the incision to absorb any moisture that may accumulate.
7. Make several sutures before applying the incision seal powder to the incision. In this manner, a "pocket" is created and the powder is retained within the incision and not spread on the surface of the body (Fig. 15–2D).
8. After suturing, apply a surface glue over the area to prevent leakage.

Suturing

Cotton or Linen Thread. Linen thread is stronger than cotton thread and is recommended for autopsy and vessel incision sutures. For restorative sutures, which are located on visible areas, dental floss is an excellent material to use.

A $\frac{3}{8}$-inch Circle Needle. The $\frac{3}{8}$-inch circle needle is used for restorative sutures and to suture incisions made to raise vessels.

Double-Curved Autopsy Needle. The double-curved autopsy needle is easy to grip with the gloved hand. It is used to close autopsy incisions, surgical incisions, and incisions made to raise vessels.

Needles come in a variety of sizes and shapes, for example, single-curved autopsy needles. Loopyt needles, circle needles. Some have a "patented eye." These eyes are threaded by merely pushing the thread against the eye portion of the needle, which eliminates the need to pass thread through the eye of the needle. Regardless of the size or the shape of the needle, it is most important to keep it sharp. Suturing can be very dangerous if the nee-

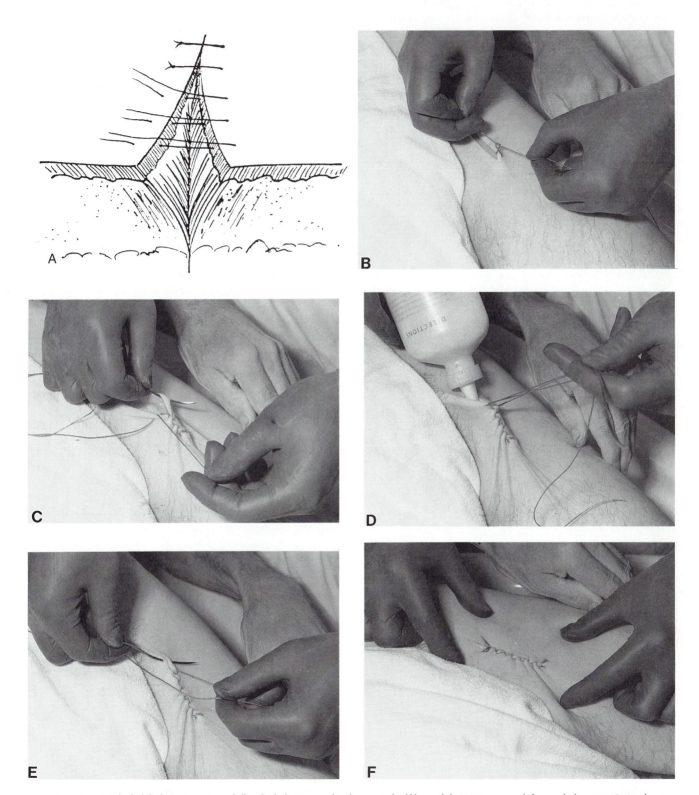

Figure 15–2. **A.** Individual (bridge) sutures. **B.** Baseball stitch. The ligature is tied in place. Knots should be avoided. **C.** Sutures are made from inside the incision. **D.** A pocket is made before the suture ends and incision seal powder is inserted. **E.** When properly sewn, no string should be visible. **F.** The completed suture. The ligature cord should not be visible. These sutures are airtight.

dles are dull, as extra pressure must be applied. In doing so, the embalmer increases the chance of the needle breaking or piercing her or his skin. A sharp needle makes suturing much easier, safer, and faster.

Keep in mind that when suturing, one should pull on the thread and not on the needle to tighten the suture. Pulling on the needle weakens the suture cord where it passes through the needle's eye. In closing long sutures, as in autopsies, this may cause the cord to break.

The embalmer can suture using single- or double-stranded thread. This depends on the strength of the suture cord or on the type of suture. It is wise to double the cord when cotton thread or three- or four-twist linen thread is used. Single-stranded suture cord works best with five- and six-twist linen thread, dental floss, and single and double intradermal and worm sutures.

Direction of Suturing

To make suturing more efficient, follow these directions for the various sutures.

Common Carotid Artery. If using the parallel incision, suture from the inferior portion of the incision superiorly. Suture from the medial portion of the incision laterally if using a supraclavicular incision.

Axillary Artery. Suture from the medial area of the incision laterally (with the arm abducted).

Brachial Artery. Suture from the medial portion of the incision laterally.

Radial and Ulnar Arteries. Suture from the distal portion of the incision medially.

Femoral Artery. Suture from the inferior portion of the incision superiorly.

Autopsies (Truck Standard "Y" Incision). Use bridge sutures to align the skin into position. Begin the trunk suturing at the pubic symphysis and suture superiorly.

Popliteal Artery. Begin the suture at the inferior (or distal) portion of the incision and suture superiorly.

Anterior and Posterior Tibial Arteries. Begin the sutures distally and suture superiorly.

Common Sutures

Individual (Bridge) Sutures. Individual sutures are used to align tissues into position prior to, during, or after embalming (Fig 15–2A). They are temporary and are later replaced by more permanent sutures.

Baseball Sutures. Considered the most secure and commonly used, the baseball suture can be airtight. In addition to the injection site incisions, it is used for autopsy stitching. To make this stitch, pass a suture needle and thread from beneath the incision up through the integument, and cross the needle from side to side with each stitch (Fig. 15–2B). This creates a strong tight closure. In the process, however, the tissues adjacent to the incision are pulled up into a ridge.

Single Intradermal (Hidden) Suture. The single subcutaneous or intradermal suture is made with one needle and a single thread (Fig. 15–3). It is referred to as the "hidden stitch," because it is used on exposed areas of the body and is directed through the subcutaneous tissue only. To begin the closure, insert the needle deep into the tissues at one end of the incision. Make a knot in the thread a short distance from the end and pull the knot to the position of the needle puncture in the integument. Keeping the needle directed through the dermal tissues only, develop a back-and-forth pattern from one side of the incision to the other. Take care to line up the margins as the thread is drawn so that there are no gaps between stitches. To complete the closure, direct the needle through the integument as far as possible from the end of the incision. Once this is completed, draw the margins of the incision together by pulling the free end of the thread. Puckering may result if the thread is pulled too tight. The excess thread is cut off close to the incision as slight pressure is applied, concealing the ends of the thread.

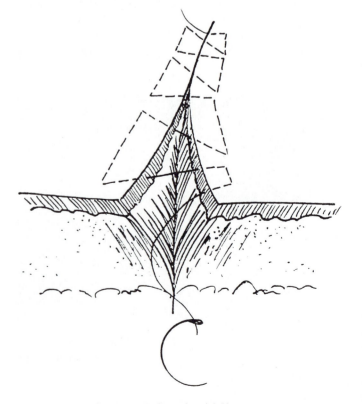

Figure 15–3. Single intradermal (hidden) suture.

Double Intradermal Suture. The double intradermal suture is made with two needles threaded with opposite ends of the same thread (Fig. 15–4A). As this suture is permanently fixed at each end, it has greater holding ability than the single intradermal suture. Pass each needle through the dermis of opposite margins so that both stitches are parallel, similar to the lacing on a shoe. Continue the process until the incision is completely sutured. After drawing the margins tight, knot the two ends together within the incision. Correct puckering by light massage or smoothing with the finger. To end the suture, insert both threads onto one needle and insert it under the skin from the end of the incision to a point ½ inch away. The excess threads are then cut as pressure is applied, resulting in the ends of the threads being hidden.

Inversion (Worm) Suture. The inversion suture is used to gather in and turn under excess tissues (Fig. 15–4B). The pattern of this suture is the same as that of the single intradermal suture, except that the stitches are made parallel to the incision edges and do not pierce the margins of the incision. The stitches are generally made as close to the margins as possible. The best results are obtained by making the stitches uniform in length. The stitches do not enter the incision except to start the suture. Each stitch should be drawn taut as sewn. The worm suture is not visible and may be waxed as needed. It is an excellent suture for closing a carotid incision or closing the scalp on the cranial autopsy (Fig. 15–5).

Interlocking (Lock) Suture. The interlocking suture creates a tight, leakproof closure. It has a disadvantage in that an unsightly ridge appears on the surface of the incision. Begin the suture at one end of the incision and direct the needle through the tissue so that it passes through both sides of the incision from the outside. Keep the thread tight with the hand not holding the suture needle. Then, lock the stitch by looping the needle through the thread. When completing the loop, pull the thread tight. Repeat this process until the incision is closed. The needed insertion should be made consistently from the same side of the incision.

Continuous (Whip) Suture. The continuous suture is generally used to close long incisions (Fig. 15–6). Frequently, it is used by the autopsy technician to close the long incisions from the autopsy. This suture prevents leakage of fluids from the body cavities during transfer from the hospital to the funeral home. The suture is also seen in people who have died during surgery; the incision has been drawn closed to prevent leakage of fluids. Organ transplant retrieval teams use the stitch to close long incisions after the removal of visceral organs. To make this stitch, anchor the suture thread. Pass the needle through both sides of the incision, starting on the outside of the tissue on one side of the incision and passing directly through and out the tissues of the opposite side of the incision. Pass the thread over the top of the incision and begin the next

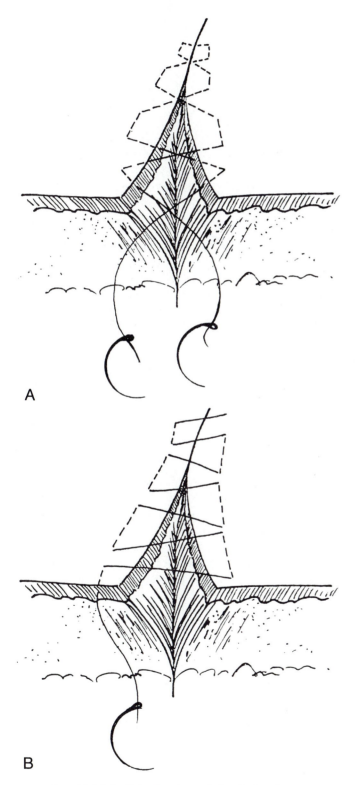

A

B

Figure 15–4. **A.** Double intradermal suture. **B.** Inversion (worm) suture.

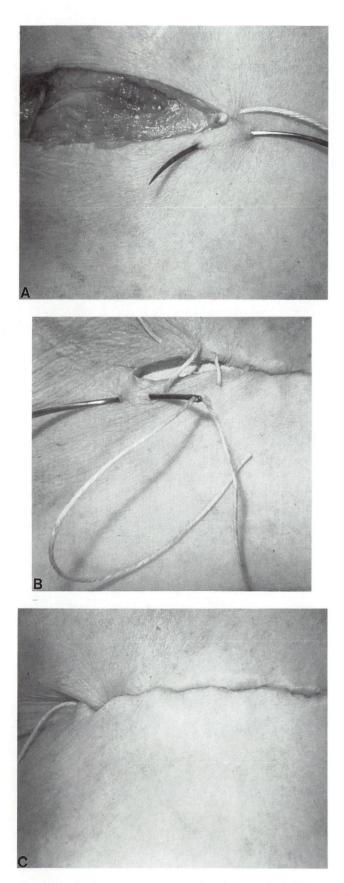

Figure 15–5. Worm suture. All stitches are made on the surface of the skin.

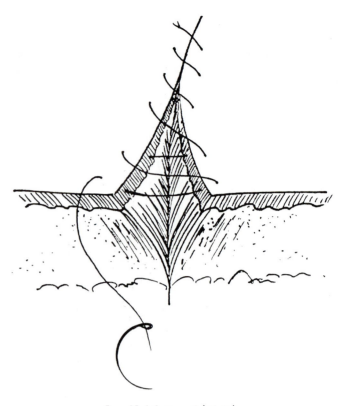

Figure 15–6. Continuous (whip) stitch.

stitch $\frac{1}{2}$ to 1 inch beyond the previous stitch. The process is completed when the incision is closed.

Adhesives

The other method of closing incisions involves the use of a super adhesive. Many brands are available today in local stores. Most super glues can work in the presence of moist tissues. These adhesives are excellent for closing jagged tears in the skin.

Many embalmers use the glues to close the incisions made to raise vessels. Some use the glues to close the scalp in cranial autopsies. Long autopsy incisions, however, are closed with sutures. As there are many uses for these glues in the embalming room, super glues should be kept in stock.

REMOVAL OF BODY INVASIVE DEVICES

Many hospitals do not remove the intravenous needles or tubes from bodies after death. It is best to leave these needles and tubes in place until *after* arterial injection. If the needle is in an artery, considerable swelling will result if the needle is removed prior to arterial injection. A similar problem arises when needles or tubes inserted into veins are removed prior to embalming. A large ecchymosis or swelling and discoloration can develop. These punctures can be sealed with a drop of super glue. Tissue builder or a phenol solution injected beneath the skin also helps to seal these punctures on visible skin areas. When the needle or tube has been placed into the subclavian or jugular vein a small incision can be made, and the area filled with incision seal powder, then sutured with a small tight baseball suture. If the area will not be seen, a trocar button may be used to seal the puncture.

Pacemakers. A pacemaker should be removed if the body is to be cremated. Certain radioactive powered units must be returned to the manufacturer. A small incision can be made over the device, which is usually located in the upper right pectoral region. The wire leading to the heart is cut. Incision seal powder is placed in the pocket and the incision sutured.

Colostomy Closures. Remove the colostomy collecting bag. Pour some cavity fluid into the bag for disinfection before destroying it. Disinfect the body area and colostomy stump with cavity fluid or a phenol solution on cotton. By placing pressure on the stump and slighlty twisting, force the piece of bowel back into the abdominal cavity. A pursestring or "N" suture can be used to close the colostomy (Fig. 15–7). Surface glue may be applied to the closure after the body is washed and dried. The colostomy opening may be closed before or after arterial injection.

Surgical Drains. Remove surgical drains and close the openings using a pursestring suture. Surface glue may be applied after the body is washed and dried to ensure against leakage.

FINAL WASHING AND DRYING OF THE BODY*

After all sutures are completed and points of leakage sealed, the body should be washed and thoroughly dried. Particular attention should be given to the removal of blood from the surface of the body. A washcloth or rough surface material will help to loosen the blood. Lukewarm water and plenty of antiseptic soap should be used. Care should be given to the washing of the hair, especially if

---

*Proper preparation room attire—gown, gloves, and, if necessary, mask and eye protection—should be worn during these postembalming procedures.

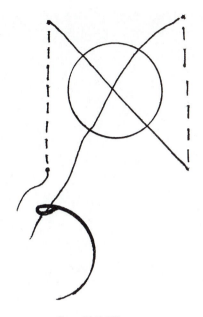

Figure 15–7. "N" suture.

the jugular vein has been used for drainage. A conditioner rinse can be massaged into the hair during washing to help eliminate tangles and deodorize the hair. If the scalp exhibits a lot of dander or flaking, wash the hair several times and thoroughly dry with a hair dryer. (This pertains to men as well as women.) Attached hair pieces, natural curly hair and permed hair should be dried with cool air so the hair does not straighten. If plats are present, especially in an African-American, it may be wise to consult with the family prior to combing them out when the hair is washed.

The body should be carefully dried. Good drying eliminates mold growth on the skin surface, especially in warm climates. Turning the body on its side gives the embalmer an opportunity to examine the posterior area. After the body has been dried, any intravenous punctures or punctures used to draw postmortem blood samples can be sealed with a super adhesive (Fig. 15–8).

TREATMENT OF ULCERATIONS, LESIONS, AND DISCOLORATIONS

After the body has been washed and dried, the sutures have been closed, and invasive devices have been removed and their punctures sealed, the embalmer should treat those lesions (e.g., decubitus ulcers) and discolorations (e.g., an ecchymosis on the back of the hand) on visible areas. Of course, decubitus ulcers should have been treated (preservative surface compresses) at the beginning of the embalming. After embalming, these ulcerations are redressed with compresses of phenol solution, accessory surface embalming chemicals, cavity fluid, or

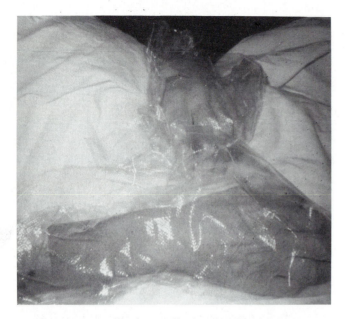

Figure 15–8. Cosmetized hands protected by plastic during dressing and casketing.

autopsy gels. This redressing helps to ensure preservation and sanitization.

Dry the tissues and deodorize the ulceration. Plastic clothing (overalls, pants, and stockings) can be placed on the body to help control odors. The buttocks may be diapered. The embalmer can inject the area around the decubitus ulcer with cavity fluid or accessory chemicals designed to combat the gas bacillus that forms tissue gas. The solution may be injected with a large-diameter hypodermic needle (6 gauge) or an infant trocar. Gloves should be worn in dressing these ulcerations. A mask is also advisable. Decubitus ulcers will be located at pressure points—the buttocks, shoulders, and heels.

Surface compresses containing phenol solution, an accessory bleaching solution, or cavity fluid can be applied to discolorations (e.g., an ecchymosis on the back of a hand). These discolorations can also be treated internally by hypodermic injection of the same chemical into the discolored areas. With this method, cosmetics may be applied without the delay needed for surface chemicals to work.

If any "raw skin areas" are present in viewable areas, the tissues should be dried at this time. Chemical compresses of a surface preservative chemical (or cavity chemical) can be applied over the areas. These compresses should remain in place for several hours. When the compresses are removed, the tissues should be cleaned with a solvent and thoroughly dried with a hair dryer. If arterial fluid seeps through these broken skin areas during injection, some embalmers simply remove all loose skin, clean with a solvent, and dry with a hair dryer.

TREATMENT OF PURGE

After arterial and cavity embalming, there always exists the possibility of purge from the anus, mouth, or nose, generally because cavity fluid is present in a position or an amount that allows its exit from one of these orifices. The injected cavity fluid may have built up enough pressure to purge materials from the upper respiratory tract, upper esophageal area, or rectum. Tightly packing the nasal passages, throat, and rectum prior to arterial injection should eliminate this problem. This will help to contain odors, prevent purging, and prevent any soiling of the clothing or casket interior.

When anal purge is present after embalming, force as much purge as possible from the rectum by firmly pressing on the lower abdominal area. Pack the rectum using cotton saturated with cavity fluid, autopsy gel, or a phenol solution. Dry packing should be inserted into the anal orifice after the moistened cotton. Leave a portion of the dry cotton so it can be seen. This will help to fully block the anal orifice.

When purge is present from the mouth or nose immediately following arterial injection and cavity treatment, it may be necessary to immediately reaspirate the body and reinject cavity fluid. Clean out the orifices and be certain they are tightly packed with plenty of dry cotton or cotton webbing.

The purge observed at the conclusion of embalming is not the same purge observed several hours after embalming (caused by the buildup of pressure from gases that form in the body cavities). This immediate postembalming purge is generally the result of cavity embalming. Prior to dressing and casketing, reaspirate the body cavities and, if gas is present, reinject the cavities.

TREATMENT OF DISTENSION

Visible areas—face, neck, and hands—that are distended often need to be reduced for viewing of the body. These treatments can be carried out during the postembalming period. Some swellings, such as edema, can be treated by specific arterial solutions during arterial injection. It is necessary to know the cause of the distension to perform a corrective treatment. Swellings present prior to arterial injection should be noted on the *embalming report*. Examples of such conditions include edema, tumors, swellings caused by trauma, distension from gases of decomposition in the tissues or cavities, tissue gas produced by *Clostridium perfringens, distension* caused by allergic reactions, distension brought about by use of steroid drugs, and gases in the tissues from subcutaneous emphysema.

Distension of facial tissues, the neck, or glandular tissues of the face or the tissues surrounding the eye orbit during embalming of the body can be caused by an excessive amount of arterial solution in these tissues. Some of the causes of this swelling are very rapid injection of solution, use of too much injection pressure, poor drainage from these tissues, breakdown of the capillaries (possibly decomposition) in these tissues, excessive massage, and use of arterial solutions that are too "weak." It is essential during embalming of the body that the embalmer is alert to any tissue distension. Injection should be immediately stopped and the situation evaluated. If correction of distended tissue involves excision of tissue (e.g., goiter, tumor), permisson must be obtained from the persons in charge of disposition of the body.

Areas of the body that contain skeletal edema should be treated during the embalming period with fluids of sufficient strength to meet the preservative demands of the tissues and, at the same time, reduce the edema. Edema of the face and hands can be somewhat corrected in the postembalming period, if adequate preservation has been achieved.

In pitting edema, excess moisture is present in the tissue spaces. In solid edema, the excess moisture is within the cells. Pitting edema can be moved by mechanical aids such as gravitation, massage, channeling of the area, and application of pressure (e.g., pneumatic collar, weights, Ace bandage, water collar, digital pressure) to move the moisture to another area. Elevation of the head and firm digital pressure slowly drain pitting edema from the facial tissues. During cavity aspiration, the trocar can be used to channel the neck, which allows the edema to drain from the facial tissues into the thorax. Edema of the eyes can be treated in several ways: (1) surface compresses using cavity fluid, phenol compound, or autopsy gel, during and after injection; (2) cavity fluid on cotton under the eyelids, during and after injection; (3) hypodermic injection of phenol compound or cavity fluid after embalming.

After preservation of the lids is accomplished channels can be made under the skin (e.g., from within the mouth, temple area): carefully applying external pressure to the distended tissues, "massage" as much of the edema from the tissues of the eyelids as possible. Drainage areas, such as in the temple area, can be sealed later with a drop of super adhesive. The primary problem that arises in removing edema from the facial tissues or hands is that the skin may become very wrinkled. Tissue preservation must always be the first concern.

Subcutaneous emphysema is frequently seen when the lung has been punctured. It may be the result of a surgical procedure (e.g., tracheotomy), a bullet wound in the thorax, or a broken rib that tears into the lung. Cardiopulmonary resuscitation can fracture a rib and

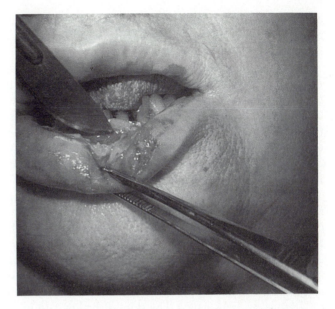

Figure 15–9. After embalming, the lips are lanced to release gases in the tissues.

tear the lung. Gas escapes into the subcutaneous tissues. As the individual struggles to breathe, more air is forced into the body tissues. Gases can easily be detected after death by palpating the tissues. The term **crepitation** is used to describe the spongy feel of the gas as it moves through the tissues when they are pushed on. Arterial injection and blood drainage remove a small portion of the gas, but gas that is trapped in the facial tissues must be removed by channeling. This channeling can be done after the body is embalmed. The lips can be opened and a scalpel, bistoury knife, or large hypodermic needle used to channel the tissues of the face from inside the mouth (Fig. 15–9). Once the channels are made the gas can be pushed out of the tissues. If the eyes are affected the lids can be everted and the underside of the lids incised with a suture or hypodermic needle. Cotton can be used to close the eyes; it will also absorb any leakage.

Subcutaneous emphysema can be differentiated from true tissue gas. True tissue gas has a very distinct foul odor that worsens progressively and is caused by an aneaerobic bacterium. Blebbing and skin-slip develop with true tissue gas. (See Chapter 24 for treatments of true tissue gas.)

RESETTING AND GLUING THE FEATURES

The features can be corrected after embalming. Additional cotton or feature posing compound can be inserted to fill out sunken and emaciated cheeks. If the cotton that was originally used to set the features becomes moist during the embalming, as a result of contact with purge or blood and fluid from the suture or needle injector used for mouth closure, it should be replaced with dry cotton.

The dentures are not always available at the beginning of the embalming. The mouth can be reopened and the dentures inserted afterward. These procedures are, of course, more difficult when the tissues are firm. Eyes, too, can be closed or reset after arterial injection. (Refer to Chapter 18 for a discussion of the postembalming procedures employed when eye enucleation has been performed.)

After the features have been properly aligned and the cavity embalming has been completed, the features can be glued. Adhesive applied to the lips and eyelids helps to avoid the separation caused by dehydration. The area where the adhesive is to be applied should first be cleaned with a solvent. Rubber-based adhesive, which is often used for the mouth and eyes, does not work well on a moist or oily surface. The skin of the lips and margins of the eyelids should be clean, dry, and free of moisture or oils. Super adhesive works very well for securing the eyelids. It ensures good closure of the inner canthus.

When glue is applied to the mucous membranes it is advised that it be kept behind the "weather line." This is not always possible. In some elderly persons or in individuals in whom blisters are removed from the mucous membranes after the gluing, the mucous membranes are not even visible. New mucous membranes can be drawn with cosmetics. Gluing helps to place tension on the mucous membranes, and this tension often "pulls" wrinkles from the membranes. Wrinkled lips can be corrected by gluing, waxing, or injecting the mucous membrane with tissue builder.

If the body was shipped, the lips may separate as a result of flight vibrations. Because of the delay, the tissues have time to become very firm. In such cases, the lips can be stretched or exercised with the blunt handled of an aneurysm needle or a pair of forceps (Fig. 15–10A). If the eyelids separate, they may also have to be "exercised" or stretched to obtain closure. Super adhesive is more effective in securing the mouth and eyes when the tissues are very firm (Fig. 15–10B).

PLASTIC GARMENTS

Prior to dressing, protective plastic garments can be placed on the body. Pants or coveralls can be placed on the trunk and plastic stockings on the legs. Embalming powder should be sprinkled into these plastic goods. The powder deodorizes the body and helps to control mold growth. Plastic sleeves may be applied to broken skin at the elbows or on the arms. Coveralls do not cover the shoulders, however. So, if edema is present in the shoulder area, place the body in a unionall. The unionall cov-

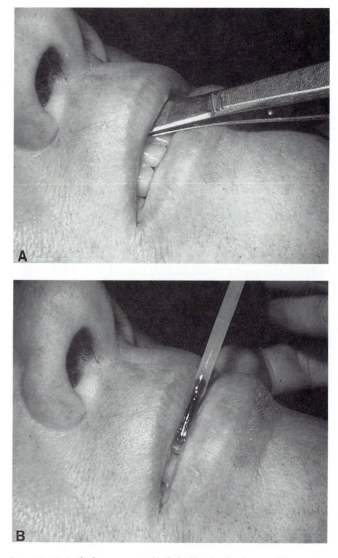

Figure 15–10. **A.** The lips are exercised with the blunt handle of a pair of forceps. **B.** A rubber-base adhesive or a super adhesive is used to seal the lips.

ers the arms, trunk (including the shoulders), and legs. Unionalls are very helpful in bodies that show advanced decomposition or extensive burns.

TERMINAL DISINFECTION

Terminal disinfection comprises the disinfection practices carried out after the embalming process to protect the environment and includes personal hygiene for the embalmer as well as disinfection of the instruments, equipment, and preparation room.

Care of the Embalming Machine

After use, the embalming machine should be flushed with warm water. Fluids that contain a humectant such as lanolin or silicon often leave a thick residue in the tank. Ammonia and lukewarm water should be flushed through the machine to remove the residue. Many embalmers prefer to flush the machines with a water softener or the powder used in electric dishwashers. Additives for machine cleaning can be purchased through fluid manufacturers. A final flush with warm water is necessary. It is recommended that the machine be filled with water at this time for the next preparation. This keeps the gaskets moist. Give the water time to release any dissolved gases such as chlorine. Adding embalming fluid (later) to an already filled machine decreases the release of formaldehyde fumes. A lid must be placed on the water tank of the machine.

Surfaces

All surfaces should first be cleaned with cool water and a small amount of antiseptic soap to remove organic debris. Torn-up sheets make good washcloths and can be disposed of after use. A preliminary wash removes organic debris and also any formaldehyde present. Remember that a number of good disinfectants contain chlorine, and this chemical should not come into contact with formaldehyde. Bleach and warm water make a very good cleaning solution. The table, countertops, and drains can be wiped clean and disinfected with this solution. Lysol products are good disinfectants and are easily available. Be certain to clean the area *under* the table surrounding the drainage outlet. Tops of overhead lighting should also be given attention. Tubing used for aspiration should be soaked in a disinfectant solution. Pay attention to handles on cabinets and drawers. Commercial products used for cleaning the preparation room contain dilution instructions. (Refer to Chapter 3 for a review of disinfection practices.)

Instruments

Clean instruments prior to disinfection. Removing organic material from the instrument makes disinfection more effective. Immerse all instruments including trocars in a solution of Bard–Parker disinfectant (8% by volume formaldehyde in 70% ethanol or isopropanol) or in 200 to 300 ppm of an iodophor for 45 minutes or longer. If possible, destroy cutting blades in a biohazard sharps container. Take special care with cutting instruments when gas gangrene or "tissue gas" has been encountered. The causative agent of this condition, *Clostridium perfringens*, is a spore-forming bacillus and can easily be passed via contaminated cutting instruments. They should remain in this solution several hours. After disinfection, instruments should be rinsed, dried, and properly stored (Fig. 15–11).

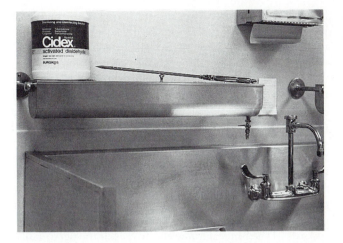

Figure 15–11. Containers of sufficient size must be provided so all instruments can be completely immersed for disinfection.

Disinfectant Checklist

In selecting a disinfectant for instruments and other preparation room paraphernalia, keep in mind the characteristics of a good disinfectant:

- Has a wide range of activity (works against viruses, bacteria, and fungi)
- Is of sufficient strength (active against spore-forming organisms of bacilli and fungi)
- Acts in the presence of water
- Is stable and has a reasonably long shelf-life
- Is noncorrosive to metal instruments
- Acts fast
- Is not highly toxic to living tissues or injurious to the respiratory system

PERSONAL HYGIENE

Terminal disinfection also concerns the embalmer. *Destroy* gloves after use; gloves are made to be used *once*. Thoroughly wash hands after removing gloves. Keep fingernails short and trimmed to prevent tears in the gloves. Numerous antiseptic preparations are available for washing or applying to the skin after the hands are dried. Consult a hospital supply catalog. Treat all cuts and punctures immediately: disinfect the area, induce bleeding, and consult a physician. Review Chapter 3 for preembalming and postembalming sanitation techniques.

DOCUMENTATION AND SHIPPING PREPARATION

After embalming, the work should be documented. The report should contain information pertaining to the embalming and to all personal property received with the body. Particular attention should be made to the list of jewelry and clothing. A report should accompany all bodies being shipped. When the body has been autopsied and is being shipped, the report should contain information indicating if viscera were returned from the hospital or morgue. Organs and tissues removed at autopsy or for donation must be noted, especially if the eyes have been removed. If the viscera were returned from the hospital and replaced in the body cavities, note how the organs were preserved and note that they have been placed in the cavities.

Later, when the death certificate is available, the cause of death and contributing causes should be added to the report. This may be valuable information for health records of the funeral home employees. If the person died of a contagious or infectious disease, properly label the body if it is being shipped to another funeral home. Bodies should never be shipped without some partial dressing. Place plastic coveralls or pants and undergarments on the body. If undergarments are not provided, clothe the body in pajamas or a hospital gown.

Place the body deep enough in the shipping container that the lid does not press against the face. Remember, in moving bodies on and off planes, the shipping container may be slightly tilted. The body should be firmly secure in the shipping container. Position casket pillows or cardboard packing at the sides, head, and foot of the body to keep it from shifting. Place a large piece of plastic under the body to protect the container from leakage or purge. Arrange cotton around the head and neck and in the nares to absorb any purge that may be released. Let the cotton stick out from the nostrils, so that flies are less likely to be attracted to the body. This practice should always be followed in the summer months when the body is in the preparation room. Careful packing of the nasal, throat, and oral passages prior to embalming is an important factor in preventing any postembalming purge.

When positioning instructions have *not* been given by the receiving funeral home, make certain one of the hands is *not* placed over the other. Hands should be placed on the abdomen. Resting one on top of another (which is a custom in many communities) can mark the covered hand.

A very light coating of massage cream can be placed on the face and hands when the body is to be shipped. Large amounts are not necessary and may be difficult to remove even with a solvent.

If they have not been given instructions by the receiving funeral home, many embalmers do NOT seal the mouth when the body is being shipped. The lips are coated with massage cream. This allows the receiving funeral home an opportunity to be certain the mouth is dry, allow any gases created by the movement of the shipping of the body to escape from the mouth, and permit tissue building to be done from inside the mouth. The body will be reaspirated by the receiving funeral home; any reconstruction work will be performed by them.

MONITORING: SURVEILLANCE OF THE CASKETED REMAINS UNTIL DISPOSITION

It is the duty of the funeral establishment having custody of the remains (either casketed or waiting to be casketed or to be shipped uncasketed) during the postembalming period to observe the appearance of the body and to correct any problems that might arise.

Detailed examinations should be made before and after each visitation period. Likewise uncasketed remains should be daily inspected for any changes.

Postembalming problems include, but are not limited to, dehydration of tissues, purge, leakage from incisions (embalming or antemortem surgical), leakage from any antemortem invasive treatments, softening and discoloring of tissues, gas formation, separation of lips or eyelids, leakage from areas where edema is present, odors, maggots, and needed cosmetic changes. If any of these conditions are noted, immediate steps should be taken to make a correction.

Cosmetic Corrections

Areas of the face, neck, hands, or arms may reveal color changes in the skin. The causes include greening of tissues affected by jaundice, darkening of the skin due to dehydration, darkening of the skin due to insufficient preservation of the area, and darkening from minor trauma. Where softening of the skin or darkening from trauma or ecchymosis has occurred, the area should first be treated by hypodermic injection of undiluted cavity fluid or application of a surface compress (it needs to remain in contact with the skin for several hours). These areas and dehydrated areas can be covered with a variety of opaque cosmetic "undercoats"; an adjustment can easily be made with cream cosmetics.

Separated Tissues

Tissues such as the lips and eyelids may separate due to dehydration, improper gluing, or motion and handling if the body has been shipped. These tissues should be "exercised" to establish good contact. The contact surfaces should be cleaned with a good solvent and a super adhesive applied. Lips may also be "filled out" with tissue builder to establish contact of the surfaces or they may be waxed.

Leakage

Potential areas of leakage could include some of the following:

- Any area of trauma to the face or hands where the skin was broken or torn
- Cranial autopsy incisions
- Autopsy sutures

- Surgical sutures
- Sutures at sites where vessels were raised for arterial injection
- Areas where edema is present
- Intravenous punctures
- Punctures used drawing postmortem blood samples
- Any point where the skin has been broken

Minor seepage (e.g., intravenous puncture) may be corrected by wiping away the accumulated liquid, injecting a phenol compound to cauterize the area, and sealing the puncture with a super adhesive. Where the skin has been torn, a phenol compound surface compress (or a cavity fluid compress) can be applied; later the area can be cleaned with a solvent, dried with a hair dryer, and sealed with a super adhesive or surface glue.

Clothing can be protected by sheets of plastic. The casket interior, pillow, and clothing should be inspected for any signs of leakage. If leakage is judged severe, the body should be removed from the casket and carefully undressed. Incisions can be opened, dried, checked to be certain vessels are ligated, and resutured using large amounts of incision seal powder within the incisions. Plastic garments can be placed on the body and, if necessary, edges sealed with duct tape. Interior damage may be severe enough to require replacement. Casket pillows can be reversed for minor leakage. Blankets and clothing may need to be replaced.

Purge

If purge has occurred it will be necessary to reaspirate the body. No doubt the body will have to be taken back to the preparation room for this procedure. Not only should the body be thoroughly reaspirated, but the cavities should also be reinjected with undiluted cavity fluid. If gases were noted when the trocar button was removed leave the body in the preparation room, if possible, for several hours and repeat the treatments again before redressing the body. The mouth and nasal cavities should be checked for dryness and tightly repacked with cotton or cotton webbing. The lips can then be resealed and recosmetized. Distended eyelids may indicate the presence of gases in the tissues. It may be necessary with this condition to aspirate the cranial cavity and inject some cavity fluid into the anterior cranial cavity. The presence of "true tissue gas" may necessitate reembalming of the body.

Maggots

Infestation of a body with maggots is a nightmare experienced by few embalmers today. In the summer months, bodies should be carefully examined for fly eggs, in particular the corners of the eyes, within the mouth, and the nostrils. If maggots are present, they can be picked from the surface of the body with cotton saturated with a dry hair wash. To stimulate maggots to emerge to the surface from areas beneath the skin or from the mouth or nostrils, the areas can be swabbed with a petroleum product (kerosene has been used by many embalmers). As the maggots emerge on the skin surface they can be removed with cotton saturated with dry hair wash. They should be placed in plastic bags before being discarded. The problem with maggots is not knowing if all have been found. If they persist it may become necessary to close the casket. Maggots in the clothing and hair can be vacuumed with a suction vacuum. The dust bag then can be destroyed.

Mold

In warm climates, mold can be a problem when bodies are being held for long periods. Bodies should be thoroughly dried to discourage mold growth. Mold needs to be carefully removed with a scalpel or spatula. The area is then swabbed with a phenol compound chemical and later thoroughly dried before cosmetics are applied. Placing embalming powder inside plastic coveralls, pants, and/or stockings helps to control mold growth.

KEY TERMS AND CONCEPTS FOR STUDY AND DISCUSSION

1. Define the following terms:
   autopsy gel
   baseball suture
   bridge suture
   coverall
   crepitation
   hypodermic embalming
   postembalming analysis
   purge
   single intradermal suture
   surface embalming
   terminal disinfection
   unionall
   worm suture
2. Describe a body area that is well embalmed.
3. Describe a body area that has not received any arterial solution.
4. Describe a postembalming treatment for a large decubitus ulcer of the buttocks.

BIBLIOGRAPHY

Grant ME. Chronological order of events in embalming. In: *Champion Expanding Encyclopedia*. Springfield, OH: Champion Chemical Co.; October 1986: No. 571.

16

Age and General Body Considerations

A factor that must always be considered in the preembalming analysis of a body is **age.** Embalmers often think only of the extremes—the techniques that will be used in the preparation of children as compared with those used for adults. If age is taken into careful consideration as a factor influencing embalming technique, four categories become evident:

Infant to child   Birth to about age 4

Child to young adult   About age 4 to approximately age 12

Young adult to adult   Approximately age 12 to about midseventies

Old age   Midseventies to late nineties

Not only does age influence the techniques used in the embalming process; age also leads the embalmer to expect certain difficulties and conditions with respect to positioning, setting of features, sites for injection and drainage, strength and volume of embalming solution, and injection pressure and rate of flow.

The hands and head of an infant are positioned differently than those of the adult. Elderly persons may present positioning problems if arthritic conditions are present. Methods of mouth closure in adults and infants differ because the bones of the infant have not yet ossified. In old age the mandible and maxillae may have undergone degenerative changes to the point where a needle injector cannot be used and the mouth must be sutured closed.

This chapter deals with some of the problems encountered in the preparation of bodies of different age groups and the techniques required. The embalmer should remember that many factors other than *age* influence technique. Size and weight of the body, cause of death, moisture conditions in the body, postmortem changes, and discolorations are a few of these other factors considered in the preembalming analysis.

The embalmer should not stereotype bodies by age. For example, not all elderly persons are thin-skinned, emaciated, and toothless. Many very elderly persons are in excellent health. Their vessels are free of sclerosis and they may have a normal or above-normal weight, good musculature, and excellent teeth. Likewise, not every middle-aged adult will have vessels free of sclerosis, good teeth, good muscular build, and normal weight.

Even in children, it is not always the rule that small quantities of a mild-strength arterial fluid should be used. Many children die from diseases that produced edema or show evidence of advanced postmortem changes. In these cases, seemingly large volumes of strong arterial solutions are needed.

Every body must be individually judged in making a preembalming analysis.

INFANTS AND CHILDREN—GENERAL CONSIDERATIONS

Infants and children require the use of several definite techniques that vary from those used in an adult or very elderly person. As defined in pediatric medicine, the infant period ranges from birth to 18 months and the toddler period from 18 to 48 months. Obviously there are considerable variations in both total weight and development between individuals in these classifications.

In embalming infants, it is important to realize the relationship of body water to body fat. Both contribute to total body weight. At birth, body water is approximately 75% of total body weight. At 1 year of age the body water declines to about the normal adult level of 60% of total body weight. It is therefore easy to understand the need for special embalming care for infants.

Similarly, body fat in the newborn is about 12% of total body weight and normally doubles to 25% at 6 months of age and then increases to about 30% at age 1.

Infant skin is much more delicate than adult skin and can easily distend and wrinkle on injection of the arterial solution. The vessels in the infant are extremely small but should be free of sclerosis. Most infants are autopsied, but infants dead from birth defects and systemic disease may not be autopsied. **It is important that the embalmer be familiar with the preparation of both autopsied and unautopsied infants.**

Several important facts should be stated at this point. The embalmer must have arterial tubes available for embalming infants. These tubes should be cleaned thoroughly after each use as they are easily clogged. They should always be tested prior to use to be certain they are in working order.

With regard to embalming solutions, it must be remembered that the infant body normally contains a large amount of moisture. In addition to this moisture, disease processes and medications can further increase moisture in the body. Renal and liver failure can bring about the accumulation of toxic wastes in the blood and tissues. This moisture and the toxic wastes can greatly increase the preservative demand of the body. It is suggested that the embalmer *not* use preinjection and weak arterial solutions for embalming infants. Many of these small bodies do not demand as much preservative as an adolescent or adult, but require a similar strength of arterial solution. **Use regular arterial fluids and strengths only slightly reduced from those for the adult.**

Certain factors characterize the different cases encountered in the embalming of infants and children:

1. Autopsied bodies
   A. Complete autopsy: cranial, thoracic, and abdominal cavities, spinal autopsy, limbs examined
   B. Partial autopsy: examination of only cranial, thoracic, or abdominal cavity, spine, or limbs
   C. Organ examination only: removal of only one organ
2. Unautopsied bodies
3. Organ donors: removal of eyes and/or any of the visceral organs or skin that may be used for transplantation
4. Infants whose embalming has been delayed but who have been neither refrigerated nor frozen
5. Infants that require restorative treatments (these bodies may or may not be autopsied)
6. Fetuses
   A. Premature infants: referred to as "preterm" in pediatric medicine today, any infant weighing less than $5\frac{1}{2}$ pounds at birth or born prior to the end of the 37th week of gestation
   B. Stillborn: fetus that dies prior to delivery from the uterus (In many states the definition of a stillborn includes a specified number of weeks of gestation, and if that specified time has passed, a death certificate and burial permit are required.)

EMBALMING THE INFANT

All treatment should begin with topical disinfection followed by a good soap and water washing of the body, cleaning of the nasal, oral, and orbital areas, and gentle extension and manipulation of the head and extremities to relieve any rigor mortis. Intravenous tubes or any other invasive connections to the arterial or venous systems should be left in place and removed *after* arterial injection. Tracheotomy tubes or any tubing placed into the mouth or nose should be removed *prior to* arterial injection.

Eye Closure

Eyecaps may be "cut down" and inserted under the lids, or cotton pads can be placed under the lids to effect closure. After embalming, the lids may be glued with rubber-based glue or affixed with super glue. Most embalmers close the eyes prior to arterial embalming, but it should be pointed out that closure can also be done after arterial preparation. In addition, some embalmers prefer to cover eyecaps or the cotton with a thin film of massage cream. Care should be taken when using massage cream that the free margins of the eyelids are cleaned with a solvent if the lids are to be glued.

Mouth Closure

In the infant, the needle injector method of closure is not possible; however, in an older child this method can easily be used. In the infant, a muscular suture can be used (passing the needle for the suture just in front of the mandible). The suture is completed by passing the needle through the septum of the nose. As the mandible and maxillae are very soft in the infant, closure can also be made by passing a sharp $\frac{3}{8}$-inch circle needle directly through the mandible. The needle can then be passed either through the septum of the nose or directly through the maxillae.

In some small infants the embalmer may wish to use a rubber-based adhesive prior to embalming as a method of closure rather than suturing. After embalming the mouth can again be cleaned and reglued with a rubber-based glue or super adhesive. Depending on the customs of the community, some embalmers leave the mouth of an infant open. When this is done, massage cream should be placed on the tongue and walls of the mouth. The corners of the mouth can be glued.

It may be difficult to create a good line of mouth closure in an infant. If a suture has been used for mouth closure the embalmer may also want to use a rubber-based glue or super glue to obtain a good line of closure. The mouth is generally glued *after* arterial and cavity embalming because air from the lungs can be trapped in the mouth. If gluing is necessary before embalming, use of a rubber-based glue is advised, as the mouth can easily be reopened by the use of a solvent or by reapplication of glue. (The glue acts as its own solvent.) After the features are set, light cover of massage cream is applied over the face, hands, and arms. Massage cream should *not* be placed over discolored areas where opaque cosmetics will later be applied.

Positioning

After washing and drying of the infant, the body is placed on a towel. The towel can be gathered to hold the head in a proper position. It later is discarded and replaced with a clean, dry one. The position of the arms and head can vary considerably. Generally, the funeral home will have a policy. In some cases the arms are arranged along the sides of the trunk, and forearms and hands are placed on the body, barely touching, so as to encircle or clasp a toy, doll, or stuffed animal. In other cases, the arms are positioned bent at the elbows, forearms flexed, and hands placed near the shoulders. One arm may be placed across the body to hold some object while the other arm is positioned upward near the head and shoulder area.

The head may be so placed that it rests upon its side (the right cheek area) or, like an adult, is slightly turned to the right. As it may be impossible to use a head block, pads of cotton or towels can be used. The infant body can firm as strongly as that of the adult. Changes in position can be difficult in the casket. Attention should also be given to the positioning of the legs. Often, the legs are

visible during viewing of the infant. If the legs are flexed, they may be straightened by wrapping them with strips of sheeting during the injection of arterial solution.

Blood Vessel Selection: Unautopsied Infants

Common Carotid Artery. The common carotid is the largest of the nonaortic arteries. It is easily accessible and very shallow. The infant has little neck musculature so the incision area can easily be concealed by the chin. This artery is accompanied by a relatively large adjoining vein (the internal jugular vein) and affords excellent drainage. A special incision is available in addition to the conventional carotid/jugular skin surface incisions. Placing support under the shoulders helps to elevate this neck area. Dropping the head backward brings the vessels closer to the surface. Keep in mind that the thymus gland can be quite large in the infant. Turn the head in the direction opposite that of the vessel being raised (i.e., to raise the right common carotid turn the head to the left). In using this variant incision, place a horizontal incision in one of the horizontal neck wrinkles present in all infants. Later, a super adhesive, a subcutaneous suture, or an inversion (worm) suture can be employed to close the incision. If, because of damage, it is not possible to drain from the right jugular vein, raise and attempt to take drainage from the left internal jugular vein. If this is not successful, use a small trocar to drain directly from the right atrium of the heart. Insert the trocar at the standard entry point over the abdomen and direct the point toward the lobe of the right ear.

Femoral (External Iliac) Artery. The second largest nonaortic vessel that can be used is either the external iliac artery or the femoral artery. The external iliac is slightly larger than the femoral. The same incisions can be used to raise these vessels as are used to raise the vessels of an adult. The accompanying veins are relatively large and may be used as points of drainage. If a small drain tube is not available, these veins can be expanded by inserting a small pair of forceps into the vessels. **Always inject the distal leg first.** This gives the embalmer a chance to observe the effects of the fluid solution on the skin of the leg and to determine if too much or too little fluid dye has been used. If drainage is difficult to establish from the femoral location, the right internal jugular vein can be raised and used as a drainage point.

Use of the axillary vessels is *not* advised in preparation of the unautopsied infant. The vessel is too small for efficient use, and establishing drainage may be very difficult. In the autopsied infant, however, it may be necessary to inject this vessel. If possible, the embalmer should try to use the larger subclavian artery for arterial injection of the arm.

Abdominal Aorta. The abdominal aorta is a large artery and is accompanied by the largest vein that could be used for drainage. The artery and vein are deep-seated, resting on the anterior surface of the spine. A 2- to 3-inch incision can be made just to the left of the midline in the middle of the abdomen. The incision is made to the left of the midline and inferior enough to avoid the liver, which is very large in the infant. The greater omentum must be opened and some of the small and large intestines either held away from the spine or removed from the cavity during arterial injection. The aorta is held in position by its parietal branches (the four pairs of lumbar arteries in particular). Once located, the aorta can be opened and a tube placed in the direction of the legs and another tube in the direction of the upper portions of the body. The vein can be opened and the blood allowed to drain into the cavity. It is not necessary to place a drainage instrument into the vein. The lower portion of the body should be injected first, then the upper portion. During injection the viscera can greatly expand. The viscera can be clipped and drained prior to return to the cavity (Fig. 16–1).

Ascending Aorta. In a variant technique involving the aorta as a primary injection point, the ascending aorta is used. Several incisions are used to reach the ascending aorta as it leaves the heart. In one incision for drainage, the right auricle of the heart (the small earlike appendage of the right atrium of the heart) is clipped open. An incision can be made directly down the midline of the sternum. As this bone is not ossified but is actually cartilage, a sharp scalpel or strong surgical shears can be used to make this incision. The difficulty is that the incision must be held open with some form of retraction. A 2-inch block can be placed in the spread incision to hold it open and to allow the embalmer to work. A second incision, a U-shaped one, is made straight down from the midclavicle to the bottom of the rib cage, where it makes a right angle across the inferior margin of the sternum to a point identical to the original midclavicle incision. From this point, the cut is directed upward to the midclavicle position. The skin is then dissected upward, thus disclosing the sternum, which is then opened by severing the sternal cartilage at its junction with the ribs.

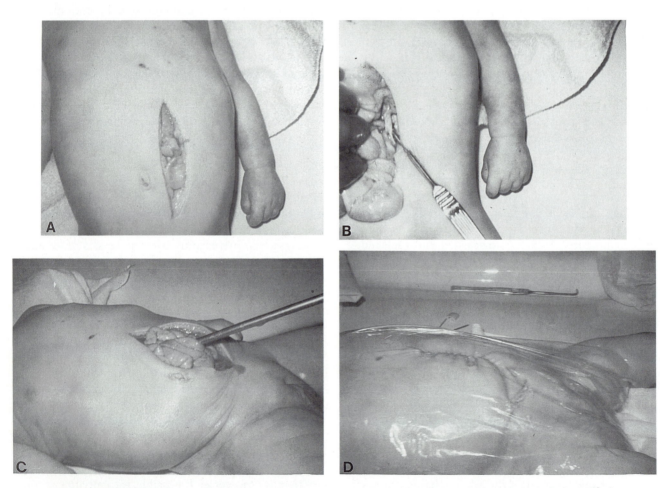

Figure 16–1. Preparation of an infant using the abdominal aorta. **A.** The incision is made to the left of the midline to raise the abdominal aorta. **B.** The abdominal aorta is exposed. Note that the small intestine has been carefully pulled out and set to the right. The small intestines are lifted out during the injection. These should not be severed. **C.** Viscera are treated after injection. **D.** Plastic is placed over the incision after preparation.

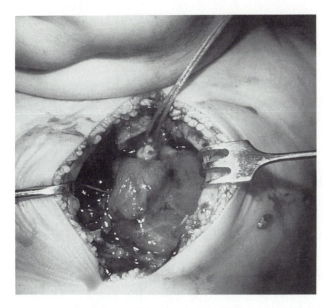

Figure 16–2. The pericardium is opened. Note the string around the ascending aorta. The right auricle is in the center; it will be incised and used for drainage.

When the sternum is severed free of its lateral attachments it can be bent upward toward the head. With this incision, the internal thoracic arteries may need to be clamped during arterial injection. Once the incision has been made and the pericardium exposed, the embalmer must cut open the pericardium and expose the heart and the great vessels (Fig. 16–2). The ascending aorta is observed as it rises from the left ventricle of the heart. It can be opened, or an opening can be made in the arch of the aorta and an arterial tube inserted. The entire body can be embalmed from this one point.

With respect to use of the abdominal aorta or the ascending aorta (or the heart) method of embalming, it is necessary to point out the possibility of legal ramifications. In many areas of the United States, all hospital deaths require hospital personnel to solicit autopsies. Obviously, in the cases just described, an autopsy has not been performed, the legal next of kin having denied consent for the autopsy. The family may suspect that an autopsy was performed without their consent and thus want to examine the body of the embalmed infant at their first opportunity. The incisions for raising the abdominal aorta or the arch of the aorta closely resemble autopsy incisions. Laypersons can arrive at a false conclusion in these circumstances and blame both the funeral home and the hospital using the mistakenly identified incisions as evidence of a surreptitious autopsy.

Infant Cavity Treatment

For aspirating and injecting the unautopsied infant, use an infant trocar. These trocars are generally about 12 inches in length with an inside diameter of at least $\frac{1}{4}$ inch.

The standard trocar point of entry or a lower point, such as the right or left inguinal abdominal area, may be used.

Cavity embalming may either immediately follow arterial injection or be delayed several hours. Injection of an undiluted cavity chemical follows aspiration. The amount of cavity chemical depends on the size of the infant. The trocar point of entry can be closed by suture or the trocar button. Reaspiration several hours later is recommended.

Preparation of the Autopsied Infant

The embalmer should try to prepare autopsied infants by arterial injection, which produces very satisfactory results. Although this process may be very time consuming, every attempt should be made to effect complete arterial distribution of embalming fluid. Those areas not reached by arterial injection or that cannot be embalmed by arterial injection can be treated in several ways. Regardless of the techniques employed, preservation is accomplished by hypodermic or surface embalming.

The proportion of infants autopsied in some large hospitals in major cities approaches 70% or more. In these communities, autopsies of infants by coroners or medical examiners may approach 100%. (It should be noted that in some areas of the country, the hospital or coroner may permit arterial embalming of the body prior to autopsy. The same is true of autopsies on adult bodies; however, the majority of hospital and medical examiner autopsies are performed prior to arterial embalming.)

Four types of autopsies are performed on infants:

- *Complete autopsy:* Cranial and trunk cavities are opened and enclosed viscera removed.
- *Partial autopsy:* Only one cavity is opened (cranial, thoracic, abdominal, or spine)
- *Special or local autopsy:* Only one organ is removed or a special examination is made of the route of blood vessels or nerves.
- *Organ donor autopsy:* Eyes may be removed, for the eye is quite large in the infant and the cornea of great value. The heart, heart/lungs, liver, kidneys, or skin may be removed as in the adult, and these donations can be treated as partial autopsies.

When viscera are removed in the autopsy, they may or may not be returned with the body. Generally, any viscera removed by a coroner or medical examiner are returned with the body. With hospital autopsies, the viscera are not always returned.*

---

*Refer to Chapter 17 for treatment of viscera.

Blood Vessel Selection: Autopsied Infants

Neither the common carotid, common iliac, or external iliac arteries and their accompanying veins, the iliac and internal jugular, of the adult and infant vary greatly except in *size*. If the autopsy pathologist has left vessels of reasonable length, the difficulty encountered is no greater than when working with an adult. If the vessels are severed excesssively short (iliacs at the inguinal ligament, carotids at thyroid cartilage), considerable extensive dissection will be required to locate the vessels and to ligate arterial tubes within them. In lieu of string for ligation, an arterial tube hemostat may be helpful. Do not attempt to locate veins. Drainage can be taken without the use of any instruments. Remember that arteries remain open when cut. This can often help in locating the tiny arteries. It is also most important that the embalmer be certain of the anatomical locations and relationships of the vessels.

If the iliac arteries cannot be located or if they are too small for the arterial tubes, supplemental methods of embalming can be used to preserve the legs. Hypodermic treatment with long large-gauge needles can be employed. Painting the surface of the legs with an autopsy gel and wrapping the painted limbs in plastic could serve to embalm the limbs. When the carotid arteries are missing the embalmer can place cotton saturated with cavity fluid in the mouth and under the eyelids. With a diluted cavity fluid, deep hypodermic treatment can be made from inside the mouth, from the scalp incisions of the autopsy, and from the opened neck areas of the autopsy. If arterial fluid is going to be injected hypodermically, one with little dye should be used. The dye can create blotches of color as the fluid spreads through the facial tissues. Likewise, the face can be painted with autopsy gel and covered with plastic for several hours. This treatment often bleaches the skin, and corrective cosmetics will be needed. The inside of the scalp and the base of the cranial cavity can also be painted with autopsy gel.

Subclavian arteries can be located at the usual adult site. If they have been cut short, the axillary artery can be raised at its largest point, as the artery passes into the axilla just at the lateral border of the first rib. To reach the axillary at this point it may be necessary to dissect the pectoralis major and minor muscles. Some embalmers prefer to raise the subclavian artery by elevating the clavicle bones. This exposes the subclavian arteries where they have been severed. An arterial hemostat may again be more useful than string ties in securing the arterial tube.

Instruments and Chemicals

Very small arterial tubes are a necessity. These can be made by filing off the tip of a hypodermic needle.

There are many suggested chemical combinations, strengths, and dilutions for infant arterial embalming. A false theory is that infants must always be embalmed with very dilute low-index arterial fluids. Infant body tissue contains a higher percentage of water than adult body tissue. In addition, disease processes and drugs may have increased tissue moisture and toxic wastes. Therefore, use of a chemical solution containing normal adult dilutions is advised. Humectant and coinjection chemicals can be added to these solutions to reduce any harsh fluid reaction. Generally, arterial fluid not containing humectants and coinjection chemicals has been found most satisfactory. A small amount of fluid dye to add color to the tissues is recommended.

In the autopsied body, the legs are embalmed before the head or arms. This allows the embalmer to adjust the fluid strengths and dyes.

The volume to be injected is best determined by guidelines similar to those for the adult. Intravascular blood discolorations should be cleared and the fluid dyes must appear uniform throughout the tissues. Generally, the tissues may plump slightly. Massage may be necessary to assist distribution of the fluid. Pinching the fingertips and lips helps to clear these areas of blood discolorations. If the eyelids wrinkle after discolorations have cleared, it is recommended that injection be stopped. If any swelling occurs, the arterial solution can be strengthened and only a minimum amount injected. In addition, all injection can be stopped and the untreated areas preserved by hypodermic and surface embalming. Keep in mind that *weak* solutions can easily distend tissues, another reason to use arterial solution at a strength close to that used in the adult.

Treatment of Areas Not Reached by Arterial Injection

Hypodermic Injection. The head may be injected hypodermically from within an incised neck area or natural openings (mouth and nostrils) or an incised scalp area; arms and legs may be injected from within the open trunk cavity.

In larger children this may entail injection of the arm from the point of insertion of the hypodermic needle or trocar from the antecubital fossa upward toward the shoulder, and then, utilizing the same point of insertion, down toward the fingers. The puncture incision is closed with a trocar button and later covered by glue, cotton, plastic sheeting, and adhesive tape.

The legs may similarly be injected by inserting the hypodermic needle or trocar from a point within the abdominal cavity or on the inner aspect of the knee area. The instrument may be directed upward first and then, when injection is completed, downward using the same point of insertion. The point of insertion may be closed in the same manner as previously described. Diluted cavity fluid can be used for injection. Cosmetic arterial fluid should not be used.

Internal Compresses. Internal compresses, sometimes referred to as inlays, are cotton or sheeting (well dampened with cavity fluid) inserted into such areas as the interior of the neck, the cranium, and the trunk cavity, when devoid of viscera. Internal packs can also be inserted under the pectoral chest flaps (over the sternum) before trunk incision closure. Autopsy gel can be used in lieu of cavity fluid.

Preservative Gels. Preservative gels are semisolid chemicals that are inserted over the calvarium as well as under the anterior chest and abdominal skin flaps before skin suturing.

External Compresses. Cotton saturated with undiluted cavity fluid or other special chemical preparations may be needed to preserve areas as small as the ears or, in other cases, the entire body. An attempt should be made to secure a smooth cotton surface, for irregular application to the skin surface impresses the unevenness onto the skin. Compresses should be left in place long enough to accomplish complete preservation.

Treatment of the Trunk Walls of the Autopsied Infant

The back, shoulders, trunk walls, and buttocks, and the scrotum and penis of the male, may require additional chemical treatments for preservation. An infant trocar, a large-diameter hypodermic needle, or a straight long arterial tube can be used to inject these areas with a strong chemical solution. This solution is injected either through the embalming machine or with a large hypodermic syringe. In addition, the inside walls may be treated with autopsy gel or embalming powder. If the viscera are not returned, cavities can be filled with sheeting saturated with cavity fluid.

Autopsy Viscera Treatments

The viscera of the autopsied body may be immersed in undiluted cavity fluid. Some prefer to place the viscera and cavity fluid together within a plastic bag and then, later, place the plastic-encased viscera in the abdominal and thoracic cavities. The organs should be clipped and freed of gases after the addition of cavity fluid. It is also recommended that the cavity fluid not be added until the bag of viscera has been positioned within the body cavity. Some embalmers also prefer to make a cut in the thick

solid organs (e.g., lungs and liver) to ensure contact with the cavity fluid.

Closure of Cavities in Autopsied Infants

In small infants the scalp has been opened by the usual transverse incision from ear to ear. Access to the floor of the cranial cavity would have been necessary to control leakage from the internal carotids and, possibly, the vertebral or basilar arteries during arterial injection. The scalp should be reflected and the floor of the cavity dried. The walls of the cranial vault can be liberally coated with autopsy gel, and the inside surface of the reflected scalp can likewise be coated with a preservative gel. To repair the area, a quantity of cotton may be used to fill the cranial cavity and to reproduce the normal contours as well as act as an absorbent for seepage. The scalp is drawn back to its normal position, and then carefully sutured.

When the fontanelles are still present, it may be helpful to fill the cranial cavity with cotton. With dental floss and a $\frac{3}{8}$-inch circle needle, the soft cranial bones are sutured together. The fontanelle areas can be filled with "mortuary putty." If this is not available, the cranial cavity must be tightly filled with cotton. If the cavity is not tightly filled, sunken areas may be noticed at the locations of the fontanelles. Many embalmers do not want the scalp to rest on the cotton at the fontanelles, so they coat the cotton with massage cream. This prevents dehydration of the scalp around the fontanelles.

For the scalp, suturing begins on the right side of the cranium and ends on the left side. The inversion (worm) suture is excellent for infants. It helps to tighten the scalp. When the autopsy incision has been made high on the head and the hair is very thin, it is recommended that the funeral director request that a bonnet be used. It is not necessary to discuss the reason unless questioned by the family. Most hospitals make these incisions low enough that the sutured incisions can be hidden by the pillow. Super adhesive can provide a closure that is not easily detected. If the embalmer prefers, a small baseball or interdermal suture using dental floss may be used for closure instead of the worm suture.

In infants in whom the bones of the cranium are well calcified and the calvaruim has been removed as in an adult case, the same procedure used for such repair in the adult is recommended.

If the temporalis muscles have been cut from the cranium or calvarium, the area can easily be filled in with "mortuary putty" to prevent a sunken appearance. Tissue building of the temple is not possible if the muscular tissue has been removed. When the calvarium has not been "notched" it may be very difficult to maintain the calvarium in correct position during and after suturing. Calvarium clamps might possibly be used to hold the calvarium in place. As the bones are not completely ossified, small holes can easily be made on either side of the calvarium and the calvarium wired into proper position.

The abdominal, thoracic, and pelvic cavities should be coated with autopsy gel or a preservative-drying powder, following aspiration and drying of the cavities. If neck organs have been removed the neck area should be filled with cotton and saturated with a preservative such as cavity fluid. The trunk cavities should be filled with an absorbent material and also saturated with a preservative chemical. The breast plate should be laid into proper position (and if necessary anchored with sutures); paper toweling can be laid over the plate and saturated with preservative chemical. The skin flaps are tacked together to ensure proper alignment. Suturing is begun at the pubic symphysis and directed upward; a small baseball suture provides a good closure. The body is bathed and the skin surfaces thoroughly dried. The sutures may be coated with a surface sealer glue. The trunk area can be covered with a thin sheet of plastic to ensure protection of the clothing.

To reemphasize, although many premature infants are autopsied and may be extremely small (less than 1 pound), there may exist a need to preserve them temporarily for funeral, burial, or cremation services.

Optional Treatments. If the premature infant has not been autopsied, arterial injection may be attempted. Some success is achieved by injection of the internal carotid artery followed by cavity aspiration and injection of a small amount of cavity fluid. Injection of the arterial umbilical vessel has occasionally been advocated, but difficulty in identifying the artery from the other two veins as well as the poor results obtained when the proper vessel is injected make this procedure unattractive. Other large vessels that could be injection sites are the abdominal aorta, the ascending aorta, and the arch of the aorta.

External compresses constitute the easiest treatment. The premature infant is wrapped in cotton saturated with cavity fluid or painted with autopsy gel.

The limbs, trunk cavity and walls, and head are injected hypodermically with a strong concentration of preservative chemicals. Cavity treatment and external compresses are additionally applied as necessary.

General Treatments. In other treatments for autopsied infants, the entire body and hair should be rewashed, the nails cleaned and trimmed, and all incisions sealed. Cosmetics should be applied in accordance with the requirements of the individual case. Trunk autopsy incisions as well as other incised or lacerated areas should be covered with plastic. Also recommended are long-sleeved dresses, shirts, and jackets, long trousers (boys), and tights (girls). This, obviously, minimizes the skin area to be cosmetized.

EMBALMING THE 4- TO 12-YEAR OLD

The second age group relative to embalming ranges from approximately 4 years to approximately 12 years. Although the special techniques used for the infant or the aged are not required, some difficulties are encountered because of the body size.

Vessel Selection

The vessels in this age group are much larger than those of the infant, but still smaller than those of the adult. The two major injection sites used in embalming the adult are also used for preparation of the child: (1) the common carotid artery and the internal jugular vein and (2) the femoral artery and femoral vein. There is no need to consider use of the abdominal aorta or the arch of the aorta in this age group. Likewise, the many disadvantages of the axillary artery and vein do not make this a good primary injection site. Many members of this age group are autopsied, so most of the embalming is done from the primary autopsy sites—right and left common carotid, right and left external and internal iliac, and right and left subclavian arteries.

In the unautopsied body, the right internal jugular vein is the largest vein that can be used for drainage. It also affords direct access to the right atrium of the heart. Whenever facial blood discolorations are present, this vein affords the best possible clearing of the facial tissues.

Some embalmers prefer the femoral vessels for this age group strictly because their location permits the use of clothing that can be opened at the neck. The possibility of leakage or visibility of the carotid incision should be of little concern if properly prepared, sutured, and sealed.

Remember that in this age group (4–12 years), if there has been any trauma to the face or head or if there has been a long delay between death and preparation, the facial tissues may swell during injection. The best control over fluid flow into the head and face is obtained by use of restricted cervical injection.

The arteries of children in this age group should all be in excellent condition with no evidence of arteriosclerosis.

Fluid Strengths and Volume

Fluid strength is determined by the condition of the body. As 4- to 12-year-olds have more delicate skin than adults, for routine embalming, a medium-index fluid in the range 18 to 25 is most satisfactory. Dilutions should follow those recommended by the manufacturer. If instructions are not given, a fluid strength of 1 to 2% should produce satisfactory results. To these solutions, a coinjection chemical or a few ounces of humectant can be added. Dye can always be used for its cosmetic effect and to indicate the distribution of arterial solution. In these bodies, however, dyes should be kept to a minimum for, no doubt, cosmetic application will be minimized to produce the most natural appearance.

In cases of trauma and the effects of diseases, such as edema and renal failure, appropriate fluid strengths should be used and, if necessary, special-purpose high-index fluids.

Four- to twelve-year-olds require a smaller volume of fluid than adults, but a greater volume than used for infants. Intravascular blood discolorations should have cleared, some firming of the tissues should be present, and there should be evidence of good distribution as indicated by the presence of dye. All of these indicators help to establish the volume of fluid to be injected.

In this age group, the causes of death include infectious and contagious diseases (e.g., meningitis and pneumonia), childhood viral diseases, and systemic diseases (e.g., leukemia and cystic fibrosis). When contagious or infectious disease is the cause of death, the arterial solution strength should be at least 2%. At this strength the tissues should be sufficiently sanitized. If the embalmer feels this strength may cause difficulties in establishing distribution or may dehydrate the skin, a 1.5% solution can be injected, but a greater volume should be used. With the coinjection and reaction-controlled chemicals available today, the embalmer should be able to work with 2% or higher solutions for the injection of children.

Pressure and Rate of Flow of Injection

The rate of flow is of greater concern than pressure to the embalmer, especially in embalming a child. If arterial solution is moved too quickly into the body, the tissues may distend. In addition, rapid injection often forces a large amount of fluid through the paths of least resistance, resulting in great loss of arterial solution to the drainage.

The embalmer must remember that sufficient force is necessary to establish good distribution, especially in distal body areas such as the hands and feet. By the use of intermittent drainage, short-circuiting of solution is reduced and retention of solution increased. Rapid injection with continuous drainage also has the tendency to remove moisture from a child's tissues. This could lead to wrinkling of the skin.

For injection of the child, a pressure setting of 5 to 10 pounds with the rate-of-flow valve closed should be sufficient. At the start of injection, the rate-of-flow valve

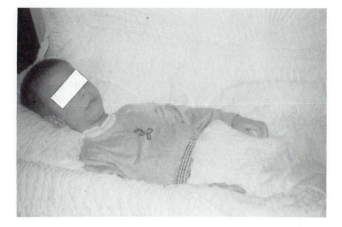

Figure 16–3. Positioning of the child. Note that the arms are placed at the sides.

can be opened almost to maximum for a moment. This tells the embalmer the maximum rate of flow possible.

If it is assumed that the starting pressure with the rate-of-flow valve closed is 10, opening the rate of flow valve to maximum shows an actual pressure reading of 5 (the differential which indicates a rate of flow of 5). To establish a uniform rate of flow for injection, divide the differential reading of 5 in half, thus reducing the rate of flow by half. If the pressure is set at 10 with the rate-of-flow valve closed, by opening the rate of flow and allowing the needle reading to drop to 8 or 7, a rate flow is established that should be sufficient to overcome the resistances of the body and to produce uniform and complete distribution.* Should the signs of distribution indicate that fluid is not being distributed to all areas, the rate of flow can be increased or the pressure elevated. If the pressure is elevated, the embalmer may wish to use pulsation during the injection.

Setting of Features and Positioning

Positioning of the child is similar to that of the adult. The arms can be a little more "relaxed" than those of the adult and, generally, are placed straighter (Fig. 16–3). The head should be slightly tilted to the right.

Facial hair must be removed for good cosmetic treatment. Some drugs stimulate growth of facial hair, and this hair can easily be removed with shaving lather and a sharp razor. It is best not to attempt to shave the forehead.

Mouth closure may pose some difficulty if the child has buck teeth or is wearing braces. For buck teeth, place a small layer of cotton over the *lower* teeth and gum. This

---

*These pressure settings or differential numbers *do not* indicate the ounces per minute (rate of flow) of fluid entering the body. Measuring devices may be added to machines. Differential only indicates that there *is* a rate of flow.

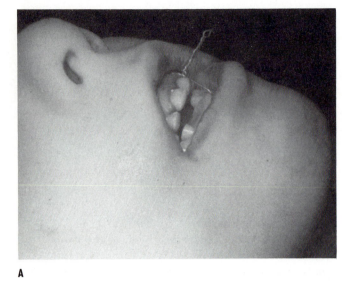

A

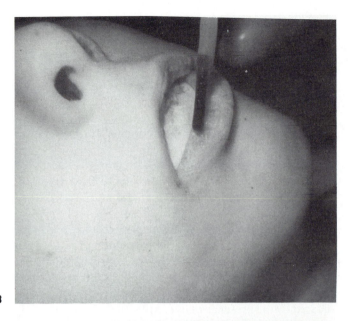

B

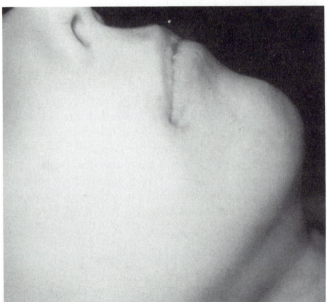

C

Figure 16–4. **A.** Note the large separation of the lips with this child. **B.** The lips are glued prior to arterial injection with a rubber-base glue. **C.** A glued closure is made prior to arterial injection.

helps to push the lower lip forward. The lips can now be glued together with a rubber-based glue prior to arterial injection (Fig. 16–4). Some embalmers prefer to inject the body with the lips slightly parted. This allows the tissues of the lips to "round out." The super adhesives can assist, after injection, with difficult closures.

EMBALMING THE ADOLESCENT AND ADULT

For embalming purposes, the adolescent/adult group comprises persons from 13 to approximately 75 years of age. As in all age categories, individual variations and exceptions exist. Because this age group is characterized by average body conditions for which average embalming treatments are practiced, embalming of the "routine" or "normal" body is outlined. For the beginning practi-

tioner, this overview is suggested in an outline of the step-by-step preparation of the unautopsied or autopsied body (see Chapter 1).

Causes of death in this group include heart disease, malignancies, and accidents. It is important that the embalmer remember that age is only one factor in the embalming analysis. Other factors are time between death and preparation, progress of decomposition, moisture content, discolorations, condition of the blood vascular system, protein and nutritional condition, traumatic or surgical considerations, time between preparation and disposition, weight, autopsy and organ donation considerations, and pathological changes.

Chapter 1 provides a recommended sequence for complete embalming of the body. Here, certain points of the chronology are discussed in greater detail.

Vessel Selection

In the embalming of the "normal" adult body, the order of injection sites would be to first employ *restricted cervical* injection, using both right and left common carotid arteries and the right internal jugular vein for drainage; second would be the use of the right common carotid artery and right internal jugular vein; third would be the use of the right femoral artery and vein. This order is based on the fact that should there be any arterial coagula in the aorta, it would be best that this material be pushed toward the legs rather than toward the head. The internal jugular vein is the largest vein that can be used for drainage, and any coagula present in the right atrium of the heart can easily be removed with angular spring forceps. Rarely does the common carotid artery show arteriosclerosis, whereas the femoral is the first vessel used for embalming to exhibit this condition. Use of both common carotids gives the embalmer control of the strength and volume of arterial solutions entering the head and trunk areas of the body.

Preinjection and Coinjection

Preinjection and coinjection may be used with the adult/adolescent age group. Preinjection is not recommended when there has been a long delay between death and preparation or when poor circulation or tissue distension is anticipated.

Coinjection fluids can be used to help coordinate almost all arterial solutions. Preinjection fluid should be used when the embalmer feels that the body should drain well and exhibit good circulation. Preinjection solutions help to ensure that the circulatory system remains in good working order. Preinjection can also be used to help clear some intravascular discolorations and mild jaundice.

Fluid Strength and Volume

Bodies aged 12 to 75+ should react very well to the firming effect of the arterial solution, especially after a sudden death, such as a heart attack, or when the body is prepared a short time after death while it still retains body heat. It is important that the embalmer inject sufficient arterial solution into these bodies. Fluid always follows the path of least resistance, which is usually through the superficial tissues. Thus, blood discolorations will clear and the skin will feel well embalmed.

It is also most important that the deep tissues and muscles receive a sufficient amount of solution. Use of large volumes of arterial solution and manipulation in the form of massage help to encourage the distribution of the arterial solution to all tissues of the body including the deep skeletal tissues. The superficial tissues of the body have a much greater blood supply, to assist in temperature and waste control in the living body. For this reason and because rigor mortis offers little resistance in these superficial areas, the fluid has a tendency to distribute well to the superficial tissues. Intermittent drainage helps fluid to penetrate the deeper tissues.

To ensure complete sanitation of the body, 2 to 3% arterial solution is ideal. In bodies dead from a contagious disease, 2.3 to 3.0% solutions are preferred. Solution strength and its effect on the sanitation of tissues are discussed in Chapter 3. In preparation of the "average" body, however, the microbial population is generally an unknown factor. To ensure that the tissues are properly sanitized, use at least a 2% solution.

Follow the dilution instructions of the manufacturer. These instructions should be contained on the labels of the fluid bottles. Many embalmers *BEGIN* injection with a milder solution (1–1.5%) and then, after the blood discolorations are cleared and drainage established, gradually increase the strength of subsequent gallons. Equal amounts of coinjection fluid may be used with all solutions. If a humectant is warranted for emaciated dehydrated bodies or to prevent dehydration, follow the dilutions recommended by the manufacturer.

Two examples follow. In the first are the volumes of the different components when a 25-index arterial fluid is used:

Solution	Arterial Fluid	Coinjection Fluid
First gallon	6–8 ounces	6–8 ounces
Second gallon	8 ounces	8 ounces
Third gallon	10 ounces	10 ounces

The second example gives the volumes when a 25-index arterial fluid and a high-index (30+) arterial fluid are used:

Solutions	Arterial Fluid	Coinjection Fluid	High-Index Fluid
First gallon	6–8 ounces	6–8 ounces	0
Second gallon	6–8 ounces	6–8 ounces	4 ounces
Third gallon	6–8 ounces	6–8 ounces	4–6 ounces

In this second example, the strength of the arterial solution is increased by use of a high-index arterial fluid to boost the preservative content of the solution.

Pressure and Rate of Flow of Injection

With most embalming machines the pressure and the rate of flow are related. The important factor is the rate of flow—how fast or in what volume the fluid enters the body.

In Chapters 2 and 3 the ideal speed of 10 to 15 minutes per gallon was recommended for the first gallon of solution. Discussion of the ideal rate of flow indicated that sufficient pressure and rate of flow should be used

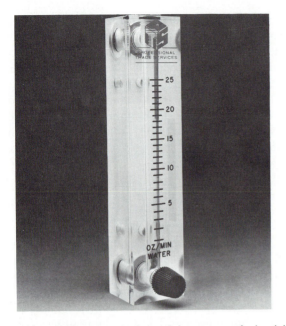

Figure 16–5. Rate-of-flow meter can be installed on any centrifugal embalming machine.

to overcome the resistances of the body and to distribute the arterial solution without causing tissue distension. The greater the resistance in a body, the greater the pressure required. A pressure setting of 5 to 20 pounds, using the centrifugal machine, should be sufficient to overcome most body resistances. This range is very wide; many embalmers prefer a low pressure, whereas others prefer a higher setting. The rate of flow can be varied with either setting (Fig. 16–5).

The first injection, while the body arteries are filling, should be slow, to prevent any arterial coagula from loosening and moving. The arterial solution can then "ride over top" of the coagula. After the first gallon, the speed of injection is increased. Many embalmers inject a gallon of solution at a rate of 10 to 15 minutes per gallon. Healthy body tissues can accept fluid at this rate of speed without distension.

The skin of adolescents is much firmer and dryer than that of adults, indicating a good protein level. Adolescent tissues are able to assimilate injected arterial solution much better than those of the elderly, in whom skin support is often weak and swelling occurs easily. For this reason, a wide range of pressures and rates of flow are used to embalm bodies in this category.

First injections should be slower, to fill the vascular system. Subsequent solutions can be injected at a faster rate of flow.

Some embalmers prefer to inject at a rapid rate of flow from the very beginning (5–10 minutes per gallon). The theory is that this places greater pressure on the arterial side of the capillaries and increases filtration of the embalming solution through the capillaries. With this method, continuous drainage is used throughout the

preparation. The body must be observed carefully to detect any facial or neck distension. This method can also loosen coagula in the arteries. Multipoint injection and hypodermic embalming may then be required to overcome the problems thus produced.

EMBALMING THE ELDERLY PERSON

Modern medicine has provided health care and control of disease with the result that the average life expectancy has increased to 72.6 years for men and 77.6 years for women. The number of persons living into their eighties and nineties is expected to double within several years. Embalmers are, as a consequence, required to prepare greater numbers of those dying in these upper age groups. Of course, certain afflictions and pathological conditions are more frequently encountered in the elderly than among the other previously described three age groups. It is useful to identify some of the more common conditions associated with advanced age and to give some general comments on them. As in all age groups, drug therapy can greatly alter the classic conditions of certain diseases, so the medications in and of themselves will play an important role in determining what postmortem conditions exist in the body.

Arthritic Conditions

Many elderly are afflicted with arthritis. This condition, which may be long-standing, may be accompanied by atrophy of many muscles. These conditions are manifest many times in a patient restricted to bedrest. Legs are drawn up and curvature of the spine is evident. Frequently the arms are drawn up onto the chest and the fingers clenched (Fig. 16–6).

These conditions create a number of positioning problems for the embalmer. Placing head blocks under the thighs helps to position the body on the embalming table. It may also be necessary to tie the body in position.

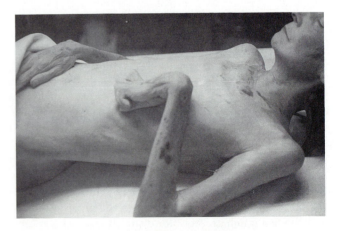

Figure 16–6. Arthritic arm and hand.

Generally, blocks under the thighs and head blocks under a shoulder provide adequate support. Turkish towels placed under the shoulders also help to achieve temporary position. After casketing, the bedding of the casket along with pillow supports places the body into a comfortable-looking position. The neck may be difficult to position. Application of firm pressure to arthritic limbs and arms may change their position. It is possible to tear tendons and atrophied muscles. It must be remembered that the person has had this arthritic condition for many months or years, so leaving the arms and legs in these positions may be acceptable to the family. It is not recommended that tendons or skin be cut to achieve good positioning. It is almost impossible to open and expand arthritic fingers. These can be left in their clenched position and partially hidden by the blanket in the casket. When the legs are drawn to one side or into the fetal position, use of the femoral vessels is limited.

The common carotid would be the best site for a primary injection. If it becomes necessary to inject the legs, an attempt can be made to raise the femoral or external iliac artery. The popliteal artery may also be a choice. If these vessels are found to be sclerotic, an attempt should be made to inject using a small arterial tube; if this is not possible the legs should then be hypodermically injected using a small trocar and a dilute solution of cavity fluid injected through the embalming machine. In addition, plastic stockings can be placed on the legs. Autopsy gel can be poured into the stockings so that the viscous preservative coats the legs.

Mouth Closure Problems

Frequently a loss of weight is manifested in the facial tissues of the elderly. After mouth closure, it is necessary to place either cotton or "mortuary putty" over the teeth or dentures. This helps to fill out the sunken cheek areas. These areas should not be overfilled, especially if it is known that the deceased did not wear dentures. In this age group there are natural depressions of the facial tissues. The biggest problem with mouth closure is atrophy of the maxillae and mandible. The mandible in particular has a tendency to atrophy, and for this reason, it is more difficult many times to use the needle injector method of mouth closure. It is necessary to suture using either a muscular or a mandibular suture. The mandibular suture holds the dentures forward and in a tight position in the mouth.

Arteriosclerosis

Although not a problem exclusively of the elderly, arteriosclerotic arteries are frequently encountered in this age group. (Persons who live into their late nineties frequently exhibit very little sclerosis. This is a factor in achieving their longevity.) The vessel that most frequently exhibits sclerosis and that would be used for embalming is the femoral artery. Many times in a very thin individual, the sclerotic condition of the femoral can be palpated. The common carotid artery is thus the best choice in embalming the elderly. Rarely is the carotid found to be sclerotic, and if there is sclerosis, it is generally not sufficient to occlude the carotid (refer to Chapter 22). Restricted cervical injection, which uses both common carotid arteries, would be the first choice.

In addition to bringing about occlusion of the arteries, arteriosclerosis can also bring about poor peripheral circulation. As a result of poor circulation, bedfast individuals tend to form bedsores (decubitus ulcers). These sores develop where there is pressure contact with the bedclothing. Bacteria invade these areas. Of first concern to the embalmer is control of the odor from these ulcerations. It is important to properly disinfect these areas. Undiluted cavity fluid can be applied on cotton compresses to the ulcerated areas. If bandages cover these areas it may be useful to saturate the bandages with undiluted cavity fluid or a phenol cautery–disinfectant during the embalming procedure. It is also wise to hypodermically treat the areas around these ulcerations using a small trocar and undiluted cavity fluid. This prevents continued bacterial activity and decreases the possibilty of tissue gas (Fig. 16–7A).

At the time of dressing, fresh cotton saturated with undiluted cavity chemical, a phenol solution, or autopsy gel is applied to the ulcerations; then the area is wrapped or, if possible, plastic garments should be used to cover these areas. Embalming powder should be placed in the garments to control odors. Some of these ulcerations are quite small, as frequently seen on the shoulders. Others are very large, often involving the entire buttocks or hip area.

Arteriosclerosis can also result in loss of a limb. If the limb was amputated recently, the stump should be treated by hypodermic injection with undiluted cavity chemical (Fig 16–7B). If stitching is still present, a plastic stocking is placed over the stitches in case there is leakage. Many times the embalmer is faced with gangrene of the leg. It is very important that these limbs be hypodermically injected with undiluted cavity chemical. They can also be wrapped in cotton saturated with undiluted cavity chemical, phenol solution, or autopsy gel. A plastic garment containing embalming powder can be placed over the leg. It is important to thoroughly hypodermically inject the tissues immediately superior to the gangrene area.

Arteriosclerosis can also lead to a ruptured aneurysm. When an aneurysm ruptures in the aorta, death results within minutes. This rupture is a site for leakage of embalming fluid during arterial injection. Many times the embalmer is unaware that a ruptured aortic aneurysm is the cause of death. On injection there is little or no drainage. The abdomen distends during injection and there are no signs of arterial fluid distribution such as the presence of dye in the tissues. A six-point injection becomes necessary. The trunk walls will have to be hypodermically injected with a small trocar as in an autopsied body for preservation.

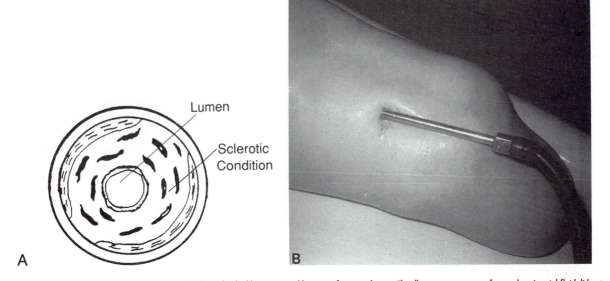

Figure 16–7. **A.** Diagram of medial sclerosis. **B.** The lower leg had been removed because of arteriosclerosis. This illustrates treatment of upper leg. Arterial fluid did not enter this area of the body.

Senile Purpura

Senile purpura (or ecchymosis) is an extravascular irregularly shaped blood discoloration that often appears on the arms and backs of the hands. The condition is brought about by fragility of the capillaries. In the elderly, drug usage, blood thinning, vitamin deficiencies, uremia, hypertension, thin skin, and slight bruising can easily bring about senile purpura. These discolorations vary greatly in size. The embalmer's concern in senile purpura lies in the fact that these discolorations do *not* clear during arterial injection. Often, these areas become engorged with fluid and swell during arterial injection. Purpural areas often darken after embalming and are prone to separate from underlying tissue, causing the tissues to tear open. Care should be taken in handling these areas. (Quite often the persons removing the body place a tight strap across the hands, and when the embalmer receives the body, skin areas on the backs of the hands are torn.)

If senile purpura is evidenced over the hands and arms (and often the base of the neck) the arterial solution should be strengthened. A fast rate of flow is *not* recommended. A slower rate of flow helps to limit further rupture of capillaries. It may be necessary to use multiple injection points. If the arms are separately injected, a special-purpose high-index fluid can be used in an attempt to dry these areas. Surface compresses of cavity fluid, phenol, or autopsy gel can be used. **If the skin over the purpural areas has been torn or broken open, all loose skin should be removed. This should be done at the beginning of embalming.** After surface compresses have had time to cauterize or bleach these discolored areas, the surface of the skin can be dried with a hair dryer and restora-

tive and cosmetic treatment performed. Unseen hemorrhaged areas can be packed with cotton saturated with a proper preservative solution (a phenol solution is preferred) and then covered with plastic. Leakage is always possible with this condition. Care should be taken to protect the clothing of the deceased.

Care should be taken when massage is used to assist in fluid distribution and senile purpura is present. This condition is often the result of the use of blood thinners. Rough handling of the tissues can bring about postmortem bruising. This bruising is frequently seen when the eyes of the elderly or of individuals on blood thinners have been enucleated.

Malignancy

Improved medical procedures have done much to lengthen the life expectancy. With the extension of life, there is also an increased probability of a malignant tumor. Cancers or neoplasms that begin as localized tumors can easily invade healthy tissues, spread via the blood vascular system, and invade organs. This can interrupt vital functions to the point where death ensues. The embalmer is concerned with the following systemic effects of a malignancy:

- Disseminated intravascular coagulation
- Disruption of metabolism by uncontrolled secretion of hormones (This can greatly affect weight control, cell membrane activity, and metabolism of sugars, fats, and proteins.)

■ Secretion of both peptide and steroid hormones by many tumors (Some of these hormones can bring about sustained hypercalcemia.)

■ Anemia

■ Cachexia (caused by the tumor's competition with the body for metabolites and resulting in a wasting away of tissues)

The local effects of a malignant tumor include invasion and destruction of normal tissues; obstruction of intestines, airways, urinary tract, and biliary tract; pathological fractures; perforation of the hollow viscera; erosion of blood vessel walls, creating acute and chronic hemorrhage; and establishment of portals of entry for infections.

Both local and systemic effects of a malignancy have an effect on the embalming. There can be a loss of weight and emaciation; often, the skin is loose and flabby and has no support. The skin can be dry because of the body's inability to take in proper amounts of water. Localized edema can result when local tumors exert pressure on veins and lymphatics. If the hormone balance has been interrupted and a condition such as sustained hypercalcemia exists, the calcium can easily create a barrier, making it very difficult for embalming solutions to enter the cell and preserve the protoplasm. Because the fluid cannot penetrate the cells, tissue firmness is difficult to establish. When there is loose, flabby tissue, what appears to be firming is only a plumping of the tissues with embalming solution (actually, distension of the tissues). After the solution gravitates away, the tissues become soft along with being underembalmed.

The malignancy in and of itself may not be the cause of death. Most often the actual cause of death is pneumonia leading to respiratory arrest. In embalming these bodies fluid solutions should be of moderate strength (at least 2% or above) and should be well coordinated. Use of a coinjection fluid is advised. The coinjection helps to increase the distribution and diffusion of the arterial solution. It is especially helpful in the passage of the arterial solution through the cell membranes.

Metabolic disturbances and renal and respiratory failure, which often accompany a malignancy, result in the buildup of metabolic wastes in the tissues. These wastes increase the demand for preservative. Use of a strong arterial solution helps to ensure satisfactory preservation. The rate of flow should be adequate to distribute the fluid throughout the entire body, but if the skin appears flabby and loose, a slower rate of injection may be helpful. Senile, flabby tissue does not assimilate fluid as well as healthy tissue and swelling can result.

If the facial tissues are emaciated, restricted cervical injection is recommended. This allows for separate embalming of the head, at which time a slightly milder solution can be used or a solution containing humectant can be used to moisturize and restore the facial tissues.

If local edema is present as in the arms or legs, it may be necessary to use multiple sites for injection. In the elderly, the femoral arteries are often sclerotic. If it is not possible to inject the femoral, the legs can receive supplemental preservation by hypodermic treatment with undiluted cavity chemical. In addition, autopsy gel can be painted on the legs and plastic stockings placed over the gel.

A colostomy may be present if there has been a malignancy in the intestinal tract. The collecting bag can remain in place during arterial injection and cavity treatment. After cavity treatment the bag should be removed and its contents disinfected with cavity fluid. Cotton saturated with cavity fluid or a phenol solution can be inserted into the colostomy opening in the abdominal wall. Closure of the opening is easily achieved with a purse-string suture.

Cardiac Disease

In some diseases of the heart the medical treatment may include surgical procedures. If the patient died shortly after surgery and if no autopsy was performed, the embalmer may be confronted with extensive incisions of one or both legs and of the anterior chest wall and possibly the abdominal wall. In addition, very pronounced amounts of edema may be present in the facial tissues, especially if death occurred within a day or so of the operation. Generally, the surgery involves bypass repair or valve repair.

The common carotid artery and the internal jugular vein would be the best primary points for injection and drainage on these cardiac patients. A moderate to strong arterial solution should be used. Addition of dye to the solution from the start helps to indicate the distribution of arterial fluid.

If local obstructions exist, sectional embalming is necessary. If there is extensive edema of the facial tissues, restricted cervical injection should be used and strong solutions for treatment of the edematous face employed. If the sutures are recent and leak during injection, the metal staples used to hold them closed should be removed with a hemostat. Dry the incisions and inject a phenol cautery agent by hypodermic needle within the open incisions. Tightly suture them closed with a baseball stitch using incision seal powder to prevent leakage. After washing and drying the body, paint the incisions with a surface glue.

Some surgical procedures, such as the installation of a pacemaker, require only a small incision. This device is generally placed in the upper lateral portion on the right side of the chest. The contacts for the pacemaker run from the device into the right internal jugular vein and then into the heart. Drainage may be difficult to secure from the internal jugular vein. The angular spring forceps is the easiest drainage device to use. A drainage tube may be very difficult to insert. The left internal jugular vein or the femoral vein may be a necessary second choice for a point of drainage. If the body is to be cremated, the pacemaker should be removed. Some hospitals also require removal and return of the pacemaker.

Diabetes Mellitus

Diabetes mellitus may be defined as both an acute and a chronic metabolic disorder characterized principally by hyperglycemia (an excess of sugar in the blood) resulting from a deficiency of insulin.

Medical authorities estimate that up to 5% of the population are afflicted with diabetes mellitus, and that over the age of 40, women outnumber men so afflicted by about 3 to 2. Individuals who are obese are more frequently diabetic than those who are not. The disease usually manifests itself during adult life at the age of 50 to 60. The exception is an acute juvenile type that has a far younger age of onset. Remember that even though the onset of the disease can be in middle age, its effects continue into old age and may contribute to a middle-age death. The affliction affords some merit to the congenital theory of the origin of the disease as researchers have observed that when both parents are diabetic, offspring have a 90% (estimated) chance of acquiring diabetes mellitus.

The principal manifestations of diabetes mellitus include *hyperglycemia,* excess sugar in the blood; *glycosuria,* sugar in the urine; and *ketosis,* acidosis characterized by the presence of ketones in the blood and body tissues.

Pathological changes resulting from the disease include poor peripheral circulation brought about by accelerated arteriosclerosis and degenerative changes in small blood vessels that result in poor circulation, particularly in the lower extremities. This often results in gangrene (Fig. 16–8). Kidney failure and enlargement of the liver (very often resulting in infestation of the liver because of the high sugar content of the tissues) and fungal infestations of the lung can also be prevalent. The skin often exhibits scratch marks and infections brought about by pruritus and itching. A strong odor of acetone may be noted, as it is present in the urine and the perspiration.

In embalming these bodies a strong arterial solution is needed. Peripheral circulation is often poor; therefore, dyes should be added so the embalmer can detect where fluid is present. Areas of the face such as the ears, tip of the nose, and cheeks often do not receive an adequate amount of fluid. Likewise, the hands and the legs should be carefully evaluated. The common carotid artery (restricted cervical) would be the best primary injection point. This artery is the least likely to exhibit arteriosclerosis.

The **restricted cervical injection** is recommended so that higher pressures and two arterial solutions can be employed. Restricted cervical injection also allows the embalmer to inject both sides of the head. This helps to ensure good circulation to all facial tissues. If the lower extremities or the stump of an amputated leg do not receive sufficient fluid by arterial injection then hypodermic and surface treatment may be needed. Plastic garments, containing surface preservatives or gels, may also be placed on the lower extremities.

If the hands or fingers do not receive sufficient fluid, a small-gauge hypodermic needle can be inserted between the fingers and arterial or cavity fluid injected to secure preservation. The hands can also be wrapped with cotton saturated with a surface preservative such as a cavity fluid compress or autopsy gel. Manufacturer's directions may inform how long compresses should be left in place. One must be certain that the preservative is applied to the palm side of the hand in addition to the back of the hand.

The following list summarizes the recommended treatment for diabetics:

1. Use the carotid vessels for primary injection.
2. Use strong arterial solutions.
3. Use fluid dyes for tracers.
4. Carefully disinfect the respiratory tract, as fungal infections may be present.
5. Institute hypodermic treatment and surface treatment for areas receiving insufficient arterial fluid.

Cavity embalming should immediately follow arterial injection. The embalmer should be certain that a liberal amount of cavity fluid is injected into the liver and lungs.

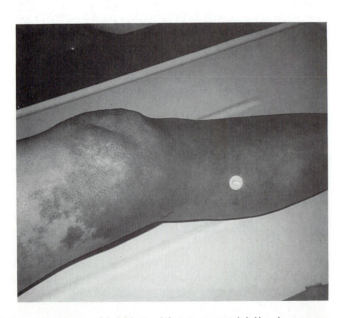

Figure 16–8. Gangrene of the left leg in a diabetic. Treatments included hypodermic injection of cavity fluid and application of surface preservative gel with a plastic stocking.

KEY TERMS AND CONCEPTS FOR STUDY AND DISCUSSION

1. Define the following terms.
   ideal fluid strength for embalming the "normal" adult body
   ideal pressure for embalming the "normal" adult body
   ideal rate of flow for embalming the "normal" adult body
   infant
   senile purpura
   stillborn
2. Describe in detail several arterial methods of injection for embalming an infant.
3. Explain why it may be necessary to use the same strength arterial solution for embalming an infant or child and an adult.
4. Discuss the following complications in embalming of the elderly:
   arteriosclerosis
   arthritis
   atrophy of the mandible and maxillae
   senile diabetes

BIBLIOGRAPHY

Bickley HC. *Practical Concepts in Human Disease.* Baltimore, MD: Williams & Wilkins; 1974:92–95.

Slocum RE. Type six classification. In: *Pre-embalming Considerations.* Boston: Dodge Chemical Co; 1969: 79.

Smith AL. *Microbiology and Pathology.* 12th ed. St. Louis, MO: CV Mosby; 1980:513–514.

Spriggs AO. Preparation of children's bodies. In: *The Art and Science of Embalming.* Springfield, OH: Champion Chemical Co.; 1963:Chap. 29, pp. 127–128.

The elderly cases. In: *Champion Expanding Encyclopedia.* Springfield, OH: Champion Chemical Co.; January–March 1971: Nos. 413–415.

17

Preparation of Autopsied Bodies

An autopsy (necropsy or postmortem) is a postmortem examination of the dead human body. There are two types of autopsy: the medical (hospital) autopsy and the medicolegal (forensic) autopsy. In some communities the pathologist prefers that the arterial embalming of the body be done prior to the autopsy. In contrast, most coroners and medical examiner offices **do not** want the body embalmed prior to the autopsy.

Before an autopsy can be performed proper permission *must be given* by the family member who has the right of disposition of the remains.

In certain autopsies, particularly hospital autopsies, the family not only must give permission for the autopsy; they also have the right to limit the extent of the autopsy. Where special instructions have been given, it is important that the pathologist follow the limitations established by the family. A family often gives permission only for what is called a partial autopsy, which consists of external examination and removal of one or two organs.

With respect to liability, the embalmer should also note in the funeral home records the type of autopsy performed. In addition, a memorandum should be made as to the disposition of the visceral organs: Were they returned with the body? *This is very important. In a number of instances a second autopsy has been ordered to support insurance claims or to confirm a cause of death. This is especially true in communities where black-lung and industrial deaths have insurance relationships.*

TYPES OF AUTOPSIES

Medical or Hospital Autopsy

Permission for the medical or hospital autopsy is obtained from a family member who has the proper authority to take charge of the body after death. Several reasons are given by the College of American Pathologists for the performance of the hospital autopsy*:

- When doctors have not made a firm diagnosis
- When death follows unexpected medical complications
- When death follows the use of an experimental drug or device, a new procedure, or unusual therapy
- When death follows a dental or surgical procedure done for diagnostic purposes and the case does not come under the jurisdiction of medical examiner or coroner
- When death occurs suddenly, unexpectedly, or in mysterious circumstances from apparently natural causes and the case does not come under the jurisdiction of medical examiner or coroner
- When environmental or workplace hazards are suspected

*Adapted from recommendations of the College of American Pathologists headed by Dr. Hans J. Peters, *N.Y. Times*, July 21, 1988.

303

- When death occurs during or after childbirth
- When there are concerns about a hereditary disease that might affect other members of the family
- When there are concerns about the possible spread of a contagious disease
- When the cause of death could affect insurance settlements (e.g., policies that cover cancer or that grant double indemnity for accidental death)
- When death occurs in a hospital and the patient comes from a nursing home and the quality of care is questioned

In addition to the preceding reasons, hospital autopsies are requested to confirm or to verify a diagnosis. Also, many of these institutions are teaching hospitals, and the autopsy serves as a tool in explaining a diagnostic technique or disease process.

Coroner or Medical Examiner Autopsy

In the coroner or medical examiner autopsy, the cause of death and the manner of death are the goals. The cases that come under the jurisdiction of a coroner or medical examiner vary from state to state and from county to county *within* a state. The following list represents typical cases that would be reported to a coroner or medical examiner. This will vary from state to state and even county to county.

- All sudden deaths not caused by readily recognizable disease or wherein the cause of death cannot be properly certified by a physician on the basis of prior (recent) medical attendance.
- All deaths occurring in suspicious circumstances, including those where alcohol, drugs, or other toxic substances may have had a direct bearing on the outcome
- All deaths occurring as a result of violence or trauma, whether apparently homicidal, suicidal, or accidental (including those caused by mechanical, thermal, chemical, electrical, or radiation injury, drowning, cave-ins, and subsidences), regardless of the time elapsed between injury and death
- Any fetal death, stillbirth, or death of a baby within 24 hours of birth, where the mother has not been under the care of a physician
- All therapeutic and criminal abortions, regardless of the length of pregnancy, and spontaneous abortions beyond 16 weeks gestation
- All operative and perioperative deaths in which the death is not readily explainable on the basis of prior disease
- Any death wherein the body is unidentified or unclaimed

- Any death where there is uncertainty as to whether or not it should be reported to the coroner's office

Death within 24 hours of admission to a hospital is not considered a reportable death unless it falls into one of the specific categories defined.

GUIDELINES TO DETERMINE WHEN AUTOPSIES ARE TO BE PERFORMED

The following list includes not only the cases that fall under the jurisdiction of a coroner or medical examiner, but **specific cases on which an autopsy must be performed.** (This list is only representative.) Autopsies must be performed on all of the following cases, which fall under the jurisdiction of the coroner; this varies from state to state and even county to county.

- Victims of homicide
- Victims of deaths in the workplace
- Motor vehicle drivers who have been involved in accidents
- Pedestrians who have been involved in accidents
- Passengers who have been involved in accidents but who lack clear evidence of trauma
- Victims of intra- and perioperative accidental deaths
- Epileptics
- Possible victims of sudden infant death syndrome
- Infants or children with evidence of bodily injury
- Inmate fatalities in correctional facilities, nursing homes, or medical institutions
- Victims of trauma
- Victims of nontraumatic, sudden, unexpected deaths
- Victims of anorexia nervosa
- Multiple victims of coincidental, unexplained death at one location
- Victims of possible poisoning or overdose deaths
- Any other case in which the pathologist holds a bona fide belief that the death is unexplained and/or an autopsy is in the best interest of the public or that it is necessary for the proper administration of the statutory duties of the office of the coroner.

GENERAL CONSIDERATIONS IN AUTOPSY TREATMENT

Order in Working

Do one item at a time in preparation of the autopsied body. In injection of the legs, that must be the only concern. Check for distribution, use intermittent drainage by clamping off the external iliac vein, massage the leg to assist distribution, and so on. Do not try to set features or raise other vessels while injecting the legs. Do one procedure at a time. In the long run this makes the work more thorough. Time is not saved by doing several things at the same time.

Fluid Strength

Preparation of the autopsied body is usually *delayed*. The delay may occur between death and autopsy or between autopsy and release of the body. Most institutions *refrigerate* bodies during these time delays. These factors combined with the pathological conditions of the body generally require that somewhat **stronger-than-average arterial solutions** be used. Delays increase the chances of **distension** during arterial injection and also increase the preservative demand of the tissues.

Use of Fluid Dyes

Delay also brings about rigor mortis and, if long enough, the passing of rigor. Rigor can cause poor arterial solution distribution and may also be a false sign of fluid firming. Fluid reactions with body proteins do not proceed normally when a body is in rigor mortis. Refrigeration can bring about hemolysis of blood trapped in the superficial tissues. This hemolysis can create an appearance similar to that of the dye present in arterial solutions. The tissue thus appears "embalmed." In addition, refrigerated tissues feel "embalmed" because the facts in the subcutaneous region have hardened. Use dye in the arterial solution, for it serves as the best sign of arterial solution distribution. Keep in mind that dyes show only *surface* distribution of arterial solutions. Massage deep tissues, such as the muscles of the legs (especially in rigor). Employ intermittent drainage to "force" fluids into the deep tissues.

Pressures and Rates of Flow

Rate of flow, rather than pressure, is generally the big cause of swelling during injection. Tissues can assimilate only a certain amount of fluid in a given period. Far too often, arterial solution is injected too fast into the body and swelling results. Or, the fluid is rushed through the capillaries and diffusion does not occur. In preparation of the autopsied body, inject each section separately. During injection into a specific body region such as an arm or leg (and not into the whole body as in a one-point injection in the unautopsied body), higher pressures and faster rates of flow can be safely used to help establish good circulation. The embalmer can vary the rate of flow for each area and, if necessary, vary the pressure to overcome the resistances of a particular body part. In addition, intermittent drainage can be used for each area to establish good distribution and diffusion.

Drainage

With the autopsied body it is **not** necessary to insert drainage devices (drain tubes or angular spring forceps) into the veins. Drainage can be taken directly from the cut vein and the drainage material can flow directly into the body cavities. Once in the cavities, an autopsy aspirator is used to keep accumulated drainage at a minimum. These instruments are useful because they are designed not to clog. These accumulated fluids can be aspirated into a sanitary sewer system. Intermittent or alternate drainage can also be used for each area injected in the autopsied body. Clamping the vein with a hemostat or applying digital pressure with a piece of cotton temporarily stops the drainage. Intermittent and alternate drainage greatly assists in fluid distribution, diffusion, and retention.

COMPLETE AUTOPSY/PARTIAL AUTOPSY

In this chapter, autopsies are divided into two categories (based on the extent of the autopsy): the *complete autopsy* and the *partial autopsy*. The hospital or forensic autopsy can be either type. The coroner or medical examiner autopsy is generally a complete autopsy. Complete examination of the body is necessary when the findings will be challenged in a court of law (Fig. 17–1).

The **complete autopsy** involves opening of the following body cavities and removal of the following organs:

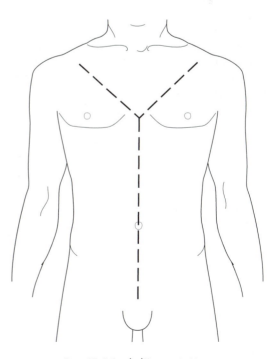

Figure 17–1. Standard Y autopsy incision.

1. Cranial cavity and its contents
   A. Possibly removal of the inner ear
   B. Brain
   C. Removal of the pituitary gland
2. Eye enucleation
3. Removal of the neck organs
   A. Thyroid gland
   B. Larynx
   C. Cervical portion of the esophagus and trachea
   D. Possibly removal of the common carotid arteries
   E. Possibly removal of the tongue (especially if a "cafe coronary" is suspected)
4. Thoracic cavity and its contents
5. Abdominal cavity and its contents
6. Pelvic cavity contents
7. Removal of spinal cord
   A. *Dorsal* approach: body is turned over and vertebral column opened (Fig. 17–2).
   B. *Ventral* approach: vertebral column is opened from within the body cavities and cervical area
   C. Removal from the foramen magnum
OR
8. Sample removal of the spinal cord, usually through the ventral approach (a "wedge" cut from the vertebral column)

In the **partial autopsy,** generally only one body cavity (cranial, thoracic, or abdominopelvic cavity) is opened to examine one specific item. This type of autopsy is most frequently performed as the medical (or hospital) autopsy.

Some institutions remove and examine only one organ, usually because they are limited by the person grant-ing permission for the autopsy. If only one organ is removed and all vessels ligated, the embalmer should have little difficulty. Many pathologists, however, remove the one organ but do not ligate the vessels. This often leads to extensive prosection of the cavity and contributes to interrupted circulation in the embalming process.

SUGGESTED ORDER FOR PREPARATION OF THE AUTOPSIED BODY

1. Unwrap the body. To disinfect, apply a topical droplet spray to the surface of the body and the orifices. Wash the body with germicidal soap and dry it. Relieve (as much as possible) any rigor mortis present. Position the head and shoulders.
2. Shave the body and set the features.
3. Open the cavities. Remove the viscera if they have been returned. Disinfect the internal surfaces of the body cavities with droplet spray.
4. Locate and place ligatures around the six vessels needed for sectional arterial injection:
   A. Right and left external-iliac arteries*
   B. Right and left axillary or subclavian arteries
   C. Right and left common carotid arteries
5. Prepare the arterial solution. Consider a variety of factors in determining the strength of the solution:
   A. Cause of death
   B. Size and weight of body
   C. Time between death and preparation
   D. Presence of decomposition changes
   E. Moisture content of tissues
   F. Protein content of body
   G. Refrigeration
   (Different solutions may have to be prepared for different sections of the body, e. g., if edema is present in the legs but not in the arms or head.)
6. Inject at rates of flow and pressures that meet the demands of the various body areas. Drainage may be concurrent or intermittent.
   A. Inject the legs first, one at a time.
   B. Inject the arms second, one at a time.
   C. Inject the head.
      a. Inject the left side *first.*
      b. Inject the right side.
7. Institute supplemental treatments: hypodermic injection of the *trunk walls, shoulders, neck,* and *buttocks.*
8. Drain all liquids from body cavities and treat internal surfaces with hardening compound or autopsy gel.
9. Prepare abdominal and thoracic cavities and neck area.

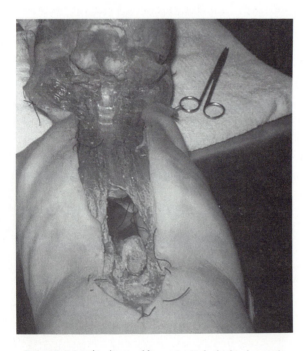

Figure 17–2. Spinal cord removed for examination by the dorsal approach.

---

*Common iliacs can be injected when present. Internal iliacs may be injected if they are present.

A. Return the bag of viscera and add preservative chemical.
B. Fill cavities with absorbent material such as sheeting or cotton and saturate material with preservative chemical.
C. Fill out neck area with cotton saturated with preservative chemical or autopsy gel.
10. Suture thoracic and abdominal cavities.
11. Dry cranial cavity. Treat walls with preservative powder or gel and attach calvarium.
12. Suture scalp.
13 Wash and dry body.
14. Apply glue to incisions of the thoracic and abdominal cavity.
15. Dress body in coveralls, adding embalming powder to surface of abdominal and back areas.

PREPARATION OF THE AUTOPSIED BODY

Carefully open the zippered pouch or plastic or cotton sheeting enveloping the autopsied remains. Liberally, using a droplet spray, disinfect the exposed surfaces and inner wrappings. Several minutes later, roll up the covering material, and gently roll the body from side to side to remove all of the wrappings. Place these immediately in a biohazard container. Next, wash the body with a disinfectant solution. Let this topical solution remain on the body for at least 10 minutes. The body can then be rinsed and dried. Relieve any rigor mortis present and proceed to position the body.

1. Remove the pathologist's stitches and lay back the flaps of skin, exposing the thoracic and abdominal and cranial cavities. Spray these cavities with a broad spectrum disinfectant droplet spray. Remove the stitches from the scalp and remove the calvarium. Disinfect the cranial cavity or better yet, swab it with autopsy gel, especially in cases of systemic infection (meningitis, hepatitis, AIDS). Support the scalp in the forehead area, especially during arterial injection, to avoid a "creased" area across the forehead and to assist distribution of fluid through the scalp.
2. Inspect the arteries needed for injection.
3. OPTION: Some embalmers prefer to shave and set the features at this time; others prefer to inject the legs and arms prior to setting the features.
4. Mix arterial solution. Remember that if there has been a delay between death and preparation or if the body has been refrigerated, or both, a slightly stronger arterial solution is needed: *either a higher-index fluid or a standard arterial solution to which 4 to 6 ounces of a high-index fluid has been added.* Add some tracer dye to indicate the distribution of arterial solution in the body.

5. Inject the lower extremities.
   A. The ideal vessels to use for injection of the legs are the right and left common iliac. Any leakage from the internal iliac branch can be clamped (vessels were severed when the pelvic organs were removed). Arterial solution will reach the legs by the external iliac and the internal iliac artery will supply solution to the buttocks, anal area, and perineal tissues. Injection of the common iliac would also supply solution to the trunk walls through branches off the external iliac artery. In some autopsies the common iliac and internal iliac arteries have been excised. In this situation the embalmer will use the external iliac artery to inject each leg. Injecting each common iliac artery or external iliac artery separately permits more control over the flow of the solution into the extremity being injected. The embalmer can control massage, pressure, rate of flow, and strength of the solution being used for each leg. Separate direct injection of the internal iliac artery accompanied by massage to the buttocks and upper thighs can bring about a noticeable amount of arterial solution distribution to these areas. It should always be attempted; leakage may need to be controlled with hemostats.
   B. Some autopsy technicians and/or pathologists sever the external iliac artery directly beneath the inguinal ligament. It is important to remember that arteries remain open when severed. In the nose of a hemostat, grasp the cut end of the artery and gently expose it sufficiently to insert an arterial tube. If possible place a tight ligature around the artery to secure the tube; if this is not possible use an arterial hemostat to secure the tube in the artery. Always attempt to place strings around arteries to hold arterial tubes in place rather than holding them in position using hemostats.
   C. If necessary, raise the femoral artery to inject the lower extremities.
   D. Allow drainage to enter the abdominopelvic cavity. If intermittent drainage is desired, use a hemostat to stop drainage for intervals.
   E. If fluid does not reach the foot, institute the following procedures:
      a. Very firmly massage the leg, pushing strongly along the arterial route(femoral, popliteal, and anterior and posterior tibial arteries). Rotate the foot medially. This squeezes all the muscles of the lower leg.
      b. Use a higher injection pressure and pulsation.
      c. Limit drainage by using intermittent drainage.

Many times, the vessels of the leg are sclerotic. If injection of the lower arteries is impossible, inject the legs hypodermically (infant trocar) with a preservative. Then paint the legs with autopsy gel and clothe them in plastic stockings.

The volume and strength of solution depend on pathological conditions, leakage, and postmortem conditions. Sometimes, ½ gallon is sufficient. With edema, 2 or more gallons might be needed per leg. *There is no set volume or strength.*

Some embalmers prefer to aspirate drainage material continuously while injecting the legs and arms. Others prefer to let the excess fluids that accumulate sit in the cavities during arterial injection, the theory being that these fluids preserve the tissues of the inner surface of the back area. The problem with the latter method is that the working environment may become quite uncomfortable for the embalmer because of the excess fumes. It is easier to aspirate the excess fluids from the cavities and thus reduce exposure to formaldehyde fumes.

6. Inject the upper extremities.
    A. If the arch of the aorta or its branches are present, use the subclavian arteries for injection. In this way fluid is distributed to the shoulders, to the back of the neck, and to the upper back regions. In the complete autopsy, however, the following vessels must be clamped if the subclavian artery is injected:
        a. Vertebral artery (if a cranial autopsy has been done)
        b. Internal thoracic artery
        c. Inferior thyroid artery (when neck organs have been removed)
        The right subclavian is a branch of the brachiocephalic artery. It can be distinguished from the right common carotid artery, because the subclavian is usually larger in diameter. Follow the direction of the insertion of an arterial tube to determine if the right subclavian artery has been entered; it heads laterally toward the arm. The left subclavian branches off the arch of the aorta. If, after clamping off the leakage from the severed branches of the subclavian, leakage still continues, it may be necessary to raise and inject the axillary artery. The problem with using the axillary is that the shoulder, upper portions of the back, and deep muscles of the neck do not receive arterial solution distribution.
    B. The axillary artery can be raised by cutting the pectoralis major and minor muscles (Fig. 17–3). It is easy to raise this artery just as it leaves the cervicoaxillary canal. This canal is bounded by the scapula, the first rib, and the clavicle. If the axillary artery is raised at this point, all its branches can be used to distribute fluid to the trunk walls and shoulders areas. In addition, the arm can be placed in a natural position. Use of the

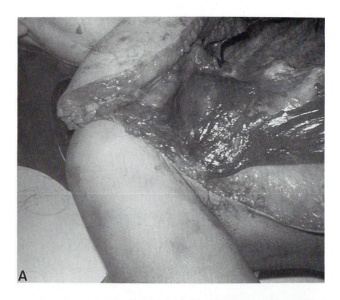

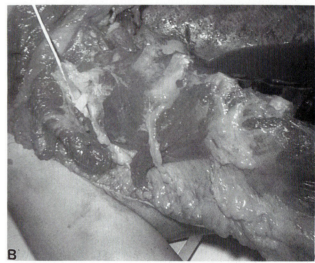

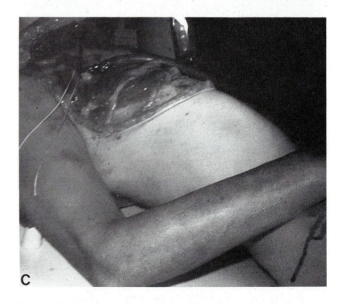

Figure 17–3. Autopsy injection of arms using the axillary artery. **A.** Note the pectoralis muscle. **B.** The axillary artery is shown; inject from this location. **C.** The arm may be positioned during injection.

axillary artery avoids many of the leakage problems seen with the subclavian artery, and the axillary can be raised from the incision the pathologist has already made (if that incision rises to the shoulder area). *If fluid does not flow easily down the arm, pull the arterial tube out a little. This usually frees the tube of any blockage.*

C. Drainage can be taken from the subclavian vein. If intermittent drainage is desired, place a hemostat on either the subclavian or the axillary vein.

D. Fluid strength and volume vary from body to body or even from right side to left side. Continue injection until the hand has cleared and distribution is evident. Manipulate the arm, flexing at the elbow and wrist, to assist distribution along with intermittent drainage. It may also be necessary to place digital pressure on the cephalic vein to increase distribution by blocking the loss of fluid from the superficial drainage route.

If fluid is not flowing into the hand, try the following: lower the hand while injecting, massage by pushing very firmly along the arterial route (axillary, brachial, radial, and ulnar arteries), increase injection pressure (using pulsation if available), and use intermittent drainage. Finally, the radial and ulnar arteries can be raised and injected. If fluid still does not enter the fingers, treat by hypodermic injection of a preservative fluid.

7. Inject the head.

A. Place arterial tubes in the right and left common carotid arteries. If the common carotid has been cut by the pathologist, try to find the external carotid. Remember that the common carotid bifurcates at the level of the superior border of the thyroid cartilage. This point is quite high in the neck. If the artery can be located, insert a small arterial tube. Clamp it in place with an arterial hemostat.

B. If the eyes have been enucleated, loosely pack the eye orbits with cotton saturated with autopsy gel.

C. If the inner ear has been removed, tightly pack the area of the temporal bone from which the tissues were removed with cotton saturated with autopsy gel. If this area leaks profusely during injection, apply a hemostat to the leaking vessels.

D. OPTION 1: Inject the left side of the head first. Certain arteries must be clamped for leakage if the left common carotid artery is injected. The *left internal carotid* is located inside the cranial cavity just lateral to the sella turcica of the sphenoid bone. Clamp this vessel after arterial injection has begun. In this way, filling of the vascular system supplied by the common carotid artery can be observed. The *superior thyroid artery* is located in the neck; this branch of external carotid artery leaks if the neck organs have been removed.

Inject the right side of the head. The left is injected first so that a certain amount of fluid flows to the right side via anastomosis. It also gives the embalmer a chance to observe the effects of the fluid and the dyes on the left side. If there is any problem, the arterial solution can be changed before the right side is injected. This method also prevents overinjection of the right side of the face. Arteries to be clamped are the *right internal carotid*, found lateral to the sella turcica in the cranial cavity, and the *right superior thyroid*, found in the neck if the neck organs have been removed.

E. OPTION 2: Once tubes are in place in the right and left common carotid arteries, attach them to a Y tube. Inject both right and left sides at the same time. Clamp all arteries, such as internal carotids and superior thyroids or any other major leaking arteries, with hemostats.

F. Observe the parotid, sublingual, and submaxillary glands for swelling. Use of a stronger solution and pulsation, a slower rate flow, and a reduced pressure during the injection helps to limit swelling of these glands. If swelling occurs, apply digital pressure against the glands. These glands can also be pierced from under the skin with a scalpel, which, together with digital pressure, helps to reduce swelling. If the swelling is too pronounced, the glands may have to be excised from under the skin by going up through the neck.

SUPPLEMENTAL HYPODERMIC INJECTION

Depending on the incisions made by the pathologist and the extent of vessel removal, only a small portion of the trunk may receive arterial fluid. It now becomes necessary for the embalmer to preserve those areas lacking fluid, as best as possible, by hypodermic embalming (Fig. 17–4). Preservative solution is injected via a trocar attached to the embalming machine. Some embalmers prefer arterial solution for this work; others use a mixture of cavity fluid and water.

It is important that all tissues be channeled: the trunk walls (anterior, lateral, and posterior), with special emphasis on injection of the buttocks, breasts in the female, and shoulder and neck regions. Channel these regions first; then turn on the machine or allow the fluid to pass through the trocar into the channels. Avoid accidents that expose the embalmer to excessive amounts of embalming solution. Universal Precautions requires eye protection during all embalming procedures; hypodermic treatments certainly demand this protection. In addition to the hypodermic treatment of the trunk walls, surface embalming can be used:

1. A scalpel can be used to cut the intercostal muscles in the thoracic area. Later, this area can be

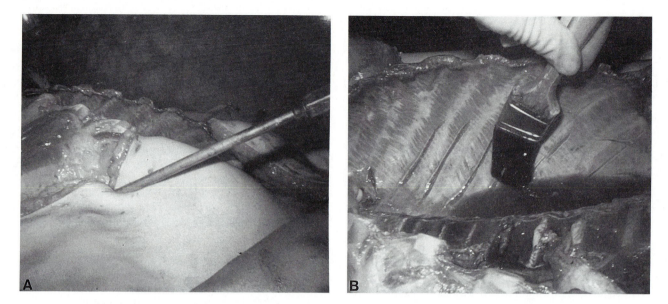

Figure 17–4. **A.** Hypodermic treatment of the walls after autopsy. **B.** After the intercostal muscles are incised, the cavity walls are painted with autopsy gel.

painted with autopsy gel, which, over time, penetrates the tissues of the back (Fig. 17–4B).

2. The trunk walls on the outside of the rib case can be cut further back (some embalmers do this as far back as the vertebral column) and then painted with autopsy gel. In lieu of autopsy gel, cotton or paper towels or strips of sheeting can be placed between the trunk wall and the rib cage and saturated with cavity fluid.

3. All inside surfaces of the cavities can be painted with autopsy gel.

4. If viscera are not returned, sheeting can be placed in the cavities and saturated with cavity fluid. This provides an "inside compress" for surface embalming.

5. Even if viscera are returned, the cavity can be lined with cotton, paper towels, or sheeting and saturated with cavity fluid before the plastic bag of viscera is placed back in the cavity. This material can be saturated with preservative or cavity fluid, in lieu of autopsy gel.

Autopsy gels are made to cling to the lateral walls. In addition, they are formulated to penetrate the tissues, so their use may be preferred to that of inlays of cavity fluid. The autopsy gels are a little easier to work with from the standpoint of formaldehyde irritation.

Care should be taken to pack the pelvic cavity so there is no leakage from the rectum. If the pathologist has removed the entire rectum, it may be necessary to turn the body over and suture the area closed. The rec-

tum, esophagus, and trachea can be tightly ligated from within the cavities.

Attention should also be given to the neck area if the neck organs have been removed. Cotton is used to replace the missing organs, and once it is in place, the cotton is saturated with some preservative fluid. This is necessary, because circulation to the skin of the neck is interrupted when the neck organs are removed. Again, all inside areas of the neck can be painted with autopsy gel before cotton is inserted.

TREATMENT OF THE VISCERA

The viscera, if returned, are usually enclosed in a plastic bag. A number of methods are used to treat the viscera.

If the viscera are to be returned to the abdominal and thoracic cavities, a new plastic bag should be used. A minimum of two bottles of cavity fluid should be mixed and poured over the viscera before the bag is returned to the cavities. It is much easier to position and "find room" for the viscera in the cavities if the preservative fluids are not poured over the viscera until the bag is in position. After being covered with cavity chemical, the hollow organs can be incised using shears to release any gases.

Some embalmers return the viscera to the cavities but *not* in plastic bags. The viscera should be soaked in cavity fluid several hours, returned to the abdominal and thoracic cavities, and covered well with absorbent autopsy hardening compound, absorbent cotton, and a piece of sheet. Then, the cavities are sutured closed.

CLOSURE OF THE CAVITIES

After *walls of the cavities* have been treated *hypodermically* and by *surface embalming* and the viscera returned (preferably in a plastic bag) to the abdominal and thoracic cavities, the next step is closure of the cavities.

If the viscera are not returned to the abdominal and thoracic cavities, the cavities should be filled with absorbent material such as sheeting, kapoc, or cotton. This material should be saturated with cavity fluid or autopsy gel to prevent it from molding or developing odor. The sheeting or cotton also serves as an internal preservative compress.

Position the breastplate, being certain it is coated on both sides with autopsy gel or preservative powder.

Begin to suture using a double-curved needle and linen suture cord. Linen suture cord is much stronger than cotton suture cord. A minimum of a five-twist (strand) linen suture cord should be used. When pulling the cord to tighten the stitches, **pull on the thread, not on the needle.** Otherwise, the thread may break as it rubs against the eye of the needle.

If cotton is used as filler for the cavities, be certain that paper toweling or sheeting is placed over the cotton. Cotton has a tendency to get caught in the suturing and can be quite troublesome to work with.

Bring all three flaps of the incision together and tie them together with one suture. From this point, if desired, sew to the shoulder area along one of the branches of the incision extending from the xiphoid process of the sternum to the shoulder (Fig. 17–5).

Start the suture for the abdominal cavity at the level of the pubic symphysis. Begin the suture by *tying the suture in place* rather than just tying a knot on the end of the suture. Knots have a tendency to pull through the skin. Use a baseball suture for closure. This suture is very tight. In fact, if properly done, it is airtight. String from the suture pattern should not be seen. If the suture looks like the lacing pattern of a baseball, it is *too loose*. Pull the sutures *very tight*. Single- or double-cord suture thread may be used. If linen is used, single-strand thread should be sufficient and not cause any breakage. [If the hole made by the suture needle appears large, double-stranded thread may be preferred to close (fill) the hole.]

If the suture thread should break, assess the situation. Rather than tearing out all the suturing and starting over, it may be more convenient to begin sewing from another direction and tie the two sutures together.

When the tie at the location of the xiphoid process is reached, continue the suture up the branch of the Y incision that was not previously closed to the shoulder. It is important, especially in the shoulder areas, to use *incision seal powder* to prevent any leakage. This is the one area of the Y incision that is most likely to leak.

The skin of bodies with certain wasting diseases may be difficult to suture because it tears easily. Try using a large inversion suture to close these incisions. In extreme cases, it may be necessary simply to wrap the trunk closed by wrapping strips of sheeting around the body.

In the female, suturing is easier if the pathologist made a Y incision over rather than under the breasts. This might be suggested to the pathologist.

During the embalming of the body, a phenol cautery chemical can be placed on cotton compresses and laid along the autopsy incision where the scalp has been opened. This will assist in drying the marginal tissues and reduce the possibility of leakage from this incision when the scalp is closed by suturing.

Arterial solution or blood that has accumulated in the posterior portion of the cranial cavity should be removed by aspirating or sponging. The walls of the cavity can be painted with autopsy gel or dusted with a preservative powder. An absorbent material should be placed in the cavity to absorb liquids that may accumulate. In addition, some embalmers place incision seal powder in the foramen magnum and the posterior areas of the cranium to absorb liquids that might leak.

Some embalmers force (by hammering) a long wedge of wood into the foramen magnum. This holds the head steady if the vertebral column has been cut open.

Next, the calvarium should be replaced. If the autopsy has been properly performed, there should be one *notch* in the area of the *frontal bone* and other *notches* laterally in the *area of the temporal bone*. If notches are present, the calvarium will not be able to move forward or backward or laterally (from side to side). If notches are not present, several methods of attachment can be used to prevent the calvarium from moving:

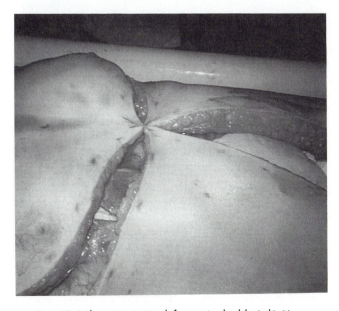

Figure 17–5. Align autopsy incisions before suturing the abdominal incisions.

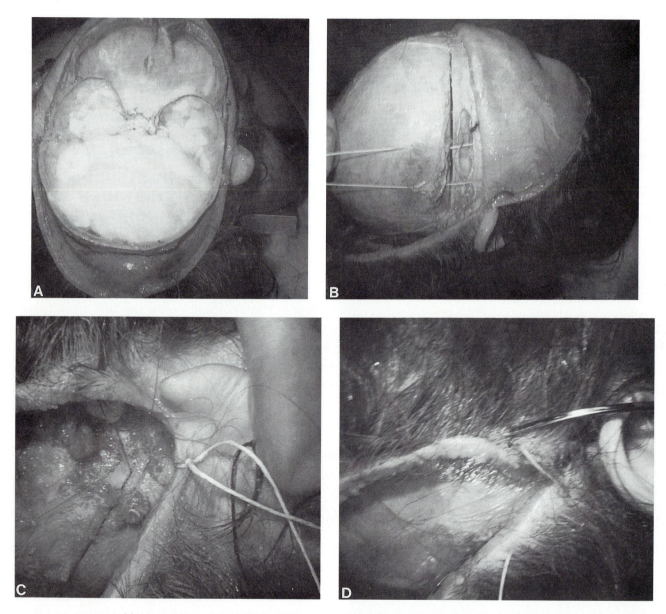

Figure 17–6. Treatment of the autopsied skull. **A.** The base of the skull is prepared using absorbent powders and cotton. Cavity walls are painted with gel preservatives. **B.** The temporalis muscle is sutured to the calvarium. The scalp is painted with a preservative gel. **C.** Begin on the right side when suturing the scalp. **D.** Use a "worm" suture for scalp closure. Spread incision seal powder along the incision.

1. Suture through the temporalis muscles and up across the calvarium. Suture through the cut portion of the temporalis muscle still attached to the temporal bone and through that portion of the muscle still attached to the calvarium.

2. Separately suture the cut temporalis muscles on either side of the head.

3. Use calvarium "clamps." Several varieties are available.

4. Drill opposing holes in the calvarium and the temporal bone and wire the calvarium into position.

5. Use super glue to help hold the calvarium in position.

6. Use plaster of Paris. This older method of attachment may have advantages if the skull was fractured. The base of the skull would be aligned and plastered into position (prior to arterial injection). Later, the cranial cavity can be filled with cotton and this covered with plaster, and the calvarium (or its pieces) can be placed into position.

7. Use needle injector wires. Use four wires on each side: two attached to the calvarium and two attached to the temporal bone. Then crisscross the wires.

After the calvarium is attached, place a small amount of "mortuary putty" along the cut line of the calvarium

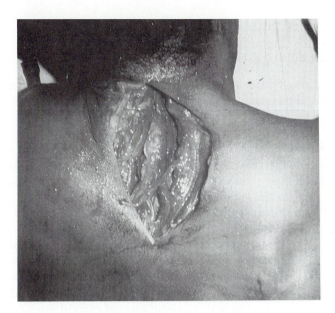

Figure 17–7. Examination of cervical vertebrae.

in the region of the *forehead*. Mortuary putty can also be used to fill in the area of the temple where some of the muscle may have been cut away.

Mortuary putty is a useful substitute for incision seal powder along the scalp incision. The putty helps to prevent leakage, especially if some of the material is pulled through the punctures made by the suture needle. If "mortuary putty" is not available and the temple muscles have been cut away, use mortuary wax as well as cotton and glue as a filler. "Tissue builder" cannot be used if the muscles are missing.

Next, coat the calvarium with autopsy gel or preservative powder (Fig. 17–6). Reflect the scalp over the calvarium. While attaching the calvarium, pull the scalp down over the face. Doing so prevents wrinkles in the area of the forehead. After reflecting the scalp, spread some incision seal powder or mortuary putty along the posterior portion of the area where the scalp meets the occipital and temporal bones, to help prevent leakage through the sutures.

Begin sutures on the right side of the head and end them on the left side.

There are many ways in which the hair can be kept out of the suture line. Comb the hair with water as the suturing proceeds. Use hair clamps to "clamp" the hair away from the sutures. Moisten the hair with liquid soap and comb the hair away from the incision line.

Using a double-curved needle, tie the first suture into place behind the right ear. *Do not use knots;* they have a tendency to pull through the scalp. Single or double linen suture cord can be used. Single is preferred and the cord should be a minimum of five-twist (strand) linen suture cord. Two sutures can be used to close the scalp incision. The *inversion (worm) suture* is made entirely on the surface of the scalp. The area between the edge on the scalp and the needle "rolls under" if each stitch is tightly pulled when the sutures are completed. Only a straight line should be seen. On a bald body the line can easily be waxed or covered with glue, and cosmetics placed over the dried glue. If a *baseball suture* is used, be sure each suture is tightly placed. No thread should be seen.

Some embalmers use *super adhesive* in place of sutures on the scalp. In the preparation of infants and in difficult circumstances (such as when surgery has been performed on the cranium), super adhesive may be advantageous.

FINAL PROCEDURES

After closure of the cranial incisions, the body and the hair should be again washed and dried. A hair dryer dries not only hair but also the incision. After skin is dried, the incisions can be covered with a surface glue. Some embalmers then cover the incisions with cotton or a cotton webbing while the glue is still wet. Others prefer to wait until the glue has dried and place the body in coveralls.

In yet another method, the incisions can be covered with glue, then cotton, and the body clothed in coveralls. An embalming powder should be sprinkled inside the coveralls to control odors, prevent mold, and assist in preservation.

If air appears to be trapped in the thoracic area, insert a trocar through the abdominal wall just under the skin surface to draw out the air. Also, use forceps to separate one of the thoracic sutures. This allows the air to be expressed through the gap in the forceps. Keep in mind that a properly sewn "baseball suture" should be airtight.

ADDITIONAL EXAMINATIONS

In some autopsies the posterior of the cervical vertebrae is opened externally and examined (Fig. 17–7). Cervical vertebrae are usually examined when a broken neck is suspected or when bleeding may have occurred along the vertebrae (as might occur in falls or automobile accidents).

For the pathologist to examine the vertebrae, an incision is made along the back of the neck, above the line where the shirt collar would pass to as high as the hairline.

Roll the body on its side or, if necessary, completely over prior to arterial injection and remove any sutures.

Pack the area with a phenol cautery chemical. Hold the edges together with bridge sutures or several strips of duct tape. After the body is embalmed again roll the body on its side or completely over. Remove the cautery packing, dry the deep tissues, fill the incision with incision seal powder or "mortuary putty," and tightly suture closed using a baseball stitch. The sutures can be coated with a thick layer of surface glue.

Tissues are sometimes taken from the knee areas. These incisions can be opened prior to arterial embalming. They should be dried with cotton and packed with a cautery agent on cotton swabs. After injection, dry out the area, fill with incision seal powder, and suture tightly closed with a baseball stitch. The incisions can then be glued. If leakage might be a problem, place plastic stockings on the body.

Death from Pulmonary Embolism

After a pulmonary embolism, the pathologist often makes incisions along the medial portions of the legs. The pathologist is looking for the source of the clot that moved into the lungs. These incisions can be filled with cotton packs dipped in a phenol cautery solution or cavity fluid while the rest of the body is embalmed. After the other incisions have been closed, the cotton packs can be removed and the incisions packed with dry, absorbent cotton. Use sufficient amounts of incision seal powder or mortuary putty when suturing these long incisions (some of these incisions may be 2 feet or longer). A baseball suture is the tightest stitch and the easiest to use. The stitching can be coated with a surface glue. Plastic stockings may be used if any leakage is anticipated.

Death from Drug Overdoses

In the autopsy of persons dead from suspected drug overdoses, the pathologist is likely to excise tissue where old keloid scars (fibrous tissue) have formed from the use of needles. Generally, a square of tissue is cut out, quite often in the bend of the elbow. **The excision cannot be closed by suturing.** It is best to cover these open areas with cotton saturated with phenol chemical prior to embalming. After arterial injection, remove the cotton, dry with a hair dryer, and paint the area with glue. Apply fresh cotton and wrap the area. If the possibility of leakage exists, place a plastic "sleeve" on the arm or self-clinging food wrap around the arm. Some embalmers cut out a portion of plastic stocking to make a sleeve, slip it onto the arm, and tape it in place with duct tape.

PARTIAL AUTOPSIES

Cranial Autopsy Only

In this partial autopsy the cranial cavity is opened and the brain is removed. The body can be embalmed by one of three procedures.

Method 1. Raise the right and left common carotid arteries. Insert tubes in both, directed upward toward the head. Insert one tube directed downward toward the trunk in the right common carotid. Tie off (ligate) the lower portion of the left common carotid.

Use the right internal jugular vein for drainage.

Inject downward *first* to embalm the extremities and trunk. Clamp off leakage in the cranium from the right and left vertebral arteries (which are branches of the subclavian arteries). Inject the left and right sides of the head, clamping off the left and right internal carotid arteries.

Method 2. Raise the right common carotid artery and the right internal jugular vein. Insert two tubes directed upward toward the head and one tube directed downward toward the trunk.

Inject downward, clamping off the right and left vertebral arteries and the left internal carotid artery. These are found in the base of the cranial cavity.

Inject up the right side of the head. Clamp off the right internal carotid artery in the base of the skull.

Method 3. Raise the right femoral artery and vein. Insert into the artery one tube directed upward and one tube directed to the foot.

Inject the right leg.

Inject upward toward the trunk and head. Clamp off the right and left internal carotid arteries and the right and left vertebral arteries. After arterial injection, dry the cranial cavity, paint it with autopsy gel, and fill it with cotton.

Attach the calvarium and suture the scalp back into position using the inversion or baseball suture. Spread plenty of incision seal powder or mortuary putty within the incision as the suturing progresses. Begin suturing on the right side of the head and end on the left side.

THORACIC AUTOPSY ONLY

In a thoracic partial autopsy, one or more organs of the cavity have been removed (assuming that the neck organs have not been removed). Drainage taken for the lower extremities and the abdomen are drained through the inferior vena cava, which is located at the lower right area of the diaphragm (Fig. 17–8).

There is only one way to prepare the head and the arms. It is similar to the technique used after a complete

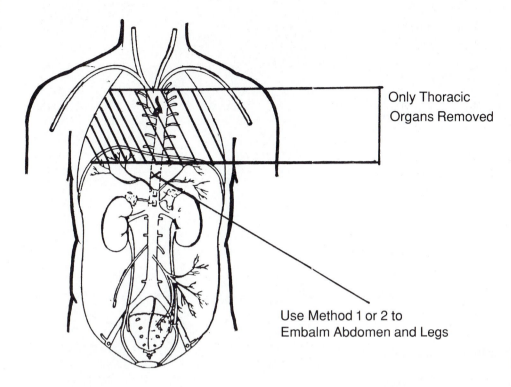

Only Thoracic
Organs Removed

Use Method 1 or 2 to
Embalm Abdomen and Legs

Figure 17–8. Thoracic autopsy only.

autopsy, when the head and the arms are separately injected. Inject the left arm using the left subclavian or left axillary artery. Inject the right arm using the right subclavian or right axillary artery. Inject the left side of the head using the left common carotid artery. Inject the right side of the head using the right common carotid artery. Two methods can be used to inject the abdomen and the lower extremities.

Method 1. Locate the terminal portion of the thoracic aorta on the vertebral column at the central posterior portion of the diaphragm. Insert a large arterial tube into the aorta. Either clamp the tube in place with an arterial hemostat or, if possible, tie the tube in place. Inject downward through the arterial tube. This embalms the abdominal walls, abdominal contents, and lower extremities. Leakage may occur from the right and left inferior or superior epigastric arteries, depending on how the pathologist made incisions.

Method 2. Raise the right femoral artery and insert a tube directed upward toward the abdomen. Also, insert a tube downward to inject the right leg. Inject the right leg first. Next, inject upward. This embalms the left leg, abdominal contents, and trunk. Ligate by tying or clamping the thoracic aorta when fluid is observed flowing from this artery into the thoracic cavity.

After arterial injection, check for preservation of the thoracic walls and the back and shoulders. If the preservation is inadequate the walls should be treated by hypodermic injection. The thoracic cavity can be painted with autopsy gel and filled with sheeting or an appropriate absorbent material. This material, in turn, can be saturated with cavity fluid or some other preservative, the breastplate put into position, and the incisions closed with a baseball suture. Aspirate the abdominal cavity and inject cavity fluid over the abdominal viscera (Fig. 17–9).

ABDOMINAL AUTOPSY ONLY

In an abdominal partial autopsy, the contents of the abdominal cavity are removed (Fig. 17–10). If only the abdominal cavity is opened and the organs are removed, two methods can be employed for arterial embalming of the thorax, upper extremities, and head. The legs can be injected from the external iliac arteries. Drainage from the arterial injection of the upper trunk, arms, and head can be taken from the *inferior vena cava,* found in the lower right area of the diaphragm, where it would be attached to the liver.

Method 1. To inject the thorax, upper extremities, and head, locate the abdominal aorta as it passes through the diaphragm. The aorta can be located at the level of the vertebral column in the central posterior position of the diaphragm. Tie or clamp an arterial tube into the aorta. Upward injection should embalm the thorax and its contents, the arms, and the head.

Method 2. Raise the right common carotid artery. Insert a tube upward for the right side of the head. Insert a tube downward. Inject downward toward the trunk; the arms, thorax, and left side of the head should receive

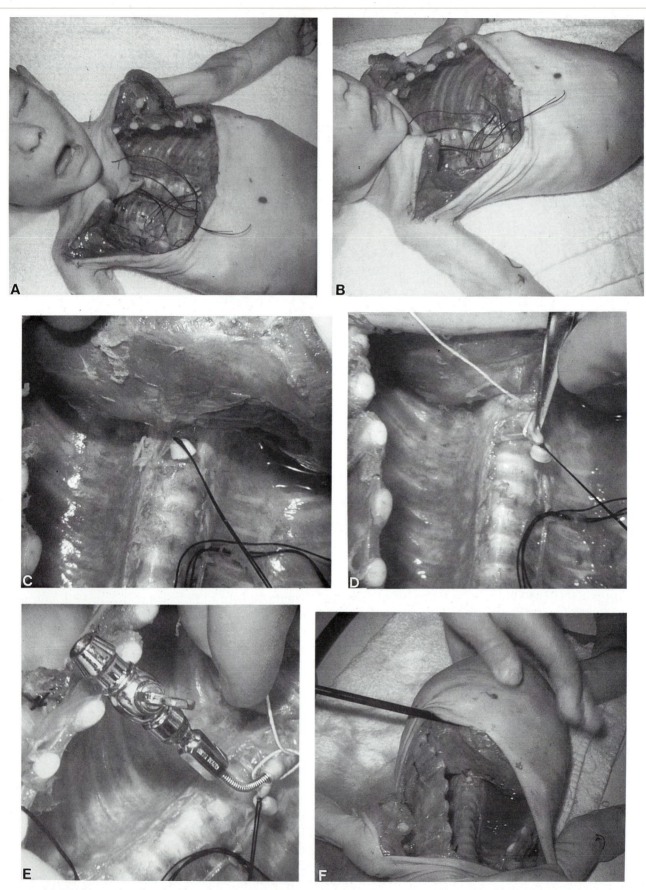

Figure 17–9. Partial autopsy of an infant (the abdominal aorta was used). **A, B.** Only the thoracic organs have been removed. **C.** The thoracic aorta is located on the spinal column. The diaphragm is at the top of the picture. **D.** The aorta being opened. Drainage is taken from the inferior vena cava located at the diaphragm. No drainage instruments are needed. **E.** The arterial tube is inserted into the aorta. **F.** Treatment of the abdominal viscera.

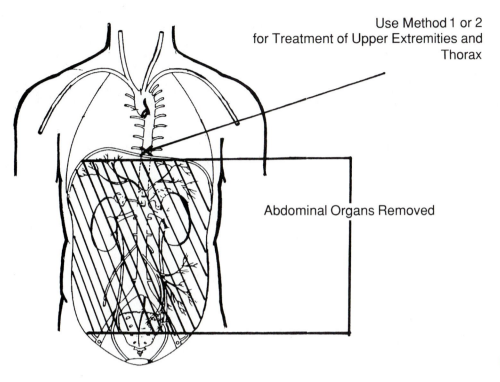

Use Method 1 or 2
for Treatment of Upper Extremities and
Thorax

Abdominal Organs Removed

Figure 17–10. Abdominal autopsy only.

arterial solution. When leakage is noted from the aorta, clamp or tie the aorta in the abdominal cavity. After the downward injection, inject the right side of the head. (The restricted cervical method of injection could also be used.)

Check the abdominal walls, the buttocks, and the back for fluid distribution. Depending on the pathologist's incision there may be leakage from the superior epigastric arteries during injection. *(Hypodermic injection can be used to preserve the abdominal walls and buttocks.)* Injection of the male genitalia may also be necessary. Direct injection of both internal iliac arteries will provide good distribution of arterial solution to the buttocks, genitalia, and upper thighs. The walls of the cavity can be painted with autopsy gel and the abdominal cavity filled with sheeting or other absorbent material. This filler can then be saturated with cavity chemical or other preservative.

Suture the abdominal incisions using a baseball suture. After washing and drying the body, cover the incisions with surface glue.

In both partial autopsies, thoracic and abdominal, the cavity *not* opened and examined should be treated by trocar. Aspiration can be done either through the diaphragm or by inserting the trocar through the rib cage for the thorax or through the abdominal wall for the abdomen. This treatment can be done *before or after* the autopsied cavity has been closed by suturing. The cavity not autopsied should also be injected with a minimum of one bottle of concentrated cavity fluid.

PROTOCOL FOR THE TREATMENT OF AUTOPSIED BODIES WHEN RESTORATIVE TREATMENTS ARE NECESSARY

Restoration of the deceased to natural **form** and **color** is directly related to *embalming*. Many restorative treatments begin in the preembalming period and some are carried out during embalming. The majority of restorative work, however, is accomplished in the postembalming period. Accidental deaths may involve *trauma*, which involves visible regions of the body such as the face and hands. As these deaths are accidental, the certification of death is under the jurisdiction of the coroner or medical examiner. In most instances the official will have the body autopsied to determine the exact cause of death.

The outline that follows suggests the order of preparation of bodies that have sustained traumatic injuries to the face and have also been autopsied. Restorative art is a subject unto itself, and this protocol involves only some of those restorative treatments that should be carried out before and during arterial embalming. Two important criteria must be achieved for good restorative work. Tissues of the body must be *firm* and completely *dry*. It is the goal of the embalmer to adequately preserve and, thus, firm the tissue. By the use of embalming chemicals, solvents, and manual aids, the embalmer can dry the tissue.

In addition to trauma, be it lacerations, abrasions, bruising, or fractures, pathological conditions may exist in the body prior to accidental death. Consideration must also be given to postmortem changes. Preparation of the body with facial trauma and a complete autopsy allows the embalmer to use a different strength of arterial solution for each area of the body injected. If trauma is in the facial tissues, a stronger solution can be injected to control swelling, and dry and firm these tissues; a milder solution may be desired for the arms and/or legs. These factors, taken together, constitute the basis for the embalming analysis.

1. Disinfect and position the body.
   A. Be cautious of shards of glass that may be embedded in the skin if glass was involved in the accident. Sometimes these shards can be flushed out with water or picked out with forceps.
   B. Use cool water and plenty of liquid soap to remove blood, grease, and oils.
2. Assess the damage to all body areas.
3. Begin with injection of the legs; then, inject the arms.
4. Prepare the head and face.
   A. Open the cranial cavity and check for fractured bones. Inspect for scalp lacerations or abrasions.
   B. Shave the body. Observe punctures, lacerations, abrasions, and hematomas. Remove all loose skin and dehydrated edges of lacerated tissues using a sharp razor or scalpel.
   C. By application of digital pressure to face, inspect for fractures of the mandible, maxillae, and nasal bones and for the presence of air (subcutaneous emphysema).
   D. Close the mouth using a method that keeps the lips in contact and align the jaw bones if they are fractured. Suturing may be required. Use several needle injector barbs. Temporarily gluing lips may help.
   E. Close the eyes using cotton support or eyecaps. Depending on the damage to the eyelids, it may be necessary to glue the lids prior to injection.
   F. Attempt to realign fractured bones and support depressed fractures.
   G. Align lacerated tissues. Temporary individual sutures of dental floss or super glue can be used. After embalming, remove the temporary sutures or glue anchors and place permanent sutures or glue.
   H. Prepare a very strong arterial solution using a high index fluid (25-index above), for example, (1) 16 ounces of fluid and 32 ounces of water or (2) 16 ounces of fluid, one bottle of coinjection, and one bottle of water. Then add the fluid dye.
   I. Inject the left side of the face first. Pulse the fluid into the head and observe the dye to check fluid distribution.

In many of these bodies there will be a great amount of fluid leakage. This leakage helps to control some of the swelling. What is important is that the tissues receive fluid, as indicated by the presence of dye.

KEY TERMS AND CONCEPTS FOR STUDY AND DISCUSSION

1. Define the following terms:
   autopsy gel
   baseball suture
   calvarium
   cranial autopsy
   forensic autopsy
   hardening compound
   hypodermic embalming
   necropsy
   partial autopsy
   surface embalming
   worm suture
   Y tube
2. Describe the general order for embalming the autopsied body.
3. Describe several methods for securing the calvarium.
4. List the branches of the external carotid artery.
5. Give the location where the common carotid artery divides.
6. In the complete autopsy (neck organs removed), name the major arteries that must be clamped if the *left subclavian artery* is injected.
7. In the complete autopsy (neck organs removed), name the major arteries that must be clamped.
8. List the branches of the internal iliac artery and the area each supplies.
9. Describe several methods for preserving autopsy viscera.
10. Discuss several treatments for embalming the trunk walls in the autopsied body.
11. Describe two methods of injection to embalm the abdomen and legs when a partial autopsy has been performed and the contents of the thoracic cavity have been removed.

BIBLIOGRAPHY

Altman LK. Sharp drop in autopsies stirs fears that quality of care may also fall. *N.Y. Times*, July 21, 1988.
Slocum RE. *Pre-embalming Considerations*. Boston: Dodge Chemical Co.

18

Preparation of Bodies of Organ Donors

LEGALITIES OF ORGAN AND TISSUE RECOVERY

The legalities of organ and tissue donation fall into three categories: (1) determination, documentation, and pronouncement of death; (2) consent from the legal next-of-kin; (3) consent from the medical examiner or coroner.

Determination, Documentation, and Pronouncement of Death

Brain death is an established medical and legal principle that has been approved by the American Medical Association and the American Bar Association as a valid diagnosis of death. Brain death may be pronounced on the basis of accepted medical standards while the patient's cardiopulmonary function is artificially supported. The primary attending physician is responsible for making the determination of death according to the criteria for brain death. Most physicians secure neurological or neurosurgical corroboration.

Many states have passed acts giving statutory recognition to brain death. These acts provide full legal acceptance of brain death as death of a person. Although these laws have been enacted, the determination of death of a potential organ donor, as with any patient, legally remains within the clinical judgment of the attending physician.

Establishment of the time of death is, by law, a medical act and therefore consent is not required from the

next-of-kin. The patient's family should, however, be given complete information concerning the determination of death. Pronouncement and time of death are recorded in the progress notes after all criteria for determination of brain death have been met. A death certificate should be completed by the physician pronouncing death except in cases in which the medical examiner or coroner has jurisdiction. In these cases, the medical examiner or coroner completes the death certificate.

Consent for Organ and Tissue Donation

The Uniform Anatomical Gift Act (UAGA) has been enacted in all states to provide statutory regulations regarding postmortem organ and tissue donation. The UAGA allows any person 18 years and older to donate all organs and tissues of his or her body for transplantation, research, or educational purposes after death has been determined. Although many people make known their desire to be an organ donor by completing and carrying a Uniform Organ Donor Card, and although such cards are legal documents, in practice consent must be obtained from legally responsible next-of-kin. The UAGA provides the order of priority for consenting persons and specifically protects physicians who act in good faith from civil liabilities and criminal prosecution. The UAGA provides for consent for organ donation from a next-of-kin in the following order of priority: spouse, adult son or daughter, either parent, adult sibling, guardian of the deceased at the time of death, any other person authorized or under obligation to dispose of the body.

If any member of the family of the same or higher priority classification as the person giving consent objects to organ donation, the donation may not be accepted. Consent from the next-of-kin for postmortem organ and tissue donation is obtained either immediately before or after pronouncement of death is made. This document requires two witnesses and is maintained as a part of the patient's permanent record. Consent is obtained primarily through the use of a specifically drafted consent form. A sample of this form is included in Chapter 1. The UAGA also permits the relative's consent to be obtained by recorded telephone message or telegram.

Discussion of the opportunity for organ donation is enhanced through direct contact with the responsible relative and every effort is made to secure consent in writing. The following principles should be considered in approaching families regarding organ donation:

1. Organ donation can be realistically considered by a family only after they have accepted that the patient is terminal or is, in fact, dead.
2. The family needs to fully understand that brain death is death of the person.
3. The person discussing organ donation with the family needs to be familiar with basic issues regarding organ donation and transplantation (e.g., how organ retrieval is accomplished, the critical need for organs, how recipients are selected).

Whenever possible, it is strongly encouraged that those who approach the family be in contact with the organ procurement staff prior to offering the family the option for organ donation. This allows the organ procurement coordinators to advise the donor institution as to the particular needs for all organs and tissues for transplantation on both a local and national basis. Additionally, it eliminates the necessity for repeated family approaches. Organ procurement coordinators are available on a 24-hour basis to assist and coordinate the necessary permissions to satisfy all legal requirements for postmortem organ and tissue recovery.

Medical Examiner or Coroner Consent. All deaths that remain unexplained or are due to other than natural causes must be reported to the medical examiner or coroner. In all such cases in which organ and tissue donation is being considered, the medical examiner or coroner must grant permission for retrieval before the organs or tissues are removed. To facilitate the process, it is recommended that the medical examiner/coroner be contacted prior to pronouncement, but after family consent has been obtained, to alert him or her to the situation and receive a tenta-

tive ruling; however, final permission must be sought and received after pronouncement.

The date, time, and name of the person in the medical examiner/coroner's office granting permission must be recorded in the patient's chart.

USES FOR DONOR TISSUES

Therapeutic transplantation of vital human organs has become a common lifesaving therapy for patients suffering from end-stage organ failure. On any given day, well more than 12,000 individuals are in need of a kidney, liver, heart, lung, or pancreas for transplantation. Bone, skin, corneas, and many other tissues can restore thousands of people to normal, productive, and active lives. This modern medical achievement has been made possible by two factors: continued medical research and the thousands of people who have donated their own or deceased family members' vital organs and tissues for transplantation purposes (Table 18–1). Through their caring and generosity, these people and millions of others who now carry organ donor cards have become active partners with medical science in offering hope and life to victims of catastrophic diseases.

The most common reasons an individual chooses to donate his own or his loved one's organs and tissues for transplantation is the comfort derived in knowing that a person will be provided an opportunity for extended life or a better quality of life. Many organ donors are previously healthy patients who have suffered irreversible catastrophic brain injury of known etiology. These deaths are tragic and untimely, and through the donation, the family finds some solace in knowing something positive can come out of this meaningless death.

Very often, when families are deciding whether to donate a loved one's organs or tissues for transplantation, they turn to their funeral director for advice. Funeral directors should be able to reassure families that organ and tissue donation causes no mutilation or adverse effect and that the family of the donor can carry out whatever burial arrangements they wish.

Every year the number of transplants performed in the United States exceeds that of the previous year. Therefore, the funeral director or more importantly the embalmer must acquire a working knowledge of the methods used in organ and tissue recovery so that he or she can apply the appropriate embalming techniques. This chapter should help the funeral director and embalmer in acquiring that knowledge.

VASCULAR ORGAN DONATION

The most common vascular organs transplanted today are kidneys. Every year, approximately 8000 to 10,000

TABLE 18–1. PRIMARY USE OF ORGANS/TISSUES FOR TRANSPLANTATION

Organ/Tissue	Use	Organ/Tissue	Use
Heart	Orthotopic heart transplantation Heterotopic heart transplantation Heart/lung transplantation Aortic valve replacement Pulmonary valve replacement Research	Long bones (femur, tibia, etc.)	Total joint revision Trauma Tumor resection
Liver	Orthotopic liver transplantation Heterotopic liver transplantation Research	Tendons (achilles and patellar)	Anterior and posterior cruciate Ligament repair
		Fascia lata	Dura replacement Tendon, ligament, and eyelid reconstruction
Lung	Single/double-lung transplantation Hearth/lung transplantation Research	Iliac crest	Spinal fusion and dental procedures
		Fibula	Trauma Tumor resection Multilevel spinal fusions
Kidney	Renal transplantation Research	Cartilage	Nasal and facial reconstruction
		Dura	Dura and eyelid reconstruction
Pancreas	Pancreas transplantation Islet cell transplantation Research	Ribs	Maxillofacial reconstruction Oral surgical procedures
		Skin	Skin replacement (burn patients)
Small bowel	Small bowel transplantation	Mandible	Mandible reconstruction
Entire viscera (liver, stomach, small and large intestine, etc.)	Multivisceral transplantation	Eyes	Corneal transplantation Sclera for trauma and reconstruction Research
Saphenous vein	Coronary and peripheral bypass procedures Arteriovenous fistula construction	Temporal bone	Audiology reconstruction
		Intervertebral disk	Disk reconstruction
Iliac artery and vein	Grafts for transplantation	Vertebral bodies	Recovery of bone marrow for bone marrow transplantation

patients receive a kidney transplant. Two types of kidney transplants are performed: (1) a *living relative* transplant, in which the patient receives the kidney of a close relative; (2) a *cadaveric* kidney transplant, in which the patient receives a kidney from someone who has died. The first kidney transplants were performed in 1954. Today heart, liver, lung, and pancreas transplants are routinely performed.

Although each organ has specific needs and some procedures vary with the organ, the initial surgical approach to recovery of any vascular organ is the same (Fig. 18–1).

The operative procedure begins when access to the peritoneal cavity is established through a long midline incision extending from the sternal notch to the symphysis pubis. With this approach, all organs, including kidneys, liver, heart, lungs, and pancreas, can easily be recovered. Brief descriptions of procedures for individual organs follow.

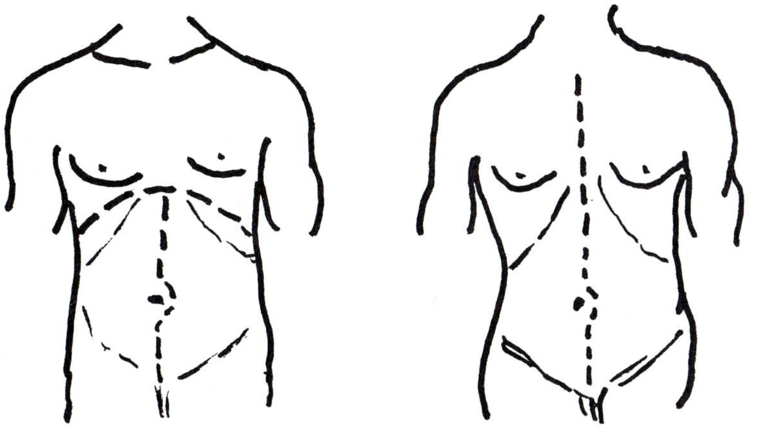

Figure 18–1. Incisions frequently used for organ transplantation.

KIDNEY—METHOD OF REMOVAL

After the initial incision is made, the abdominal contents are examined for evidence of penetrating wounds, hematomas, or lacerations within. The next step in performing a bilateral en bloc nephrectomy (kidney recovery) is incision of the posterior parietal peritoneum in the area of the cecum and dissection of the attachments to the bowel. The inferior and superior celiac vessels are identified, ligated, and divided, and the lateral attachments to the kidneys freed. The aorta and vena cava are identified and freed just below the diaphragm. Umbilical tapes are then placed around these structures.

The next step is to identify the abdominal aorta and vena cava proximal to the common iliac arteries. These vessels are freed and both are encircled with umbilical tapes. The lumbar vessels are then identified, ligated, and divided. Both ureters are freed from deep within the pelvis. At this point, the donor is administered heparin (approximately 300 units per kilogram body weight), and cannulas are introduced into the aorta and vena cava just above the bifurcation. The distal aorta and vena cava are ligated and divided. At this point, approximately 2 liters of cold Collins solution (an isotonic solution) is infused. The kidneys are then lifted out of the abdomen and placed in containers for transport to the transplant centers.

Lymph nodes from the small bowel mesentery or pruritic region are recovered. These lymph nodes, along with the spleen which is also recovered, are used for tissue typing. Finally, the iliac arteries and veins are dissected out and taken as vascular grafts.

LIVER—METHOD OF REMOVAL

Removal of the liver requires some modification of the procedure used for kidney recovery. The peritoneal cavity is accessed as in kidney recovery. First, the left triangular ligament is identified and divided. The gastrohepatic ligament is then divided and the hilum encircled. Hilar structures are carefully dissected out and identified. The common bile duct is then divided. The gallbladder is opened and bile washed out with a saline solution. The gastroduodenal artery is then identified and ligated distally. The splenic artery is identified, encircled, and divided distally. Similarly, the left gastric artery is identified, encircled, and divided distally. If the pancreas is not to be recovered, the pancreatic tissues are swept inferiorly, identifying the splenic vein and superior mesenteric vein, which are both ligated and divided.

Next, the portal vein is lifted to identify any apparent right hepatic artery branches arising from the superior mesenteric artery. The superior mesenteric artery is identified and cleaned down to the aorta, making sure not to injure the renal vessels. The inferior mesenteric vein is isolated and cannulated. Heparin is also administered prior to this step. At this point, the dissection of the vessels needed for kidney recovery takes place. Approximately 5 liters of cold Collins solution is introduced into the aorta and portal vein. Then, the diaphragm around the liver is divided to mobilize the liver. The infrahepatic vena cava is identified, encircled, and divided superior to the takeoff of the renal veins. The remaining tissues attaching the liver posteriorly are carefully divided and the liver is carefully removed.

HEART—METHOD OF REMOVAL

The same incision employed for liver and kidney recovery can also be used in a cardiectomy. Removal of the heart for transplantation is a relatively simple procedure. The ascending aorta is identified and dissected to the aortic arch. Limited dissection of the heart is carried out at this point to free all attachments. After administration of heparin, a 12-gauge angiocath is inserted into the aortic arch and sutured in place (using a pursestring suture). The superior vena cava is stapled and the heart allowed to partially empty.

The aorta is included in a cold cardioplegic solution [1 liter containing 5% dextrose in water (D_5W), mannitol, sodium bicarbonate, and potassium] which is then infused. The inferior vena cava is transected to prevent escape of the cardioplegic solution. Subsequently, the left and right pulmonary veins, the left and right pulmonary arteries, and the distal aorta are transected. The distal portion of the aorta is stapled as was the superior vena cava. The remaining attachments for the heart are transected and the heart is removed.

HEART/LUNGS—METHOD OF REMOVAL

Excision of the heart and lungs for a combined heart/lung transplant requires slight modification. Limited dissection of the heart and lungs is performed to separate the aorta from the pulmonary artery and to isolate the inferior vena cava. A pursestring suture is placed in the pulmonary artery, through which an 18-French sump pump drain is inserted after anticoagulant is administered. Again, a cardioplegic needle is inserted into the ascending aspect of the aorta. After anticoagulant is administered, the cardioplegic solution is infused. The inferior vena cava is transected to prevent distension of the heart. After approximately 500 milliliters of cardioplegic solution is infused, the infusion into the pulmonary artery is begun.

At this point, the tip of the left atrial appendage is excised also to prevent distension of the heart. The aorta is transected distal to the cardioplegic needle. First the inferior pulmonary ligaments and then the inferior vena cava are divided. The dissection is carried out along the anterior aspect of the esophagus to the middle of the ascending aorta. The ascending aorta is then transected.

The superior vena cava is stapled and then transected. Dissection is carried along the trachea to a point three rings above the carina and the trachea is transected. Other attachments holding the heart and lungs in place are transected and the heart and lungs removed.

PANCREAS—METHOD OF REMOVAL

Recovery of the pancreas for transplantation is carried out similarly to recovery of the liver. The spleen is freed from its parietal attachments and the tail of the pancreas is dissected free, including division of short gastric vessels. The diaphragmatic crura are divided, which permits control of the aorta above the celiac artery. Nerve tissue and lymphatic structures are divided to the left of the aorta. Next, a full Kocher maneuver is performed and the entire head of the pancreas is freed so the pancreas and superior mesenteric vessels can be elevated from the retroperitoneum.

The structures in the portal hepatis are dissected and the common bowel duct is ligated, leaving the hepatic artery and portal vein intact. Dissection is carried out along the right side of the aorta. The mesenteric vessels are dissected free. The duodenum is carefully dissected off the pancreas, taking care to ligate all the small vessels. As with all other procedures, the donor is administered heparin and cannulas are placed in the aorta and vena cava. Before the aorta is tied off, the hepatic artery distal to the gastroduodenal artery and the superior mesenteric artery and vein are ligated below the branches to the pancreas. The aorta is clamped above the iliac artery, and the vena cava is clamped just below the liver. The portal vein is divided at its bifurcation. The duodenum is divided below the pleuras between a row of staples, preserving a short duodenal segment. The pancreas, spleen, and duodenal segment are removed. The incision is closed using a running suture.

TREATMENT AFTER VISCERAL ORGAN REMOVAL

Bodies in which one or more organs have been removed from the thoracic or abdominal cavity must be considered separately, in the light of several factors:

1. Heparin has been run through the vascular system. This decreases postmortem clotting.
2. There has been a delay between death and embalming. Generally, a stronger-than-average arterial solution is required.
3. Circulation may be interrupted. Strong arterial solutions containing tracer dyes are needed.

TREATMENT AFTER HEART/LUNG REMOVAL

An embalmer may use the following protocol in embalming a body following heart/lung removal:

1. Inject, from inside the thoracic cavity, the right and left subclavian arteries to prepare the arms and shoulders.
2. Inject the right and left common cartoid arteries to prepare the head.
3. Inject down the abdominal aorta to preserve the abdominal viscera, trunk walls, and legs. **Or,** inject the right femoral artery distally to embalm the right leg and then inject toward the trunk. Clamp off the abdominal aorta in the thoracic cavity. This embalms the left leg, abdominal contents, and trunk walls.
4. If the walls of the thoracic cavity require additional fluid, use hypodermic injection.
5. Fill the thoracic cavity with absorbent material saturated with cavity fluid. The walls may also be painted with autopsy gels. Suture the incision closed.
6. Aspirate and inject the abdominal cavity.

TREATMENT AFTER ABDOMINAL CAVITY ORGAN REMOVAL

In the removal of organs from the abdominal cavity, when the liver, kidneys, or pancreas has been removed, two major techniques are employed (Fig. 18–2):

Method 1. The body is injected sectionally from the right and left femoral, right and left axillary, and right and left common carotid arteries. Trunk walls are treated by hypodermic injection and the sutures closed. Then, the thoracic and abdominal cavities are aspirated and injected.

Method 2. In most removals of organs from the abdominal cavity, the abdominal aorta and common iliac arteries are also removed. The following protocols may be used:

1. Inject the abdominal aorta toward the head to embalm the arms, head, and chest and trunk areas.
2. Separately inject the legs from the femoral or external iliac arteries (from inside the abdominal cavity); if the internal iliac arteries are present these should be injected to preserve the buttocks and anal and perianal areas.

OR

1. Ligate the thoracic abdominal aorta. Inject the right common carotid artery toward the trunk. This embalms the left side of the head, the arms, and the chest and trunk areas. Inject the right common carotid artery to embalm the right side of the head.
2. Raise and inject the femoral arteries to preserve the legs.

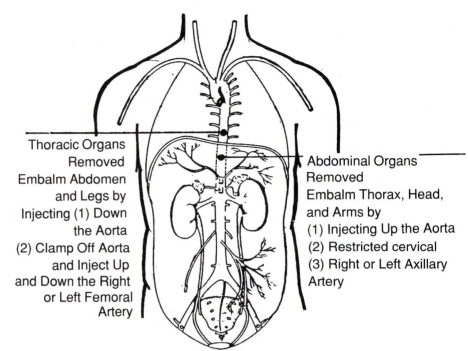

Thoracic Organs Removed
Embalm Abdomen and Legs by Injecting (1) Down the Aorta (2) Clamp Off Aorta and Inject Up and Down the Right or Left Femoral Artery

Abdominal Organs Removed
Embalm Thorax, Head, and Arms by (1) Injecting Up the Aorta (2) Restricted cervical (3) Right or Left Axillary Artery

Figure 18–2. Embalming sites in bodies from which organs have been removed.

3. Treat the abdominal walls by hypodermic injection.
4. Close the abdominal incision. Aspirate the cavities and inject cavity fluid.

TREATMENT AFTER EYE ENUCLEATION

One of the tissues most commonly transplanted today is the human cornea. Approximately 30,000 individuals undergo corneal transplantation every year. The need for corneal tissue, like all other organs and tissues, continues to grow. Although the cornea itself can be removed from the organ donor, most frequently the eye is enucleated.

The first step in excising the eye is separation of the conjunctiva from the eyeball. Next, the four rectus muscles and the two oblique muscles that control eyeball movement are cut. The final step in removing the eyeball from its socket is to cut the optic nerve. This procedure can be carried out under nonsterile conditions and is one of the few procedures carried out in this manner. The eye is then placed in a container, refrigerated, and immediately delivered to an eye bank.

Swelling is the most common problem encountered in treatment of the enucleated eye. In addition, ecchymosis may be present, and there is always the possibility of small lacerations.

To help control swelling of the eyelids during embalming, the following procedures are recommended:

1. Use restricted cervical injection to control arterial solution entering the head.
2. Avoid preinjection fluid use.
3. Do not use "weak" arterial solutions; use solutions slightly stronger than average.
4. Avoid excessive manipulation of the lids prior to and during embalming.
5. Let the eye "drain" embalming solution during arterial injection.
6. Avoid rapid rates of flow and high injection pressures during arterial injection.

The following treatments have produced very satisfactory results:

1. Remove packing from the eye.
2. Saturate pieces of cotton with "autopsy gel" and *loosely* fill the orbital cavity. Autopsy gel on the outside of the eyelids will not create additional problems.
3. Fill the eye with sufficient cotton to recreate the normal appearance of the closed eye.
4. Embalm the body; use the procedures previously suggested to avoid swelling. If swelling does begin, strengthen the arterial solution so only a minimum amount can be injected. Stop injection if swelling becomes excessive, and, if necessary, use surface embalming.
5. After arterial injection, remove the cotton saturated with autopsy gel and dry out the orbit.

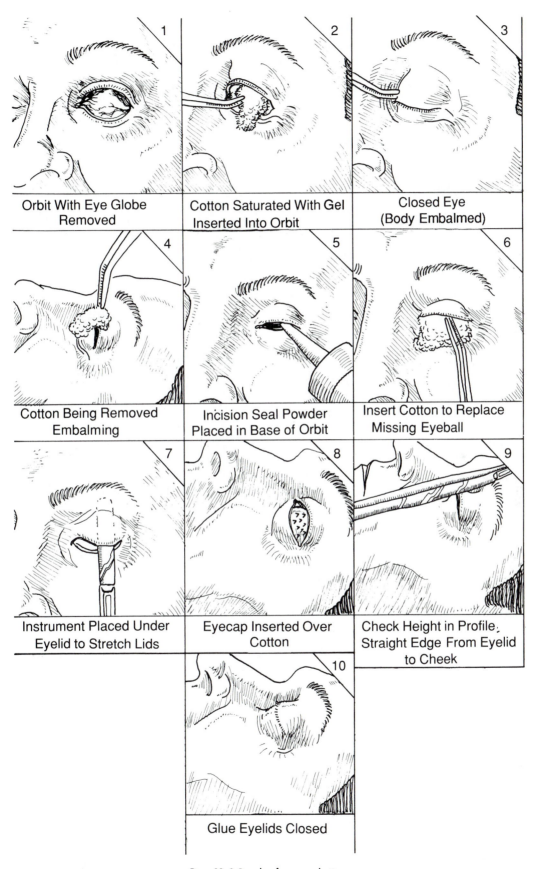

Figure 18–3. Procedure for eye enucleation.

6. Carefully place a small amount of incision seal powder or mortuary putty in the base of the orbit.
7. Pack the eye globe with cotton, kapoc, or mortuary putty.
8. Exercise the eyelids and insert an eyecap over the filler.
9. Glue the eyelids closed.

In this method, major treatment of the eye occurs *after* the arterial injection (Fig. 18–3).

TREATMENT AFTER CORNEA REMOVAL

When only the cornea has been removed, the preparation work is greatly reduced. The body can be embalmed using whatever injection technique and arterial solution strength the embalmer feels necessary. The eyes can be set after the arterial injection.

As the front of the eye is opened when the cornea is removed, the embalmer may find it necessary to aspirate the fluids from the eye to prevent leakage. A large-diameter hypodermic needle can be used to aspirate these fluids, as can the standard aspirator. The needle is inserted through the opening created by the removed cornea. The eye is then filled with "mortuary putty" by passing the nozzle of the gun used to inject this material through the opening in the eye (incision seal may also be used). A cap can then be placed over the eyeball to prevent the eye from appearing sunken. The eyelids can be secured with super glue.

TREATMENT AFTER VERTEBRAL BODY REMOVAL FOR BONE MARROW

After vascular organs are removed, and before closure, vertebral bodies (L-5/S-1) are sterilely recovered from the abdominal cavity. Using curved Mayo scissors, dissect all muscle attachments away from the vertebral bodies bilaterally from L-5 to S-1.

Starting at L-5/S-1, the middle of the intervertebral disk space is transected using a straight lambotte osteotome. Three disk spaces to L-4/L-2, the disk is also transected.

Using a curved lambotte osteotome, transect the pediculus bilaterally. Using curved Mayo scissors, dissect all remaining attachments along the vertebral bodies to be removed. The same procedure is used to remove vertebral bodies T-12 to L-1.

Removal of the lumbar vertebral bodies does not present a difficult problem for the embalmer. If portions of the large and small intestines are still located within the abdominal cavity, it may difficult to identify the vertebral bodies. As removal of the bodies interrupts circulation to the surrounding tissues, the embalmer can en-

sure preservation by hypodermic treatment of these lower back tissues with cavity fluid. The hypodermic treatment is carried out most successfully from within the abdominal cavity.

Care should be given to treatment of the large psoas muscles and the quadratus muscles. If abdominal organs remain in the cavity, the embalmer should suture the incisions made for removal of the transplant organs and the vertebral bodies. Then, the cavity should be aspirated and cavity fluid injected. The cavity fluid assists in preserving the tissues of the lower back. If all the organs have been removed from the abdominal cavity along with the vertebral bodies, then the lower back can be painted with autopsy gel. These gels penetrate and preserve the tissues. Hardening and embalming powders have neither the penetrating ability nor the preservative action of autopsy gels.

If autopsy gels are not available, the embalmer can place cotton saturated with cavity fluid in the posterior portion of the abdominal cavity. The cavity can be filled with sheeting and the sheeting soaked with cavity fluid. This ensures preservation of the trunk walls.

LONG BONE RECOVERY AND TREATMENT

As already mentioned, tissue recovery for transplantation is increasing, and more than 200,000 individuals every year are in need of some type of cadaveric tissue for transplantation.

The following procedure is used to remove the ilium, femoral head, femur, tibia, Achilles tendon, and fibula for transplantation: An initial skin incision is made from the posterior third of the ilium along the crest, down the vertical aspect of the thigh extending distal to below the ankle, laterally circumventing the patella. Using blunt dissection, the anterior fascia is separated from the skin while the posterior is separated from the muscle. With sharp dissection, the fascia is transected just superior to the knee and just distal to the lesser trochanter. Dissection is continued along the lateral edge at the table level. The fascia lata is removed (Fig. 18–4).

With a scalpel, the quadriceps muscles are dissected to expose the femoral shaft superior to the condyles. The quadriceps tendon is dissected superior to the patella. The hamstring muscle group is dissected to completely expose the femoral shaft. The femur is disarticulated from the tibia and the femoral head is disarticulated from the acetabulum. The entire femur is then removed. All muscles are transected from the tibia with a scalpel. The capitular and anterior tibiofibular ligaments are transected along the tibia, patella, and patellar ligament to be removed.

A procedure similar to that for the tibia is used to recover the fibula and remove it from the field.

The Achilles tendon is separated from the muscle with a scalpel, and a straight osteotome is used to cut the

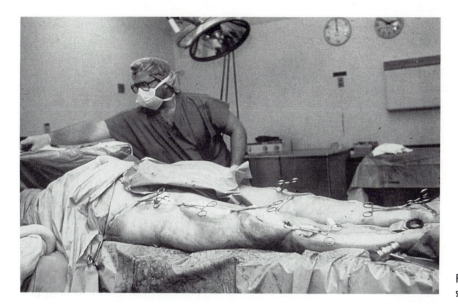

Figure 18–4. Removal of long bones from the legs. Performed under sterile conditions.

anterior portion of the ankle. This portion, along with the Achilles tendon, is recovered intact and removed from the field.

By sharp and blunt dissection, the muscles and tendons are separated from the ilium on the interior and posterior sides down to the sacroiliac junction. With a curved osteotome, the ilium is separated at the sacroiliac junction. By use of a straight osteotome, an osteotomy is made from the interior inferior spine of the ilium to join the other osteotomy at the sacroiliac joint and acetabulum. The ilium is removed.

An additional skin incision is made to remove the entire humerus. A surgical incision is made on the ventral aspect of the shoulder, originating at the level of the acromion process and extending to the elbow. Sharp dissection is used to separate the deltoid and biceps brachii muscle groups from the humerus. The humeral head is disarticulated by dissecting the rotator cuff free of the glenoid fossa. The humerus is disarticulated at the radical head. Remaining muscles and ligaments are transected and the humerus is removed.

After these tissues are removed, a wooden dowel approximately 1 inch in diameter is inserted. On the lower extremities one end of a plastic prosthetic dowel is placed in the extraterritorial region against the superficial aspect of the peritoneum in the right and left pugilistic area. The lower end is placed against the talus. A No. 2 cotton and a cutting needle are used to close the quadriceps muscle groups around the dowel. The skin incision is closed with a tight running baseball stitch. A similar procedure is used to reconstruct the humerus.

Long bone recovery is the most dramatic of all tissue recovery. It involves a great amount of time, not only for the removal but for the treatment by the embalmer. When the body is received by the funeral home, the long incisions on the arms, shoulders, thighs, and lower legs are sutured. The body has form because the bones have

been replaced with wooden dowels by the recovery team at the hospital. If there has been an autopsy or if other visceral organs have been removed for transplantation, sectional injection is necessary. If there has been no autopsy and no other organs have been donated, standard embalming injection can be used.

Because of the delay and the large interruption of circulation, fluid strength should be increased. *These bodies should not be preinjected.* The increased strength of the arterial solution does two things: (1) The small volume of fluid that is distributed to the tissues and muscles of the arms and legs provides satisfactory preservation. (2) As so much fluid is lost in the tissues of the arms and legs, while the incisions are still closed, the fluid acts as an osmotic solution to help preserve the tissues. Two methods of preparation of the legs are discussed. In the first technique the incisions are opened; in the second, if the sutures are tight they are not opened.

Method 1. Supports, such as head blocks, can be placed along the medial and lateral sides of the legs in preparation for removing the sutures. This work practice helps to create a "channel" to drain blood and embalming chemicals down to the foot of the table, thus allowing the embalmer to maintain a cleaner work area.

In those cases where the donor's legs have been sutured, ALL suture lines are removed from the extremities, followed by removal to the prosthesis. This provides unobstructed access to the tissue beds. The embalmer then locates and identifies the ligatures of the obturator, lateral femoral circumflex, and popliteal arteries that were put in place by the procurement team.

The embalmer dissects and ligates the left and right femoral arteries to isolate each extremity for injection separately from the rest of the body.

The trunk, hips, head, neck, and upper extremities of the body can be injected by using cervical and/or femoral vessels as injection and drainage sites. If necessary, the embalmer can choose other injection sites as needed to complete this portion of the preparation.

Care is taken to ensure that embalming solution *does not* free flow into either of the lower extremities during injection of the trunk, hips, head, neck, and upper extremities.

The thigh and leg areas are injected by using the left and right femoral arteries. Care is taken to clamp off other vessels, as loss of embalming solution becomes apparent. Particular attention is paid to the multiple branches of the genicular arteries found just above the knee, because they will likely have been cut during sharp dissection. A large number of hemostats may be required.

The leg and foot are injected by using the left and right popliteal arteries. In some instances, the popliteal may not be accessible and the embalmer uses the superior aspects of either the anterior or posterior tibial artery for injection. Care is again taken to clamp off other vessels, as loss of embalming solution becomes apparent.

Here, also, the multiple branches of the genicular arteries found just below the knee will likely have been cut during sharp dissection. A large number of hemostats may be required.

Hypodermic injection may be required to supplement arterial injection. The embalmer must carefully assess the success of arterial injection to determine where hypodermic supplement might be required.

At the conclusion of the arterial and hypodermic injections, the embalmer dries the tissue bed with absorbent cotton.

The prosthetic device is then placed back into position.

A light coating of hardening compound is applied to the tissue beds. It is to the embalmer's advantage to use a substance that has both preservative and absorptive qualities.

The incisions are then sutured closed. Care is taken by the embalmer to make the sutures tight. Additional hardening compound may be added during the suturing process.

Following suturing, the body is thoroughly bathed.

Cotton and liquid sealer are then applied to the incision to provide an additional barrier to leakage.

Finally, plastic stockings are placed on the legs as a further barrier to leakage.

The body is now ready for dressing and casketing.

Method 2. There is a second method of preparing the lower extremities when the long bones (femur, tibia, and fibula) have been removed. This method leaves the transplant surgeon's sutures in place. If tight baseball stitches have been used to close the incisions, leakage from these sutures should be minimal. Raise the right and left external iliac arteries (or right and left femoral arteries) and insert arterial tubes directed down the legs in each vessel. Prepare an arterial solution of very strong concentration: a high-index arterial fluid with equal parts of wa-

ter or 100% arterial fluid. Inject each leg using at least a half-gallon of solution. The tissues of the leg will distend slightly. Be certain the solution has reached portions of the leg below the knee. Stop the injection and let the fluids saturate the tissues while the arms and head and trunk areas of the body are embalmed. After the solution has had time to thoroughly saturate the tissues of the legs, with a scalpel, place a puncture in the area of the heel. Insert a drain tube or trocar and force as much of the solution as possible from the leg. The transplant surgeons have placed dowels into the legs and heavily padded them with gauze sponges. The concentrated arterial solution will be soaked up by the sponges. These will now act as an internal compress. The recovery surgeon's sutures can be coated with a surface glue and the leg placed in a plastic stocking containing preservative powder or autopsy gel.

When bones have been removed from the shoulder, the arms can be injected through the axillary or brachial arteries. These sutures (for shoulder–bone removal) should always be opened and the area drained following arterial injection of the arms. Local hypodermic treatment using a concentrated arterial solution may be necessary. A liberal amount of incision seal powder can be placed in the cavity created by the removed bones and the incisions sealed with a tight baseball suture. A surface glue should be applied after the body is washed and dried.

SKIN RECOVERY AND TREATMENT

The entire area to be used is shaved and disinfected. Generally, skin is recovered from the nipple line area to midthigh on both the anterior and posterior sides of the body. An instrument called a **dermatome** is used to peel off very thin layers of skin (Fig. 18–5), approximately 1/15,000th inch thick and approximately 3 inches wide. These layers are about as thick as layers of skin lost in sunburn. Occasionally, after skin recovery, the donor appears to have a sunburn.

The recovery of skin from the dead human body for transplantation is not as dramatic as may be inferred. The skin removed is "tissue paper" in thickness. Skin recovery presents two major problems for the embalmer: (1) drying of the areas from which the skin has been removed and (2) control of leakage from the areas where the skin has been removed. The body should be unwrapped and the surface sprayed with a disinfectant. Next, the body should be washed with a liquid soap and warm water. This solution removes sterilant that was swabbed on the body areas from which the skin was removed. In addition, it removes fluid or blood that may have seeped through the regions where the skin was removed (Fig. 18–6).

Next, the body is positioned on the table. This may be difficult, as bodies have a tendency to "slip" when skin has been recovered from the back, buttocks, or backs of

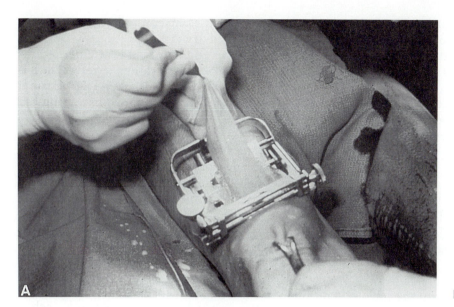

Figure 18–5. Skin recovery.

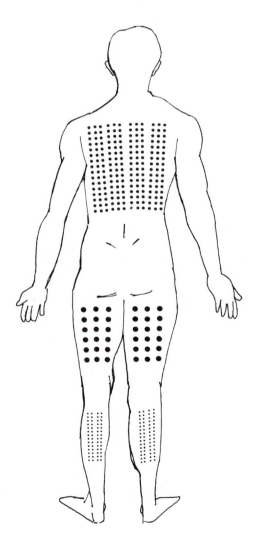

Figure 18–6. Areas from which skin is most often removed.

the legs. A towel can be placed beneath the body to help position it. In addition, the degree of slant of the embalming table can be changed to stabilize the body.

Body conditions dictate the fluid strength, but to dry the tissues, a stronger-than-average solution should be used. A special-purpose high-index fluid can be used along with a suitable coinjection chemical. Lanolin fluid as well as humectant coinjections should be avoided. If restricted cervical injection is used, a separate, milder solution may be injected to embalm the head. During injection, some of the fluid may seep through the areas from which the skin has been taken. This ensures good preservation and drying of the tissues.

After arterial injection is complete several techniques, depending on the chemicals available, can be utilized to treat the raw tissue areas:

1. Paint the raw tissue with a phenol cautery. This chemical works very rapidly to dry tissue. The area should be cauterized in 20 minutes. It can be painted on or applied in surface packs.
2. Cavity packs can be applied to the raw skin areas. Undiluted cavity fluid can be difficult to work with because of the formaldehyde fumes. Cover the saturated cotton with plastic to reduce the fumes. These packs should remain in place several hours.
3. Autopsy gel can be painted over the raw skin or applied on a cotton surface pack. The gel should be given time to work.

In all the preceding treatments, the tissues should be dried after surface applications. A hair dryer can be used to speed the drying. This drying helps to prevent further leakage. Simply exposing the raw skin areas to the air (after removing surface packs) helps them to dry. Plastic coveralls and stockings should be placed on the body, and an embalming powder can be sprinkled inside these plastic garments. The plastic garments serve as added protection against leakage.

After drying, some embalmers prefer to cover the raw skin with a surface glue, over which they place cotton. This is not necessary if the plastic garments are used.

MANDIBLE RECOVERY

At present, because the prostheses available for reconstruction are not exact fits, human mandibles for transplantation are recovered usually from patients who will not be viewed.

No external incisions are made to remove mandibles. Both blunt and sharp dissection is used to free the mandible from all muscle and ligament attachments. It is disarticulated at the temporal bone and removed. A prosthetic mandible is implanted and tac sutured in place.

RIB RECOVERY

Ribs are usually recovered through the same incision used for vascular organ recovery. After organ recovery, a scalpel is used to peel back the skin from the rib cage area. Only every other rib is removed. The rib, with cartilage attached, is disarticulated from the sternum. Sharp dissection is used to separate the rib from muscle tissue.

A rib cutter is used to cut the rib approximately 10 to 15 centimeters from the rib cage. After recovery, the cartilage is separated from the rib and processed separately from the rib. As only every other rib is removed, no reconstruction is carried out.

TEMPORAL BONE RECOVERY AND TREATMENT

Two techniques are employed to recover the temporal bone: an exterior approach and an internal approach. The internal approach is most commonly used to recover the bone during autopsy procedures. This ensures that no disfigurement appears. The recovery process, however, in both procedures is almost identical. Soft tissues and periosteum are scraped from the mastoid with a chisel. All tissue forward of the external auditory canal is elevated. After the external auditory canal is identified it is transected. Soft tissue is further elevated from the bone around the open ear canal.

A plug cutter is placed on the mastoid bone so that it is centered over the external auditory canal. It is moved posteriorly so the front of the blade is at the anterior edge of the external auditory canal. The plug cutter is angled

20° backward so that it points toward the opposite temple. Pressure is applied to a drill attached to the plug cutter, and the drilling is continued until the plug cutter is completely embedded in the incision. After drilling is complete, chisel cuts must be made around the temporal bone specimen to sever the deep bony attachments. At this point, any soft tissue attachments can be cut by sharp dissection. As the temporal bone becomes more mobile, a twisting motion frees it from its last attachment.

If an internal approach is used (Fig. 18–7), there should be no problems with embalming. If the external approach is used, the technique begins with a curved incision 1 inch behind the ear crease that extends from above the ear to the mastoid tip. This poses some additional challenges for the embalmer.

The major problem encountered after removal of the inner ear bone by the internal approach is that the upper portions of the face and the eyes do not receive sufficient arterial fluid. The embalmer can use tracer dye to check circulation to the various facial regions. Care should also be taken to check for arterial fluid leakage from the base of the skull, where the temporal bone was removed.

Generally, leakage can be controlled with hemostats or by placing a ball of cotton into the area where the temporal bone has been removed and applying hand pressure. After embalming, mortuary putty or incision seal powder can be placed in the area from which the bone was removed. Some embalmers prefer plaster of Paris as a filler for this cavity. These measures ensure against further leakage from the external ear and also from the scalp. Plenty of absorbent cotton filler can be placed in the cranial cavity prior to suturing the scalp.

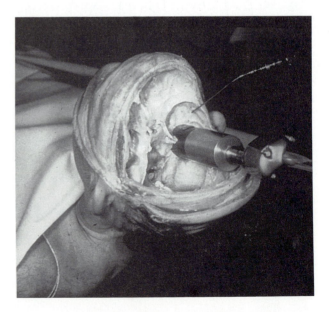

Figure 18–7. Temporal bone recovery—internal approach.

It is wise to pack the external auditory meatus with cotton and some incision seal powder to prevent leakage from the external ear.

If the bone was removed by the external approach and the ear has been partially excised after embalming, the temporal area should be packed with a phenol cautery agent. This material should be left in place for a time, then replaced with dry cotton and incision seal powder. Mortuary putty could also be used as a filler. The ear can be reattached with interdermal sutures or super glue.

CONCLUSIONS

Organ and tissue donation is becoming everyday practice in the United States and other countries. Almost everyone can donate some organ or tissue for transplantation or research. Although most organ donors are under the age of 65, bone, skin, and eye donors can be well beyond that age. It is imperative that funeral directors and embalmers recognize that they play an important role in the donation process. If families are concerned that funeral wishes cannot be carried out, they will be reluctant to donate organs and tissues for transplantation. This will jeopardize thousands of lives and cause many patients unneeded excess pain and expense.

KEY TERMS AND CONCEPTS FOR STUDY AND DISCUSSION

1. Describe the embalming of a body from which only the heart has been removed.
2. Describe the embalming of a body from which only the eyes have been removed.
3. Describe the embalming of a body from which the abdominal organs have been removed.
4. List procedures that can be used to help prevent or control swelling of the eyelids in the embalming of a body from which the eyes have been removed.
5. Describe treatment for the legs when the long bones have been removed.
6. Describe treatment when skin has been removed.

BIBLIOGRAPHY

A Killer Among Us. Audiovisual. Boston: Dodge Chemical Co.

Community Participation Manual. Birmingham: Alabama Regional Organ Bank, 1983.

Helen Keller Memorial Hospital Lions Eye and Temporal Bone Bank, 1985 Protocol. Sheffield, AL.

Klitzke K, Kroshus JM, Stroud DE. Embalming techniques in long bone donation cases. *The American Funeral Director* 1995;118:26.

Koosmann S. Bone transplantation. In: *Champion Expanding Encyclopedia.* Springfield, OH: Champion Chemical Co.; 1984: Nos. 549 and 550, pp. 2210–2217.

Mayer RG. Enucleation restoration. In: *Champion Expanding Encyclopedia.* Springfield, OH: Champion Chemical Co.; 1987: No. 577, pp. 2322–2325.

Organ and Tissue Procurement Manual. Pittsburgh; 1986.

Pittsburgh Transplant Foundation, 1986 protocol, Pittsburgh; 1986.

Sawyer D. Split skin homografts. *Dodge Mag* 1977;69:2.

Starzl TE, Hakala TR, Shaw BW, et al. A flexible procedure for multiple cadaveric organ procurement. *Surg Gynecol Obstet* 1984;158:1–8.

19

Delayed Embalming

The postmortem period between death and preparation of the body plays an important role in determining the proper embalming technique. It is during this period that the postmortem changes occur within the body. These changes include algor mortis, hypostasis of the blood, livor mortis, dehydration, increase in blood viscosity, decomposition, change in body pH, rigor mortis, postmortem stain, postmortem caloricity, and hydrolysis.

These changes do not always occur in a uniform manner in the tissues of the body. For example, rigor may be present in some muscles but will have passed in others. Also, tissue pH varies and heat is retained by some tissues (e.g., viscera) but rapidly lost from others (e.g., extremities). Decomposition may be present in a gangrenous limb but not in other body areas. These changes are greatly influenced by the length of time between death and preparation and the temperature of the environment during that period.

As a general rule, most postmortem changes are speeded by a warm environment or by the presence of heat. An exception is algor mortis. The longer the period between death and embalming the more changes can be expected to occur. From an embalming standpoint, the longer the delay the more problems the embalmer may expect to encounter. As time passes, the preservative demands of the various tissues increase.

Figure 19–1 illustrates the gradual increase in the demand for preservative. Increased temperature increases the preservative demand, because the higher temperature speeds the decomposition of the proteins. A shift to a more alkaline pH increases preservative demand. Autolysis and putrefaction produces an increased number of sites for the union of preservative and the products of protein decomposition. Bodies from which rigor has passed and those showing early signs of decomposition have a very high preservative demand. Bodies in a state of rigor mortis have very little preservative demand, for the proteins are engaged in such a manner that they are not free to make contact with the preservative. After the rigor passes, however, the demand increases. Thus, in preparing a body in which most of the muscles are in a state of rigor, the embalmer must saturate the tissues with a strong arterial solution so that the preservative is available to make contact with the protein as the muscle fibers begin to pass from this contracted state of rigor.

Bodies in three postmortem states are discussed in this chapter: (1) bodies in a state of intense rigor mortis, (2) bodies from which rigor has passed and in which early signs of decomposition are observed, (3) bodies refrigerated for long periods. The techniques used to prepare all of these bodies are almost the same. The embalmer must understand the specific problems presented by each body type as well as the reasons for using the prescribed technique. These techniques vary with other body factors, such as age, weight, general body nutrition, and the effects of diseases or medications.

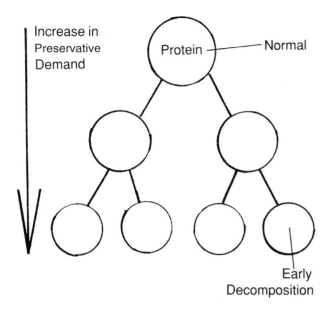

Increase in Preservative Demand

Protein — Normal

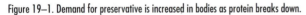

Early Decomposition

Figure 19–1. Demand for preservative is increased in bodies as protein breaks down.

The three body types listed all show some degree of delay. Generally, the longer the period between death and preparation, the more problems can be anticipated. Temperature also affects all three categories. Elevation of environmental temperature speeds both rigor mortis and decomposition cycles. Low temperatures can also slow these cycles, but during refrigeration, *autolysis* and bacterial enzymes continue tissue breakdown. Low temperatures can slow arterial solution diffusion but increase capillary permeability. Increased capillary permeability can result in tissue distension during arterial solution injection. Lowered temperature affects all chemical reactions, so bodies can be expected to firm more slowly after refrigeration.

Preservative absorption by tissue proteins is usually greatest immediately after injection. Most bodies exhibit some degree of firming during the injection process. One reason for this early fixation is that the concentration of preservative (fixative) is greatest when the arterial solution is first introduced into the tissues. If a sufficient amount of preservative has been injected, complete firming of the body will occur several hours to a day later. Degree of decomposition, tissue pH, and temperature and concentration of arterial solution all play a role in determining the speed and degree of fixation. Cool temperature slows these reactions, alkaline pH above 7.4 slows fixation, and decomposed protein demands more concentrated preservative.

Arterial fluids vary. Some are buffered to act slowly (slow-firming fluids) and others are buffered to fix tissues rapidly (buffered-acid fast-firming fluids). It is imperative that the embalmer provide sufficient preservative to

the tissues to meet the total preservative demands of the tissues. **It is better to overembalm than to underembalm body tissues.**

All these bodies have a high preservative demand. This increased fluid need is brought about by the breakdown of tissues. As circulation is impaired in most of these bodies, distribution problems can be anticipated. As these bodies are all subject to distension, use *of a minimum amount* of *a stronger* arterial solution best establishes good preservation and minimizes tissue distension. Strong (hypertonic) arterial solution help to minimize swelling of the tissues.

INJECTION PROTOCOL

The suggested order of arterial treatment for the bodies discussed in this chapter follows.

Injection and Drainage Sites

For injection and drainage, *restricted cervical injection* is the first choice in the embalming of the unautopsied body. *Both* the right and the left common carotid arteries are raised. A tube is placed in each artery directed toward the head, and the tubes are left open. Another tube placed in the right common carotid is directed toward the trunk. The trunk is injected first. The head is injected through the left common carotid and then the right common carotid. Drainage may be taken from the right internal jugular vein.

The second choice would be to begin the preparation using a six-point injection.

The third choice is use of the right common carotid artery for injection and the right internal jugular vein for drainage.

Use of the one-point injection is not recommended. It affords no control over the amount of arterial solution entering the head or over swelling of neck or facial tissues.

Arterial Solution Strength

As previously stated, a stronger-than-average arterial solution is needed for the bodies discussed in this chapter, especially when signs of decomposition are evident. A *high-index special-purpose fluid* is best for the preparation of these bodies. If this fluid is not available, an arterial fluid of 25 index or higher should be selected.

In preparing the arterial solution the first recommendation is to follow the suggestions of the manufacturer. Many labels carry dilution instructions for delayed, refrigerated, or decomposed bodies. Preinjection fluids should be avoided. Use of a coinjection would be a better choice.

The first half-gallon may be made milder in an attempt to clear blood discolorations in the unautopsied body, but should be followed by stronger fluid solutions, 2.0% strength or higher. In the treatment of bodies that show evidence of decomposition, 100% arterial fluid with a coinjection fluid may be required. If a body is exhibiting advanced signs of decomposition and restricted cervical injection or a six-point injection is used, the head can be injected using a waterless embalming technique. For extreme situations, the instant tissue fixation method may be helpful. This helps to minimize swelling of the face and establishes maximum fluid distribution throughout the facial tissues.

Volume of Arterial Solution

The amount of solution injected depends on the size of the body and the success in distributing the arterial solution.

Order of Injection

The following order of injection is recommended when there has been a delay between death and preparation, when intense rigor is present, when the body has been refrigerated a long time, or when decomposition is evident:

1. Raise the right and the left common carotid arteries.
2. Use the right internal jugular vein for drainage.
3. Place tubes directed toward the head into the right and left common carotid arteries; leave these tubes open. Place one tube directed toward the trunk.
4. Slowly inject about 1 gallon of arterial solution toward the trunk using extra fluid dye.
5. Evaluate the distribution of fluid. If the extremities of the body are not receiving arterial solution, separately arterially inject those areas needing arterial solution.
6. Inject strong arterial solutions by using sufficient pressure and rate of flow to distribute the solution and minimize swelling. Increased pressures and rates of flow can be used for sectional embalming. Pulsation injection is usually helpful. Use firm massage and manipulation to encourage fluid distribution.
7. Embalm the head last, first the left side and then the right side, using a strong arterial solution. Use dye to trace the fluid. For extreme conditions, consider using waterless solutions and instant tissue fixation injection techniques.
8. Evaluate the body and use hypodermic and surface embalming for areas not receiving arterial solution.

Pressure and Rate of Flow

When there has been a long delay between death and embalming, the unautopsied body should be very slowly injected. This minimizes abdominal distension and helps to prevent purge. In addition, slow injection helps to prevent clots in the arterial system from moving (solution flows over the coagula). Rapid injection can easily cause abdominal distension, which can create purge. Even in embalming the "normal" body, the first gallon of arterial fluid is slowly injected; then, the process may be speeded to facilitate distribution of the arterial solution.

In the injection of arms or legs of the autopsied body, higher pressures and faster rates of flow may be needed to establish distribution. Pulsation may be helpful in distributing fluid to the extremities, and higher pressures can be used with pulsation.

A pulsed flow can be created in several ways: use an embalming machine with a pulse setting; manually turn the rate of flow valve on and off; turn the stopcock valve on and off; bend the delivery hose, starting and stopping the flow of fluid.

PREPARATION OF BODIES IN RIGOR MORTIS

One of the most difficult preparations is that of the body in the intense state of *rigor mortis*, in particular, the body that is well nourished and has a well-developed musculature. The death may have been accidental or sudden as in a heart attack or fatal stroke. These bodies with well-developed musculature develop a very intense rigor mortis. It may be impossible for the embalmer to remove this rigor by manipulating the body prior to injection of the arterial solution. Thin bodies, bodies that demonstrate the effects of wasting disease, and bodies in which the musculature is not well developed undergo as complete and intense rigor as the body with good musculature, except that the muscles are not as large and the rigor can be relieved prior to injection.

Rigor is first observed in the average body approximately 2 hours after death. Depending on cause of death, environmental temperature, and activity prior to death, the rigor can occur sooner or be delayed beyond the 2 hours. (See Chapter 5 for further details concerning the rigor mortis cycle in the dead human body.) Rigor comprises three general stages: (1) primary flaccidity, the period in which the rigor develops and is hardly noticeable; (2) the period of rigor; (3) secondary flaccidity, in which the rigor passes from the body. The most problems are

TABLE 19–1. PRESERVATIVE DEMAND OF THE MUSCLE TISSUES DURING RIGOR

Prerigor	Great preservative demand	The protein centers to which preservative attaches and crosslinks the proteins are readily available. Tissue pH is slightly alkaline and fluids work best in this pH range.
Rigor	Little absorption of preservative	The protein centers to which preservative attaches are engaged in maintaining the state of rigor mortis; vessel lumens are reduced so distribution is decreased. Muscle protein is contracted so fluid does not penetrate the muscle fibers well. The acid pH retards the absorption of preservative.
After rigor	Great absorption of preservative	Proteins have disorganized (or broken) and many centers are available for preservative attachment. The alkaline pH increases preservative absorption; nitrogenous wastes increase the need for preservative.

encountered when the body is to be embalmed while in intense rigor.

Table 19–1 summarizes the preservative demand of the muscle tissues during the stages of rigor.

As noted in Table 19–1, a body in rigor requires or absorbs a very small amount of preservative. The problem, however, arises in that once the rigor passes, the demand for preservative increases greatly. **It is imperative that the embalmer saturate the tissues with a well-coordinated solution of sufficient strength to meet the preservative demands of the body when the rigor has passed.** Otherwise, the body will soften not only from the passage of rigor, but from the decomposition processes that break down body proteins. Therefore, bodies embalmed prior to the onset of rigor should be injected with a sufficient strength of arterial solution to meet the preservation needs as determined from body weight and effects of disease or drugs; bodies embalmed during and after rigor mortis need a strong arterial solution.

Problems Associated With Embalming Bodies in Rigor

Rigor may be relieved by physical manipulation of the muscle tissues. Firmly massaging, rotating, flexing, and bending the joints help to relieve the rigor condition. Once broken, the condition does not recur. As previously stated, rigor may be broken when the musculature is not well developed. In well-developed individuals, it may be very difficult to attempt to relieve rigor in areas such as the thighs or upper arms. The following problems may be encountered in the preparation of the body in intense rigor:

1. Positioning may be difficult.
2. The features may be difficult to set if the jaw is firmly fixed.
3. Distribution of fluid may be poor because of the pressure on arteries and the narrowed arterial lumens resulting from contraction of muscle cells in the arterial walls.
4. Drainage may be poor because of the pressure exerted by contracted muscles on the small veins.
5. Tissues tend to swell, because fluid does not pen-

etrate muscles during rigor but flows to surface areas where there is little resistance.
6. The pH of the tissues is not ideal for fluid reactions.
7. Tissues may not firm well after the passage of rigor, because it may not have been possible to inject sufficient quantities of the arterial solution.
8. Firmness of rigor can be a false sign of tissue fixation.

Features. In setting the features of a body in intense rigor, use a towel to firmly manipulate the jaw. Begin by raising the jaw, even if the lips are firmly pressed together. Massaging the temporalis muscles may also be helpful. Firmly push the chin, covering the chin with a towel and pressing firmly with the palm of the hand. Cotton may also be forced into the mouth to help open it. As soon as the lips can be properly aligned, suture or use a needle injector to ensure that the lower jaw remains in the proper position.

Positioning. Firmly rotate, bend, flex, and massage the joints and muscles of the neck, arms, and, if possible, legs. This may be necessary to position the body properly. Relieve the rigor in the arms by first rotating the shoulder joint. Next, flex the elbow and wrist areas. Grasp all the fingers and gently pull them into a straightened position if the hand is firmly closed. To relieve rigor in the legs, exercise the hip joint first. Next, flex the knee joint. Finally, rotate the foot inward very firmly. These manipulations help to relieve some of the rigor present.

Injection. Both common carotid arteries should be raised for the injection of bodies in intense rigor mortis. The right internal jugular vein can be used for drainage. A medium to strong arterial solution should be used. Follow the manufacturer's recommendations for dilutions. Dye and coinjection fluid can be added to the solution. The extra dye not only serves as a fluid tracer, but helps to prevent the tissues from graying. In the embalming of these bodies, blood drainage is often minimal and formaldehyde gray can easily develop hours after the embalming. The coinjection fluid assists in fluid penetration and adjustment of tissue pH. Keep in mind that the dye merely indicates that surface tissues have received fluid; there is no indicator for the deeper tissues.

Some embalmers prefer to begin the injection of most bodies with a mild arterial solution (1.25–1.50%) until surface blood discolorations are cleared. Subsequent injections are then made using stronger arterial solutions. Avoid the use of preinjection fluids with the body in intense rigor condition. Whenever distribution difficulties are expected, preinjection should not be used.

Inject slowly. During arterial injection, massage and manipulate the limbs to encourage distribution. When drainage is established, the injection speed can be slightly increased to encourage better distribution. Inject the trunk first. Both arterial tubes directed toward the head should be left open and no fluid should enter the head or facial tissues while the trunk is being injected in the unautopsied body.

Frequently, the autopsied body exhibits intense rigor, because the delay for the autopsy allows the rigor mortis to become firmly established in the body muscles. As each area of the body is separately injected, a faster rate of flow may be used. This is an excellent opportunity for the embalmer to use pulsation injection.

Using a mild to strong arterial solution, inject the head separately in the unautopsied body, first the left side then the right. Remember that swelling may be a problem, so a minimum amount of arterial solution should be injected. Injection should be stopped as soon as fluid dye is evident or if there is any distension in the eyelids, neck or glandular areas of the face, or neck. If parts of the face require additional treatment, hypodermic or surface embalming can be employed. **Use of a minimum amount of a strong solution helps to control swelling and achieve good preservation and tissue fixation.**

Injection of Limbs in Rigor. Physical manipulation of the limbs removes some of the intense rigor. The muscles should be manipulated before arterial injection is begun. As an example, take the healthy, well-developed, well-nourished man who dies as the result of trauma or sudden heart attack. Delay has resulted in intense rigor. If the arms and legs are to be separately injected, try first to relieve some of the rigor. This will be very difficult; more success will be possible with the arms than with the legs. Attempt to manipulate the arms so they can be positioned as they will appear in the casket. Inject from the brachial, axillary, or subclavian artery in the autopsied body. The brachial artery is most frequently used in the unautopsied body and the axillary in the autopsied body. The femoral artery can be used to inject the legs in the unautopsied body, and the external iliac artery can be used to inject the legs in the autopsied body.

The arterial solution used for injection should be stronger than the "average" arterial solution. A high-index arterial fluid can be used or several ounces of a high-index fluid can be added to the standard arterial solution. When injecting the arms or the legs, begin at a slow rate of flow (i.e., set the pressure with the rate-of-flow valve closed at 20 psi; open the valve until the pressure drops to 18 psi). By lowering the arms and using gentle but firm massage, attempt to distribute the fluid into the hands and fingers. Once distribution is established, a higher rate of flow can be used. If slow injection is not very successful in establishing distribution, use pulsation. Try pulsing the fluid into the limb (inject, pause, inject, pause, etc.) until distribution is established. Pulsation allows the use of higher pressures but also greater rates of flow.

Keep in mind that some swelling of the arms can be expected. Again, the stronger fluid helps to limit the swelling because less fluid is needed. Inject until blood discolorations clear and dye is present in the tissues. Intermittent drainage helps to achieve penetration of the fluid. The same procedure can be used to inject the legs. If distribution to the legs is unsuccessful, use hypodermic treatment to ensure thorough preservation of the leg tissues. If the hands do not receive adequate fluid, raise and inject radial or ulnar artery. Individual fingers can be treated by hypodermic injection of a preservative solution.

Other Considerations for Bodies in Rigor Mortis. During the period in which rigor occurs, the pH of the tissues is slightly acid. It has been found that the preservative–protein reaction occurs most readily at slightly basic pH, about the same as that of normal, healthy tissues (7.38–7.4). **Rigor mortis does not occur in all muscles simultaneously.** Rigor may pass from those muscles where it first occurs (the face and upper extremities) while it is still very intense in the lower areas of the body, such as the leg muscles. Also, pH will not be the same in the various muscles. Where rigor has passed from the muscles, autolysis and hydrolysis have proceeded to a point where protein has decomposed and the pH has become increasingly alkaline (basic).

Increase of tissue pH into the alkaline pH range after rigor mortis indicates that the muscle proteins have begun to break down or decompose. There are now additional sites for reaction with preservative. During rigor there are few sites for the reaction of preservative and proteins. A body being embalmed while in rigor should be saturated with sufficient preservative, so that it will be available later as the state of rigor passes.

Rigor and varying pH combine to make it very difficult for the embalmer to obtain uniform preservation of the body. Some of the factors that contribute to this lack of uniform embalming are outlined in the following chart:

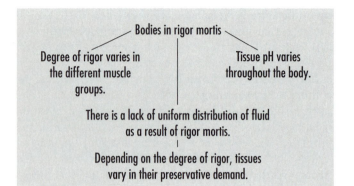

Bodies in rigor mortis

Degree of rigor varies in the different muscle groups.

Tissue pH varies throughout the body.

There is a lack of uniform distribution of fluid as a result of rigor mortis.

Depending on the degree of rigor, tissues vary in their preservative demand.

been torn, which would also account for the swelling of muscles and tissues during arterial injection. Tissues also swell because fluid follows the path(s) of least resistance. These paths lead to surface areas, as the deep muscle tissues, because of the rigor, resist the flow of fluid.

Causes of Swelling in Bodies in Rigor

1. Capillary beds are torn when muscles are flexed, bent, rotated, and massaged.
2. Fluid flows to surface areas because the deep muscles and tissue in rigor offer resistance to flow.
3. Drainage is limited because muscles in rigor exert pressure on veins.

PREPARATION OF REFRIGERATED BODIES

Today, almost all bodies removed from hospitals and other institutions have been refrigerated for some period. It is difficult to set an exact length of time after which refrigeration would pose special problems for the embalmer. Up to approximately 6 hours after death, few problems should be encountered. The cool environment slows the progress of rigor mortis and decomposition. In addition, the cold environment helps to maintain blood in a liquid state. Because the blood remains liquid, livor mortis can be expected to be more intense.

There are three advantages of short-term refrigeration: (1) the rigor cycle is slowed, (2) the decomposition cycle is slowed, and (3) the low viscosity of the blood is maintained. Long-term refrigeration, however, can cause a number of problems for the embalmer.

For years, one effect of refrigeration has been a major subject of discussion—*dehydration;* however, this situation is gradually changing. When bodies were wrapped in cotton sheets and refrigerated, surface dehydration occurred easily. Lips and eyes soon showed the brown discolorations associated with drying of the tissues. The blood gradually thickened as the moisture was removed from the surface tissues. Movement of water out of the surface tissues forced the liquid portion of the blood into the dry tissues, causing a postmortem edema. Gradually, this moisture also worked itself to the skin surface. If the body were exposed to the cool, dry air for a sufficient period, the tissues mummified as a result of dehydration. Today, however, most bodies are wrapped in plastic, and many are also placed into large zippered plastic pouches. Dehydration is no longer a problem. The plastic wrapping does cause other problems for the embalmer. Plastic traps heat and moisture, and refrigerated bodies show signs of decomposition and skin-slip because of the moisture trapped on the skin.

Remember that there is a slight elevation of body temperature after death (postmortem caloricity) because metabolism continues until the oxygen trapped in the

As the absorption of preservative results in firming, there is a relationship between the rate of preservative absorption by tissues and the rate of firming. This is why bodies embalmed prior to the onset of rigor rapidly firm; preservative is rapidly absorbed and rapidly attaches to the proteins. During rigor the proteins are "locked" together, and it is difficult for the preservative to attach to the proteins. As a result, there is little absorption of preservative by muscles in the state of rigor mortis. Most of the firming that occurs during the injection of a body in rigor is caused by the swelling of the tissues. If a mild or weak arterial solution is used, these tissues soften later. After the passage of rigor, demand for preservative increases greatly.

As well as a need to use strong solutions in the preparation of bodies in rigor, there is a need for a coinjection chemical. This chemical helps to adjust tissue pH as the various areas of the body are at different pH. The buffers in arterial fluids help to achieve the uniform pH necessary for the action of the preservative. It is easily seen that distribution is not uniform in these bodies, dyes are not evenly distributed, firming is not uniform, and the preservative needs of the tissues vary throughout the body.

PRESERVATIVE ABSORPTION AND FIRMING

Prerigor	Good absorption	Firming is good
Rigor	Little absorption	Firming is due to the rigor present and swelling
Postrigor	Great need for preservative	Firming is difficult to achieve

Firmness cannot be relied on as a test of preservation, for the firmness may be a result of the rigor present in the muscles. Firmness can also result from the distension of tissues during injection of arterial solution. In addition, if the embalmer attempted to relieve the rigor by manipulating the muscles, many capillary beds may have body is exhausted. As the blood no longer circulates, the heat produced by the catabolic phase of metabolism is trapped in the body. Therefore, the body temperature slightly increases. Heat speeds rigor mortis and decomposition as these are both chemical reactions. Because of this trapped heat, it is not unusual to find green discolorations on abdominal areas when the bodies are removed from refrigeration. Autolysis and bacterial activity continue while the body is in refrigeration, faster at first while the body is still warm and then slower as the tissues gradually cool.

Figure 19–2 illustrates some of the problems associated with refrigeration.

When bodies have been refrigerated for long periods and wrapped in plastic or placed in a plastic pouch, the embalmer can expect some of the following problems:

- Increased capillary permeability
- Easy rupture of the capillaries during arterial injection
- Tissue structure breakdown as a result of the slow, continuous processes of autolysis and bacterial enzymes
- Increased coagula in the vascular system
- Gravitation of blood and body liquids into the dependent body tissues, resulting in an increase in moisture in these tissues
- Intense livor mortis
- Rapid hemolysis resulting in postmortem extravascular stain
- Moist clammy tissues caused by the plastic wrapping of the surface tissues; possibly skin-slip
- Decomposition signs (e.g., abdominal discoloration, purge, and skin-slip)

- Rapid distension of abdominal organs during injection, resulting in stomach and/or lung purge

Blood gravitates to dependent areas. As the body cools, hemolysis easily occurs, causing the blood cells to rupture and release **heme** into the tissues. This results in *postmortem staining*. This type of blood discoloration cannot be removed by arterial injection and blood drainage. If the head has not been raised, these discolorations may be present in the facial tissues. Some bleaching is possible with the use of a strong arterial solution, a bleaching coinjection fluid, and surface bleaches. This stain can, however, be lightened but *not* removed. Opaque cosmetics are needed to hide the discoloration.

If the body has been refrigerated for a long period and wrapped in cloth sheeting, dehydration will be a problem. The amount of moisture in the dependent tissues increases because of hypostasis of the blood and settling of the liquids in these areas. The upper areas of the body may be browned from dehydration. Of particular interest to the embalmer are the drying and browning of the lips, eyelids, fingers, and base of the nose. The cheeks and forehead may also exhibit the brown discoloration of dehydration. This discoloration cannot be removed by arterial injection. Opaque cosmetics are used to hide the discolorations. Loss of water also results in a loss of moisture from the blood vascular system. There will be increased numbers of coagula in the vascular system, making distribution of the arterial solution very difficult.

During refrigeration, the progress of rigor mortis slows, but still occurs. Rigor usually passes 36 to 72 hours after death. Because it is slowed by cooling, it may still be present in some muscles at the time of embalming. Decomposition is what breaks rigor, and it too is slowed in a body that is cooled.

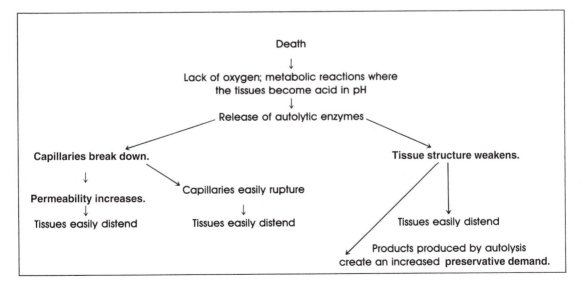

Figure 19–2. Problems associated with refrigeration: time–temperature effects.

Arterial Preparation

Swelling is not the only concern. The viscera can easily distend, which can lead to *purge*. There is an increased demand for preservative, as the processes of autolysis and decomposition slowly continue. If rigor is present there is additional need for stronger arterial solutions. Blood discolorations can be bleached with strong arterial solutions. Distribution may be difficult to achieve, so strong solutions would again be the best type. There is an increase in moisture in the dependent tissues and, thus, an increased demand for preservative.

As strong arterial solutions are necessary, the best vessels to use as a primary site of injection are both common carotid arteries (restricted cervical injection). Drainage may be difficult to establish because of large numbers of coagula; therefore, the right internal jugular vein would be best choice for the primary drainage site. Multipoint injection should be used for arms and legs not receiving sufficient arterial solution. Injection should be slow to prevent abdominal distension and to keep arterial coagula from moving and blocking smaller arteries.

Because of tissue distension, it is not possible to use large volumes of a mild arterial solution. Use of limited quantities of a strong solution produces the best results. The volume of fluid, of course, is determined by the size of the body and the embalmer's satisfaction that the tissues have received sufficient preservative solution. Because such a variety of arterial chemicals are available, the best advice that can be given with respect to fluid dilution is to follow the instructions of the manufacturer. Some manufacturers recommend the use of a coinjection fluid. Others advise that when their arterial chemicals are used to make strong arterial solutions, no coinjection fluid be used (Fig. 19–3).

Extra amounts of fluid dye should be used to trace the distribution of arterial fluid. When postmortem stain is present, the tissues can easily gray several hours after embalming. The dye helps to cover the gray discoloration produced when formaldehyde and hemoglobin combine. Most refrigerated bodies appear pink prior to embalming. This is caused by the hemolysis of red blood cells trapped in surface tissue capillaries. The tissues appear to be embalmed. In addition, the cold has a tendency to solidify the fatty tissues of the body, so the tissues may also feel embalmed.

Dependent areas of the trunk, buttocks, and shoulders that do not receive sufficient fluid can be treated by hypodermic injection. Cavity fluid can be injected (by infant trocar) into these areas through use of the embalming machine. These dependent areas are very moist and, thus, may be sites of bacterial activity. Thoroughly hypodermically inject these areas. Surface treatment is of little or no value in these high-moisture areas.

Cavity Embalming

If restricted cervical injection is used the cavities can be aspirated before the features are set and the head and facial tissues are embalmed. If purge develops during embalming of trunk areas, aspirating *before* setting of the features eliminates the need to reopen the mouth and remove *purge*. Cavity embalming should be thorough. A minimum of one bottle of concentrated cavity fluid should be injected into each major body cavity. Reaspiration is always advised. If any gases escape when the trocar button is removed for reaspiration, if the abdomen appears distended, or if the large surface veins of the neck appear distended, the cavities should also be reinjected with concentrated cavity fluid after reaspiration.

Cosmetic Treatment

Application of cosmetics may pose some problems if the tissues are still cold after arterial treatment. Condensation from the air is possible and the skin surface will feel moist to the touch. Cosmetic application may be delayed until the tissues have had time to warm and condensation has stopped.

Desquamation

Desquamation (skin-slip) has been mentioned several times as a problem in bodies that have undergone long refrigeration. Such bodies should be massaged carefully, for desquamation can easily be caused by the embalmer. Run as little water as possible over the skin of these bodies. Pat rather than rub the surface dry with toweling. Keep water from running over the skin surfaces during injection. Water should run along the sides of the table, not onto the skin surfaces.

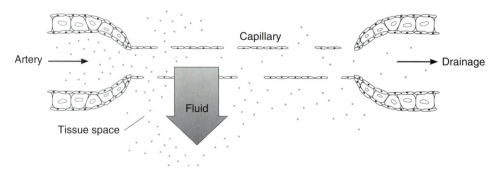

Figure 19–3. Refrigerated bodies and bodies in which decomposition has begun easily swell because of capillary breakdown and increased capillary permeability.

Loose skin should be removed prior to embalming. Apply surface compresses of autopsy gel or cavity fluid or surface embalming agents over these areas to help ensure preservation. After embalming remove the surface compresses and force the tissues to dehydrate with a hair dryer. If there is a sufficient delay between embalming and cosmetic application, enough air may pass over the body to dry the areas of nude skin. When skin-slip occurs on areas that will not be viewed, apply surface compresses and later plastic garments.

Frozen Tissues

Some refrigeration units may freeze body tissues. It is very important to remember that ice crystals form in these tissues. These crystals tear tissues. The body should not be warmed by pouring warm water over it. Allow the body to warm gradually by letting it sit in the preparation room several hours. Manipulation of the tissues while ice crystals are still present will cause more tearing. Try to manipulate the body as little as possible.

Restricted cervical injection is vital. Some embalmers prefer to inject these bodies as soon as it is possible to raise an artery and a vein. There will be little or no blood drainage. A strong arterial solution should be used and injected very slowly. The blood acts as a vehicle for the arterial solution as it does in bodies from which blood is not drained. Some embalmers prefer to use a strong arterial solution prepared with warm to hot water.

The facial tissues will, no doubt, be thawed so a stronger-than-average solution can be used to inject the head. If the embalmer feels that distension of the face will be a problem, he should use the instant tissue fixation method of injection to achieve preservation of the face.

Additional fluid dyes should be used in embalming these bodies.

PREPARATION OF BODIES THAT SHOW SIGNS OF DECOMPOSITION

Heat speeds chemical reactions. In the period between death and embalming, the cycles of rigor mortis and decomposition are speeded if the body is not cooled, but left in a warm environment. If the environment is warm and moist (conditions present during summer months), decomposition can be very rapid. After passage of rigor, tissues begin to break down, and many changes are noted (Fig. 19–4).

Color Changes

Trunk Areas. The right quadrant of the abdomen turns green; in a short time, the outline of the large intestine

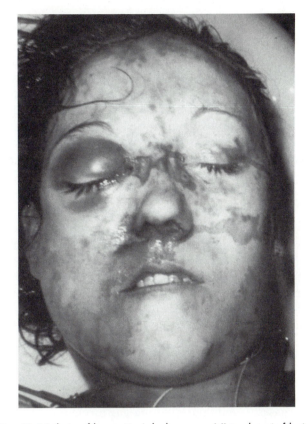

Figure 19–4. Early signs of decomposition (color changes, purge). Note ecchymosis of the right eyelid.

can be identified by the green discoloration over the abdominal wall. Hydrogen sulfide produced in the colon after death reacts with hemoglobin breakdown products to produce the greenish discoloration seen in the bowel and the structures that contact the bowel. The color change proceeds up the anterior abdominal and thoracic walls to the neck and chin.

Vascular Changes. Early decomposition color changes can affect the small veins in almost any area of the body. The blood in these superficial vessels breaks down and the coloring matter of the hemoglobin makes the veins appear as brown lines over the surface of the skin.

Livor Mortis and Stain. Livor mortis is completely established in the dependent tissues of these bodies. Some of these purple discolorations clear during injection of the arterial solution. The majority, however, become postmortem stains. Stain develops as the hemoglobin breaks down (hemolysis) and allows the heme portion of the molecule to pass from the capillaries into the tissue spaces. This light red discoloration cannot be removed by arterial injection. At best it may be bleached, which will aid in the cosmetic treatment if the stain occurs in facial tissues or tissues of the back of the hand.

Odors

As autolysis and putrefaction occur, some products of protein breakdown emit very foul odors. Foul amines and mercaptans combine with ammonia and hydrogen sulfide to produce the odors of decomposition. Embalming converts the amines, mercaptans, and hydrogen sulfide to odorless methylol compounds. Formaldehyde converts ammonia to odorless hexamethylene. Nutrition, body weight, and presence of bacterial disease prior to death all contribute to the extent of these odors.

Purges

If gases have developed in the abdominal cavity and products of partial digestion were present in the stomach at the time of death, purge can be expected (Fig. 19–5). Ruptured capillaries and congested lung passageways may also create a "lung" purge (i.e., pneumonia, tuberculosis, influenza). Abdominal pressures may also cause purging from the rectum through the anal orifice.

Gases

In some bodies, especially those in which bacterial activity increased after death, the tissues and cavities may contain gases. Conditions favoring gas formation are heat and humidity; those hindering formation are cold and dry environments. Gas can cause bloating and swelling of the body, protrusion of the tongue and eyes, and distension of the male genitalia. The pressure resulting from distension of the abdominal cavity creates lung, stomach, and anal purges.

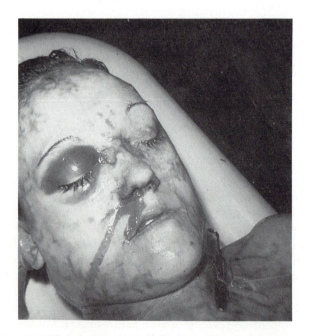

Figure 19–5. Early decomposition. Purge, discolorations. and distension from gases are evident.

Desquamation

The autolytic changes that begin immediately after death weaken the superficial layer of the skin. Gas can easily move into the weakened superficial tissues, resulting in blisters and separation of the skin layers. Frequently, the embalmer encounters skin-slip when there are no gases in the tissues. Then, mere handling of the body causes the epidermis to loosen and separate.

Dehydration

Some of these bodies exhibit local dehydration in the fingers, lips, nose, eyelids, and ears.

Chemical Changes

Although not visible postmortem changes, important chemical changes occur in the tissues that the embalmer must be concerned about. Autolytic and proteolytic decomposition of the body proteins results in numerous nitrogenous products. These products greatly increase the preservative demand of the body. Their presence also shifts the body pH to alkaline (basic). Embalming solutions react best with proteins under slightly (not strong) alkaline pH conditions.

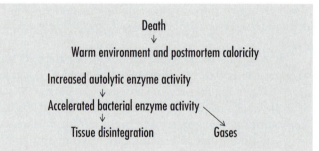

These classic signs of decomposition may also be accompanied by rigor mortis in some muscles. Rigor can be found in bodies that show early signs of decomposition in the hands, legs, and jaw muscles.

Embalming Protocol

The following factors concerning the body enter into a **preembalming analysis:** (1) general conditions of the body, (2) effects of disease on body tissues, (3) effects of drugs on body tissues, and (4) postmortem changes. The postmortem changes may be the most important factor in determining the embalming techniques to be used.

The protocols for embalming the bodies discussed in this chapter are similar, because all of these bodies have undergone a delay between death and preparation and all have a high preservative demand. Some of the complications encountered during embalming of the body with early signs of decomposition follow:

1. Fluid distribution is poor, because coagula are present in the arterial system.
2. Drainage is poor because blood elements have decomposed.
3. Tissues easily swell, for capillaries have broken down or are easily torn by the pressure of the fluid; tissue structure has been weakened by autolytic and putrefactive changes.
4. Ammonia and nitrogenous products in the tissues greatly increase the preservative demand.
5. Little or no firming is exhibited because of protein breakdown.

Maximum-strength fluid can be used to prepare these bodies—25 to 30 index or higher. For this type of body, maximum-strength arterial solutions are necessary. Supplemental chemicals can be used to increase the working ability of these arterial solutions. Again, follow the instructions of the manufacturer. The goal here is to use a minimum amount of a very strong arterial solution. **Do not preinject these bodies.** Only a strong arterial solution should be injected into the vascular system. Use additional fluid dye, because firming cannot be used to judge distribution or preservation. Remember, the dye only indicates the presence of fluid in the surface tissues.

Two protocols can be used for injection. Drainage can be taken from each injection site or from the right internal jugular vein. Little or no drainage can be expected from these bodies.

The purpose in using *injection protocol 1* is to minimize the number of arterial coagula that may move into the smaller arteries. Keep in mind that the aorta may contain a number of large coagula. If these coagula move, they will block small arteries.

1. Raise the right and left common carotid, right and left axillary (brachial), and right and left femoral (external iliac) arteries.
2. Inject the right femoral artery.
3. Inject the left femoral artery.
4. Inject the right axillary artery.
5. Inject the left axillary artery.
6. Inject the right common carotid artery through the tube directed toward the trunk. Be certain the left common carotid is tied off and a tube has been inserted and directed upward to the left side of the head; leave this tube open.
7. Aspirate the body after the trunk is injected.
8. Set the features.
9. Inject the left side of the head.
10. Inject the right side of the head.
11. Aspirate the cavities again and inject them with a suitable undiluated cavity chemical.
12. Evaluate the distribution of fluid and use hypodermic and surface embalming treatments where fluid has not been distributed.

Injection protocol 2 makes use of restricted cervical injection.

1. Raise the right and left common carotid arteries; drain from the right internal jugular vein.
2. Inject down the right common carotid to embalm the arms, legs, and trunk. The left common carotid should be tied off and a tube directed toward the head inserted; this tube should remain open.
3. Evaluate the distribution of arterial solution. Inject the arms and legs separately if these areas lack fluid.
4. Aspirate the body cavities.
5. Set the features.
6. Inject the left side of the head.
7. Inject the right side of the head.
8. Reaspirate the cavities and inject a suitable undiluted cavity chemical.
9. Evaluate the distribution of arterial solution and treat area needing fluid with hypodermic and surface embalming.

If the abdomen is distended tightly with gas prior to arterial injection, introduce a trocar into the abdominal cavity to relieve this pressure. The trocar should be kept just beneath the anterior wall. An attempt can be made to puncture the transverse colon and the distended stomach.

The trunk should be injected at a very slow rate of flow to prevent swelling of the abdominal viscera and purge. Limbs can be injected slowly at first, and then at a higher pressure and faster rate of flow to secure distribution. Pulsation is recommended. If desired, each extremity can also be injected by the instant tissue fixation method (100% arterial fluid injected in pulses under high pressure) or by using waterless embalming.

If sectional arterial embalming has produced unsatisfactory results, sectional hypodermic injection will be necessary. Undiluted arterial or cavity fluid may be injected by machine through an infant trocar. To inject the arms, insert the trocar into the area of the bend of the elbow; from this point the upper as well as the distal portion of the arm can be reached, possibly as far as the palm of the hand. To inject the legs, insert the trocar on the medial side of the leg either above or below the knee; from this point fluid can be injected as far as the buttocks and as far as the foot. An alternative point of entry is the base of the foot. From this point of entry, fluid could be injected as far as the knee. The trunk walls can be injected from points of entry on the lateral walls of the trunk at approximately the level of the midaxillary line. It may be necessary to insert the infant trocar into the upper shoulder area to inject the posterior portions of the back, shoulder, and neck. All of these points of entry can be closed with trocar buttons or, if necessary, sutured closed with a purse-string suture. Glue can be applied over the trocar button or suture to ensure against leakage. Fingers and the foot can be separately injected with a hypodermic syringe and a small gauge needle. The use of super adhesive helps to ensure against leakage from each point where the needle is inserted.

It is most important that these bodies be reaspirated several hours after embalming. Reinjection is strongly advised, especially if any gases are evident during the reaspiration. If desquamation is present, the loose skin should be removed at the beginning of the embalming. Surface compresses can be applied to help dry these areas. Air drying also helps to dry the raw skin after the compresses have been removed.

Plastic garments can be used, but embalming powder or moisture-absorbent kitty litter should be placed inside these garments. This powder produces some surface preservation but, more important, helps to control odors. Odors can be reduced by bathing the surface of the body with a solution prepared by mixing 2 pints of hydrogen peroxide with $\frac{1}{2}$ cup of baking soda and adding a tablespoon of liquid soap. This solution is left on the skin surface for several minutes before rinsing and drying.

Treatment of the Features

In preparing a body in which decomposition is evident, the embalmer may wish to vary the technique used to set features.

The man can be shaved after arterial injection to limit skin removal on the facial areas. Facial skin that appears easily removable can be painted with autopsy gel during embalming of the body, or the face can be covered with surface compresses of cavity fluid. Use shaving cream to lather the face. Avoid the use of warm water to soften the beard. A new, sharp razor blade makes the shaving much easier and puts less tension on the skin. Several blades may be needed to shave dense facial hair growth.

The mouth can be closed after arterial injection. As the lips and areas around the mouth may swell, it may be easier to obtain a proper closure after injection. Firming is not a problem in these bodies, because it is delayed. Also, if purge develops during arterial injection, the mouth can be properly dried and packed after cavity treatment.

The embalmer should evaluate the preservation of tissues surrounding the mouth. It may be necessary to place cotton in the mouth and saturate it with concentrated cavity fluid to help ensure preservation. Dehydration should not be a concern. The lips can be secured with a super adhesive.

Eyes can also be closed after arterial injection. In this way, the embalmer has an opportunity to observe if the eyelids have received sufficient fluid. Cotton can be used for closure, and this cotton can be saturated with some concentrated cavity fluid to help ensure preservation of the lids. Be very careful in handling the eyelids, for this skin is very easily removed. A super adhesive can be used to secure eye closure. Let the cavity fluid remain under the eyelids. It helps to secure preservation and to bleach the tissues. Dehydration is not a concern in the preparation of these bodies.

Areas of the face that appear not to have received sufficient arterial solution can be reached by hypodermic injection from inside the mouth. Cavity fluid should be used to treat these areas. Do not dilute the cavity fluid; use the concentrated fluid. Make all injections from inside the mouth, because cavity fluid, unlike tissue builder, has a tendency to leak from the tissues. This leakage occurs on the inside of the closed mouth. The sides of the nose can be reached as well as the cheeks and the lower eyelids from inside the mouth. A 19-gauge needle is excellent for this work.

In bodies dead for a long period, the submaxillary, sublingual, and parotid glands tend to swell during injection. If this happens, apply very firm digital pressure to these areas immediately after arterial injection. If the swelling is not reduced, make a flap incision at the base of the neck. Using an infant trocar as an operative aid, lance the glandular tissue several times and apply digital pressure again. If this treatment is unsuccessful, another operative correction—excision of the swollen tissues—may be necessary.

In bodies exhibiting decomposition, the tongue often protrudes and is swollen. Attempt to force the tongue back into the mouth by using firm digital pressure prior to arterial injection. The protruding tongue can be covered with a piece of cloth and firm pressure applied to the cloth. When teeth or dentures are present, try to force the tongue behind them and then secure the jaw shut. This helps to contain the tongue. Excision of the tongue should be a last resort.

Advanced Decomposition

There should be some preparation of the body in advanced stages of decomposition. If removing the body from a residence, use rubber gloves, masks, a plastic or rubber pouch, and disinfectant and deodorant sprays. In an emergency, wrap the body in a wool blanket to help absorb liquids and odors. These bodies should not be removed until they are placed in a zippered pouch. As much soiled clothing and bedding as possible should be removed from the residence and the family should be informed that these soiled articles will be destroyed.

If the embalmer thinks it is possible, raise and inject the right common carotid artery with about 1 gallon of undiluted high-index fluid. Coinjection fluids are made for such cases (decomposition, burns, etc.). One or two bottles of the coinjection fluid can be added to undiluted arterial fluid (at least 30 index). Some cavity fluids (undiluted) can be injected arterially in special situations. Do not attempt to drain.

The abdominal and thoracic cavities should be aspirated and filled with three or more bottles of undiluted cavity fluid. The extremities and trunk walls can be treated by hypodermic injection of undiluted cavity fluid by use of an infant trocar and the embalming machine. The primary purpose here is to diminish some of the odor and slow the progress of decomposition.

The body can be wrapped in one or more sheets and placed in a clean, zippered pouch. Before wrapping the blankets around the body, sprinkle embalming powder over the surface of the body. The entire body surface may also be painted with autopsy gel. Place the wrapped body in the pouch. If desired, saturate the sheets surrounding the body with cavity fluid or an external preservative solution. Any chemical used to saturate the sheeting should be concentrated and not diluted.

Before zippering the pouch, sprinkle additional embalming powder over the sheeting and the inside of the pouch. Placing moisture-absorbent kitty litter inside the pouch will assist in the control of odors. Some embalmers prefer to place a surface glue along the zipper of the pouch to help control the escape of any odors. A double pouch may be necessary to ensure that the odors are contained and the pouch does not rip when it is lifted. To prevent the pouch from tearing, place a sheet under it; the pouch can be lifted and moved with the sheet.

KEY TERMS AND CONCEPTS FOR STUDY AND DISCUSSION

1. Define the following terms:
   autolysis
   decomposition
   dehydration
   postmortem stain
   purge
   restricted cervical injection
   rigor mortis
   special-purpose high-index fluid
2. List the postmortem changes.
3. Explain why restricted cervical injection should be used when strong arterial solutions are to be injected?
4. Describe the effects of rigor mortis on the embalming process.
5. Describe the postmortem pH changes in the unembalmed body.
6. Describe the effects of cooling on the body.

BIBLIOGRAPHY

Boehringer PR. *Controlled Embalming of the Head.* Westport, CT: ESCO Tech Notes; Feb–March, 1969, No. 57.

Jones, H. A chemist looks at embalming problems. *Casket and Sunnyside,* May 1968.

Pervier NC. *A Textbook of Chemistry for Embalming.* Minneapolis: University of Minnesota; 1961.

Sanders CR. Refrigeration (Parts 1-2-3). *Dodge Magazine,* March/April/May 1987.

Slocum RE. *Pre-embalming Considerations.* Boston: Dodge Chemical Co.

Strub CG. Why bodies decay. *Casket and Sunnyside,* February/March 1959.

Weber DL. *Autopsy Pathology Procedure and Protocol.* Springfield, IL: Charles C Thomas; 1973:69–70.

20

Discolorations

The embalmer soon learns that hardly any body embalmed today does not have some discolorations. They might be localized, such as an ecchymosis on the back of a hand, or generalized, such as a simple condition of livor mortis or a complex condition as jaundice. Even intravenous lines begun when a body is received "DOA" (dead on arrival) at the emergency room in an attempt to resuscitate can create a postmortem bruise.

Discolorations are of utmost concern to the embalmer. These deviations from normal skin coloration may require a change in the embalming technique, the chemicals employed, and the cosmetic and restorative techniques. The embalmer should be able to identify any and all discolorations present on the body. Quite often, a family member asks questions concerning the antemortem discolorations and if they will be visible after the preparation. The embalmer should also recognize those discolorations that necessitate notification of the proper authorities if a doctor was not in attendance at the time of death or did not examine the body after death. The embalmer should be able to recognize the *cause* of a discoloration, know which *can* and *cannot* be cleared by arterial injection, know which can be altered or bleached by proper chemicals, and know which will have to be treated by opaque cosmetics to hide the discoloration.

A discoloration is defined as any abnormal color in or on the skin of the human body. In embalming, discolorations are classified according to the time at which they appeared and the cause.

There are two classifications of discolorations by time of occurence: antemortem (before death) and postmortem (after death). A discoloration that was present during life and remains after death is classified as antemortem.

There are six classifications of discolorations by cause that the embalmer can identify:

1. Blood discolorations are discolorations resulting from changes in blood composition, content, and location (Blood discolorations, in addition to being classified as antemortem or postmortem, are also classified as **intravascular** or **extravascular**)
2. Drug or therapeutic discolorations are antemortem discolorations resulting from the administration of drugs or chemotherapeutic agents
3. Pathological discolorations are antemortem discolorations that occur during the course of certain diseases
4. Surface colorating agent discolorations are antemortem or postmortem discolorations that occur prior to (or during) embalming as the result of the deposit of matter on the body surface.
5. Reactions to embalming chemicals are postmortem discolorations present before embalming

that become more intense, change in hue, or evolve as a result of the embalming

6. Discomposition changes are postmortem discolorations brought about by the action of bacterial and/or autolytic enzymes on the body tissues

The following charts summarize the classifications of the various discolorations. Examples are given for each category. Some brief explanation should be made regarding discolorations labeled as blood, pathological, and drug discolorations. Keep in mind the classification is by cause of the discoloration. Thus, "ecchymosis" is a blood discoloration if caused by trauma, is a pathological discoloration if it occurs during a disease, and is a drug discoloration when brought about by a drug. Jaundice can be classified as a drug or a pathological discoloration depending on its *cause*.

Classification of Discolorations According to Cause

1. Blood discolorations
   A. Intravascular
   B. Extravascular
2. Drug and therapeutic discolorations
3. Pathological discolorations
4. Surface coloring agent discolorations
5. Reactions to embalming chemicals on the body
6. Decomposition changes

Classification of Discolorations According to Time of Occurrence

1. Antemortem
   A. Blood discolorations
   B. Drug and therapeutic discolorations
   C. Pathological discolorations
   D. Surface coloring agent discolorations
2. Postmortem
   A. Blood discolorations
   B. Surface coloring agent discolorations
   C. Reactions to embalming chemicals on the body
   D. Decomposition discolorations

Examples of the various classifications follow.

I. Blood discolorations
  1. Antemortem blood discolorations
     A. Intravascular
        a. Hypostasis of blood (blue-black discoloration)
        b. Carbon monoxide poisoning (cherry red coloring)
        c. Capillary congestion (hypostatic, active or passive)
     B. Extravascular
        a. Ecchymosis: a large bruise caused by escape of blood into the tissues
        b. Purpura: flat medium-sized hemorrhage beneath the skin surface
        c. Petechia: small pinpoint skin hemorrhage
        d. Hematoma: swollen blood-filled area within the skin
  2. Postmortem blood discolorations
     A. Intravascular: livor mortis
     B. Extravascular: postmortem stain
II. Drug and therapeutic discolorations: There are many discolorations under this classification. Some are specific to a particular drug. Large amounts of drugs, in time, affect the vascular, renal and hepatic systems. Frequently, drug discolorations such as echymosis and purpura result from the breakdown of capillaries by the drugs. Often, the capillaries are fragile and bruising occurs easily. A second frequently encountered drug discoloration is jaundice, a result of the toxic effect of drugs on the liver. All drug discolorations are antemortem and are caused by specific drugs or combinations of drugs. These discolorations are very common. Usually, the arms are affected by hemorrhagic discolorations, and the entire body is affected by jaundice.
III. Pathological discolorations: These discolorations, all antemortem, are brought about by specific diseases.
  1. Gangrene
     A. Wet: infected tissues red to black in color
     B. Dry: caused by arterial insufficiency; a dark red-brown to black color
     When gangrene occurs in a facial area or affects the fingers, it becomes of cosmetic concern to the embalmer. Frostbite and diabetes can be responsible for this condition in the facial areas and hands. Arterial preservation is difficult to establish, and surface and hypodermic preservation are necessary.
  2. Jaundice: caused by many disease processes, for example, diseases of the liver, a bile problem, or a blood problem
  3. Specific diseases
     A. Addison's disease: a bronze discoloration produced in the skin
     B. Leukemia: petechiae
     C. Meningitis: rashes on the skin surface
     D. Tumors: discolorations in and around the tumor itself may be caused by pathological changes
  These are only some of the discolorations resulting from pathological disorders. Discolorations may also be brought about by a reaction to drugs or radiation therapy
IV. Surface coloring agent discolorations: These may be antemortem or postmortem depending on when

the agent was applied to the skin surface. Examples include blood, adhesive tape marks, gentian violet, paint, Mercurochrome, mold, and tobacco tars. This list could be more extensive as the embalmer encounters many surface discolorations. Most can easily be removed with soap and water or with a solvent such as the dry hair washes and trichloroethylene.

V. Reactions to embalming chemicals: These are postmortem discolorations that occur before, during, or after embalming of the body. Examples are razor burns, dehydration of tissues, formaldehyde gray, and conversion of yellow to green jaundice.

VI. Decomposition discolorations: These postmortem color changes occur during decomposition and may be yellow, green, or blue-black to black. Examples are progressive skin color changes and mottling of the veins on the skin surface.

GENERAL TREATMENT OF BLOOD DISCOLORATIONS

Intravascular Blood Discolorations

Intravascular blood discolorations respond best to arterial injection and blood drainage. These discolorations include antemortem hypostais, cyanosis, carbon monoxide poisoning, capillary congestion, and livor mortis. A preinjection fluid can be used to flush the vascular system if the body has been dead a short period and the embalmer feels distribution and drainage will be good. A mild arterial solution could also be used as a beginning injection in an attempt to flush the vascular system of the discoloration.

Very strong solutions should be avoided, as they may convert an intravascular discoloration into an extravascular stain. Many of the high-index arterial fluids today do a fine job of promoting distribution and drainage without creating postmortem stains. Concurrent drainage also promotes clearing of the intravascular discolorations. Many of these discolorations can be gravitated from visible areas by elevation of the face, neck, and hands. Massage many also be helpful in removal of intravascular discolorations. Once surface discolorations have cleared, intermittent drainage may be the preferred method for effecting the best diffusion of the embalming chemical.

If these intravascular discolorations are localized, such as in the legs, arms, or side of the face, and do not respond to injection and drainage, then local injection may be necessary to clear the discoloration. In essence, failure of the discoloration to clear is a very good sign that fluid has not entered the area. Therefore, selection and injection of an artery closest to the discoloration may be necessary. If a condition such as arteriosclerosis exists in the femoral arteries and the discoloration in the legs does not clear, use of the femoral or external iliac arteries may be impractical for arterial injection. Hypodermic and surface embalming of the legs is then necessary (Table 20–1).

TABLE 20–1. EMBALMING CONSIDERATIONS AND BLOOD DISCOLORATIONS

Antemortem Hypostasis	Postmortem Hypostasis	Time ⟶	Livor Mortis	Time ⟶	Postmortem Stain	Time ⟶	Formaldehyde Gray
Occurs prior to death or during the agonal period	Begins at death		Seen as soon as blood fills superficial vessels; begins approx 20 minutes after death; depends on postmortem/ antemortem hypostasis		Normally occurs about 6 hours after death; rate varies with cause of death and blood chemistry		Occurs after embalming
Intravascular	Intravascular		Intravascular		Extravascular		Intravascular or extravascular
Movement of blood to dependent tissues	Movement of blood to dependent tissues		Postmortem blood discoloration as a result of postmortem/antemortem hypostasis		Postmortem blood discoloration as a result of hemolysis		Embalming discoloration
Antemortem physical change	Postmortem physical change		Postmortem physical change		Postmortem chemical change		—
	Speed depends on blood viscosity		Color varies with blood volume and viscosity and amount of O$_2$ in blood		May occur prior to, during, or after arterial injection		Seen after arterial injection
Antemortem	Postmortem		Postmortem		Postmortem		Postmortem
—	—		Clears when pressed on		Does *not* clear when pressed on		Seen as a gray stain
—	—		Removed by blood drainage		Not removed by blood drainage		Methemoglobin (HCHO+blood)
—	Arterial injection stops progress		Arterial injection (mild) clears with drainage		Strong solutions bleach and "set" livor as stain		—
—	Speeded by cooling of body, low blood viscosity		Speeded by cooling, blood "thinners," low blood viscosity, CO deaths		Speeded by cooling, rapid red blood cell hemolysis, CO deaths		Speeded by poor drainage, small amount of arterial fluid
							Vascular system not well cleared of blood

Livor mortis is a postmortem intravascular blood discoloration. It is also a postmortem physical change, a discoloration brought about by the gravitation of blood into the dependent capillaries (Fig. 20–1). It is first observed approximately 20 to 30 minutes after death and is well established by the sixth hour after death. Refrigeration and drugs such as blood thinners speed the onset and increase in intensity of livor mortis. If the darkened area is pushed on and the area clears, this is an indication that the discoloration is intravascular. Livor mortis can be gravitated. If a body is laid on a flat surface, the heart is slightly higher than the head. Blood, thus, has a tendency to gravitate into the facial and neck tissues.

The head and shoulders should always be elevated to help drain blood from these upper tissues. While the body is shaved, the face and hair washed, and the features set, most of the blood gravitates from facial and neck tissues if the shoulders and head have been elevated. If the discoloration does not clear, this may be an indication that there is blockage (e.g., a coagulum) in the right atrium of the heart or in the right or left internal jugular veins. The best vessels for injection and drainage of this body would be the right and left common carotid arteries and the right internal jugular vein. The internal jugular allows access to the right atrium of the heart. Any coagula present can be removed with an angular spring forceps.

Preinjection fluids were developed to help clear blood discolorations such as livor mortis. If the body has not been dead very long, the embalmer may wish to inject a preinjection fluid solution. A large enough volume

of solution should be injected to clear the livor mortis. If a preinjection fluid is not used, a mild arterial solution may be used to clear the blood discolorations. Subsequent injections can be stronger. This method helps to prevent setting of the livor mortis as a stain. Most of the fluids manufactured today are of such a nature that strong solutions can be injected and the fluid will clear the blood discolorations without setting the livor mortis as a stain. Many of these fluids are labeled "reaction controlled fluids," meaning that they are able to be distributed throughout the body and diffuse into the tissue spaces before the chemical reaction with the proteins of the body. *Note:* In attempting to clear livor mortis, the drainage used should be concurrent (or continuous) until the livor has cleared. Then, intermittent or alternate methods of drainage can be employed.

Livor mortis can also be an advantage for the embalmer. The breaking and clearing of the livor mortis indicates that fluid has been distributed into those tissues. Most bodies exhibit some degree of livor mortis. Some, however, are quite dramatic and the face may be almost blue-black. Elevation, continuous drainage, use of the internal jugular veins for drainage, and a mild arterial solution all help to clear the discoloration of livor mortis.

In making an embalming analysis, the nail beds should be observed for livor. This is especially important in the embalming of African-Americans in whom the livor in the skin tissues is not always evident. Clearing of the nail beds indicates distribution of the fluid.

Areas such as the trunk and buttocks where livor does not clear should be treated hypodermically to ensure preservation. When livor does not clear from the limbs or head, arteries should be raised and sectional embalming performed.

Antemortem as well as the postmortem intravascular discoloration should respond to arterial injection and subsequent blood drainage.

Carbon monoxide discolorations are antemortem blood discolorations classified as intravascular and, thus, should be cleared by arterial injection. Remember, however, that many times there is a delay between death and preparation. The body might not be found for a while or the death must be investigated by the coroner or medical examiner. Quite frequently the *intra*vascular condition becomes an *extra*vascular condition because of the delay. The blood in these bodies rapidly breaks down allowing for hemolysis and staining of the tissues. The embalming is routine, but the bright discoloration may not clear. Care should be taken to use a dye with the arterial solution to be certain of the distribution of the arterial fluid.

To summarize, the embalmer must consider several factors in embalming the body with livor mortis:

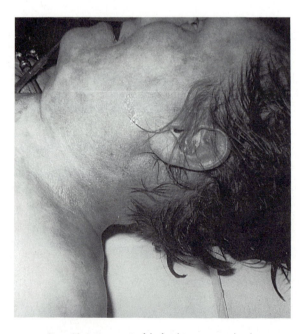

Figure 20–1. Livor mortis of the facial tissues, ear, and neck.

1. It is a postmortem physical change.

2. It appears in dependent tissues.

3. It is speeded by refrigeration and blood thinners, carbon monoxide deaths, low blood viscosity, and large blood volume.

4. Sometimes it begins even before death and is seen rapidly after death.

5. It is an intravascular condition.

6. It may be cleared by arterial injection and blood drainage.

7. It may be gravitated and massaged from a body region.

8. Color varies from light pink to almost black depending on blood volume and viscosity.

9. When pushed on (or palpated), tissues clear.

10. It is cleared best by the use of mild arterial solutions or preinjection solutions.

Extravascular Blood Discolorations

Extravascular blood discolorations do not respond well to arterial treatment. Examples of these discolorations are ecchymosis, purpura, petechia, hematoma, and postmortem stain. Specific treatments for ecchymosis, hematoma, and postmortem stain are discussed later. Injection of a stronger arterial solution assists in bleaching some of these discolorations. Keep in mind that livor mortis and postmortem stain can both be present in a dependent area. The livor might be "washed out" but the stain remains. The stronger solution helps to bleach and to preserve these affected areas. Local treatment such as surface compresses and hypodermic treatment are frequently needed. No preinjection, coinjection, or "special

arterial" fluids can completely remove these extravascular discolorations. Some may be lightened by the bleaching action of these fluids.

Ecchymosis, purpura, and petechia are all extravascular. They are classified as blood discolorations but can also be classified as pathological and drug discolorations, for they can be *caused* by diseases as well as by extended use of many drugs. A good example of both is the ecchymosis caused by use of the drug thinner coumadin. The disease leukemia produces hemorrhagic petechiae on the body surface. The treatment of these extravascular conditions can involve all three types of embalming: arterial, hypodermic, and surface.

Compared with ecchymoses, purpura and petechiae are smaller discolorations, and very frequently, simple arterial embalming satisfactorily bleaches and preserves these discolorations. Ecchymoses are of concern when they occur in a visible area such as on the face or the back of the hands, the most frequently seen areas. If the ecchymosis was caused by a needle puncture, the area may distend during arterial injection (Fig. 20–2A).

Let us assume that a large ecchymosis on the back of the hand was caused by a hypodermic puncture (Fig. 20–2B). Three things can happen during arterial injection of this body: (1) Arterial solution will profuse the area, there will be little distension, and the area will be well preserved and may even bleach a little. (2) The area will distend, oftentimes very dramatically. (3) Nothing will happen. The area will not receive arterial solution. It will be neither preserved nor bleached. The ecchymosis must now be treated by hypodermic or surface embalming, or both.

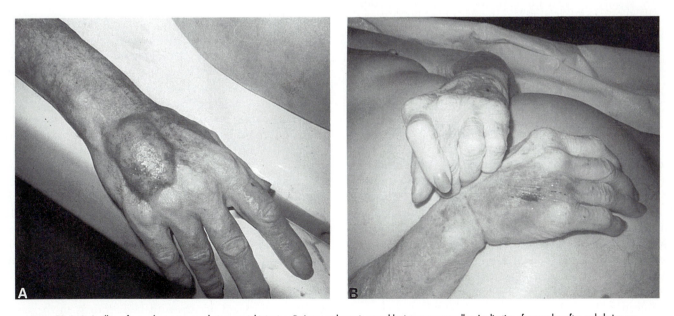

Figure 20–2. **A.** Swelling of an ecchyomotic area during arterial injection. **B.** Large ecchymosis caused by intravenous needles. Application of super glue after embalming can easily prevent leakage.

Hypodermic Treatment. (After Arterial Injection). Two chemicals can be used: a phenol cautery solution or formaldehyde (a cavity fluid). The phenol solution is a better bleaching agent. It also works much faster and cauterizes as well as preserves and disinfects the area.

1. Insert a hypodermic needle between the fingers.
2. Repeatedly push the needle through the discolored tissues prior to injecting any of the solution.
3. Inject the solution and massage the area to uniformly distribute the chemical beneath the skin.
4. Some of the chemical will leak out of the points of entry between fingers; some may also exit from the needle puncture on the back of the hand.
5. Let the chemical remain for 15 to 20 minutes. Then, massage as much of the chemical as possible through the punctures in item 4.
6. Seal the needle punctures with a drop of super adhesive.

Surface Embalming. In addition to formaldehyde and phenol solution, a variety of surface preservatives are available. The autopsy gels are quite popular for surface embalming. Surface treatments can be done before, during, or after arterial injection.

1. Coat the surface of the ecchymosis with autopsy gel. Or, saturate cotton compresses with the preservative chemical and apply the cotton packs to the ecchymosis.
2. Cover the cotton compresses with plastic. This helps to decrease odors and prevent dehydration of the chemical.
3. Allow sufficient time for these chemicals to penetrate and preserve the ecchymotic tissues. Several hours will, no doubt, be required. Keep in mind that phenol solutions work very fast. Autopsy gels have a good penetrating ability.
4. Later, remove the surface compresses. Clean the area with a solvent and dry the tissues.
5. If a puncture to the skin is present (i.e., from an intravenous line), the puncture can be sealed with a drop of super adhesive.

Ecchymosis or Hematoma of the Eye. In treating an ecchymosis or hematoma of the eye (Fig. 20–3), commonly known as a "black eye," it is wise to raise and separately inject both the left and the right common carotid arteries. A stronger solution can be employed and the embalmer can control the amount of solution entering the head. The solution that is injected will be strong, so a smaller volume can be used in the event that the eye (or eyes) begin to distend. Do not inject the head of these bodies with a preinjection fluid.

In addition to surface embalming or hypodermic treatment of the eyes, a preservative such as cavity fluid

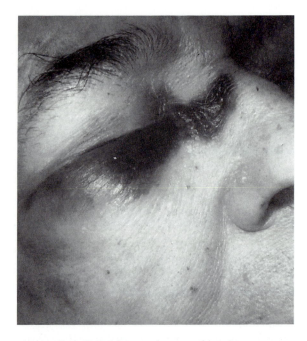

Figure 20–3. Ecchymosis or hematoma of the right eye.

can simply be placed underneath the eyelid. Use cotton to close the eyes. Place a few drops of cavity fluid on the cotton, then glue the eyes closed. This acts as a compress under the eyelids and assists in preserving the tissues and bleaching some of the discoloration. This method is also good for routine embalming when the embalmer feels the eyelids have not received enough preservative. The eyes can be glued and dehydration need not be a concern. The important factor is preservation. Cavity fluid does not contain dye; over time, fluids with dyes could stain the tissues.

Another approach can be taken to the treatment of swollen black eyes. Inject the tissues around the eyes and the lids with a phenol cautery chemical prior to arterial injection. Wait about 20 minutes for the chemical to cauterize the tissues; then proceed with the arterial injection. This method cauterizes the tissues and does not permit arterial solution to flow into the area. Many phenol chemicals are accompanied by specific directions for their use. Follow the time periods set by the manufacturer.

Postmortem Stain. Postmortem stain, an extravascular blood discoloration, occurs in tissues where livor mortis was present or in surface tissues from which blood could not be drained. With postmortem stain, a period has elapsed between death and embalming. Actually, postmortem stain indicates decomposition or breakdown of the red blood cell. The coloring matter (heme) has moved through the capillaries and into the tissue spaces. Often, postmortem stain occurs with livor mortis in the same tissue regions. When pushed on (or palpated), the skin does not clear.

When embalming bodies with stain, use stronger solutions than used for routine preparation. Keep in mind that stain indicates that the blood has begun to break down. Expect poor distribution of fluid, a tendency for the capillaries to be broken down, and a tendency for the tissues to distend on injection. Thus, the embalming solution used should be of sufficient strength so that a minimum volume effects preservation but at the same time minimizes distension.

Some dye should be added to this solution, because when formaldehyde and the coloring portion of the blood mix to produce a gray hue, the extra dye not only indicates surface distribution of the fluid but also acts to counterstain the adverse discoloration.

Avoid using preinjection solutions in the preparation of these bodies. Bodies dead for long periods require strong, well-coordinated solutions. A preinjection treatment would only fill the vascular system with a weak and often nonpreservative solution and possibly cause distension.

Several factors must be taken into consideration with respect to embalming the body with postmortem stain:

1. A number of hours (approximately 6 or more) have elapsed since death.
2. It is speeded by refrigeration and carbon monoxide death.
3. Pressed on skin does not clear.
4. It is extravascular.
5. It cannot be removed by arterial injection and blood drainage.
6. It is a postmortem chemical change.
7. It is caused by hemolysis and is not blood in the tissues.

TREATMENT OF JAUNDICE

There are three general types of jaundice: toxic jaundice, hemolytic jaundice, and obstructive jaundice. Within each category are a large number of diseases that bring about the antemortem discoloration.

Healthy human blood serum contains approximately 1.0 to 1.5 milligrams of the bile pigment bilirubin (which is yellow in color) per 100 milliliters as a result of the breakdown of red blood cells. Most red blood cells live about 120 days. Because of a variety of diseases that result in *hepatic failure, excessive blood hemolysis,* or *obstruction of the contents of the gallbladder,* the level of bilirubin reaches above 1.5 milligrams per 100 milliliters of blood serum and the tissues of the body begin to take on the yellow jaundiced condition (Fig. 20–4).

In embalming, yellow jaundice (bilirubin) can be converted to green jaundice (biliverdin) by the use of strong arterial solutions. The following statement by

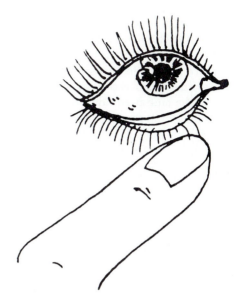

Figure 20–4. Yellow or mild jaundice is often first detected in the sclera (white) of the eye.

Mr. Lee Rendon for Champion Chemical Company points out what is thought to be the actual cause of this conversion. Remember that formaldehyde is a chemical *reducing agent* and the conversion of yellow jaundice to green jaundice is an *oxidation* chemical reaction.

When aldehydes react with proteins, one of the chemical reactions that occurs is said to be that of release of hydrogen ions which, of course, results in a low pH (acid) that is acid in nature. A given amount of formaldehyde or aldehyde can unite with a given amount of protein to form a given aldehyde condensation resin (fixed protein). Once the proteins have received the necessary amount of aldehyde to form these condensation resins, any excess aldehyde tends to become more acid in character and, therefore, causes oxidation changes. From another point of view, aldehydes, in combining with protein or amino acid, increase the local acidity in the tissues by proton release. The hydrogen (H⁺) ions which produce the acid condition result from the chemical action between aldehyde and protein. This acid medium, in turn, results in oxidation changes. The yellow (bilirubin) is converted to green (biliverdin). *It is not the formaldehyde* which causes the oxidation (formaldehyde is a reducing agent). It is the chemical reaction (oxidation) as a result of the acid present.

Five methods for treatment of the jaundiced body are discussed in this chapter. Each method employs a different chemical. Many funeral homes do not stock all of the chemicals discussed; however, every embalmer should have at his or her disposal the proper chemicals to clear the mild jaundiced condition.

Each method is based on the assumption that the embalmer uses a small amount of formaldehyde so that yellow jaundice is not converted to green jaundice. *These treatments work best on the body with a mild jaundice.*

As the primary concern of the embalmer in the preparation of the jaundiced body is the clearing of the discoloration present in the face and hands, the preparation of these bodies could entail restricted cervical injection, wherein both common carotid arteries are raised and remain open during injection of the lower body. Then the head is treated separately, much the same as in the autopsied body. Therefore, the embalming solution intended to clear the jaundiced discoloration would be needed only for injection of the head. The embalmer should remember this point when she or he encounters a jaundiced body in which preservation may be a problem. A different, much stronger arterial solution can then be used to inject the trunk region than would be used for the head.

In the embalming of all jaundiced bodies, preservation takes precedence over clearing of the discoloration.

Method 1: Use of a Jaundice Fluid

Almost every chemical manufacturer produces a jaundice fluid. Most of these fluids are very low in formaldehyde. Some even substitute other preservatives for formaldehyde. For the most part, these fluids are not strong preservatives. Therefore, always follow dilutions recommended by the fluid company. Also, inject the volume of fluid (as minimum) recommended in the instructions.

When in doubt about preservation, reinject the body with a stronger preservative solution of standard embalming fluid. Most jaundice fluids contain a large amount of dye and companies recommend that additional dye be added. The dyes not only indicate to the embalmer where the fluid has distributed, but even more important, they serve to counterstain the jaundice and, thus, cover the discoloration.

Method 2: Use of a Preinjection Solution

In the treatment of mild jaundice a preinjection fluid can be injected prior to the arterial preservative. The theory here is to wash out as much of the discoloration as possible. Enough preinjection fluid should be used to thoroughly rid the body of as much blood as possible. After the preinjection solution has remained in the body for a short period, inject a mild arterial solution containing dye. Again, sufficient volume should be injected to satisfy the preservative demands of the body. Dye can be added to the preinjection solution.

Method 3: Use of Mild Arterial Solution

If preinjection fluids are not used and jaundice fluids not purchased, treat the body by injecting a mild arterial solution and adding extra dye to the solution. Run enough solution to satisfy the preservative demands of the body.

Method 4: Use of Cavity Fluids as Arterial Fluids

Some manufacturers state on the labels of their cavity fluids that they may be used as arterial fluids for specific treatments. One of these treatments is the embalming of jaundiced bodies. It is the bleaching chemicals in the cavity chemical that clear the jaundice. Also keep in mind that many cavity fluids are not of high index, so their formaldehyde content is not high. Again, dye should be added to these arterial solutions.

Method 5: Use of Bleaching Coinjection Solutions

Instructions for several coinjection fluids state that they may be used for the treatment of bodies with extravascular discolorations such as postmortem stain, ecchymosis, gangrene, and jaundice. It is the bleaching property of this fluid that acts on these discolorations. The fluid is injected along with a preservative arterial solution. Dilutions are indicated on the labels of these coinjection fluids. They tend to work best on *mild jaundice.* They lighten the dark jaundice but the remaining discoloration must be covered with opaque cosmetics.

In conclusion, it is most important to again state that above all, preservation is most important in the preparation of a jaundiced body. These bodies can always be treated with opaque cosmetics to successfully hide the discoloration. A good foundation even for cosmetic treatment is good preservation.

TREATMENT OF THE PATHOLOGICAL DISCOLORATION OF NEPHRITIS

One of the signs of chronic renal failure is a "sallow yellow color" to the skin resulting from the presence of urochrome in the tissues. This antemortem pathological discoloration takes on the appearance of mild jaundice. Remember that in chronic renal failure, urea in the blood system is converted to ammonia. Ammonia in the tissues and the blood acts to neutralize formaldehyde. The discoloration is generally treated easily by adding additional dye to the arterial solution. Treatment of bodies with renal failure requires strong arterial solutions to establish firming and good preservation.

Chronic renal failure often accompanies diabetes mellitus. One of the major problems for the embalmer in the preparation of bodies with diabetes mellitus is poor peripheral circulation. Again, this calls for stronger arterial solutions with a good coinjection fluid to help increase distribution and diffusion of the chemical. In many of these bodies gangrene has already been established in the lower limbs. A good dye is recommended to indicate fluid distribution.

Should a preinjection solution be used to rid the blood vascular system of the nitrogenous wastes prior to injection of the preservative arterial solution? Here, the embalmer needs to use extreme caution. When it is felt that the circulation and drainage will be good, this preinjection treatment can be used. If, however, there is evidence of poor circulation and drainage may be difficult to establish (if the body has been dead for a long period, gangrene is present, or there is heavy clotting and ischemic necrosis is present), avoid the preinjection treatment and employ a good strong arterial solution, possibly using a coinjection fluid to assist in distribution and diffusion of the preservative.

TREATMENT OF SURFACE DISCOLORATIONS

Surface discolorations may be antemortem or postmortem. They result from the application of some product (e.g., antiseptic such as betadine) to the skin. They can also be the result of a stain applied for surgical or treatment purposes (e.g., gentian violet is used to mark an area where radiation treatment is to be applied), simple discolorations such as marks made after adhesive tape is pulled away, paint, and tobacco stains on the hands.

Blood is, no doubt, one of the most common discolorations and it can be treated very simply by washing the skin surface with cold water. A mild liquid soap is also of help, and an abrasive cloth such as cheesecloth or gauze pad assists in the removal of dried blood.

Most of the discolorations described above (gentian violet, adhesive tape, surface antiseptics, etc.) respond well to a cleaning with the "dry" hair wash solvents or trichloroethylene (a dry cleaning solvent). Mold, which may occur when the body has been stored for a time, should be scraped away and the area swabbed with a 1% phenol, 1% creosote solution or a mixture of half methyl alcohol and half acetic acid. The majority of surface discolorations respond very well to cleaning with cool water and liquid soap or a mortuary solvent such as the "dry" hair washes.

Surface discolorations should be cleaned away prior to arterial injection. The pores of the skin are easier to clean at this time. After arterial injection the pores close and it is more difficult to completely clean off the discoloration. A second reason is that the embalmer must see the skin to evaluate if arterial solution is present in a particular location. For example, cleaning blood, dirt, and grease from the fingers prior to embalming allows the embalmer to observe the presence of livor mortis in the nail beds. During arterial injection the embalmer can then observe the clearing of the nail beds and the replacement of the livor by the dye of the arterial solution.

TREATMENT OF DISCOLORATIONS RESULTING FROM EMBALMING

Postmortem embalming discolorations and abrasions include dehydration, green jaundice, formaldehyde gray, flushing, razor abrasion, and postmortem bruising. Each should be discussed, because many of these arise as a result of the embalming treatment. A discoloration present prior to embalming, such as yellow jaundice, may be intensified by the embalming. In this case the yellow jaundice is converted to green jaundice.

Dehydration

Dehydration is a drying of the skin. The classic colors of this discoloration are yellow, brown, and black. There are a variety of reasons the dead human body becomes dehydrated. Use of too much and too strong a fluid through a particular area is one reason. Dehydration can also be the result of loss of the superficial layer of skin (e.g., abrasion) or the drying of cut edges of skin (e.g., laceration). Remember that this discoloration cannot be bleached and usually progressively darkens. The application of opaque cosmetics is the best treatment for this discoloration. The embalmer must be able to distinguish this darkening of the tissues from a similar darkening caused by decomposition. Dehydrated skin areas are generally very hard to the touch, whereas a skin area that has decomposed is generally very soft and on touching, skin-slip may be evidenced (Fig. 20–5).

Dehydration of the fingers should be mentioned. This condition is frequently seen when the body has been shipped from another location. If strong dehydration chemicals were employed, the ends of the fingers may have wrinkled and darkened because of dehydration. To prevent this from happening, a small amount of tissue builder can be injected into each finger at the conclusion of the embalming. Another area of the hand that frequently darkens as a result of dehydration brought about by the embalming is the tissue between the thumb and the index finger. Again, filling out this area with some tissue builder after arterial injection will hide the discoloration. The arterial solution may also bring about a loss of moisture from the lips. Wrinkling and, possibly, separation can occur. Tissue builder (after arterial injection) can be injected, from the end of each mucous membrane, to round out the lips and restore their natural fullness.

Many embalmers add a humectant coinjection fluid to the arterial solution for the purpose of adding (or retaining) moisture in the tissues of the body. When using a humectant, however, the embalmer should carefully follow the instructions of the manufacturer, because adding this viscous fluid changes the osmotic balance of the arterial solution. The humectant adds large colloid molecules to the solution. Now, the osmotic pressure of the solution can be reversed and can pull the moisture out of the tissues and into the blood drainage. Only a small

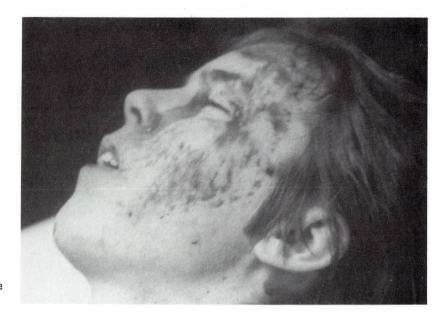

Figure 20–5. Abraded tissues and small lacerations of the left side of the face.

amount of humectant coinjection should be used and intermittent or alternate drainage employed.

Green Jaundice

The second embalming discoloration is the conversion of yellow jaundice to green jaundice. Refer to the section of this chapter on the embalming of jaundiced bodies. This conversion of bilirubin to biliverdin is an oxidation reaction. Formaldehyde, being a strong reducing agent, is only indirectly the cause of this reaction. The excessive use of formaldehyde is the cause. This gradually brings about an acid condition in the tissues, and it is the acid condition that converts the yellow jaundice to green jaundice. The most important point is the *preservation* of the body. This is more important than clearing the yellow jaundice. Treatment can be accomplished by the use of dye in the embalming solution. If this fails to cover the jaundice condition, an opaque cosmetic treatment will be necessary.

Embalmer's (Formaldehyde) Gray

Embalmer's gray, a graying of the tissues, can be seen about 6 hours after embalming. In essence, it is due to failure of the embalmer to wash as much of the blood out of the body as possible. The remaining blood gravitates and mixes with the preservation fluids in the tissues, and the resulting color is a dark gray. This condition can be avoided by the injection of a large volume of arterial solution accompanied by thorough drainage and complete aspiration of the heart. Be certain the head and shoulders of the embalmed body are kept elevated. This elevation prevents blood present in the heart after embalming from moving into the facial and neck tissues, and, thus, prevents embalmer's gray. The discoloration can create a

cosmetic problem, especially when the body has been shipped to another city for final preparation. The firmness of the tissues combined with the dark coloring can create a need for the use of opaque cosmetic treatment.

Flushing

Flushing is seen in those body areas into which the embalmer has been able to distribute arterial solution but has been unable to secure good drainage of blood. Take as an example the body in which the femoral artery is used for injection and the accompanying femoral vein for drainage. If drainage is poor because of clotting in the right atrium of the heart or in one of the internal jugular veins or because of abdominal pressure, arterial solution will quite often flow into the facial tissues. Blood will not be able to rapidly drain from these tissues. The facial tissues and neck look cyanotic. Establishing drainage from another point such as the right internal jugular vein will clear this problem. Some embalmers place a trocar in the right atrium of the heart and drain directly from this point. Relieving gases or edema in the abdominal cavity may solve the problem. If there is edema of the pleural sacs, as seen in some pneumonias, drainage from the jugular will help to remove blood from the facial tissues and the neck. Flushing can result from leaving the drainage closed too long when using intermittent drainage. The establishment of drainage should clear the problem.

Razor Abrasion (Razor Burn)

Another form of dehydration, razor abrasion, occurs when a moist abrasion dries during or after embalming (Any abraded area, area of desquamation, or area of skin where superficial layers of tissue have been torn or scraped away will bring about this condition). Air drying alone turns these areas dark brown. With razor abrasion, application of a light layer of massage cream during embalming helps to prevent the nicked area from dehydrating and browning. If cream cosmetics are to be used and a small layer of wax is placed over the area, the discoloration should not darken or be noticed. The darkening may also be considered an advantage, because it indicates that the areas have dried, and an opaque cosmetic can be used to cover the discoloration. Dried tissues accept cosmetics and, when necessary, wax very well. The embalmer can promote the drying of these areas by using a hair dryer for a few minutes. This ensures that there will be no further leakage, and establishes a good surface for cosmetics

Postmortem Bruising

Postmortem bruising is rare; it occurs if sufficient pressure is applied to tissues to damage capillaries. This condition is particularly noted in persons who have been on blood thinners and in elderly people whose skin is thin. This discoloration is also observed after eye enucleation, because the skin around the eyes is ecchymotic. In fact, the person appears to have had a "black eye" before death. In these situations, the tissues can easily distend when the face is injected. It is wise to raise both common carotid arteries and employ restricted cervical injection. Use a preservative solution that is a little stronger than that normally used so only a minimum of solution need be injected to ensure preservation. Avoid preinjection treatment of the head and facial tissues in these bodies. (Restricted cervical injection is recommended). A hypodermic injection of a phenol solution may help preserve and reduce the distension. Surface compresses of a phenol solution or other preservatives such as cavity fluid or the autopsy gels may also be used during or following arterial injection to reduce distension, bleach the discoloration, and ensure preservation.

TREATMENT OF DECOMPOSITION DISCOLORATION

Decomposition discolorations are brought about by the action of autolytic and bacterial enzymes, as well as the hemolysis of red blood cells.

Decomposition is evidenced by five signs: odor, desquamation, gas, purge, and color changes. The first external sign of decomposition is a color change, usually a green discoloration of the right inguinal or iliac area of the abdomen. This green discoloration enlarges over a period and outlines on the abdominal wall the ascending, transverse, and descending colon. The green then proceeds upward over the chest area into the tissues of the neck and face. A color change is also evidenced throughout the skeletal tissues. Generally the color changes from yellow to green to blue-black to black. In addition, the blood in the veins begins to break down.

This discoloration progresses from the red of the postmortem stain to a black, and follows the course of the particular vein. The pattern thus forms a "spider web" and the veins are described as being mottled.

Both the general progression of color changes resulting from decomposition and the mottling of the veins are discolorations that can be bleached with external compresses such as phenol solutions, cavity fluid, or autopsy gel. These discolorations can be lightened but not to normal skin color. Hypodermic treatment can also be used to lessen the discolorations and to help ensure preservation.

CONDITIONS RELATED TO DISCOLORATIONS*

As previously defined, a discoloration is simply any abnormal color appearing in and on the human body. The discolorations already described involved color changes and possibly some swellings. There were no breaks or tears in the skin surface with the exception of the razor abrasion. In the following conditions, a discoloration is present but, in addition, there is some form of disruption of the skin surface (Fig. 20–6). The emphasis is not so much on the pathological origins of these conditions, but rather on the treatment of these conditions from an embalming standpoint. Restorative treatment is not discussed beyond the extent of those treatments begun in the embalming phase of the restoration.

A *skin lesion* is any *traumatic* or *pathological* change in the structure of the skin. The objective of the embalmer is to properly sanitize skin lesions, clean them of debris, remove skin that cannot be used in the restorative treatment, and secure adequate preservation and drying of the tissues. There are four categories of skin lesions: (1) unbroken skin, (2) skin scaling, (3) skin that is broken or separated from the body, and (4) pustular or ulcerative lesions.

Unbroken but Discolored Skin

Skin may remain unbroken but discolored for a variety of pathological and traumatic cases, for example, allergic reaction, inflammation, trauma, and tumors. Generally, a discoloration will result from an increase in blood flow into the tissues of the affected area and some swelling. If this area is to be viewed (face, neck, or hands), a strong arterial solution can be used to help decrease further swelling or surface compresses can be used to help bleach the area and possibly reduce some of the distension. A phenol solution can be injected beneath the skin after arterial injection to preserve, bleach, and reduce the swelling.

---

*Conditions discussed relating to discolorations and lesions pertain to those conditions located on the face and/or hands of the deceased or other areas of the body that will possibly be viewed.

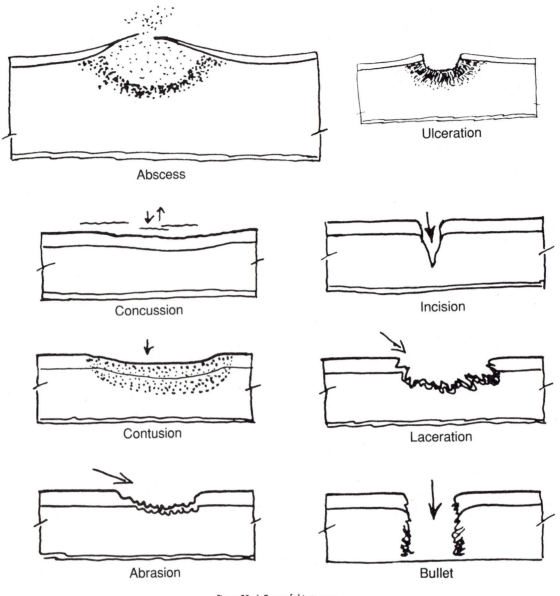

Figure 20–6. Types of skin trauma.

Scaling Skin

Exanthematous diseases such as measles and chickenpox can result in small discolored skin eruptions. Dry skin and large amounts of medications can result in extensive scaling of the skin on the face and hands. Some of the skin breaks away, as in the healing of sunburn. The embalmer must make certain that as much of the loose skin as possible is removed. This is necessary for a good cosmetic treatment on the affected area. Sometimes, a razor can be used to shave the loose skin. Take a solvent (e.g., trichloroethylene and the dry hair washes) and, applying pressure, clean off as much of the loose skin as possible. Apply massage cream to the area, leave it on during the embalming process, then wipe off with solvent. This helps to remove skin debris.

All eruptive and scaling skin conditions should be treated as if they were infectious and/or contagious. Thoroughly disinfect these areas prior to any treatments.

If there is any question as to preservation, brush autopsy gel over the affected area for several hours or apply compresses of a surface preservative. The gels work well because they can be evenly applied and are not harsh bleaching agents. Surface compresses or gels should always be covered with plastic to reduce fumes.

Broken Skin

Three types of broken skin are discussed: abrasions, blisters, and skin-slip.

An **abrasion** is defined simply as skin rubbed off. When the raw skin is exposed to the air and dries, it dis-

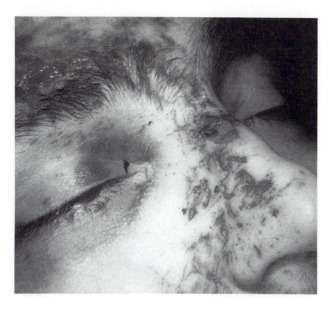

Figure 20–7. Minute lacerations and abrasions, once dried, turn dark brown.

colors to a brown (Fig. 20–7). An abrasion must be dried before restorative treatment commences. This may be cosmetic application, wax application, or surface glue treatment. When an individual falls at the time of death, the moist abrasion might not be noticed by the family. After drying, however, the abrasion is very noticeable.

The embalming treatment is quite simple. During injection, the surrounding tissues can be protected with massage cream. **Do not apply massage cream to the abrasion.** Let the fluid flow through the broken skin. After embalming use a hair dryer to dry the tissues. The tissues will darken and will be firm and dry and ready for restorative treatment. Abrasions on areas that will be viewed must be dry. If there is a preservation problem and fluid did not reach the abraded tissue, a surface compress of phenol cautery solution will help promote preservation and drying of the tissues. Abraded tissue cannot be bleached with surface packs because it is dehydrated.

Blisters are elevations of the epidermis containing a watery liquid. The embalmer must make some decisions here. When blisters are present on an area of the face and preservation has been adequate, they could be coated with a preservative gel for a period, then merely treated with cosmetics. On the lip, however, where glue must be applied, blisters can be "glued under," and no treatment is needed except the creation of a new lip line with cosmetics. If the embalmer feels that blisters should be opened and drained, this can be done prior to arterial treatment. Be certain to remove all loose skin. A phenol cautery solution compress can be used to help dry the raw tissue (Fig. 20–8), or after embalming, a hair dryer can be used to force-dry the tissue.

Tissues must be dry before they are treated with cosmetics, waxes, or surface glues.

Blisters that have been opened and drained prior to death can pose a problem. If the scab is noticeable, it can be removed. A scalpel may be needed to remove the scab, and this should be done prior to arterial injection. The area can be cleaned with a solvent and disinfectant then force-dried with a hair dryer. Drying may also be accomplished with the use of a concentrated phenol cautery compress.

Blisters are characteristic of second-degree burns. In most second-degree burns, the individual lives for a time during which the blisters are opened and drained as part of the treatment. When present on the face, these lesions should be cleaned of loose skin with a sharp razor. A stronger than average solution should be used to embalm the affected area. Then the lesions would be force-dried with a hair dryer, or phenol solution would be used to dry and cauterize the opened blisters.

TREATMENT

1. Lance and drain.
2. Remove all damaged skin.
3. Cauterize.
4. Dry.

Desquamation (Skin-Slip)

Desquamation, separation of the upper layer of skin (the epidermis) from the deeper dermal layer, can be a sign of decomposition. The embalmer's goal is to achieve good

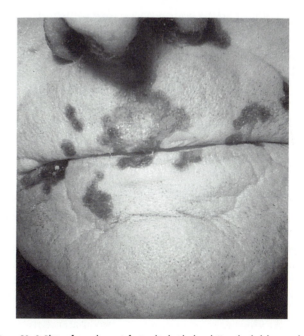

Figure 20–8. Blisters from a herpes infection dried with phenol. Note the dark brown color.

preservation and make sure the areas are dried. Remove all loose skin prior to arterial injection. Peel all loose skin away then use a scalpel to cut at the point where freed skin joins attached skin. For exposed areas with desquamation the following protocol is recommended:

1. Apply a topical disinfectant.
2. Open and drain vesicles if present.
3. Remove all loose skin.
4. Apply surface compresses of cavity fluid or phenol solution to the "raw" tissue or coat the "raw" tissue with autopsy gel.
5. Sectional embalming may be necessary. Use a strong arterial solution.
6. Check preservation. Compresses can be continued or hypodermic treatment instituted with cavity fluid or phenol solution.
7. Clean away all preservative chemicals with a solvent (e.g., dry hair washes or trichloroethylene).
8. Dry the area with a hair dryer to ensure no further leakage.

If desquamation is present on the eyelids or in the vicinity of the eye orbit, cotton can be used to close the eye. Saturate the cotton with a few drops of cavity fluid and glue the eyelids closed. This will serve as an additional internal compress to help establish good preservation. Leave it in place and use cosmetics over the affected skin areas when dried.

Desquamation in unexposed body areas can be treated in the following manner:

1. Apply a topical disinfectant.
2. Open and drain any vesicles that are present.
3. Remove all loose skin.
4. Embalm the body with a strong well-coordinated arterial solution.
5. If possible apply a cavity or phenol compress to the raw tissue or paint it with an autopsy gel.
6. Check for preservation. If not complete, hypodermically treat the area with cavity fluid.
7. Paint again with autopsy gel, cover with embalming powder, or do both.
8. Cover the area with absorbent cotton.
9. Use plastic garments over the affected area.

Pustular and Ulcerative Lesions

Examples of pustular or ulcerative lesions are ulcerations, pustules, herpes fever blisters, chickenpox lesions (Fig. 20–9), boils, carbuncles, and furuncles. These lesions are pustular and contain dead tissue. Treat these lesions in the following manner:

1. Disinfect the surface of the lesion.
2. Open and drain or remove any material in the lesion; clean the lesion and coat with autopsy gel

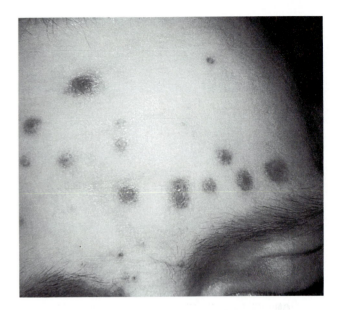

Figure 20–9. Chickenpox lesions on the forehead.

or compress with cotton saturated with cavity fluid or a phenol cautery solution.
3. Embalm the body.
4. Check for preservation. Hypodermic treatment with a preservative or surface compress may be necessary.
5. Dry the area with a solvent and force-dry with a hair dryer.

Decubitus Ulcers (Bedsores)

Because of their size and the fact that most occur on body areas that are not visible during viewing, decubitus ulcers bear special mention. These lesions are the result of a constant inadequate blood supply to the tissues overlying a bony part of the body against which prolonged pressure has been applied. These ulcerations can be very large and are most frequently seen over the sacrum, heels, ankles, and buttocks. In addition, bacterial infections often occur at these locations. Not only does the skin break and drain, but an odor is emitted because of the infection, usually Staph infections. Be certain proper barrier attire is worn when treating all skin lesions.

Routine treatment of these ulcerations (when present on body areas that are not visible) can be summarized:

1. Disinfect the surface. Remove all bandages and apply a droplet spray.
2. Temporarily pack the area to reduce odors and to promote surface preservation.
   A. Autopsy gel can be painted over the ulceration.

B. A cavity or phenol solution compress can be placed over the ulcer. When the lesions are located on the sides of the body, it may be helpful to leave taped bandages in place and soak them with cavity fluid.

3. Embalm the body.

4. Hypodermically inject cavity fluid (via infant trocar) into all the areas surrounding the ulceration.

5. Apply new surface compresses of cavity fluid or autopsy gel to the ulceration.

6. Clothe the body in plastic garments (stockings, pants, coveralls, etc.). If plastic garments are not available for the buttocks, make a larger diaper.

7. Spread embalming powder in the plastic garments to control odors.

CONDITIONS RELATED TO DISCOLORATIONS: UNNATURAL CAUSES OF DEATH

The unnatural causes of death are briefly discussed at this point. In most instances, these causes are related to discolorations (Table 20–2). Although it is not a cause of death, refrigeration does result in some special discoloration problems. Suggestions are given for preparation of bodies dead from unnatural causes.

Almost all deaths from unnatural causes are investigated by legal authority, either the coroner or a medical examiner. Some of these deaths may be work related

and the subject of workmen's compensation and insurance claims. Investigation by the coroner or medical examiner, in most states, leads to autopsy. The autopsy presents its own set of problems for the embalmer. Many of these deaths occur in the absence of other individuals, and there may be a considerable delay between death and finding of the body.

Because of these two factors (investigation and delay), specific directions as to how the body should be prepared are not given here. In the face of a long delay, two actions are recommended: the use of a strong arterial preservative solution (special-purpose high-index arterial fluids) and injection of the right common carotid artery and accompanying internal jugular vein. Injection of both common carotid arteries (restricted cervical injection) is recommended when problems are anticipated in preservation or circulation.

Preservation must be the most important goal in embalming these bodies. Discolorations can always be masked with opaque cosmetics.

Refrigerated Bodies

From a discoloration standpoint, intense livor mortis can be expected in bodies that are refrigerated shortly after death. The cooling process helps to keep the blood liquid. When the body has been stored 6 to 12 hours prior to preparation, the dependent tissues can turn a variety of dark hues from red to blue-black. It is important to elevate the head and shoulders of refrigerated bodies to avoid intense livor mortis in the tissues of the neck and face.

Postmortem stain is also prevalent in these bodies. Hemolysis is speeded by cooling. In addition, the capillaries are more porous. Thus, stain can be expected in areas where livor is present if the body has been refrigerated more than 12 hours.

If the body has been refrigerated several days, expect surface dehydration of the body. The lips and fingertips darken because of dehydration, as does the remaining skin, after a long period of refrigeration.

The means of storing bodies have changed in the past several years. Many hospitals and institutions now place the body in zippered plastic pouches or wrap the body in plastic. Years ago, the body was wrapped in cotton sheeting. The plastic bags cause the body to retain some heat and tend to trap moisture, thus slowing the dehydration process. This accelerates decomposition—sometimes extensively!

No treatment for refrigerated bodies is given at this point, but several items should be remembered:

1. No one condition such as refrigeration should dictate the method of embalming. Other factors

TABLE 20–2. UNNATURAL CONDITIONS RELATED TO DISCOLORATIONS

Burns	First degree—redness of the skin
	Second degree—blistering and redness
	Third degree—charred tissue
Carbon monoxide poisoning	Bright red color to the blood
	Low blood viscosity, intense livor
	Rapid postmortem staining
Drowning	Low blood viscosity, intense livor
	Head faced downward, livor and stain
	Possible abrasions and bruising
Electrocution	Point of contact, burn marks can be present
Exsanguination	Little livor mortis, paleness to skin surfaces
Gunshot wounds	Eyelids can show ecchymosis, swelling of eye area when injury is to face or head
Hanging	Intensive livor in facial tissues; some capillary rupture showing petechial discolorations; no blood present in facial tissues
Mutilation	Loss of blood—little livor mortis
	Ecchymosis and bruising at affected areas
Poisons	Variable—from generalized conditions such as jaundice and cyanosis to localized discolorations such as caustic burns and petechiae
Refrigeration	Low blood viscosity, intense livor
	Postmortem stain speeded
	Dehydration of mucous membranes and skin surface after long exposure to cold air

are equally as important (e.g., manner of death, time between death and preparation, effects of conditions such as edemas and jaundice, and effects of drugs).

2. Today, if death occurs in an institution, the body is usually refrigerated for some period. Refrigeration slows, but does not stop, postmortem changes such as decomposition and rigor mortis. These processes continue at a slower pace in these bodies.

3. Hemolysis also occurs in blood trapped in superficial nondependent tissues. The tissue looks as if it has already been embalmed; it is a light pink. Close observation and tracer dyes should be used in the preparation of these bodies to ensure the presence of embalming solution in all tissues.

4. Refrigeration can also solidify subcutaneous fatty tissues so that they feel firm to the touch. This can falsely signal that a reaction has occurred between the preservative solution and the body proteins.

5. All chemical reactions slow in colder environments; thus, the reaction between body proteins and preservative solution is not as rapid as that in bodies that have not been refrigerated.

6. Remember that after death, blood is trapped in the large arteries of the body, particularly the aorta. This blood thickens and agglutinates during refrigeration, and, on arterial injection, these large blood masses can be loosened and pushed along with the fluid. The common carotid artery (arteries) is a wise choice of vessels in the preparation of bodies refrigerated for long periods.

7. If the body has been refrigerated longer than 24 hours, expect a high moisture content in some body tissues because the serum portion of the blood leaves the blood vascular system and gradually makes its way to the surface of the body as a result of surface dehydration. This increase in tissue fluids is called postmortem edema.

Hangings

Self-inflicted, accidental, or intentional hanging can result in two different situations. First, extensive discoloration may appear on the face as a result of the pressure placed on the jugular veins in the last moments of life, when blood was able to enter the facial tissues via the common carotids and vertebral routes, but was unable to drain from these tissues. The eyes and tongue may also protrude. The discoloration can be intense enough that the face appears almost black.

Second, no blood is present in the facial tissues because the blood was able to drain from the tissues.

Many cyanotic and blood discolorations in the fa-

cial tissues clear after the pressure has been relieved from the neck. Additionally, almost all of these bodies come under the jurisdiction of the coroner or medical examiner and most would be examined by autopsy. During autopsy a great amount of blood is drained from the facial tissues. It is wise in the preparation of bodies dead from hanging on which no autopsy has been performed that both common carotid arteries be raised and the head separately injected (restricted cervical injection).

The strength of the solution depends on the time between death and preparation, pathological conditions, and so on. As in most cases of delay, a medium to strong 2.0 to 2.5% well-coordinated arterial solution should be used.

Expect some postmortem staining if there has been a delay. In addition, there is a possibility of some small capillary hemorrhages. Preinjection fluid should be avoided. Use of a medium to strong arterial solution is advised as is the use of a coinjection fluid. The head should be injected separately, left side first then right side. Use a minimum amount of fluid, for there is a good possibility of swelling. Remember, strong solutions help to bleach discolorations (minimum amounts are needed) and to prevent swelling.

Burned Bodies

Burns may be caused by heat (thermal burns), electrical shock, radioactive agents, or chemical agents. It is not always the local effect of the burn that should concern the embalmer, but rather the systemic effects brought about by major burns: bacterial infections, lack of blood flow to peripheral areas of the body, and kidney failure and the resulting buildup of wastes in blood and tissue fluids.

Many victims of burns will have lived for a period between the injury and their death. The blistering of second-degree burns is rarely seen. These blisters are opened, drained, and treated long before the death. It is the systemic effects that the embalmer must keep in mind. Burned bodies have a very high preservative demand. Circulation may be very difficult to establish, unless the cause was electrical shock. Very strong arterial solutions are used to prepare these bodies. Dye is added to trace the distribution of solution. Sectional injection, if the body has not been autopsied, is often needed. The skin must be dried:

1. Remove all loose skin before arterial injection using a good sharp razor (on visible areas).

2. Apply surface cavity (or phenol) compresses or paint the visible areas with autopsy gel. These gels can be painted over damaged skin areas that will not be viewed. (It is not necessary to clean these areas as they will be covered with plastic and clothing.)

3. Clean the skin surface with a good solvent.
4. Air-dry or force-dry with a hair dryer.

Burns are classified into three categories:

■ *First degree:* The skin surface is red (erythema); only the surface epithelium is involved.
■ *Second degree:* The skin blisters and edema is present. Blisters beneath or within the epidermis are called *bullae*. There is destruction of the deep layers of the epidermis and the upper layers of the dermis (Fig. 20–10).
■ *Third degree:* The tissues are charred. The epidermis, the dermis, and epidermal derivatives such as hair follicles and glandular inclusions are destroyed.

Often, burns (and scalds) affect large regions of the body but not the face or hands. The affected areas may emit an odor. Painting these unseen areas with an autopsy preservative gel helps to ensure preservation and reduce odors. Edema and swelling are often present with second-degree burns. To prevent leakage and again to control odors, use of a *unionall* garment is recommended. This plastic garment covers all of the body except the face and hands. Unionall garments cover the arms and shoulders, areas not covered with other plastic garments such as coveralls or sleeves. Ample embalming powder should be spread in the unionall, especially over the burned areas. The autopsy gel may be left in place. The sprinkled

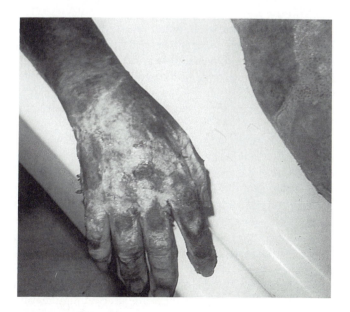

Figure 20–10. Second-degree burns. Burned bodies often have a very high preservative demand because of kidney failure.

powder adheres to the gel surface. Moisture-absorbent kitty litter can be liberally sprinkled over the burnt tissues to help control odor.

The need to achieve preservation cannot be overemphasized in the preparation of burned bodies. Many of these bodies should be embalmed with 100% high-index arterial fluid using no water. Coinjection fluid may be added to help dilute.

Many bodies cannot be viewed because the facial tissues are severely swollen. All the embalmer can do is obtain some preservation and control leakage and odors.

Another problem arises in suture of the incision used for embalming. Application of super glue may help. There is no question that the best vessels to inject and drain in burned bodies are the common carotid artery and the internal jugular vein.

Use restricted cervical injection whenever possible so the maximum preservative solution can be injected. There is one exception. If only the neck area is affected by the burns, it might be wiser to inject and drain from an area of the body not affected by the burn.

Electrocution

Electrocution is related to discoloration because of the burn that results from contact with the electrical source. Many times the palms of the hands are burned. Remember, however, the body is embalmed on the basis of a number of conditions (e.g., time between death and embalming, pathological problems, body size and weight, presence of rigor mortis).

The cause of death, the electrical contact, should present no problem to the embalmer. Restoration of the burn area is a restorative art problem only if the burn exists in a viewable area. Often, these bodies are autopsied, as the death must be investigated by a coroner or medical examiner. For the preparation, the routine autopsy protocol is followed. In some instances the coroner or medical examiner may have excised the area of tissue where the electrical burn occurred. If so, a strong cautery phenol solution should be applied to the raw tissue to dry and firm the area.

Carbon Monoxide Poisoning

The primary concern in discolorations associated with deaths from carbon monoxide poisoning is the classic "cherry-red" color. Students of mortuary science who have not viewed these bodies often mistakenly believe that the entire body turns bright red. The "bright red" color is found in the dependent areas of the body to which

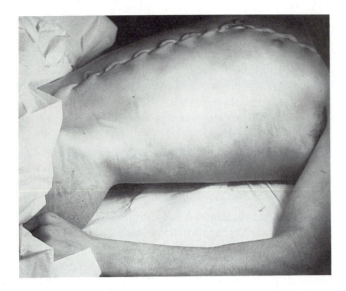

Figure 20–11. Dependent areas are bright red in this unembalmed autopsied body. The cause of death was carbon monoxide poisoning.

the blood gravitates after death—the areas where livor mortis is present (Fig. 20–11).

Most areas of the body where livor mortis is not present appear normal, although some blood is usually trapped in the anterior surface tissues. It looks as if the tissue was well embalmed and fluid dye was employed.

The bright color of the blood is due to carboxyhemoglobin, a component of blood. In addition, if the body is prepared a short time after death, the blood has a very low viscosity, very few clots are present. Of course, as time progresses so do the problems of distribution.

This blood discoloration is classified both as an antemortem discoloration and as an intravascular discoloration. It should clear during arterial injection and subsequent blood drainage; however, there are usually some time delays between the death and the preparation of the body. As most of these deaths must be investigated by a coroner or medical examiner, preparation is delayed and the blood rapidly undergoes hemolysis. Therefore, in the majority of these bodies, some, but not complete, clearing of the discoloration occurs.

Solution strength should be based on the postmortem changes, the length of the delay, and the size and weight of the body. Delay and refrigeration necessitate use of a stronger-than-average solution. Extra dye should be used to indicate solution distribution and diffusion. Once circulation is established, the solution strength can be increased further. Individuals who commit suicide by carbon monoxide poisoning often may have been suffering from some disease process. Again, such complications as jaundice, edema, and circulatory problems, as well as drug therapies, influence the strength of the solution used.

With regard to the selection of vessels, if there are no major problems or delays, any vessel is appropriate. Where there has been a delay, pathological problems, and so on, the best vessels are the common carotid artery and the internal jugular vein. If the embalmer feels that large volumes of solution are needed, as in the preparation of obese bodies with generalized skeletal edema, or decomposed bodies, restricted cervical injection is recommended.

Carbon monoxide poisoning in and of itself should not be a big problem for the embalmer. In many cases, the blood is quite thin and there is minimum clotting. If the facial tissues and neck are dependent, however, intense livor and staining can be expected. When some discoloration exists after embalming, a semiopaque or opaque cream cosmetic is advised, as the tissues tend to gray over time. Again, counterstaining with extra dye in the arterial solution helps to overcome this graying.

Most of these bodies are autopsied for medicolegal purposes. In these situations, follow the normal autopsy preparation protocol.

Drownings

In a victim of drowning, the most noticeable discolorations are intense livor mortis and possibly cyanosis. The livor mortis is due to the low temperature of the water, similar to refrigeration; the blood remains liquid and rapidly settles to the dependent tissues. If enough gas is generated to bring the body to the surface, the body floats face downward. Therefore, the livor and the resulting postmortem stain are intense in the facial areas. The cyanosis would be the result of the asphyxia (from the water in the respiratory system).

Each case must be handled on an individual basis. Preparation of some bodies has been delayed months because the drowning occurred in winter but the body was not recovered until spring. These bodies were viewable. Other drowned bodies that have been in the water for a matter of hours have been so decomposed that they could not be prepared for viewing.

In addition to livor, postmortem stain, and cyanosis, some bodies may be dragged by currents along a river or ocean floor and bruised (lacerations). Large abrasions are frequently seen. Cool water preserves the body. Warm water speeds decomposition. In addition, fish and marine animals may desecrate the body.

A constant problem in the preparation of a drowned person is the possibility of **purge**, either lung or stomach purge. Selection of vessels should be based on the condition of the body. If the embalmer has any doubts, use of the common carotid artery and the internal jugular vein is recommended. The ideal is restricted cervical injection. The strength of the fluid again depends on the extent of decomposition, the size of the body, pathological complications, and other factors in the case analysis. Aspiration should be thorough, with a minimum of two to three bottles of cavity fluid used on adult bodies.

Be certain a thorough amount of cotton or cotton webbing is packed into the throat and respiratory passageways. These bodies should be reaspirated, and if gases are evident or the viscera do not appear firm, at least one more bottle of cavity fluid should be injected.

Gunshot Wounds

Death from gunshot wounds poses a number of problems for the embalmer. Some gunshot wounds are barely noticeable. Many embalmers have seen bodies where a pistol was discharged in the mouth but there was no exit wound. In other cases, the bullet exited through a small hole in the forehead. Still others present great amounts of trauma. These deaths must be handled individually. The conditions most likely to be found are ecchymoses and possible swelling of the eyelids. Bones of the face and cranium are often fractured. Purging is quite likely from the nose and the ears (Fig. 20–12).

Again, most of these bodies are autopsied. Difficulty arises in reshaping of the cranium when the bones are fractured. Plaster of Paris may prove helpful in realigning and reshaping the cranium after embalming.

To minimize swelling, especially if facial bones are fractured and the eyes are ecchymotic and swollen, use a very strong, well-coordinated arterial solution. The **instant tissue fixation** method of embalming has proven very useful in embalming these bodies. In this method almost 100% arterial fluid is injected in short spurts under

high pressure. With this method, the fluid is distributed as far as possible, but only a minimum amount of fluid is needed. As this method is so valuable in the preparation of bodies with gunshot wounds, whether autopsied or not, it is outlined here:

1. Realign the features as best as can be done.
2. Raise the right and the left common carotid arteries and insert tubes directed upward on both the right and left sides. Direct one tube downward on the right side.
3. Prepare a solution for injection into the trunk.
4. Inject the trunk. Be certain that the tubes directed toward the head remain open and that the lower portion of the left common carotid is ligated.
5. Prepare a solution for injection of the head: two bottles of 25-index or stronger fluid, one bottle of coinjection fluid (or one bottle of water), and fluid dye.
6. Set pressure on a centrifugal machine to 20 pounds or more with the rate-of-flow valve closed.
7. Inject the left side of the head first. Open and immediately close the rate-of-flow valve so the fluid is injected in spurts. Do this until you are satisfied that the tissues are preserved.
8. Repeat injection on the right side of the face.

If the eyelids are distended, a phenol-reducing and bleaching agent can be hypodermically injected using "hidden points of entry." It is possible for this solution to leak out of the hypodermic needle punctures; the hidden points provide a location where leakage is least likely to be seen. The following points of entry are suggested:

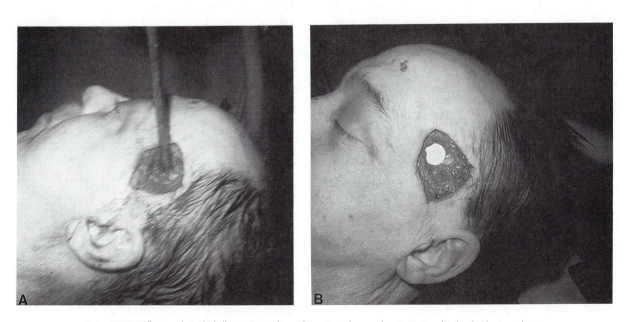

Figure 20–12. Bullet wound. **A.** The bullet entry wound is used to aspirate the cranial cavity. **B.** Wound is closed with a trocar button.

1. Lower eyelid and surrounding tissues
   A. Inside the mouth
   B. Inside the nostril
   C. Behind the ear or in the hairline
2. Upper eyelid and surrounding tissues
   A. Eyebrow
   B. Hairline

Let the phenol solution remain undisturbed for 20 to 30 minutes; then apply pressure to decrease swelling. Remove excess liquids through the needle punctures.

Surface compresses (of cavity fluid or a surface bleaching compound) may be applied to add weight to help reduce the distension as well as to preserve and bleach tissues. These compresses take more time to work and are much less effective than injection of a phenol solution into the tissues. If there is doubt about preservation, cotton may be used to close the eyelids; it can be saturated with cavity fluid and then the lids glued.

In some cases, the eyes are so distended that the eyelashes cannot be seen. The protocol just explained has been quite successful in treating such distended eyes and reducing and bleaching them to a point at which opaque cosmetics can be applied.

With black eyes or distended eyes, always encourage the use of glasses on the deceased. The lights over the casket or on either end of the casket reflect off the lenses and hide some of the problem areas.

Not all gunshot wounds affect the head or face. When the bullet enters thoracic or abdominal areas, a large amount of blood may be lost. Livor mortis is minimal in such bodies. If the body is not autopsied, use the right common carotid and the accompanying internal jugular vein. If there is drainage and signs of distribution are evident, continue the injection, but use a slightly stronger-than-average arterial solution containing plenty of tracer dye.

There may be abdominal swelling or blood purge through the mouth or nose. The abdominal distension may be blood and fluid draining into the abdomen if a large vein was affected by the gunshot. If the arterial system is intact look for signs of distribution. Blood purging from the mouth or nose during injection may indicate that a vein in the stomach was severed by the gunshot. As long as there are signs of arterial solution distribution, continue the injection. Standard drainage from the selected vein may be very decreased.

If the abdomen begins to swell immediately after the artery is injected and there is no drainage or signs of arterial solution distribution, it is obvious that a large artery has been affected by the gunshot. Stop injection and begin sectional arterial injection. The following order of injection is suggested: legs, arms, left side of the head, right side of the head. The trunk walls may be treated by hypodermic injection with an infant trocar. Several points of entry are needed to reach all of the tissues.

As previously stated, each body with gunshot wounds must be treated on an individual basis. Most of these bodies are autopsied, so the standard autopsy routine can be followed. If the eyes are affected, as has been described, instant tissue fixation may be used to control swelling and maximize preservation.

Poisoning

A variety of discolorations are associated with poisoning deaths. Some poisons act in a very short time. Others have a cumulative effect on the body. The latter poisons may affect the liver, which, in turn, leads to jaundice. Some poisons induce shock; the blood is drawn into the large veins and the body exhibits very little livor mortis.

A large number of poisons act on the nervous and muscular systems. Respiration becomes difficult and the body becomes cyanotic. Other poisons are corrosive and burn areas such as the mouth and hands with which they come into contact. In addition, the corrosive agent destroys tissues of the gastrointestinal tract, causing the rupture of veins and arteries in these organs. Some poisons cause petechiae on the skin surface. Others bring about anaphylactic shock, causing the skin to redden and swell.

Most of these bodies are autopsied. Dyes can be used to counterstain discolorations. Preservation should be the first concern. Areas burned by corrosive poisons need to be cleaned and dried before restorative treatment begins.

Mutilations

The conditions caused by the various types of mutilation could fill an entire book. An automobile accident involves mutilation; a stabbing involves mutilation; accidental deaths can involve mutilation; even some extensive surgical procedures might be classified by laymen as mutilation; the results of poor autopsy technique and some medicolegal autopsies may be viewed as mutilation.

These bodies cannot be embalmed by the "one-point" method of arterial embalming. Most require sectional arterial embalming. In addition, hypodermic and surface embalming is necessary to achieve adequate preservation of the body (Fig. 20–13).

In these bodies discolorations usually manifest as ecchymoses and antemortem and postmortem bruises. As with most unnatural causes of death, an autopsy is likely, but even with the autopsy, additional sectional and regional arterial injection may be necessary.

Remember that in the preparation of mutilated remains, arteries remain open when they are severed. An embalmer familiar with the arterial pathways can easily dissect to locate the arteries. These vessels can be used for the injection of embalming solution. Drainage need not be a concern as many of these bodies have sustained a major blood loss and drainage will be minimal. Strong

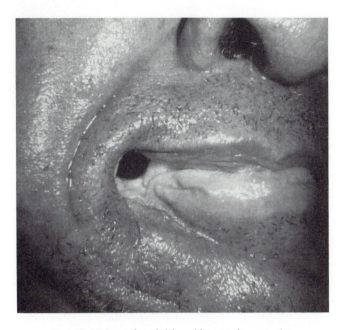

Figure 20–13. Corner of mouth deformed from use of a gastric tube.

When necessary, sectional arterial embalming should be employed. The most difficult area to embalm, when there has been a "break" in the circulatory system, is the trunk. Legs, arms, and the head pose no difficulty as these can be directly injected. The trunk may absorb some solution, but if an artery such as the aorta has ruptured, the trunk walls will have to be embalmed hypodermically, using a small trocar attached to the embalming machine.

A strong solution should be used for the hypodermic injection. A solution of cavity fluid and water is a good mixture and probably less costly than arterial fluid; however, some embalmers prefer the arterial fluid. This work must be thorough, as areas not reached by the hypodermic treatment stand little chance of contact with fluid by gravitation or diffusion from other areas. Several points will have to be used to introduce the trocar into the trunk. Special emphasis should be placed on the buttocks and shoulder areas.

arterial solutions should be used. Such cases constitute an excellent example of the type of body for which special-purpose high-index fluids can be used. Use dyes to trace arterial solution distribution.

Exsanguination

Exsanguination is excessive blood loss to the point of death. The blood loss is not always external, as in massive hemorrhage. It can be internal, for example, rupture of a blood vessel caused by ulceration of an area or rupture of an aneurysm in one of the large body cavities. Blood loss can also occur without a break in the blood vascular system, as seen in shock. Here, the blood flows to the large, deep veins of the body, draining the capillaries of needed blood.

Exsanguination deaths are characterized not so much by discoloration as by a lack of color. Whether blood is lost externally, internally, or into the deep veins, very little livor mortis is evident. In cases of shock, the blood tends to congeal in the large veins and drainage may be difficult to establish. The largest vein possible should be employed in the preparation of these bodies. That would be the right internal jugular vein, which leads directly into the right atrium of the heart.

In injecting bodies that have sustained a large blood loss, a slightly stronger arterial solution should be used, for there is likely to be a loss of arterial solution depending on the cause of blood loss. Additional dye should be added to the arterial solution to trace the distribution of arterial solution.

KEY TERMS AND CONCEPTS FOR STUDY AND DISCUSSION

1. Define the following terms:
   abrasion
   antemortem extravascular blood discoloration
   antemortem intravascular blood discoloration
   blood discoloration
   decomposition discoloration
   discoloration
   drug and/or therapeutic discoloration
   ecchymosis
   embalming discoloration
   formaldehyde gray
   hypostasis
   livor mortis
   pathological discoloration
   postmortem extravascular blood discoloration
   postmortem intravascular blood discoloration
   postmortem stain
   skin lesion
   skin-slip
   surface discoloring agent
2. Discuss the embalming treatments for a body with "mild" jaundice.
3. Discuss the arterial solutions that can be used to help clear livor mortis in embalming a body that still retains heat.
4. Discuss the problems that can be encountered, with respect to discolorations, in the preparation of a drowned body, a body dead from hanging, and a body dead from carbon monoxide poisoning.

5. Discuss the differences between postmortem hypostasis, livor mortis, and postmortem stain.

BIBLIOGRAPHY

Adams J. Embalming the jaundice case—Part IV. *Dodge Magazine*, Jan–Feb, 1995.

Bedino JH. Waterless embalming—An investigation. *Champion Expanding Encyclopedia*. 1993; 619–620.

Embalming Course Content Syllabus. American Board of Funeral Service Education, 1991.

Kazmier H. *Essentials of Systemic Pathology.* Dubuque, IA: Kendeil-Hunt Publishing Co; 1976.

Mayer JS. *Color and Cosmetics.* (3rd ed) Dallas: Professional Training Schools, Inc; 1986.

Mayer JS. *Restorative Art.* (6th ed) Bergenfield, NJ: Paula Publishing Co, Inc; 1974.

21

Moisture Considerations

There are three objectives of embalming: preservation, sanitation, and restoration of the body. Water plays an important role in achieving these objectives. A properly embalmed body should not show evidence of dehydration. Bodies that have died from conditions that resulted in edema (or high moisture content) should be treated in such a manner that the excess moisture is removed or controlled. Similarly, dehydrated bodies should be treated in such a manner that water is added to the dry tissues. The control of moisture is a major concern for the embalmer. **A major objective of the embalming process should be to establish or to maintain a proper moisture balance in the dead human body.**

Three conditions characterize the dead human body with regard to moisture: normal moisture, dehydration, and edema. It is important that the embalmer recognize that all three of these conditions can occur generally or locally in a body.

In this chapter, bodies with normal water balance are considered first. It is important that this normal water balance be maintained during the funeral. It is the job of the embalmer to prevent bodies with normal tissue moisture from dehydrating. Dehydration is discussed next, as are the methods the embalmer can employ to moisturize tissues. Finally, localized and generalized edema is discussed together with methods that can be employed to reduce moisture.

Embalming analysis involves many components and choices. Examination of the body determines what embalming chemicals are to be used and in what manner these chemicals should be injected. Body moisture plays a very large role in these decisions. Some examples of chemicals and injection techniques the use of which is determined by the moisture condition of the body follow:

- Arterial fluid (index, firming action, etc.)
- Dilution of the arterial fluid
- Volume of arterial solution to inject
- Use of coinjection or humectant fluid and its dilution
- Vessel or vessels for injection and drainage
- Injection and drainage techniques to add, maintain, or remove moisture
- Speed of arterial injection
- Use of special techniques and fluids that add or remove moisture.

NORMAL BODY MOISTURE

For the healthy, average, 160-pound male adult, *total body water* constitutes 55 to 60% (for normal to obese bodies) and approximately 65% (for thin bodies) of *total* body weight. For the female adult, the proportions are, on average, 10% less than those for the corresponding male body types. **Edema is said to be established when there is a 10% increase in total body water.**

After death, several factors bring about dehydration. Storage of the body in a refrigerator is one of the leading causes of a postmortem loss of moisture. Dry, cool, or warm air moving across the body promotes dehydration. Between death and embalming, the blood and tissue fluids begin to gravitate into dependent body regions, increasing the moisture levels in the dependent tissues but reducing the moisture in the elevated body areas.

The embalming process itself can either add or greatly reduce moisture. The primary ingredient in embalming fluids is formaldehyde, and formaldehyde dries tissues. During arterial injection the skin becomes dry to the touch. The lips and the area between the thumb and index finger rapidly indicate if the arterial embalming is producing dehydration. This dehydrating effect can be evidenced before arterial injection is completed.

The embalmer must see that a good moisture balance is established or maintained. The well-embalmed body should not show signs of wrinkled, dark dehydrated tissue during the funeral. **Well-embalmed tissues dehydrate LESS than underembalmed tissues.** Today, many bodies are shipped to other locations for funeral services and disposition, so there are delays. It is most important that the body change little in appearance during these delays.

Some embalming techniques can dehydrate a body that was normal at the beginning of the embalming process. Persons who die suddenly (e.g., accidental death or heart attacks) usually have normal moisture levels.

An article published many years ago (by Philip Boehinger in *Esco Review*) cited some interesting relationships dealing with the loss of moisture from the dead human body:

> If a pint of water weighs approximately 1 pound, consider the following: If the embalmer injects 3 gallons of arterial solution, 24 pounds of liquid is injected.
>
> The following liquid losses were estimated: $1\frac{1}{2}$ gallons of drainage = 12 pounds moisture lost; 1 quart of liquid aspirated = 2 pounds moisture lost. Up to 3 pints can be lost per day by dehydration; funerals average 3 days = 9 pounds moisture lost.

One pound of moisture remains (or was added) by the preceding example. This body should not have evidenced any dehydration during viewing. These are conservative figures, but they do present an interesting challenge for the embalmer.

A simple way to maintain the proper moisture level during the embalming process is simply to follow the dilution recommendations on the label of the arterial fluid. Almost all fluid manufacturers recommend dilutions based on the moisture conditions of the body. Many times, they recommend the volume to be injected, the type of drainage, and the rate of flow at which to inject the arterial solution. The temperature of the water is also often stated on the label. For example, a typical fluid label might state the dilution for "normal bodies," the dilution for "dehydrated" bodies, and the dilution for "edematous" bodies.

The dilution rule also applies to the use of coinjection and humectant fluids. Improperly used, these fluids can act in an opposite manner. A humectant can act as a dehydrating chemical as well as a moisturizing chemical.

The following techniques can help to maintain a good balance of moisture in the body:

1. Avoid the use of astringent or hypertonic arterial solutions. Follow dilutions recommended by the manufacturer. Hypotonic solutions penetrate better, and their diffusion and retention will be increased. Strengths of 0.75 to 1.5% help to add moisture to the tissues. Most manufacturers recommend dilutions for dry, moist, and normal bodies.
2. Avoid the use of concurrent or continuous drainage after surface discolorations have cleared. Intermittent or alternate drainage helps to distribute and diffuse the arterial solution. These methods also help the body to retain arterial solution.
3. Avoid rapid arterial injection and drainage. A slower injection helps fluid to penetrate the tissues and reduces "short circuiting" of fluids, so the solution is better distributed. Less tissue fluid is withdrawn from the tissues.
4. The delay of aspiration, if just for a short time, assists in diffusing arterial solution into the tissues. For best results, the final portion of arterial solution should be injected with the drainage closed. If aspiration is then delayed for a short time, the solution will have ample time to properly diffuse into the tissues.
5. If refrigerated prior to embalming, the body should be covered with plastic sheeting to prevent the surrounding air from dehydrating the surface tissues.
6. Strong alkaline or acid fluids can alter the reaction between protein and preservative. Formaldehyde has a drying effect on the tissues. Acid or rapid-acting arterial fluids often produce very firm and dry tissues. Old (outdated) fluids should be avoided. These fluids cause the tissues to dehydrate rapidly.
7. Disinfectants should not dry and bleach the surface tissues.

8. Use of cotton to set features can cause tissues to dry. Massage cream and cream cosmetics help to slow the dehydrating effect of cotton. Nonabsorbent cotton can be used as a substitute.

9. Fumes from the injection of cavity fluids into the neck area can dehydrate the mouth and the nose. These areas can be packed tightly so fumes cannot enter.

10. Short circuiting of arterial solution causes dehydration of the areas in which the solution is circulating. Distribution is uneven and the short circuiting regions are very firm and dry.

11. Warm water solutions increase fluid reaction. Follow the manufacturer's recommendations for water dilution temperatures. Cool solutions slow the formaldehyde reaction, thus allowing better distribution and diffusion of the arterial solution throughout the entire body.

12. After embalming, the body should be covered to prevent circulating air from dehydrating the surface. Application of cream cosmetics and massage cream to the surface tissues helps to reduce moisture loss to the atmosphere (Fig. 21–1).

It is important that the embalmer maintain the moisture present in the "normal" body. Because of drainage and the arterial fluid itself (remember that formaldehyde dries tissues), the embalmer must actually *add* moisture to the normal body. This is why so much water is used to dilute arterial fluid. Almost 20 ounces of water is added for each ounce of arterial fluid!

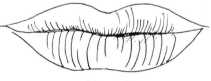

Normal

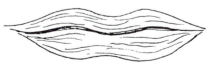

Dehydrated

Figure 21–1. Dehydration causes horizontal wrinkles to form on the lips. With the disease processes seen today it is necessary that the body be properly sanitized. A moderate arterial solution by today's standards is 1.5 to 2.0%. Many fluids are reaction controlled and do not release the preservative ingredients until they come into contact with body cells.

PREPARATION OF THE DEHYDRATED BODY

Antemortem Dehydration

Dehydration may have occurred while the person was alive. A number of disease processes result in a loss of fluid from the body cells and tissues: slow hemorrhage, febrile diseases, kidney diseases, diabetes, some cancers and localized neoplasms, and some first-degree burns. All these antemorten conditions contribute to a loss of body moisture. The classic example of a disease process that can cause dehydration is tuberculosis, especially tuberculosis of the lungs. Drug therapy, intravenous fluid injection, and stomach tube feedings are employed to maintain a normal moisture level in the living person. Therefore, today, tuberculosis may not always produce the characteristic signs of dehydration. Drug therapy and chemotherapy can result in dehydration in the living body.

Postmortem Dehydration—Preembalming

After death, a major cause of dehydration is refrigeration. Dry, cool air moves around the body and gradually draws the moisture in the tissues to the surface of the body and from the surface into the surrounding air. (Refrigerated bodies are discussed in Chapter 19.) Refrigeration keeps the blood in a fluid state. Thus, the blood and tissue fluids slowly gravitate to the dependent tissues of the body. The upper areas of the body lose moisture because of surface evaporation and the gravitation of fluids.

Embalming Treatments to Control Dehydration

The skin on a dehydrated body is very dry. Often, the skin is quite "flaky" and small pieces of tissue easily come loose. These small scaly flakes of skin must be removed from the facial areas or they will create a problem when cosmetics are applied. A liberal application of massage cream helps to control the flaking. The massage cream can be firmly wiped off with a gauze pad saturated with solvent, completely removing the loose skin. A second application of massage cream can then be applied.

The skin of dehydrated bodies is often very dark. A condition similar to a suntan may exist. It may be difficult to trace the distribution of arterial solution through these skin areas. Dehydrated skin is very firm to the touch. The skin feels as if it has already been embalmed. Additional fluid dye is needed to be certain of arterial solution distribution.

Desiccation

Regardless of the antemortem or postmortem conditions that have brought about the condition of dehydration, there is only one positive benefit to the embalmer. Dehydrated bodies tend to decompose more slowly, as water is necessary for decomposition. Likewise, in embalming, the reaction of the preservative with the proteins leads to the drying and firming of tissues. Extreme dehydration is called *desiccation*. Desiccation is a form of preservation; however, desiccated bodies are not viewable.

Often, certain areas are desiccated in bodies that have been frozen or refrigerated for a long period. For example, desiccated lips appear black, very wrinkled, and shrunken. The lips are drawn back and the teeth exposed. When the tips of the fingers are desiccated, the skin becomes parchmentlike and turns a yellow brown. Other body areas easily desiccated are the thin skin areas such as the ears, nose, and eyelids. Arterial injection or hypodermic injection cannot correct this condition.

LOCAL DEHYDRATION PROBLEMS

An abrasion is defined as "skin rubbed off"; the epidermis has been removed. At first, the tissue is quite moist, but as the skin dries a "scab" forms. This is also true of abrasions that occur at the time of death. Such an abrasion may not even be noticed. Air passing over the body during or after embalming dries the abraded skin, which turns dark brown and hardens. This type of discoloration does not respond to bleaching and must be covered with an opaque cosmetic. Abrasions are often incurred after falls on pavement or carpeting.

When the body has been roughly shaved and small nicks have occurred on the skin surface, surface drying, in time, turns these areas into small, dark brown marks. These small discolorations are referred to as razor abrasions. They are easily covered with an opaque cosmetic or waxed.

The drying of the tissues in the preceding two examples is actually desired by the embalmer, for the skin surface is now sealed and there is no leakage from these areas. Opaque cosmetics (or waxes) can be applied over these dried areas. To speed the drying of abraded tissues, following arterial injection, a hair dryer can be used. Massage cream should not be applied to these areas, because it slows the drying of tissues.

ARTERIAL EMBALMING PROBLEMS

Dehydration occurring during the antemortem, agonal, and postmortem periods prior to arterial embalming can result in a thickening of the blood. Satisfactory blood removal is essential to establish uniform distribution and even diffusion of arterial solution. Drainage may be difficult to establish in these bodies. A more important prob-

lem, however, may be congealing and clumping of this thick blood in the arterial system. On arterial injection, the heavy arterial blood and any clots may be forced into small arteries, thus cutting the flow of arterial solution into tissues supplied by these small arteries.

Blood should be drained from the best location possible, the right internal jugular vein. Likewise, arterial injection from the right common carotid artery or restricted cervical injection pushes arterial coagula toward the legs. A secondary injection point (e.g., femoral vessels) may be necessary, and if this is not successful, hypodermic and surface treatment of the legs can be used to establish preservation.

It is unwise to inject from the femoral or external iliac arteries if clots are present. The arterial clots can be pushed into the carotid arteries, making embalming of the face a most difficult task. Slow injection will minimize arterial coagula from being dislodged and moved to block smaller arteries.

From an arterial chemical standpoint, preinjection fluids, coinjection fluids, and dilute arterial solutions can be used to prepare the dehydrated body (Table 21–1).

TREATMENTS THAT MINIMIZE OR PREVENT POSTEMBALMING DEHYDRATION

Every body that is embalmed dehydrates to a certain extent. Formaldehyde solutions not only firm tissues but *dry* them. Drainage removes a large amount of moisture from the body tissues. These factors account for a great amount of dehydration during and after embalming. Some treatments can be used to maintain the level of moisture in or add moisture to these dehydrated bodies:

TABLE 21–1. PROBLEMS ASSOCIATED WITH DEHYDRATION

Darkened skin	Corrected by cosmetic application; use fluid dyes to ensure fluid distribution to all body areas
"Flaking" or peeling of skin, especially in facial areas	Apply massage cream and then clean with a solvent to remove all loose skin; mortuary cream cosmetics further reduce skin drying
Firm feel to the skin	Skin feels embalmed; additional dye helps to trace the distribution of fluid
Desiccated lips, eyelids, or fingertips	May need correction with restorative waxes; opaque cosmetics needed to hide discolorations
Thickened blood	May be diluted with a preinjection fluid; use right internal jugular as drainage point; inject from the carotids to push arterial coagula toward the lower extremities
Dehydration created by the embalmer; wrinkled lips, fingertips; facial areas	Use correct dilutions for arterial and humectant fluids; areas may be filled out with tissue builder after embalming
Dehydration of large facial area from embalming and passage of air over body	Use massage cream on exposed areas prior to cosmetic application; if skin is discolored, opaque cosmetics will be needed; cream cosmetics further reduce dehydration; fingertips and facial areas may also be treated with tissue builder to reduce dehydration

1. Use a moderate arterial solution. A moderate arterial solution by today's standards is 1.5 to 2.0%. Many fluids are reaction controlled and do not release the preservative ingredients until they come into contact with body cells. Many arterial fluids contain antidehydrants in their formulations. Large volumes of a mild solution can be used to moisturize and to secure preservation. Follow the recommendations of the manufacturers of the arterial fluid. They generally recommend dilutions for dehydrated bodies.

2. Use a coinjection fluid with the arterial solution. The coinjection fluid helps to reduce the astringent dehydrating action of the arterial solution and also adds moisture to the tissues. It is recommended that equal amounts of coinjection and preservative arterial fluids be used.

3. Use a humectant coinjection fluid along with the arterial solution. These fluids are designed to maintain or add body moisture. It is very important that the dilution recommended by the manufacturer be used. If improperly used, humectants can hydrate the body.

4. Run large amounts of fluid through these bodies to replenish the lost moisture.

5. Intermittent or alternate drainage can be used to help the tissues retain the arterial solution and also to reduce short circuiting of fluids and, thus achieve more uniform embalming. This type of drainage also helps the arterial solution to penetrate the deeper body tissues (Fig. 21–2).

6. Apply massage cream, petroleum jelly, lanolin, or silicone to exposed skin surfaces of the face and the hands during and immediately after arterial injection to retard water loss to the surrounding atmosphere. In the preparation of infants, the arms and legs should also receive treatment. It is not necessary to use a large amount of lubricant. A light layer is sufficient. Cream cosmetics also retard surface dehydration.

7. Avoid excessive massage of the hands, neck, and face. Massage is often necessary to distribute fluid through these regions, but excessive massage not only draws additional fluid into these areas but also removes tissue and arterial solution from these areas.

8. Do not expose reposing or stored bodies to air currents. Forced-air heating and air-conditioning currents quickly dehydrate the exposed areas of the body.

EDEMA

Edema in a body, whether localized or generalized, creates many problems for the embalmer. This condition is one of the most frequently encountered problems in embalming today. **Edema is defined as the abnormal collection of fluid in tissue spaces, serous cavities, or both.**

Interstitial or tissue fluids enter and leave the bloodstream (in a similar manner to embalming fluids) through the walls and pores of the capillaries, the small vessels connecting the smallest arteries (arterioles), and the smallest veins (venules). If more fluid leaves the blood vascular system and enters the tissues than is absorbed from the tissues into the blood, the tissues become filled with moisture; this condition is called *edema*.

The condition can be local, for example, when surgery has involved the axillary area and the lymph and venous channels have been obstructed; the arm swells with edema. It may be generalized and present in all the dependent tissues, as is seen in bodies dead from congestive heart failure.

From an embalming standpoint, the embalmer can identify edema in three body sites: within the individual cells, in the intercellular spaces, and within the body cavities.

A number of diseases and conditions can cause edema: diseases that affect cardiac function and result in increased venous pressures, diseases that affect the renal system and result in small amounts of plasma proteins, capillary damage or inflammation and allergic reactions, and obstructive diseases that interfere with venous or lymphatic circulation.

In addition, long-term use of drugs can damage such vital organs as the liver and kidneys and the circulatory

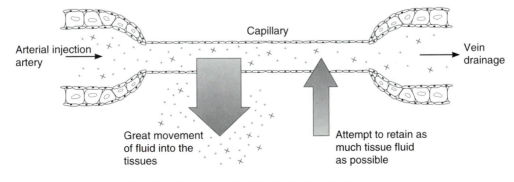

Figure 21–2. Hypotonic arterial solutions help the tissues to retain moisture.

system. Failure of these organs or systems can lead to edema. Drugs also act on cell membranes, causing cells to retain or take up moisture, thus creating a condition of edema within the cell.

It is not the purpose of this writing to explain the disease processes that bring about edema. The embalmer should have an understanding of pathology and microbiology to recognize the relationship between certain conditions and edema. The following diseases/conditions are often associated with edema. The embalmer should be able to relate the cause of the edema with the condition.

- Alcoholism
- Burns
- Cirrhosis of the liver
- Carbon monoxide poisoning
- Congestive heart failure
- Allergic reactions
- Inflammatory reactions
- Extended drug therapy
- Renal failure
- Trauma
- Lymphatic obstruction
- Steroid therapy
- Venous obstruction
- Phlebitis
- Malnutrition
- Hepatic failure and/or obstruction
- Surgical and transplant procedures

CLASSIFICATION OF EDEMA BY LOCATION

Cellular (Solid) Edema

When moisture is retained by the cell, or abnormal amounts of moisture are allowed to pass into the cell, a condition called solid edema results. The tissues appear swollen and, when pushed on by the embalmer, feel very firm. Indentations are not made by pushing on these tissues. Frequently, this condition arises when large doses of corticosteroids have been administered over a long period. This form of edema, often seen in the facial tissues, does *not* respond to embalming treatments. The swelling and distortion remain. The only possible, although not practical, method of reducing the swelling is excision of the deep tissues after arterial treatment is completed.

Intercellular (Pitting) Edema

In intercellular edema, fluids accumulate between the cells of the body. When these swollen areas are pushed on by the embalmer, the imprint of the fingers remains for a short period after the fingers are withdrawn. This form of edema, also known as **pitting edema** (Fig. 21–3), responds well to embalming treatments and can be gravitated to dependent body areas. It can be drained from

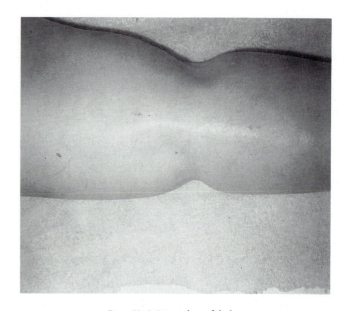

Figure 21–3. Pitting edema of the leg.

the tissues into the circulatory system and removed with the blood drainage. This edema may be localized, as is frequently seen in bodies dead from cardiac diseases where only the legs are distended, hydrocele (edema of the scrotum) and pulmonary edema (edema of the alveolar spaces in the lung tissue). Or, it may be generalized, as is frequently encountered after death from liver or renal failure. Generalized edema is referred to as **anasarca.**

Edema of the Body Cavities

Ascites is edema of the abdominal (or peritoneal) cavity; the edema is found within the cavity and surrounds the abdominal viscera. **Hydrothorax** is edema of the pleural cavity; it may involve one or both pleural cavities. **Hydrocephalus** is edema of the cranial cavity, and **hydropericardium** is edema of the pericardial sac surrounding the heart.

> Edema of the cavities does not dilute the arterial solution. If the body being prepared has ascites, it is not necessary to increase the strength of the arterial solution because of the edema in the abdominal cavity. Edema of the cavities does not mix with the arterial solution. The embalmer's concern is that the edema in the abdominal cavity might dilute the cavity fluid when it is injected.

EMBALMING PROBLEMS CREATED BY EDEMA

Generalized edema presents a number of problems for the embalmer. The tissues in which edema is present are swollen. When this involves the face and the hands, measures must be taken to reduce the distortion. Edema of the skeletal tissues has a tendency to gravitate into the dependent body areas, during life as well as after death.

In the bedridden patient, the edema is found largely in the back, buttocks, shoulders, and backs of the legs. The embalmer must understand that this movement or gravitation of edema into the dependent areas eventually leads to the passage of this fluid through the skin. This exit of fluid from the body can dampen the clothing of the deceased and the casket bedding, unless precautions are taken (e.g., use plastic garments to trap and hold the fluids).

Bodies with large amounts of edema also exhibit leakage from intravenous punctures and small openings such as those made with hypodermic needles. Any surgical incisions or openings resulting from other invasive procedures are possible sites of leakage. Another major concern with edema is that the excess moisture in the tissues will hasten the decomposition cycle. A good, moist environment for bacterial growth is provided. Autolytic enzymes will have an ample source of water for their role in decomposition, and embalming fluid is thoroughly diluted by this excess fluid.

EMBALMING PROBLEMS CREATED BY ANASARCA

1. Affected tissues are swollen with fluid.
2. When edema gravitates or moves from a region, the skin can wrinkle and appear distorted.
3. Fluid can leak from intravenous or invasive punctures, through the skin surface by gravitation, through hypodermic needle punctures, through surgical incisions, and through incisions made for embalming purposes.
4. Arterial fluid is diluted (secondary dilution).
5. Decomposition is speeded.
6. The possibility of separation of the skin layers (skin-slip) is increased.

When the face is affected by edema, the embalmer must first determine whether *solid* or *pitting* edema is involved. This can be done by gently applying digital pressure to the swollen tissues. Solid edema *cannot* be indented by pressure from the fingers. With solid edema, the extra fluids are located within the individual cells of the tissues. This type of edema is seen in allergic reactions and as the result of certain drug therapies, such as the extended use of corticosteroid drugs. Solid edema cannot be removed by arterial or mechanical means. It would not be wise to attempt to reduce the swelling by surgical removal of subcutaneous tissues after arterial embalming. Leakage would be a major problem.

In pitting edema the fluid is in the interstitial spaces (between the cells). Pitting edema can be gravitated. Merely elevating the head helps to drain some of the fluid

from the tissue spaces. Solid edema, especially of the facial tissues, is not as frequently encountered as pitting edema. It should also be mentioned the facial tissues are not as frequently affected by edema as are other body tissues, probably because the head is almost always elevated.

When a general facial edema exists in the unautopsied body, the trocar, on aspiration, can be passed into the tissues of the neck to make channels for drainage of the edematous fluids. Pressure can be applied to the face in a downward motion to squeeze the edema from the facial tissues into the neck and finally into the thorax. The carotid incisions can be left open several hours after embalming to drain fluid from the face. Following arterial injection and cavity treatment some embalmers place the body onto the removal cot and secure the body to the cot. The head end of the cot is then fully elevated, thus placing the body in a standing position. The body remains in this position for several hours to encourage as much edema as possible to gravitate from the head, face, and neck.

Edematous arms and hands (especially hands) can be elevated. Leaking intravenous punctures on the backs of hands can be sealed with super adhesive after embalming. Super adhesive is the one type of glue that can be used to seal a moist area. The embalmer may also want to squeeze as much edema as possible out of any intravenous punctures on the back of the hand. Elevation and firm massage of the tissues help to move the edema from the hand to a point above the wrist where it will not be visible. An edematous arm can be wrapped in plastic or a plastic sleeve to cover the swollen areas. It would be unwise to lance and drain the edema after embalming, as closure of the incision may be quite difficult.

ARTERIAL TREATMENT FOR GENERALIZED EDEMA

Generalized edema presents a number of problems for the embalmer. First and foremost is the increased rate of decomposition resulting from the presence of a large amount of body moisture. Water is necessary for decomposition. In generalized edema, vast quantities of water can be found in almost all the dependent skeletal tissues. In addition, the excess moisture causes a great secondary dilution of the arterial fluid, reducing the ability of the embalming solution to dry, sanitize, and preserve. The edema will, in time, seep through the skin, soiling the clothing and the casket interior. The large blebs that can form at edematous sites can break open and release fluids.

The objectives of the embalmer are to (1) inject an arterial solution of sufficient strength and volume to counteract the secondary dilution that occurs in the tissues, and (2) to remove as much of the edema from the tissues as possible. **It is very important that the embalmer know what condition caused the edema.**

For example, generalized edema can be the result of heart disease or renal failure. With renal failure, in addition to the edema, there is a buildup of nitrogenous wastes in the tissues. The nitrogenous wastes have the ability to neutralize the preservative solution. Therefore, very astringent solutions should be used.

Edema also coexists with nitrogenous wastes in bodies dead from second-degree burns, especially when the patient lived several days or weeks after being burned. These bodies demand large amounts of preservation solution.

Edema can be present in all body types. Edema can and does quite often exist in emaciated bodies. The first concern, even in an emaciated body, is to achieve preservation and dry the tissues. Overdehydration of the face and features is best avoided by raising both common carotid arteries at the beginning of the embalming and injecting the head separately.

Frequently in cases such as cancer of the liver, the body with generalized edema may also be jaundiced. Again, of primary importance are the preservation and drying of the tissues. The discoloration is secondary. Only the face and hands will be viewed. The restricted cervical method of injection allows the head to be embalmed separately. A jaundice fluid could be employed for embalming the head and a strong arterial solution in large amounts for the preparation of the trunk.

When arterial methods have not been completely successful, hypodermic injection of cavity fluid (or concentrated arterial solution) via the embalming machine can be used to inject local body areas. A small trocar can be used for the injection. The puncture is easily closed with a trocar button. Application of super adhesive around the trocar button helps to prevent leakage. The body is clothed in plastic garments. This technique works well with edematous legs.

Methods of Arterial Treatment

In treating the body with generalized edema, the embalmer should realize that often large amounts of arterial solution must be injected. Generally, the facial tissues are not affected by the edema, so to control the amount of arterial fluid entering the facial tissues it is wise to use restricted cervical injection. In this method, both right and left common carotid arteries are raised at the start of the embalming. The left artery is opened and a large tube is inserted toward the head; the lower portion of the artery is ligated. A tube directed toward the head is placed in the right artery, as is a tube directed toward the trunk. Both tubes directed toward the head remain open during the injection of the trunk.

In some of these treatments, several gallons of arterial solution are injected. Fluid that enters the head and

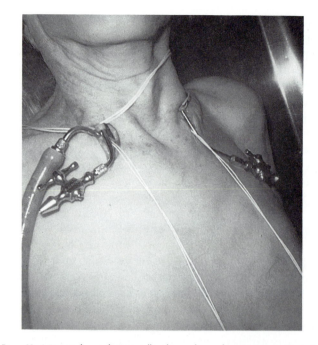

Figure 21–4. Restricted cervical injection allows large volumes of very strong arterial solution to be injected without overembalming the head.

facial areas exit through the open tubes while the lower portion of the body is being injected (Fig. 21–4). After satisfactory injection of the lower portion, the head can then be injected using a strength and quantity of arterial solution desired by the embalmer. In many instances, this solution is much milder than that used to inject the portions of the body where edema was present.

In bodies where the head and facial tissues are affected by edema, the restricted cervical injection is still recommended. The embalmer can inject the head separately with arterial solution of sufficient strength and quantity to ensure proper preservation of the facial tissues. The embalmer may wish to employ a specially prepared arterial solution with osmotic qualities that assist in removing the excess fluids from the facial tissues.

When edema affects the head and facial tissues, the tongue and eyes may be grossly distended. Digital pressure on the scalp (especially the dependent portions) reveals the presence of pitting edema. Elevation of the head and shoulders is necessary. In addition to employing a strong arterial solution for the injection of the head, the embalmer may wish to channel neck tissues during cavity embalming to provide a route for fluids to drain from the face, scalp, and neck into the thoracic cavities. Reaspiration helps to remove some of this excess fluid. Downward massage of the facial tissues also assists in draining the excess fluids from these regions.

Local areas such as the eyes can be treated by a variety of techniques to restore swollen tissues. The first concern for the embalmer should be the complete preservation of these tissues. By injecting the left and right sides of the face separately, the embalmer can control the quantity of arterial solution entering the facial tissues. If, the eyelids exhibit large amounts of edema and do not seem to be adequately embalmed, cotton can be placed under the eyelids and saturated with undiluted cavity fluid to ensure their preservation.

If areas of the face appear to lack adequate arterial solution, surface compresses of undiluted cavity fluid can be applied and left in place several hours. If preferred, autopsy gels may be applied to facial surfaces to assist in preservation. These, too, should remain in position, covered with cotton or plastic, several hours. Facial areas can also be preserved hypodermically, but the points of entry must be carefully considered, as the edema may leak through the entry points. Most of this work should be done from within the mouth. When the head has been autopsied, a long hypodermic needle can be introduced from within the margins of the cut scalp areas.

In summary, arterial treatment for facial edema consists of injection of both common carotid arteries with a solution of sufficient strength and quantity to ensure complete preservation. Keep the shoulders and the head elevated. Use fluid dyes to locate areas of the face not receiving adequate arterial solution. These areas can then be treated by hypodermic or surface embalming methods. To drain fluid from the face and neck, channel the neck with the trocar during aspiration of the body cavities. Reaspiration as well as cavity fluid reinjection of bodies with edema is always recommended.

Several types of arterial solutions can be used to treat bodies with generalized edema (Fig. 21–5): a very large volume of an average-strength solution; a sufficient volume of a very strong "hypertonic" solution; a special "high-index" dehydrating arterial solution; an average to strong arterial solution accompanied by a salt coinjection (Epsom salts); an average to strong arterial solution accompanied by a vegetable humectant to help draw moisture out of the tissues into the capillaries.

Most bodies with generalized edema exhibit very good circulation. Few clots are found in the drainage from these bodies. There should be good distribution of the arterial solution, probably because the blood was diluted and thinned by the edema during life and after death. Therefore, formation of coagula in the blood vascular system postmortem is minimal.

In the majority of bodies with generalized edema, the embalmer can expect copious drainage and good fluid distribution and, thus, can inject large volumes of arterial solution. There are two means by which the preservative demand (or formaldehyde demand) of the body is met: by injection of strong arterial solution or by injection of a large volume of mild (average) arterial solution.

Injection Site. In the body with generalized edema, it is recommended that both common carotid arteries be raised at the beginning of the embalming. This allows saturation of the trunk without overinjection of the head and separate injection of the head after the trunk has been embalmed (the body can be aspirated prior to injection of the head; features may be set after the trunk has been embalmed and after aspiration).

Drainage Site. The center of blood drainage is the right atrium of the heart. If the right internal jugular vein is used for drainage, instruments can be inserted directly into the right atrium and the head and neck drained from this site. Some embalmers prefer to drain from both the right and the left internal jugular veins when preparing a body with severe facial edema. Continuous drainage encourages removal of edematous fluids from the body.

Rate of Flow. All embalming should begin at a slow rate of flow. Once distribution has been established the embalmer can increase the rate of flow to ensure good distribution to distal body areas.

Interrupted Injection. It is very important in removing edematous fluids from the tissue spaces to allow the embalming fluid, once injected, time to bring about osmotic exchange wherein the edematous fluids move into the capillaries and the preservatives move from the capillaries into the tissue spaces. After injecting $1\frac{1}{2}$ to 2 gallons, stop injection for one-half hour to allow these physical exchanges to occur. Then inject about $\frac{1}{2}$ to 1 gallon and

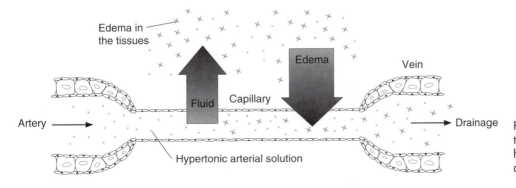

Figure 21–5. Hypertonic arterial solutions and arterial solutions containing large colloid molecules help to draw the edema from the tissues into the circulatory system.

again stop and allow the physical exchange. Massage and squeeze the limbs from their distal portion toward the heart to encourage drainage of the edematous fluids from the veins into the blood drainage. Elevation of the arms and legs also encourages the edematous fluids to move into the large veins. The injection of additional arterial solution after a rest period helps to force edematous fluid out of the vascular system into the drainage.

Arterial Solutions

Arterial Solution 1. A very large volume of a mild or average (standard) arterial solution is used. By today's standards, the strength of this solution would be 1.5 to 2.0% formaldehyde (approximately 8 ounces of a 25-index arterial fluid is used to make a gallon of arterial solution). Continuous drainage is established with the injection of the solution. It is recommended that fluid dye be added to the last gallons to trace the distribution of the arterial solution. It is not uncommon to inject at least 2 to 3 gallons of arterial solution into each leg of the autopsied body with generalized edema. The theory is that injection of large volumes of mild solution ensures good distribution of the solution and instills into the body a large volume of preservative, but at the same time washes as much of the edema as possible out of the tissues. To accomplish the fluid removal, a steady to fast rate of flow is recommended along with continuous or concurrent drainage. If the embalmer feels that preservation is inadequate, it is recommended that he or she add several ounces of a high-index special-purpose arterial fluid to the embalming solution and make use of intermittent drainage to ensure that a sufficient amount of preservative solution remains in the tissues.

Arterial Solution 2. A very strong (or astringent) arterial solution is used. Some of the high-index fluids are accompanied by instructions on their use for embalming bodies with edema. The solutions for edema are generally quite strong, and dilution occurs when the arterial solution mixes with the edema in the tissue spaces. Arterial solution 2 should be used when the embalmer feels that circulation will not be good. As previously stated, circulation is generally good in bodies with generalized edema. There may be long delays, however, between death and embalming, and decomposition may already be taking place. Use of large volumes of mild solution is not advised for these bodies. It is important to establish preservation first, then to dry the tissues. These strong solutions help both to preserve the tissues and to remove the edema. As these solutions are hypertonic relative to the moist tissues, the edematous fluids in the tissues are drawn back into the capillaries and, thus, removed with the drainage. It has been stated that use of these strong or astringent solutions is advised when the body with edema has been dead for a long period. Many of the cap-

illaries are broken, so it is very difficult to inject arterial solution without causing even more swelling than already exists. Therefore, the strongest fluids possible should reach the tissues to establish preservation; injection of a large fluid volume would result in distortion from the swelling caused by the broken circulatory system. The embalmer's goal is delivery of the least amount of the strongest arterial fluid. Knowledge of the cause of the edema is also important (e.g., renal failure, or burns). Kidney wastes in the tissues neutralize preservative and necessitate use of strong solution. Concurrent drainage can be instituted with this solution. The embalmer, however, may wish to use some form of restricted drainage during injection of the last gallon to ensure solution retention. Cavity embalming can be delayed a short time to ensure fluid diffusion and saturation of the tissues. Again, fluid dye is recommended so the embalmer can see where the arterial solution has distributed. Firming may be minimal in these preparations. Firming of the tissues and drying of the skin are not dependable signs of arterial distribution. Areas that do not receive adequate solution should be arterially embalmed separately or treated by surface or hypodermic embalming techniques.

Arterial Solution 3. Some fluid companies manufacture special-purpose high-index fluids designed specifically to preserve and dry tissues with edema. Some companies further describe these arterial fluids as either dehydrating or nondehydrating. For treatment of the body with generalized edema, the dehydrating fluid is preferred. These high-index fluids are especially useful in the embalming of bodies dead from second-degree burns or liver or renal failure. Directions on the bottle should be followed to ensure proper dilution of the arterial solutions. The quantity of fluid injected depends on the size and weight of the body, the dilution effected within the body by the edema present, the amount of edema present, and the distribution of embalming solution. Fluid dyes can be used to trace the distribution of arterial fluid. Use of coinjection fluid depends on the recommendations of the fluid manufacturer. Because these special fluids are strong, have a dehydrating effect, and must be injected in a large volume, it is strongly urged that the restricted cervical injection be implemented (raising both right and left common carotid arteries). If the head and the facial tissues have not been affected by the edema the embalmer will, no doubt, want to use a standard arterial solution to embalm the head. Keep in mind that renal failure also affects the facial tissues; these tissues will contain nitrogenous waste, which neutralizes formaldehyde. Be certain that an adequate amount of sufficient-strength arterial solution is injected into the head.

Arterial Solution 4. Arterial solution 4 works to reduce the swollen condition brought about by the edema. It is made using Epsom salts, which create a hypertonic solution. This hypertonic solution sets up an osmotic gradient that draws the edema from the tissue spaces toward this concentrated salt solution in the capillaries. The embalmer may wish to begin the embalming and clear the blood vascular system with either strong or average arterial solution. Injection continues until the blood drainage clears and the distribution appears uniform. When strong dehydrating solutions such as this arterial mixture are used, it is very important that both common carotid arteries be raised as the primary injection site. In this manner, the head can be separately injected. If the head is grossly distended by the edema, arterial solution 4 should help to remove it. The following arterial solution is suggested.

Fill a container with half a gallon of cool water; add as much Epsom salts as can be dissolved. Thoroughly stir this solution. Next, add 4 to 6 ounces of a high-index (25–35) arterial fluid. Pour this solution into the embalming machine but do not pour any of the undissolved salt that may have settled to the bottom of the container.

Inject this solution into the area affected by the edema. Massage the tissues (after they are injected). Assume that the head and face are grossly distended with edema (often seen after cardiac surgery or aortic repair). First inject the left side of the head; then inject the right side. Massage the swollen tissues downward to encourage the edema to drain through the veins. (Some embalmers allow this solution to remain in place approximately one-half hour and then reinject with a strong arterial solution. Thus the Epsom salt solution remains in the capillaries long enough to draw the edematous fluid from the tissue spaces. This edematous fluid is then flushed away by the reinjection). Massage plays a very large role in the success of this process. This is an excellent technique to use on an arm or leg grossly distended with edema. Care should be taken to keep the solution thoroughly stirred, for it is easy to clog the delivery lines of the embalming machine. If this should occur, flush the machine with warm water to dissolve the Epsom salt crystals. An aspirator hose can be attached to the delivery line to pull the crystallized materials out of the machine. After using a solution containing Epsom salts, always flush the machine with warm water. This very old technique is quite effective. Actually, the special-purpose high-index arterial solutions function in the same manner as the Epsom salts by creating a hypertonic arterial solution. Some coinjection fluids are manufactured that act like Epsom salt solutions. They are sold expressly for drying moist tissues and are, of course, added to preservative arterial solution. Follow the manufacturer's instructions carefully (Fig. 21–6). The Epsom salt solution works best on the facial tissues, especially when the edema is recent (e.g., recent surgical patients, heart or aortic surgery). This process does not work well when the edema has been present for a long period (e.g., trauma cases, drug therapy cases).

Arterial Solution 5. Arterial solution 5, like the previous solutions, makes use of the osmotic gradient between the fluids in the capillaries and the edematous fluids in the tissue spaces. Arterial solution 5 consists of a preservative arterial fluid and a coinjection humectant. Humectants, when used in small quantities, add or maintain moisture in the tissues. When large quantities of humectants are used, the arterial solution becomes very viscous. The large molecules of the humectant draw the moisture from the tissue spaces into the capillaries. Once there, the edematous fluids exit with the drainage. The humectant must be a *vegetable* and not a lanolin (or animal) humectant. The fluid manufacturers should be consulted for specifics. One suggestion is to use 6 to 8 ounces of 20- to 25-index preservation to make a gallon of arterial solution. To this solution add 20 to 24 ounces of humectant. Inject at a moderate rate of flow, thus allowing time for the exchange to occur. Continuous drainage is necessary. Stopping the drainage could waterlog the tissues if the humectant is forced from the capillaries into the tissue spaces. Before this solution is injected it is best to establish good fluid distribution by injecting a well-coordinated arterial solution of sufficient strength; a 2% arterial solution (or slightly higher) should distribute well. If desired, a coinjection chemical can also be used in equal amounts with the arterial fluid. Fluid dye added to the solution will be a good indicator of fluid distribution. After the blood vascular system is perfused with this first injection, the humectant solution can follow to dehydrate the edematous tissue.*

LOCAL TREATMENT FOR EDEMA

Legs

One of the most frequently affected areas is the legs. When only the legs are affected by edema, it is best to embalm the body with a standard-strength arterial solution. This, of course, depends on the general condition of the body. The important point is not to prepare a strong arterial solution for the entire body based on the fact that edema is present only in the legs.

After embalming the body, raise the femoral or iliac vessels and separately inject the legs using one of the arterial solutions just discussed. If the edema is severe, after arterial injection use the trocar to pierce the upper thighs beneath the inguinal ligaments while embalming the cavities. Elevate the legs and, if desired, wrap with an

*Several articles published in the 1930s indicate success with the removal of edema using glycerine and even Karo syrup to make a solution that promotes dehydration of tissues.

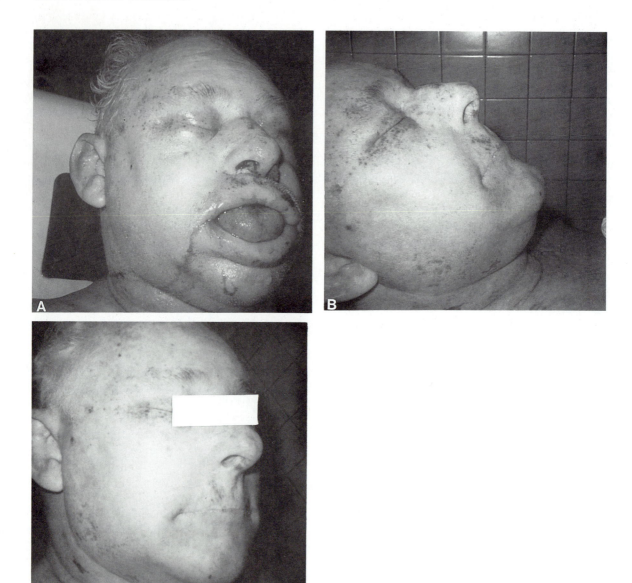

Figure 21–6. Facial edema after repair of an aortic aneurysm. The swelling was reduced by the addition of Epsom salts to the arterial solution.

Ace bandage beginning at the foot and moving up the leg. This pushes some of the edema into the pelvic cavity from which it can later be aspirated. The legs should be elevated several hours to make this treatment effective.

The legs can also be injected with cavity fluid using a trocar. This is done *after* arterial injection of the legs. The cavity fluid is placed (undiluted) in the injection machine, and the delivery tube is attached to an infant trocar. The inside of the calf is a good point of entry. From this point, the lower leg and thigh can be reached. Saturate the leg with the cavity fluid and place a plastic stocking on it to ensure surface preservation. The leg can first be painted with autopsy gel and embalming powder sprinkled inside the stocking. The powder and the gel assist in preservation of the leg. When edema is more extensive and affects the hips and buttocks, plastic coveralls or pants should also be used. When shoulders and trunk

walls are affected along with legs and arms, use of a unionall is advised, for it covers all these areas.

Arms

When only the arms and hands are affected with edema (as found after any surgery in the axillary area) the arm can be separately injected after the body has been embalmed. The hand and arm can be elevated to gravitate some of the edema into the upper arm. Wrinkling of the back of the hand now becomes a problem.

A wide piece of duct tape can be placed across the palm of the hand to "pull" the wrinkles from the back of the hand. If distal areas such as the fingers become badly wrinkled, a small amount of tissue builder can be injected into each finger. Some wrinkling may be removed by the injection of tissue builder; good points of needle entry would be between the fingers. If there are intravenous or needle punctures on the back of the hand, the embalmer can remove a considerable amount of edema through these openings by squeezing and then seal the openings with a drop or two of super adhesive.

Edema of the Trunk

After death, edematous fluid gravitates to the dependent areas. To achieve adequate preservation, insert an infant trocar into the lateral walls of the body. The point of entry can be along the right or left midaxillary line in the soft tissues inferior to the rib cage. From this point of entry, the trocar should be able to reach as far up as the axilla and also as far down as the buttocks. Cavity fluid can be injected through the embalming machine. This added embalming measure, of course, is done after arterial injection of the body. Coveralls or a unionall can be placed on the body, and a liberal amount of preservative powder can be sprinkled into the plastic garment. Remember that eventually this edema will pass through the skin of the back and dependent trunk walls. This exit of fluid can occur even before disposition of the body. It is essential to protect the clothing and the interior of the casket by use of the plastic garments.

Ascites (Edema of the Abdominal Cavity)

Ascites can exist almost unnoticed until the embalmer begins to aspirate the cavity or it can severely distend the abdominal cavity, because the edematous fluid is located within the cavity and around the visceral organs. It is unaffected by arterial fluid treatment or blood drainage. Ascites will not dilute arterial fluid, because arterial solution and the edema in the abdominal cavity do not come into contact.

When ascites is present and noticeable, do not mix arterial solutions in the belief that ascites will be a secondary dilution for arterial fluid. Ascites *will* be a diluting factor for cavity fluid. When ascites is present and the abdomen is very tense prior to arterial embalming, the pressure in the abdominal cavity may be sufficient to interfere with arterial distribution. More importantly, the pressure can interfere with blood drainage. This pressure is created not only by the enormous amount of fluid in the abdominal cavity (often several gallons) but also by possible gases in the intestinal tract. The pressure should be removed prior to arterial injection. Several techniques can be used:

1. Using a scalpel, make a small opening in the abdominal cavity and insert a drain tube or a trocar from which the point has been removed. Many embalmers prefer to make this incision in the inguinal or hypogastric area of the abdominal wall. At this lower point more liquid can be removed from the cavity. Attach the aspirating hose to the drainage tube or trocar for delivery of the edematous fluids directly into the drainage or collection system.
2. Insert a trocar keeping the point just under the anterior abdominal wall. Pierce the transverse colon to release gases. Attach the aspirating hose to the trocar.
3. Make a small incision over the area of the transverse colon, exposing the colon (which can be opened). The incision is an outlet for the edema. This technique is most unsanitary and, if possible, should be avoided.

When the distension of the abdomen is not severe enough to restrict the flow of arterial solution or interfere with blood drainage, the ascites can be removed during the normal period for aspiration of the abdominal cavity.

Hydrothorax

In hydrothorax, edema is present in the space between the wall of the thoracic cavity and the lung. This condition is not easy to recognize because the rib cage cannot expand like the abdomen does when edema is present. This condition can be expected in bodies dead from heart disease or pneumonia. Often, there is some distension of the neck, and, very frequently, both the face and neck exhibit a great amount of livor mortis after death. Aspiration of the thoracic cavity removes the fluid. Aspiration is generally done after arterial embalming. The trocar should be directed to the posterior portions of the thorax, where the fluid will have gravitated. It is possible to remove one or more gallons of fluid from the thorax when this condition is present.

If it is necessary to relieve some of this pressure prior to or during arterial injection, a trocar can be introduced from the standard point of trocar entry and guided along the lateral wall of the abdomen into the thoracic cavity. This provides a drainage outlet for the fluid, but does not rupture any large arteries or veins. When hydrothorax is suspected, use the common carotid artery for injection and drain from the right internal jugular vein. This is the best location from which to drain the head and arms. Aspiration should immediately follow arterial injection. There is a very good chance that the distension of the neck will diminish and any swelling that may have occurred in the facial tissues will disappear.

Hydrocele

In the male, the scrotum can become distended with edematous fluid. Quite frequently, insufficient arterial solution reaches the tissues of the scrotum, which can be a site for decomposition. This condition is treated during aspiration and injection of the body cavities, after arterial injection. During aspiration pass the trocar over the pubic symphysis and pubic bone and enter the scrotum. Place a towel around the scrotum and apply pressure. This forces the edematous fluid through the channels that have been made with the trocar and into the pelvic cavity. The scrotum can then be filled with undiluted cavity fluid to ensure preservation. Care should be taken not to puncture the scrotum with the trocar. It can be difficult to close the puncture and to stop the drainage of edematous fluids. Use super glue or a closure with a trocar button. If the leakage cannot be stopped, drain the edematous fluids and the cavity fluids that were injected. Let the drainage continue several hours.

Hydrocephalus

When edematous fluid fills the cranial cavity during fetal development, the head is grossly distended. Some individuals survive after birth and live many years with this condition. In the unautopsied infant, it is necessary to drain some of this fluid, or very rapid decomposition of the brain and fluids of the cranial cavity may occur. Drainage can be established by passing a large hypodermic needle through the nostril and directing it through the anterior portion of the cribriform plate of the ethmoid bone. This process should be done after arterial embalming.

Several ounces of undiluted cavity fluid or phenol solution can be injected in the same manner as the fluid was aspirated. The nostrils should be tightly packed with cotton to protect against leakage. When there has been ossification of the bones of the cranial cavity, it is not always necessary to aspirate and inject the cavity. Leakage must always be considered when the cranial cavity is aspirated.

SPECIAL CONDITIONS

Burned Bodies

Edema accompanies burns, especially second-degree burns. Generally, these victims live days or weeks after the burns. Blistering of the skin is characteristic of second-degree burns. The embalmer, however, very rarely sees the blistering condition. The blisters have been opened and drained and preparations placed on the denuded skin area to encourage cellular growth and skin replacement. Death usually results from renal failure. Because of the skin damage, many waste products that normally leave the body via the skin are retained in the blood. As a result, the kidneys overwork and cannot handle the wastes that rapidly build up in the body. These

bodies are often so grossly distended with edema that the face is not recognizable.

The first concern of the embalmer is preservation. These bodies have a very high preservative demand. Restricted cervical injection with drainage from the right internal jugular vein is recommended for these bodies when they are not autopsied. Astringent arterial solutions should be injected. Fluid dye can be added to the arterial solution to identify those body areas receiving arterial solution. Areas not reached by the arterial solution are best treated by hypodermic injection of cavity fluid or an astringent arterial solution. These bodies are very difficult to handle as they are often covered with various ointments. Washing the skin surface with a good disinfectant soap removes surface medications and debris.

Long open incisions are the result of one method used to treat burn patients. The embalmer cannot suture these long incisions. The surface can be thoroughly dried after it has been bathed with a soapy solution. Exposure to air also helps to dry the skin surface. These bodies can be placed in a unionall; this plastic garment covers all body areas except the hands, neck, and face. The body surface can be liberally covered with embalming powder. In addition, the skin surface can be painted with autopsy gel, or cavity compresses can be applied before the body is clothed in the unionall. Strips of sheeting or gauze can be used to wrap extremities when long incisions are present.

Leakage can be a big problem with these bodies. Allowing the body to drain as much as possible and to air-dry prior to placing plastic garments on the body diminishes the amount of leakage into the plastic garments after the body is casketed. Frequently, these persons have had a tracheotomy. It may be very difficult to close the tracheotomy opening if the neck area was affected by the burns. In these cases, after aspiration of the body, fill the opening with cotton and incision seal powder and liberally apply surface glue over the opening.

Renal Failure

Chronic renal failure brings about an increase in toxic wastes (urea, uric acid, ammonia, and creatine) in the blood and tissues of the body. Retention of these wastes results in acidosis (the tissues become acidic). Over time, there is a decrease in cardiac function leading to congestive heart failure and pulmonary edema. Gastric ulcerations occur and gastrointestinal bleeding can be expected. The patient becomes anemic and the skin turns sallow as a result of the retention of urochrome.

This condition is very important to the embalmer. Bodies with renal failure rapidly decompose. The edema present dilutes the arterial solution. The waste products in the bloodstream and tissues neutralize the formaldehyde. The color can deepen after embalming and become more pronounced, creating a cosmetic problem. Tissues do not firm normally, for the proteins of the body have been altered. Such bodies have a very high preservative demand. It is important that the embalmer use strong arterial solutions. Special-purpose high-index fluids are recommended. Preinjection should be avoided if there has been a delay between death and embalming or if the embalmer feels circulation may be difficult to establish. Restricted cervical injection with drainage from the right internal jugular vein is recommended.

The strength of the arterial solution should be at least 2.5 to 3.5% (12 ounces of a 30-index arterial fluid makes a gallon of arterial solution with a strength of 2.81%). Dye should be added to the arterial solution not only to trace the distribution of fluid, but also to counterstain the sallow color produced by the urochrome in the tissues. In many bodies that have been in chronic renal failure, other visceral organ damage has taken place. The body may be very jaundiced, and ecchymoses from disease and medications may be seen on the skin surface. Emaciation and protein damage may have occurred in the tissues. The embalmer will have problems with discolorations, firming, and preservation.

The most important objective in embalming these bodies is good preservation. Firming is not always necessary. Tissue can be preserved without being intensely firmed. Discolorations are secondary and can always be treated with cosmetics.

Cavity embalming is very important after renal failure. Frequently, bleeding has occurred in the gastrointestinal tract, providing an excellent medium for bacterial proliferation and a good site for the formation of gas. It may also be a source of purge. Thorough aspiration of the cavities is necessary. The embalmer may note arterial solution in the cavities or hollow viscera where bleeding occurred in life. A minimum of two to three bottles of undiluted cavity fluid should be injected. Several hours later, the body should be reaspirated and reinjected with cavity fluid. Renal failure is a condition that the embalmer must learn to recognize. If it is not detected, the body can rapidly decompose. **Check the death certificate carefully if available for references to renal involvement.** Areas not receiving adequate arterial solution should be sectionally injected. If necessary, undiluted cavity fluid can be injected hypodermically, or compresses of undiluted cavity fluid or autopsy gel can be applied to the surface to ensure preservation.

TABLE 21–2. SUMMARY OF EDEMA

Edema	Definition	Problems	Treatment
Solid	Edema within body cells	Swollen tissues; difficult preservation	Must be excised for reduction Strong arterial solutions, coinjection fluids
Pitting	Edema in tissue spaces, between the cells	Distension; fluid dilution; leakage; difficult preservation	May be gravitated; use strong arterial solutions; may be punctured and drained; use plastic garments to protect from leakage
Anasarca	Generalized edema in all body tissues	Leakage; distension; arterial fluid dilution	Strong arterial solutions; hypodermic and surface embalming; plastic garments; gravitation; puncture and drain
Edema of face	Edema in facial tissues	Swollen tissues, eyelids, and tongue	Restricted cervical injection; strong coordinated arterial solutions; possible use of salt or high-index solutions to reduce swelling; elevate head; channel with trocar neck area for drainage into thorax; surface weights for eyes and lips; surface embalming and hypodermic to ensure preservation with cavity fluid
Edema of hands	Edema in tissues of the backs of the hands	Swollen tissues; possible leakage from intravenous punctures; wrinkles after removal	Sectional injection from axillary artery; surface packs with cavity fluid to ensure preservation; bleach any discolorations; elevate to gravitate edema into arm
Edema of legs	Edema in thighs and lower legs	Dilution of arterial fluid; leakage	Sectional injection of legs from femoral or external iliac artery; use of strong arterial solutions; use of salt solutions of dehydrating solutions to remove edema; hypodermic injection with undiluted cavity fluid; surface treatment using autopsy gel; plastic stockings containing embalming powder and autopsy gel; elevate to gravitate edema into abdominal cavity; puncture and drain.
Pulmonary edema	Edema in the alveoli of the lungs	Purge	Aspiration and injection of lungs
Hydrothorax	Edema in the thoracic cavity	Purge; dilution of cavity fluid; pressure can cause venous congestion of neck and face; facial distension	Aspiration; injection of cavity fluid; careful draining prior to arterial injection
Ascites	Edema of abdominal cavity	Pressure can cause purge of stomach contents; anal purge; dilution of cavity fluid	Aspiration and injection of undiluted cavity fluid; preembalming draining via trocar or drainage tube; reaspiration and reinjection
Hydropericardium	Edema of pericardial cavity	Dilution of cavity fluid Pressure could cause drainage problems	Aspiration and injection of undiluted cavity fluid
Hydrocele	Edema of scrotum	Leakage; dilution of arterial fluid; distension; problems in dressing	Channel with trocar to drain into abdominal cavity; inject via trocar undiluted cavity fluid; surface coating with autopsy gel; use of plastic garments and embalming powder.
Hydrocephalus	Edema of cranial cavity	Purge in infant	Drain in infant via ethmoid foramen; inject cavity fluid via ethmoid foramen

The embalming complications associated with chronic renal failure can be summarized:

1. Decomposition occurs rapidly.
2. Acidosis alters the reaction between proteins and the preservative.
3. The body appears sallow because urochrome is present in the tissues.
4. Sites of gastrointestinal bleeding may be sites of arterial fluid loss and sources of purge.
5. Edema dilutes the arterial fluid.
6. Uremic wastes in the blood and tissues neutralize preservatives.
7. Skin infections may be caused by uremic pruritis.

See Table 21–2 for a summary of edema.

KEY TERMS AND CONCEPTS FOR STUDY AND DISCUSSION

1. Define the following terms:
   anasarca
   ascites
   concurrent drainage
   dehydration
   edema
   hydrocephalus
   hydrothorax
   hypertonic arterial solution
   hypotonic arterial solution
   intermittent drainage
   osmosis
   pitting edema

2. Discuss what treatments can be employed to help restore moisture to a body that is badly dehydrated during embalming.
3. List some of the conditions, both antemortem and postmortem, that cause dehydration.
4. Discuss some of the complications created by the presence of skeletal edema.
5. Discuss the arterial solutions and embalming techniques that can be used to remove edema from the skeletal tissues.
6. Discuss the complications that arise in the preparation of a body dead from renal failure.

BIBLIOGRAPHY

Elkins J. Major body elevation as a technique for the reduction of swelling in the face and hands of embalmed bodies. In: *Champion Expanding Encyclopedia.* Springfield, OH: Champion Chemical Co.; 1985:No. 554.

Henson RW. Controlling the moisture content of the tissues. *Professional Embalmer* November 1940.

Henson RW. Controlling the moisture content of the tissues. *Professional Embalmer*, October 1940.

Regulating the Moisture Content of Tissues. Wilmette, IL: Hizone Supplements; 1938:11.

Sheldon H. *Boyd's Introduction to the Study of Disease.* 10th ed. Philadelphia: Lea & Febiger;1988.

Shor MM. Can magnesium sulfate be safely used to rid body of fluid in lower extremities? *Casket and Sunnyside*, July 1965.

Sturb CG. Distribution and diffusion. *Funeral Directors Journal*, May 1939.

22

Vascular Considerations

The blood vascular system is the distribution route for the embalming solution. Any pathological change that obstructs this delivery system either completely blocks or reduces flow of fluid to a body region.

As people age, many degenerative changes can occur in the circulatory system. Although the immediate cause of death may not be heart or blood vessel disease, such a condition can greatly influence the embalming procedure. Likewise, drugs given for the treatment of heart or vascular diseases may have more influence on the embalming procedure than the condition of the diseased vessels.

The embalmer is concerned primarily with intravascular conditions, diseases or tissue changes in the walls of or within the blood vessels. The arteries are the vessels that carry the embalming solution to the capillaries. At the capillaries some of the arterial solution will leave the vascular system to enter the interstitial spaces, where it will come into contact with the body cells and cellular proteins. Arteries have three layers:

- *Intima:* the inner lining of endothelial cells, which continue to form the walls of the capillaries and then the inner walls of the veins and arteries (this endothelial layer of cells lines the entire blood vascular system)
- *Media:* the middle layer composed of muscle cells and elastic tissue

- *Adventitia:* the outer layer composed mostly of connective tissue

The cavity of the vessel is called the *lumen.* Narrowing or obstruction of the lumen is of great concern to the embalmer, because it can decrease or stop flow of arterial solution to a body area. Intravascular problems can also result in breaks or tears in vessels. These can be very small ruptures such as petechiae or major ruptures such as aortic aneurysms.

Table 22–1 lists intravascular arterial conditions that can limit the distribution of arterial solution to various body areas. Arteriosclerosis and arterial coagula are the problems most frequently encountered by the embalmer.

Preinjection fluid should not be used when it is thought it will be difficult to establish arterial solution distribution. Swelling could result later when the preservative solution is injected, as the system would be filled with the preinjection solution. Preinjection fluid should be used only if circulation is thought to be good; in such cases, it maintains the good distribution and drainage. Many persons who had vascular diseases were given blood thinners and anticoagulants. These bodies generally exhibit good arterial solution distribution and few or no clots in the drainage.

385

TABLE 22–1. CONDITIONS RESULTING FROM INTRAVASCULAR DISEASE PROCESSES

Vascular Condition or Injury	Description	Embalming Concern
Advanced decomposition	Breakdown of the body tissues	Arteries are one of the last "organs" to decompose. Some circulation may be possible. Expect a large number of intravascular clots. Distribution is very poor. Capillary decomposition causes rapid swelling of the tissues.
Aneurysm	Localized dilation of an artery	If aneurysm ruptures, fluid cannot distribute.
Arteriosclerosis	Hardening of the arteries	Vessel may not be suitable as an injection site. Narrowed arteries may easily trap arterial coagula.
Arteritis	Inflammation of an artery	Artery may narrow, resulting in poor distribution of arterial solution. Artery may also weaken and rupture from pressure of injection.
Asphyxiation	Insufficient oxygen supply	Right side of heart is congested (poor drainage). Purging can result as blood flows back into lungs instead of draining. Tissue is cyanotic. Intense livor mortis is present in neck and facial tissues. Blood may remain liquid. Capillary permeability is increased. Swelling could easily occur.
Atheroma, atherosclerosis	Patchy or nodular thickening of the intima of an artery	Flow of arterial solution may be restricted or occluded. Arterial coagula may be easily trapped during injection. Vessel is poor injection site.
Burns	Local or general damage to tissue from heat	Capillaries constrict resulting in extensive coagulation. Distribution of arterial solution may be reduced. Large burns can result in kidney failure, with retention of nitrogenous wastes, thus increasing the preservative demand of the tissues.
Cerebral vascular accident	"Stroke" caused by a clot or the rupture of a small artery in the brain	Vasoconstriction may occur on one side of the body, reducing the distribution of arterial solution.
Clots or coagula	Antemortem or postmortem clumping of blood elements	Arterial clots can block or reduce fluid flow to a body region, and may *not* be removed through drainage. Venous clots may often be removed; if clots are unmovable, swelling and discoloration can result.
Congestive heart failure	Decreased heart function	Venous congestion and clotting and cyanosis occur. Legs and feet are edematous. Capillary permeability increases. Tissues can easily swell.
Corrosive poisons	Toxic and corrosive chemicals	If poisons are swallowed, purge can usually be expected. Corrosive action may destroy blood vessels causing loss of solution or blood into the gastrointestinal tract.
Diabetes	An endocrine disease affecting the control of blood glucose levels	Poor peripheral circulation can reduce solution distribution. Gangrenous areas require surface and/or hypodermic embalming treatments. Dehydration frequently occurs. Breakdown of protein results in poor firming of tissues.
Emboli	Detached blood clot	Blockage of a small artery interrupts solution distribution. Venous emboli can block drainage.
Esophageal varices	Swollen, tortuous veins caused by a stagnation of blood and generally seen in the superficial veins	Drainage may be difficult to establish. Rupture and massive purge may occur.
Extracerebral clot (stroke)	A clot, usually in the carotid artery, that stops blood supply to the brain	The clot can occlude the artery, making it impossible for arterial solution to flow to one side of the face. Blockage may occlude the carotid so it cannot be used as an injection site. Resulting stroke may cause vasoconstriction on one side of the body, reducing arterial solution distribution.
Febrile disease	A disease or condition accompanied by an elevation of body temperature	Decomposition may be speeded. Dehydration is possible. Blood coagulates and causes congestion. Distribution and drainage may be hard to establish.
Freezing (postmortem)	Cooling of the body to the point where ice crystals form in body tissues	Small vessels and tissues easily swell on injection of solution.
Gangrene (dry)	Poor arterial circulation into an area of the body, causing death of body cells	Distribution of arterial solution into the affected area is impossible to establish. Surface and hypodermic treatment is needed.
Gangrene (moist)	Occlusion of veins draining a body area that becomes the site of bacterial infection	Very strong fluid must be injected into the general area arterially. The affected necrotic tissues require hypodermic and surface treatments.
Gunshot wounds	Entry of a foreign missile into the body	Arterial system may rupture. Multisite injection may be needed. Conditions vary depending on location of wound. Blood loss may result in very little drainage. Bodies are usually autopsied.
Hanging	Asphyxiation resulting from exertion of pressure against the large vessels of the neck	Livor mortis is intense *or* absent in facial tissues. Vessels may be damaged or severed. Restricted cervical injection and jugular drainage are recommended.
Hemorrhage	Loss of blood caused by a break in the vascular system	Blood volume may be quite low so there is little drainage. Livor mortis may be minimal. If hemorrhage is the result of a ruptured artery, arterial solution may be lost to body cavities. Multisite injection may be necessary. If a vein has ruptured, much of the drainage may collect in the body cavity where the hemorrhage occurred. If the stomach or esophageal veins are affected, stomach purge can be expected.
Ischemia	Lack of blood supply to an area, frequently resulting in tissue necrosis	Arterial solution cannot reach the affected tissues. Hypodermic and surface embalming treatments are needed.
Leukemia	Cancer of the tissues that form white blood cells	Purpura are observed over the thorax, arms, and abdomen. Edema may be present. Circulation of arterial solution and drainage may be difficult to establish.
Mutilation	Traumatic tissue injuries	Severed arteries may result in difficulty in establishing distribution. Multipoint injections may be needed.
Phlebitis	Inflammation of a vein	Edema may be present in the area. Blood does not easily drain from the area and discolorations may result.
Pneumonia	Acute inflammation of the lung	Broken lung capillaries can result in lung purge. Fever speeds the onset of rigor and decomposition. Congestion may lead to hydrothorax. Distension of the neck can easily occur. Body should be aspirated immediately after arterial injection.
Shock	Sudden vital depression, reduced blood return to the heart	Vasodilation may be present, which can cause swelling. In other types of shock, capillaries constrict and blood congestion occurs in the large veins, making drainage difficult to establish. Capillary congestion may interfere with the distribution and diffusion of arterial solution.
Syphilis	Venereal disease caused by the spirochete *Treponema pallidum*	Aneurysms may occur in arteries. Rupture can make distribution of arterial solution impossible.

TABLE 22–1. *Continued*

Vascular Condition or Injury	Description	Embalming Concern
Thrombosis	Blood clots attached to the inner wall of a blood vessel	Arterial solution distribution may be difficult. If occurring in a vein, drainage may be hard to establish from the affected tissues.
Tuberculosis	Infection of the lungs by *Mycobacterium tuberculosis* that may spread to other organs (e.g., bone, brain, kidney)	When the lungs are affected, cavitation may result; this causes small vessels and capillaries to rupture. There may be a great loss of arterial solution through purging. Purge can be expected. Untreated dehydration and emaciation may be observed.
Tumor	Benign or malignant growth of cells	Pressure may be exerted on the outside of an artery or vein. Distribution to and drainage from an area may be difficult to establish.
Vasoconstriction	Narrowing of a blood vessel	When arteries are affected, as in a "stroke," it may be difficult to supply sufficient arterial solution to the affected side of the body. Multisite injection may be necessary.

ARTERIOSCLEROSIS

Almost any body over the age of 30 may exhibit arteriosclerosis. Most people think of this degenerative condition as occurring in old age. Many persons who die from heart disease in their midfifties exhibit more sclerosis than the 90-year-old. Of the vessels used for embalming, the femoral artery is the most likely to be affected by arteriosclerosis. Thus, use of the common carotid artery as the primary site for injection is recommended.

The embalmer encounters three types of arteriosclerosis (Fig. 22–1):

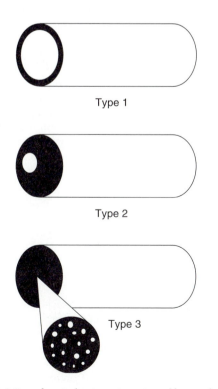

Figure 22–1. Types of arteriosclerosis seen in arteries used for arterial injection.

- **■** *Type 1:* The inner wall of the artery is hardened and thickened but the lumen is well defined and large. These vessels can usually be used for arterial injection. This condition is frequently observed in the autopsied body when the common iliac arteries are exposed.
- **■** *Type 2:* The lumen is quite reduced in size and pushed to one side of the artery. The lumen can usually be identified and a small arterial tube can be used for injection.
- **■** *Type 3:* The artery is completely occluded. If ischemia or gangrene is *not* present in the area supplied (e.g., the leg), the collateral circulation may have increased to supply blood to the limb, *or* there may be minute paths in the occluded artery through which the blood can pass. The formation of these paths or canals is called **canalization**. These arteries *cannot* be used for injection.

In the presence of sclerosis, the strength of the arterial solution can be increased if distribution is poor or slow. Use of a stronger solution ensures that sufficient preservative reaches the tissues even if a large amount of solution cannot be injected. Coinjection chemicals may be used to help distribute the preservative solution. Dye can be added to the solution; it will help to indicate what tissues are receiving the arterial solution.

Lowering the hands over the sides of the table and gently but firmly massaging the limbs help to distribute fluid in sclerotic bodies. Begin injection using a very slow rate of flow. After the vascular system is filled, rate of flow can be increased. When multisite injection is used, higher pressures and pulsation can be used to establish local distribution. Once circulation is established, the pressure and the rate of flow can be reduced.

If a femoral vessel must be used, avoid cutting into the artery where an atheroma can be felt. Make the in-

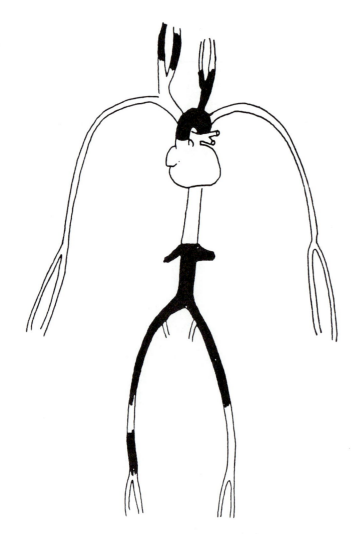

Figure 22–2. Common sites of arteriosclerosis. (Courtesy of H. E. Kazmier.)

cision a little larger at a point where the vessel is softest. Avoid raising these sclerotic arteries to the surface. Work with them from within the incision. Ligate the arterial tubes in place with an arterial hemostat or thick cotton ligature. Thin linen ligatures may separate and tear the vessel. Use an arterial tube small enough that it easily slips into the lumen.

A large arterial tube can damage the lumen of the artery and make it unusable as an injection point. If this happens, it will be necessary to hypodermically embalm that portion of the body. A surface preservative and plastic garment can also be applied to the area (Fig. 22–2).

AORTIC ANEURYSM

A ruptured aortic aneurysm can seriously affect fluid distribution in the unautopsied body. If surgical repair of the vessel was performed, extreme facial edema can often accompany this surgical repair. In the unautopsied

body, determine whether fluid can be distributed from a single-site injection. Inject from the right common carotid artery or use restricted cervical injection.

Often, the femoral vessels in these bodies are sclerotic. Use a strong arterial solution (2.0–2.5%) with additional fluid dye as a tracer. Inject slowly. If drainage is established, continue to inject. **If there is no drainage and the abdomen begins to swell, stop the injection** and institute a multipoint injection to embalm the various body areas. The trunk walls may have to be injected by use of an infant trocar with cavity fluid. Often, when the death certificate cites the immediate cause of death as a ruptured aortic aneurysm, it may be possible to embalm the entire body from one injection site.

VALVULAR HEART DISEASES

The following article, "Damage to Aorta May Bring Embalming Problems," written by Murray M. Shor, describes how disease or malformation may prevent the aorta from being the center of arterial solution circulation.

Because of the position of the aortic semilunar valve, embalmers generally consider the aorta as the center of arterial fluid circulation. In most cases this seems to be true. In the absence of damage to the circulatory system or the heart, it is only after the aorta is filled with fluid that its branches can be expected to receive fluid under any appreciable pressure.

Were it not for the position and construction of the aortic valve, fluid would pass from the ascending portion of the aorta into the left ventricle. Under those conditions the aorta would not be considered the center of embalming fluid circulation. If because of disease or malformation of the aortic semilunar valve fluid did pass into the left ventricle and was confined there by the proper functioning of the mitral valve, the problem would be merely academic. It is when other heart valves are impaired concurrently that embalming problems are created.

Anatomy of the Heart

Let us pause here for a brief review of the anatomy of the heart. The functioning valves are the left atrioventricular or mitral, which allows blood to pass from the left atrium to the left ventricle; the right atrioventricular or tricuspid, which opens from the right atrium into the right ventricle; the pulmonary semilunar, a tricuspid valve which opens to allow blood to flow from the right ventricle into the lungs via the pulmonary artery; and the aforementioned aortic semilunar, a tricuspid valve which opens into the aorta from the left ventricle.

During life any one or any combination of these valves can be affected by the same degenerative diseases that affect the arteries. They can also be attacked by bacteria and damaged irreparably or suffer a congenital malformation. In all of these conditions the circulation of blood during life and of the preservative during embalming is substantially altered.

The great strides made by the medical profession in the fields of infant mortality and infectious diseases leave an older population; one more likely to die of degenerative diseases. Also, because of better medical care, some of the infectious diseases that damage the heart, such as diphtheria and rheumatic fever, have been controlled to such an extent that victims of these diseases survive the infectious stage and live many years afterwards, often with a damaged heart valve or valves.

In the United States we have reached a point where one of every two deaths is attributable to cardiovascular disease. Therefore, it behooves the embalmer to become thoroughly familiar with embalming problems associated with these diseases.

In situations where the mitral and aortic semilunar valves are damaged, embalming fluid under pressure will pass from the aorta into the left ventricle and from there into the left atrium. The left atrium receives the pulmonary veins from the lungs. These veins have no valves. Therefore, a fluid in the atrium, under pressure, would pass back into the capillaries of the lung.

Lung Purge

During most embalming procedures the pulmonary capillaries also receive fluid from the bronchial arteries, coming from the descending thoracic aorta. When the two fluid masses, one from the bronchial arteries and the other from the pulmonary veins, meet, their collective volume and pressure create a lung purge by virtually squeezing the contents of the hollow portions of the lung out through the trachea.

This event should not cause too much apprehension. The matter thus emanating from the mouth or nostrils is the material the embalmer seeks to remove during routine cavity work.

CONGESTIVE HEART FAILURE

Frequently, death certificates cite congestive heart failure as the primary cause of death. Some complications of the end stage of congestive heart failure are of particular interest to the embalmer:

1. Blood is congested in the right side of the heart.
2. The neck veins are engorged with blood; the facial tissues are dark because of the congestion of blood in the right side of the heart and the veins of the neck.
3. Lips, ears, and fingers are cyanotic.
4. Generalized pitting edema may be present. Edema of the legs and feet is pronounced in most bodies. Ascites may be present.
5. Blood may be more viscous because of an increase in red blood cells (polycythemia).
6. Salt is retained in the body fluids.

The carotid artery is used for injection and the right internal jugular vein for drainage, or restricted cervical injection is employed. This helps to ensure good drainage from the head and the right atrium of the heart. The first gallon of arterial solution is made mild to clear the blood congestion and discolorations. If edema is present, the subsequent gallons should be stronger to meet the preservative demand of the body. If the ascites is severe, some of the fluid can be drained with a trocar or drain tube inserted into the abdominal cavity.

Lowering the arms over the table at the start of arterial injection helps to establish good distribution so the discolorations of the hands and fingers can be cleared. The facial tissues may need to be massaged to clear the blood discolorations. It may be necessary to inject both common carotid arteries. When there is extensive discoloration of the face some embalmers prefer to drain from both the right and left internal jugular veins.

Begin injection at a high enough pressure and rapid enough rate of flow to establish good distribution. Continuous drainage should be used to clear the congested blood. Pressure and rate of flow may be increased as the embalming progresses; the pressure and rate of flow should be sufficient to move arterial solution through the entire body. In the presence of generalized edema, distribution and drainage can be expected to be good.

The liver may be enlarged and its functions decreased. This should improve drainage, as the level of clotting factor in the blood will be low.

Pulmonary edema, often observed in cases of congestive heart failure, may cause lung purge. The purge should be allowed to continue during the embalming process. Cavity treatment and repacking of the nasal cavity with cotton after embalming should correct this condition.

Thorough aspiration is necessary to remove distension in the neck tissues resulting from the engorgement with blood. Remove (as much as possible) the edema that led to the ascites. This edema dilutes cavity fluid. It is best to reaspirate and, if necessary, reinject the cavities several hours after the first treatment. Bodies dead from congestive heart failure should be aspirated immediately after arterial injection to help reduce distension in the neck and facial tissues.

VASODILATION AND VASOCONSTRICTION

Sometimes, the dye used to trace the distribution of arterial solution indicates that one side of the body has received a large amount of solution and the other side a small amount. This difference is often evident down the midline of the body. This unequal distribution of arterial solution frequently occurs after death from cerebral vascular accident. The vessels on one side of the body have undergone vasoconstriction. In an effort to supply more oxygen to the tissues in life, the vessels on the opposite side of the body have undergone vasodilation. Multisite injection may be necessary, but in most bodies injection of a sufficient quantity of solution should overcome the problem. This condition may be seen when the deceased has suffered a stroke.

ARTERIAL COAGULA

At death, some blood remains in the arteries, especially in the large aorta. During the postmortem period, this blood can congeal (Fig. 22–3). Injection of the arterial solution may loosen and push coagula into the smaller arteries. By injecting the common carotid arteries these coagula would be moved toward the legs.

If the femoral artery is used as the primary injection point, coagula can be moved into the common carotid arteries and stop the flow of arterial solution into the facial tissues. When the femoral artery is injected upward arterial coagula, most frequently, flow into the left subclavian artery, and it becomes necessary to raise and inject the axillary or brachial artery of the left arm. When the common carotid is used as the primary injection site, arterial coagula are moved into the iliac and femoral arteries. The femoral arteries can be raised to embalm the legs; should this prove unsuccessful, the legs can be treated by hypodermic or surface embalming, or both.

If embalming is begun at a slower rate of flow and the use of preinjection fluids (which may loosen arterial coagula) is avoided, the arterial solution can pass *over* but not loosen coagula.

Venous Coagula

As veins enlarge toward the drainage site, venous coagula do not pose as serious a problem as arterial coagula. Failure to move the coagula, however, can block a vein, and this blockage can lead to tissue distension and discoloration. Massage from distal points toward the heart. Use the right internal jugular vein for drainage, as coagula in the right atrium can be easily reached with angular spring forceps and removed. Intermittent drainage helps to increase venous pressure and loosen coagula from the veins. Multisite injection and drainage may be warranted. When this condition is encountered in a localized area, use a stronger arterial solution to ensure that a minimum amount of arterial fluid delivers the maximum preservative.

DIABETES

A variety of problems arise in the embalming of a diabetic. Of primary concern to the embalmer is the establishment of good fluid distribution. Diabetics tend to develop arteriosclerosis, especially in the smaller vessels, and poor peripheral circulation can be anticipated (Fig. 22–4). These persons are also subject to increased bacterial and mycotic infections; all these conditions require use of a strong arterial solution (2.0–2.5% or higher). The first gallon can be slightly milder than subsequent gallons. To assist in establishing distribution and clearing of blood discolorations, the first gallon of arterial solution can be milder than subsequent injections. Some embalmers prefer to use a coinjection fluid to assist in the clearing of discolorations. Restricted cervical injection is suggested, and the embalmer should use moderate to high pressure to help distribute the solution. Massaging the extremities and using intermittent drainage also facilitate fluid distribution. High pressure and pulsation promote flow to the peripheral tissues (fingers, toes, ears, nose, and lips). Fluid dye can be used to trace the distribution of solution in the tissues.

The tissues of the diabetic may exhibit abnormal pH values. This may result in difficult tissue firming. Use of a moderate to strong solution accompanied by a coin-

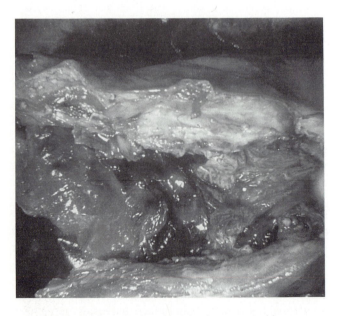

Figure 22–3. Dark areas are large clots in this sclerotic segment of the aorta.

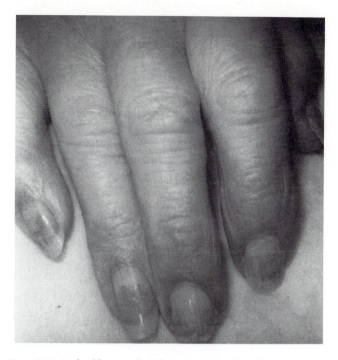

Figure 22–4. Discolored fingertips of a diabetic. Poor peripheral circulation often is seen in the diabetic.

jection fluid and dye should meet the preservative demands.

Many obese individuals are diabetic. Restricted cervical injection and drainage from the right internal jugular vein ensure tissue saturation. A large volume of solution can be injected without concern that the face may be overembalmed. The large volume of solution also promotes better fluid distribution.

Cavity embalming should be thorough. Mycotic infections are often found in the lungs of diabetics. A minimum of 16 ounces of cavity fluid should be used for each major cavity. Abscesses, necrosis, and gangrene may be present in the pancreas and liver. Arterial solution may not have reached these tissues. The cavity fluid is the only preservative that will be available to halt the decomposition that occurs in the tissues of these diseased organs.

Gangrene may also be present in distal tissues such as the fingers and toes. These areas will *not* receive arterial solution when the body is injected. Cavity fluid should be injected into these areas by hypodermic injection or injection with an infant trocar. The surface of feet affected by gangrene should be painted with autopsy gel or cavity fluid compresses should be applied and the leg clothed in a plastic stocking.

Diabetics are also subject to decubitus ulcer. These lesions should be disinfected topically and the tissue around them injected hypodermically with cavity fluid or a phenol cautery solution. Surface compresses of autopsy gel, cavity fluid, or phenol cautery solution should be applied to the necrotic surface tissues.

Restricted cervical injection allows the injection of a milder arterial solution into emaciated and dehydrated facial tissues. Coinjection chemicals and humectants may be used to help restore some moisture. After arterial preparation, tissue builder can be used to restore emaciated and sunken facial tissues.

EXTRAVASCULAR RESISTANCE

Pressure on the outside of an artery or vein is referred to as **extravascular resistance,** and may restrict the flow of arterial solution into a body region or may restrict drainage through a vein.

A slightly stronger well-coordinated arterial solution should be used as distribution may be limited. Multisite injection may be necessary if extravascular resistance is present. Use of higher embalming pressures may promote distribution. Stopping the injection and allowing time for drainage may help to prevent blood discolorations: inject–drain without injecting–inject. Use concurrent drainage throughout the entire operation. Massage and manipulate the tissues to promote both fluid distribution and blood drainage.

Sources of extravascular resistance and suggestions on how to overcome the resulting problems are listed here:

- *Rigor mortis:* Relieve as much rigor as possible by manipulation prior to arterial injection.
- *Ascites:* Relieve the abdominal pressure by draining prior to or during arterial injection.
- *Gas in cavities:* Puncture the abdomen and relieve gases prior to or during arterial injection.
- *Bandages:* Remove tight bandages prior to injection.
- *Contact pressure:* Massage these areas.
- *Tumors:* Excise, with permission, if absolutely necessary. Sectional injection may be necessary.
- *Swollen lymph nodes:* Sectional injection may be necessary.
- *Hydrothorax:* Drainage may be possible prior to injection, but can be difficult.
- *Visceral weight:* Above- and below-heart injection and drainage points can be employed.

KEY TERMS AND CONCEPTS FOR STUDY AND DISCUSSION

1. Define the following terms:
   aneurysm
   arterial coagula
   arteriosclerosis

canalization
embolus
extravascular
extravascular resistance
intravascular
intravascular resistance
lumen
vasoconstriction
vasodilation
venous coagula

2. Describe the vascular problems created by diabetes.
3. Discuss the problems created by congestive heart failure.

BIBLIOGRAPHY

Day DD, Poston G. Embalming the diabetic case. In: *Champion Expanding Encyclopedia.* Springfield, OH: Champion Chemical Co.;1985:No. 560, pp. 2254–2257.

Mulvihill ML. *Human Diseases: A Systemic Approach.* 2nd ed. Norwalk, CT: Appleton & Lange;1987.

Sheldon H. *Boyd's Introduction to the Study of Disease.* 9th ed. Philadelphia: Lea & Febiger;1984.

Shor MM. Damage to aorta may bring embalming problems. *Casket and Sunnyside,* June 1960.

23

Effect of Drugs on the Embalming Process

The contemporary professional embalmer practices this art and science in an age that has often been referred to as the *Chemotherapy Era.* (**Chemotherapy is the treatment of disease with chemical agents and drugs.**) The aims of modern medicine are to cure disease and alleviate pain via the long-sought-for "magic bullet" of Dr. Paul Ehrlich. Today, there is not a single case on which the embalmer works that has not been injected, dusted, or made to ingest some type of chemical substance or substances (drugs) prior to death. In many cases, particularly those received from medical facilities and institutions, many different types of drugs were used prior to the patient's death. Although the Chemotherapy Era began with Ehrlich's "magic bullet" for the treatment of syphilis, today we live in an age of *multiple-agent* chemotherapy.

The way antibiotics are used today exemplifies the multiple-drug approach common to the medical profession. It is very unlikely nowadays that a single antibiotic is prescribed for the treatment of an infection. Usually, two or more antibiotics are administered. In cancer chemotherapy, the multiple-drug approach is also common. It is not unusual for an oncologist to administer both a *cytotoxic* drug (one that kills the cancer cell directly) and an *antimetabolite* (one that slowly "starves" the cancer cell by depriving it of a needed nutrient). One result of this multiple-agent approach has been an increase in the number and types of embalming problems.

Before the embalming problems caused by chemotherapeutic agents are discussed, "normal" embalming must be defined. There is *no* "ideal case." It is probably impossible to find a person who has not been treated by one or more doctors with one or more drugs prior to death. So, in addition to the problems caused by the pathological processes resulting in death, the chemotherapeutic agent or agents administered for various intervals prior to death have physiological effects. The longer the drug was taken before death, the more intense are the embalming problems likely to be encountered.

Another problem may arise from the chemical reaction between the administered drugs and the components of the embalming fluid. For example, are there any components of arterial embalming fluid that form insoluble precipitates when they react with antibiotics? If so, the circulatory path may become blocked, thus preventing the preservative components of the arterial fluid from reaching the tissues for preservation (see p. 497).

THE CHEMISTRY OF PROTEINS

To discuss the chemistry of embalming, it is essential to understand the chemistry of proteins. These materials form the physical structures of the body. They give the body form. **The professional embalmer must achieve the absolute preservation of these structures.** This means that

393

the proteinaceous materials forming portions of the various tissues and organs of the human body must be rendered chemically inert. Essentially, these structures must be frozen in time and space!

Proteins are labile substances. The molecules break down quite rapidly even without bacterial action. There exist proteins that break down other proteins. These specialized proteins, called *enzymes,* are endowed with a physicochemical structure that allows catalytic activity. These enzymes can speed up decomposition reactions. It must be realized that even if a cadaver were completely sterile, the proteolytic enzymes in the cells and tissues of that body would still be fully active and capable of causing the breakdown of tissue proteins.

One goal of embalming must be to render the proteins resistant to attack by catalytic enzymes. There are two ways to do this: (1) The proteins themselves can be treated so that they are no longer susceptible to the action of proteolytic enzymes. (2) The enzymes themselves can be so changed or inactivated that they cannot exert catalytic action on other proteins. Modern embalming chemicals are formulated to do both.

To determine how both of these goals can be achieved in a so-called "ideal" case, a brief mathematical formula is helpful.

What this means in terms of actual chemicals used to embalm a case should be discussed from a practical standpoint.

AVERAGE BODY PROTEIN

The average body = 150 pounds = 65.3 kilograms.
A 65.3 kg body contains 10.7 kg of protein = 10,700 grams of protein.

FORMALDEHYDE DEMAND

100 grams of soluble protein requires 4.4 grams of formaldehyde for preservation.
The average body contains 10,700 grams of protein.
Therefore,
$$\frac{10,700}{100} \times 4.4 = 470.8 \text{ grams of formaldehyde needed.}$$

SOLUTION NEEDED

Given: Standard 30-index arterial fluid contains 16 ounces of 30% formaldehyde = 142.08 grams of formaldehyde.

Need: 470.80 grams of formaldehyde.
$$\frac{470.80}{142.08} = 3.31 \text{ sixteen-ounce bottles of a 30-index fluid needed, or approximately 53 ounces of arterial fluid!}$$

For a nonideal case (as practically all cases today are), the conclusion that some of the formaldehyde will be lost in embalming seems obvious. For example, many chemotherapeutic agents are nephrotoxic and, therefore, cause a breakdown of kidney function. As the kidneys are the main organs responsible for elimination of nitrogenous wastes, these waste materials (ammonia, urea, uric acid, etc.) are retained by the body. There is no better way to neutralize formaldehyde than to react it with ammonia, and this is exactly what happens in the body. If there has been a buildup of nitrogenous waste materials as a result of chemotherapy-induced kidney dysfunction, a standard dilution of arterial embalming fluid will not be sufficient. A large proportion of the formaldehyde in the embalming fluid will be neutralized when it encounters the nitrogenous wastes in the body. The remainder is insufficient to preserve the tissues, and the body starts to decay.

Normally, arterial embalming fluids are supplied as 16-ounce concentrates. These are diluted with water and additives prior to injection into the body. An embalming fluid containing 30% formaldehyde supplies 142 grams of formaldehyde per bottle. To embalm the "average" or "ideal" body containing 10.7 kilograms of protein, 470 grams of formaldehyde is needed, that is, a minimum of three bottles of arterial embalming fluid. (If the body has been dosed with drugs, more than double this amount of formaldehyde may be necessary!)

THE CHEMOTHERAPY CASE

All chemotherapeutic agents are toxic. This is the one axiom universally applicable to all drugs. Cellular and tissue changes occur when drugs are used. It does not matter what drug is administered; even the seemingly innocuous aspirin tablet has its effects. Drug-induced changes may be relatively minor, perhaps limited to slight skin discolorations, which, in the deceased, readily respond to cosmetic treatment. When drugs cause major problems, such as acute jaundice, or saturate the body tissues with uremic wastes, the fixative action of the preservative chemicals in the arterial embalming fluid is seriously impaired.

The chemotherapeutic agents common to modern medicine exert their effects in many ways. They may impair function of the liver, the circulatory system (heart and blood vessels), the kidneys, the lungs, and the skin. These drugs can inactivate the embalming fluid by caus-

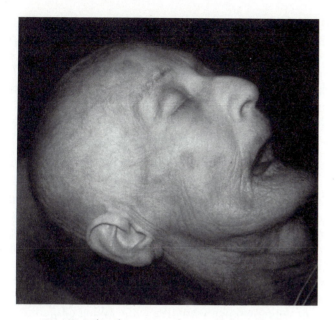

Figure 23–1. Chemotherapy patients showing weight loss and hair loss.

ing the buildup of nitrogenous wastes or decreasing the permeability of the cell membrane (Fig. 23–1).

Because the *liver* is the main detoxification center, every drug eventually enters the hepatic circulation. While in the liver, the drug may be changed to an innocuous form by hepatic enzymes, or the drug may cause profound changes in the liver itself. When the liver is damaged, the embalmer may have to cope with a jaundiced body.

All drugs ultimately pass through the kidneys. Even those that accumulate in other body areas must pass at least once (and often more) through the kidneys. If the drugs cause extensive changes in this organ, renal insufficiency follows, resulting in the buildup of nitrogenous wastes in body tissues. Saturated with urea, uric acid, ammonia, creatinine, and other wastes, the tissues become spongy and difficult to preserve. In such cases, preservation is almost impossible to achieve unless the treatment is modified.

Drugs also change the biochemical constituents of the blood. Some drugs damage even the connecting blood vessels themselves extensively. The circulatory system may become impaired as a result of extensive clot formation, lysis of the blood cells, or extensive damage to the walls of the arteries and veins.

The effects on *skin* are closely associated with the changes in the circulatory system and may include the formation of widespread areas of discoloration stemming from lysis and release of blood pigments from red blood cells. Lesions on the skin surfaces may also result from use of the nitrogen mustards.

Pharmacologically, the dividing line between the beneficial effects and toxic effects of drugs is very slender. The professional embalmer must learn to cope with these effects.

INACTIVATION OF PRESERVATIVE AGENTS BY DRUGS

The problems likely to be confronted while embalming a body administered chemotherapy do *not* result from the reactions of formaldehyde or other preservative aldehydes with the drug or drugs. Much too little drug is present, even after aggressive therapy. **It is the physiological effect of the drug that is culpable.** A drug that causes nephrotoxic changes enhances the accumulation of nitrogenous waste products in the body. These waste products, which result indirectly from the physiological effect of the drug, are responsible for the inactivation or, more specifically, the neutralization of the formaldehyde:

$$4NH_3 + 6CH_2O \rightarrow (CH_2)_6N_4 + 6H_2O$$

This neutralization reaction, whereby formaldehyde is converted to hexamethylene, is probably at the root of at least 90% of the contemporary embalmer's problems.

A change in permeability of the cell membrane is another effect of most systemically administered drugs. It is through this membrane that everything must pass, either to enter or to leave the cell. Preservative chemicals such as formaldehyde must pass through this membrane if they are going to inactivate the intracellular enzymes that decompose the proteins there.

If a chemotherapeutic agent reduces or destroys membrane permeability, preservative solutions may not be able to enter the cell. The antibiotic tetracycline is a case in point. Although most antibiotics exert their effects on bacteria they also have an effect on the human cell. They are chelating agents and tend to lodge in the cell membrane, causing calcium to form an impenetrable layer around the cell. "Chelating" means they have an affinity for metallic ions, particularly calcium and magnesium. Antibiotics appear to act selectively on cell membranes. After they are entrenched in the membrane, they start chelating or sequestering calcium and magnesium ions. [There is generally no shortage of calcium in the body; it is present in all biological fluids (secretions, excretions, etc.).]

Eventually, as more calcium and magnesium ions become lodged in the chelate in the cell membrane, the permeability of the membrane changes; the membrane becomes less permeable. It becomes increasingly more difficult for some chemicals to enter such a cell. As the goal of embalming is to inactivate the intracellular enzymes present, it is essential that the preservative enter the cell. If it does not, the proteolytic enzymes inside the cell can proceed to break down the proteinaceous materials in the cell, and the tissue is subject to decomposition and lysis of its structural features. In essence, it turns into a puddle of fluid.

To study these effects, Fredrick (1968) devised a histological method based on a chemical method of Gomori (1939). Gomori observed that if an enzyme were supplied with a substrate, it would release a material (phosphate) that could be precipitated in situ. Using this technique, one is able to determine the location of active enzymes.

There has recently come into use a group of antibiotics that exert their effects in the kidney, hampering its ability to dispose of nitrogenous wastes—the aminoglycosides, represented by kanamycin and, most recently, gentamicin. These antibiotics cause nitrogenous waste products to be retained, and if the so-called standard dilution of arterial fluid is used, embalming will fail.

COMBINATION ANTIBIOTIC CHEMOTHERAPY

Today, it is routine procedure for physicians to prescribe two or more antibiotics at the same time. This, of course, intensifies the embalming problems. The embalming problems resulting from synergistic combination chemotherapy are not new, only more intense. Use of a combination such as gentamicin and a synthetic penicillin (e.g., methicillin) makes preservation and firming difficult to achieve. These bodies are usually saturated with ammoniacal and other nitrogenous wastes. The arterial fluid in such cases must be very concentrated if any embalming is to be accomplished.

CORTICOSTEROIDS AND ANTIINFLAMMATORY DRUGS

If antibiotics are the most widely used drugs, then cortisone and its derivatives constitute a close second. The antiinflammatory drugs have many uses (e.g., itching caused by allergies) and are the drugs of choice for arthritic and rheumatic conditions. Corticosteroids are also widely used in the chemotherapy of cancer.

With regard to specific embalming problems caused by these drugs, the chief effect is blockade of the cell membrane. **Corticosteroids decrease the permeability of this membrane** and thereby block passage of liquids into the cell. On a gross macroscopic level, liquids are retained by the cells and tissues, resulting in an increase in cell turgor and waterlogging of tissues.

The use of cortisone for the treatment of chronic diseases (over long periods) may result in **gastrointestinal ulcerations with possible perforations of the gut.** Prolonged use in the treatment of ulcerative colitis has also resulted in dehydration of the body.

Corticosteroids have been shown to exert a "protective" effect on proteolytic enzymes. This is demonstrated by the difficult task one has in trying to denature these enzymes in cortisone-treated bodies. Even if these enzymes are extracted from such cortisone-treated tissues and are obtained in an almost pure form, they are still difficult to inactivate. They retain the "protective" effect originally conferred by the corticosteroids. This means that more undenatured proteolytic enzymes remain in the body after embalming. Such bodies tend to "go bad" (decompose) very rapidly after an apparently trouble-free embalming.

What has so far been described with respect to corticosteroids can also occur as the result of the use of oral contraceptives by women. Progesterone and its derivatives have chemical structures similar to that of cortisone. It has long been known in pharmacology that similar chemical structures elicit similar biological reactions. Many of the embalming problems observed after use of corticosteroids are identical to those encountered in bodies of young women who died while taking oral contraceptives.

Another problem encountered when corticosteroids have been administered for some time prior to death is of a more insidious nature. These persons have been shown to have disseminated tuberculosis. The antiinflammatory action of the corticosteroids results from their suppression of immunity. In cases of "arrested" (or so-called "cured") tuberculosis in which large doses of cortisone were administered before death, it is not uncommon to find that because immunity was suppressed the mycobacterium was reactivated and spread throughout the body. Such cases offer hidden hazards to the embalmer's health and sanitation precautions should be observed.

To secure preservation in these bodies, some permeability should be restored to the cell membranes so that preservatives can enter the cells. This can be done through the use of adjunct fluids. Preinjecting such a body restores some of the permeability; and the surface-active chemicals in such preparations facilitate entry of the preservative components of the arterials into cells. At the same time, a stronger-than-normal arterial injection should be used together with a coinjection fluid. (It is also possible to use some coinjection fluids as a preinjection.)

CANCER CHEMOTHERAPEUTIC AGENTS AND THEIR EFFECTS

Various drugs are used to treat malignancies, but generally they fall into two main classes. *Cytotoxic* drugs act directly on the tumor cells to bring about their death. *Antimetabolite* drugs substitute for an essential metabolite required by the cancer cell for growth. It is not unusual for both types to be given to the cancer patient. This multiple-agent chemotherapy creates tremendous problems for the professional embalmer.

Cytotoxic drugs (e.g., nitrogen mustards, alkylating agents) kill both malignant and normal cells. (A "magic bullet" for cancer has not yet been found.) When cells die, proteins break down and large amounts of nitrogenous wastes are released. Therefore, the tissues in these bodies, besides containing a small amount of protein as a result of the extreme cachexia associated with cancer, are saturated with nitrogenous waste products. Achievement of preservation under these conditions is a herculean task in itself, but the embalming problems that arise from the coadministration of antimetabolites must be added. These are sure to cause symptoms of extensive vitamin deficiency. Such bodies may exhibit everything from scurvy to brittle ricketslike bone disease. If radiation therapy has been administered, there may be extensive skin and circulatory problems (e.g., purpura and body clots).

RADIOACTIVE ISOTOPES AND THEIR EFFECTS

Because radioactive materials are used for cancer therapy, it is not amiss to discuss the radiation-treated body. An embalmer should not attempt to embalm a radiation-treated body unless a radiation safety officer has certified the body as safe because of the possibility of gamma radiation. The main radioisotopes used to diagnose and treat malignancies are cobalt-60, iodine-131, phosphorus-32, radium-226, gold-198, and strontium-89. Beta rays are stopped much more readily than gamma rays, which are similar to x-rays and require lead shielding. In addition, tiny needles or "seeds" of gold-198, as well as radon needles, are implanted in tissues to treat metastatic tumors in the abdomen and lungs. These bodies, if declared safe, may be embalmed as would any cancer case.

A second source of radiation exposure is an occupational accident. Radioactive materials are measured in *millicuries*. A millicurie (mCi) is defined as that amount of radioactive material in which 37 million atoms disintegrate each second. Medical institutions must "tag" bodies, warning that radioactive isotopes are present in the body or that the body has had a high exposure to radiation by accident. The medical institution is not permitted to release the body until the level of radioactivity has dropped below 30 millicuries, for unautopsied bodies. Autopsied remains are not to be released until the radiation level drops to 5 millicuries or below. It is necessary for the embalmer to follow any instructions issued by the radiation protection officer. If embalming is permitted when when radiation levels are above the figures cited, the preparation should occur at the hospital under the strict supervision of the radiation officer.

When radiation levels are below 30 millicuries for unautopsied remains and 5 millicuries or below for au-

topsied remains, standard embalming procedures can be used which would be determined by the conditions present in the dead human body. There are certain recommended precautions the embalmer should exercise. These precautions can be summarized in the words *protection, time of exposure,* and *distance.* During the preparation of bodies that have been exposed to high doses of radioactivity, the embalmer should wear rubber gloves, if possible two pairs, and a heavy rubber apron. In addition, of course, standard Universal Precautions attire should also be worn. The shortest time of exposure should be employed. Time of exposure can be shortened, when possible, by working in pairs; two embalmers can work together performing different tasks (e.g., one embalmer raises vessels and a second sets features). This helps to reduce the exposure time. Having instruments ready and fluids mixed, as soon as the body is observed, again reduce the time spent in preparation. It would be most wise to avoid raising vessels in a body region where tissues have been seeded with the radioactive isotope; for example, if seeds are present in tissues of the neck, use of the femoral vessels would reduce contact with the seeds.

Distance also plays a large role in reducing exposure to radiation. For every 3 feet of distance from the body, exposure is reduced by a substantial amount. When not actually performing a procedure, the embalmer should stand at a distance from the body (e.g., during injection of the arterial solution when massage may not be necessary). There should be a constant flow of water under the body. New tables allow the body to be positioned on slats, which allow water to flow beneath the body without coming into contact with the body. The constant flow of water is necessary to dilute and flush away all drainage matter as it exits the body. Care should be taken to cover the area around the preparation table with sheeting, which can be destroyed by incineration or placed in a biohazard container after the embalming; this ensures that all waste matter is removed from the areas surrounding the preparation table. Gloves should be frequently flushed with soap and water during the embalming procedure. Any spillage should be removed immediately with the use of forceps or tongs and new sheeting or a portion of the sheeting draped onto the floor.

Final cleanup should include the following:

- Instruments should be thoroughly flushed with running water, then soaked in a good soap or detergent and rinsed well with running water.
- Disposable waste matter should be collected in a suitable biohazard container and disposed of (if permitted) by incineration.
- Gloves (if they are to be reused) should be thoroughly washed before being removed from the hands, then placed in a container of soap and water and allowed to soak. Next they should be re-

moved and dried and stored in a suitable place until the radioactivity has decayed to a safe level.
- Gowns, towels, clothing, and so on should be monitored and stored for suitable decay before being sent to the laundry (consult the radiation officer of the medical facility for assistance in this matter).
- If the embalmer suffers any introduction of material from the body into lesions on his or her hands, the injured area should be washed with copious amounts of running water and a physician or radiation safety officer consulted.

The embalmer should follow any instructions that have been made by the radiation safety officer with regard to preparation of the body. An example would be if the officer stated that aspiration and injection of the cavities should not be carried out until a certain time. Strengths of arterial solutions, volume of fluid injected, and so on do not directly affect radiation exposure. Some examples of radioactive isotopes employed in disease diagnosis and treatment are cobalt-60, iodine-131, radium-226, gold-198, and strontium-89. A more detailed discussion of radioactive isotopes can be found in the text *Thanatochemistry* by James M. Dorn and Barbara Hopkins, published by Reston, a Prentice–Hall company, Reston, Virginia, 1985.

TRANQUILIZERS AND MOOD-ALTERING DRUGS

It is not easy to discuss prescribed legal drugs without venturing into the field of drug abuse. No matter what the drug is, if it is taken beyond the period prescribed, or if more than the dose prescribed is taken, it becomes "abused." For example, if amphetamines are prescribed for dietary or psychiatric reasons and are taken longer than necessary to alleviate the condition, they become illegal or abused drugs. It should be realized that such components of the drug culture as benzedrine, dexedrine, and methedrine were all at one time (and some still are) rigorously and ethically prescribed by physicians to treat specific ills. The same holds true for such tranquilizers as phenothiazine and its derivatives.

There are roughly five classes of tranquilizers and mood-altering drugs. In general, they have one common characteristic: they result in a loss of weight of the abuser. Embalming these bodies is very frustrating because of the lack of protein (most of the protein stores have been depleted). A person on a "trip" does not care about nutrition.

- *Sedatives:* barbiturates [amobarbital (Amytal),

secobarbital (Seconal), etc.]; meprobamate (Quanil, Miltown, etc.)
- *Stimulants:* amphetamines (Benzedrine, Dexedrine, etc.); cocaine; phenmetrazine (Preludin)
- *Tranquilizers:* phenothiazines [chlorpromazine (Thorazine), prochlorperazine (Compazine), etc.]; reserpine (Serpalan, Serpasil); chlordiazepoxide (Librium); diazepam (Valium)
- *Narcotics:* opiates (opium, heroin, morphine, etc.)
- *Antidepressants:* methylphenidate (Ritalin); imipramine (Tofranil)

The continued use (or abuse) of tranquilizers can also result in such embalming problems as jaundice because of the destructive effect of these drugs on liver cells. In addition, tranquilizers may cause hemolysis of the red blood cells and thereby add to the jaundice problem because pigments are released from these red blood cells. Also common to abusers of all five classes of drugs is the depletion of protein stores resulting from their neglect of nutrition. Protein depletion results in the release of large amounts of nitrogenous waste products. If kidney function is impaired (particularly in heroin addicts in whom both constipation and anuresis occur), these waste materials cannot exit the body. They are retained in the tissues and rapidly neutralize formaldehyde (or any aldehyde).

PROBLEMS CAUSED BY ORAL DRUGS THAT CONTROL DIABETES

A group of chemotherapeutic agents with broad-spectrum effects comprises those drugs used to control diabetes, the oral diabetic agents. Use of such drugs as tolbutamide (Orinase) and chlorpropamide (Diabinese) to control adult (type II) diabetes is increasing. These drugs certainly are more convenient (for those who can use them) than the daily (or more frequent) self-injections of insulin.

Tolbutamide was used widely until recently, when it was replaced with another second-generation sulfonylurea called chlorpropamide. Both may cause jaundice. Most of the sulfonylureas can induce changes in the voluntary muscles (site of glycogen storage and breakdown) and the liver (main glycogen storage organ of the body). Continuous use of oral diabetic agents has been linked with circulatory problems, which can result in poor distribution of the arterial chemicals. (This has been observed to be the result of extensive clot formation in the cadaver). Acidosis sometimes occurs as a result of the altered carbohydrate metabolism and leads to the formation of high concentrations of lactic acid in muscle tissue. Such bodies firm very rapidly unless an alkaline coinjection is used with the arterial embalming fluid.

In general, although oral diabetic agents may cause a large variety of embalming problems, they do not cause as severe embalming problems as do other drugs.

NEUTRALIZING CHEMOTHERAPEUTIC AGENTS

It must be understood that chemotherapeutic agents cause embalming problems not through their reactions with embalming chemicals but through their physiological effects on the body prior to death (Table 23–1). No drug, no matter how often, how long, or in what concentration it is used, could ever be administered long enough during life to react significantly with the components of an arterial chemical injected after death. As has previously been stressed, **it is the physiological reaction the drug induces that causes the problem.** For example, the nephrotoxic effect of the aminoglycoside antibiotics is produced not by the reaction between formaldehyde and kanamycin (even if a few grams of the antibiotic were present), but rather by the reaction between formaldehyde and the nitrogenous waste products released into the tissues through the action of the antibiotic.

Once absorbed into the bloodstream, a drug is rapidly diluted. An average body contains about 6 liters (1 liter is equivalent to 2.1 pints) of blood. This volume of blood circulates once per minute. It comes into contact with 35 additional liters of liquid. (Fifty-eight percent of the body weight of an average 150-pound man is water). *Therefore, there is a total of 41 liters of liquid (including blood volume) in the average body.* Any drug, usually given in milligram doses, would be so diluted as to have no significant effect in a direct chemical reaction with formaldehyde or any component of embalming fluid.

In the event of a nuclear accident, in addition to the obvious protective equipment required, massive preinjection of the cadaver is necessary (with a chelating agent containing pre-/coinjection fluid). All drainage must be collected in lead-lined containers and disposed per directions of the Nuclear Regulatory Commission.

POSSIBLE SOLUTIONS TO CHEMOTHERAPY PROBLEMS

The problems arising from chemotherapy vary in severity, but can be divided into a few broad categories. Several preventive and ameliorative treatments are available that have been shown to work in the majority of cases. **The professional embalmer must consider each case as unique.** Just as a physician does not prescribe the same dosage of a medication for all patients, so must the embalmer vary procedures (and preservative fluids) to meet the requirements of the particular case.

In Table 23–1, five different embalming treatments are recommended to combat most chemotherapy-derived

TABLE 23–1. PROBLEMS CAUSED BY CHEMOTHERAPEUTIC AGENTS[a]

Key to Table: The embalming treatment recommended is designated by a code number interpreted as follows:

1	Preinjection required
2	Coinjection required
3	Increase arterial concentration
4	Use less water for total injection
5	Use restorative or tissue builder

Note: The chemicals cited in this table pertain to one particular chemical manufacturer.

Drug	Problem	Embalming Treatment Recommended
Antibiotics (penicillins, synthetic penicillins, aminoglycosides, tetracyclines)	Cottonlike circulatory blockages (fungal overgrowth); jaundice; bleeding into skin; poor penetration	1,2,3,4
Corticosteroids (cortisone)	Cell membranes less permeable; retention of fluids; mild to severe waterlogging of tissues; "protects" proteolysis enzymes, resulting in more rapid breakdown of body proteins	1,2,3,4
Cancer chemotherapy (antimetabolites, cytotoxic agents, radioisotopes)	Emaciation and dehydration; extensive purpura; jaundice; low protein (because of anorexia and vomiting); perforation of gut; brittleness of bone; nitrogenous waste retention	2,3,4,5
Tranquilizers (phenothiazines)	Dehydration; weight loss and emaciation; low protein; kidney dysfunction and retention of nitrogenous waste products	2,3,4,5
Stimulants (amphetamines, cocaine)	Weight loss; emaciation; low protein; mucous membranes bleed easily; other problems as for tranquilizers	2,3,4,5
Sedatives (barbiturates, meprobamate)	Emaciation; dehydration; low protein; difficult to firm	2,3,5
Oral antidiabetic agents (tolbutamide)	Muscle atrophy; mild to severe jaundice; some emaciation and edema	1,2,4,5
Circulatory drugs (antihypertensives, anticlotting agents)	Blood clots; impairment of circulation; poor distribution of fluids; purpura; urine retention and spongy nitrogenous waste-filled tissues	1,2,3,4

[a]Table has been adapted and summarized from many published works. It is neither complete nor exhaustive. It is designed to point out categories of chemotherapeutic agents in use now. It is hoped that this table will stimulate both the student of embalming and the licensed professional to read about the latest developments in journals and trade magazines. As new chemical agents are introduced so frequently by the medical profession, it is impossible to publish up-to-the-minute tables. Keeping up with the literature is of the utmost importance.

problems. Obviously, these cannot solve all the problems the professional embalmer will face. They do, however, serve as a springboard for further research and, therefore, offer the embalmer an opportunity for experimentation and learning—both the marks of professionalism.

CONCLUSION

Mistaken ideas about the specificity of a particular chemotherapeutic agent are quite common. For example, one may believe that a drug known to have a pronounced effect on a particular organ will be found only in that organ. This is not so. That a drug shows a more dramatic effect on a particular tissue does not mean that the effect is limited only to that tissue.

In general, no matter what chemotherapeutic agent is used, it is concentrated, metabolized, and detoxified in the liver and excreted via the kidneys (and, sometimes, the lungs and skin). But before it reaches these organs, it passes through other tissues of the body, which is contrary to the "magic bullet" concept. Actually, there is no magic bullet! It is impossible for a drug to bring about a single reaction in a single organ or tissue. It should not be surprising then that a single drug can cause a plethora of embalming problems. Simultaneous use of two or more drugs, as is common in medical practice today, intensifies the problems.

In the body, a drug is subject to great dilution. The problems it causes do not result from its direct reaction with components of the embalming fluid, but from the chronic physiological effects it produces.

On the basis of both laboratory studies and field work, five embalming treatments for the problems encountered in bodies that have undergone chemotherapy have been recommended. It is the responsibility of the embalmer to modify the treatment to suit the particular case.

KEY TERMS AND CONCEPTS FOR STUDY AND DISCUSSION

1. It is known that elderly persons present chemotherapy-derived embalming problems because the ability of the body to circulate, detoxify, and excrete drugs decreases with age. Discuss, on this basis, the possible effects of an aminoglycoside antibiotic such as gentamicin when the "usual" dilution is used.

2. If approximately 58% of the human body is composed of water, is it defeating the purpose to embalm the body that has undergone chemotherapy, particularly if there is little protein (as in the drug addict) in that body, by further diluting the embalming fluid with water before it is injected? Discuss how use can be made of this intracellular water as a diluent for concentrated arterial fluid. As this "tissue" water is known to be high in calcium, should it be conditioned with a water softener or conditioner?

3. It is a fact that a body treated with antibiotics usually contains all types of fungi. Certain fungi may pose a hazard to the embalmer. Discuss the possibility of contracting *Candida*, *Cryptococcus*, and *Histoplasma* infections from cadavers. What can be done to protect the embalmer?

4. It has been shown that to embalm an "average" body, at least three to four 16-ounce bottles of a 30% formaldehyde arterial solution are necessary. Discuss whether enough preservative is contained in this amount of arterial fluid to embalm a body treated with corticosteroids. What adjunct embalming chemicals should be added to the arterial injection?

5. A young housewife is killed in an automobile accident. The embalmer is told that she has been taking a fertility drug (progesterone) because she was childless and wanted a family. What types of embalming problems can be expected?

6. A chronic diabetic is brought to the preparation room. The embalmer discovers that instead of insulin, the man had taken tolbutamide (Orinase) two times daily for the past 3 years. What embalming fluids should be used on this case, taking into consideration dilution of arterial chemicals, rapidity of firming, and use of preinjection fluid, water conditioners, and other fluids?

7. After arterial injection, the drainage is observed to contain small wads of greenish "cotton." The patient had been taking massive doses of penicillin prior to death. What could these "cotton wads" be?

8. If the professional embalmer knew what medications were used on a case prior to death, he or she could be better informed as to what embalming problems to expect. Discuss how a funeral director can secure the cooperation of the pathologist and other hospital authorities in obtaining this information.

9. Discuss why an embalmer cannot use one type and one concentration of arterial embalming fluid in all cases.

10. A particular drug exerts its effect on only one specific organ. Therefore, after a patient treated with cortisone for an arthritic condition dies, high concentrations of cortisone will be found only in the joints. Discuss the fallacy of this type of thinking.

BIBLIOGRAPHY

Brozek J. *Body Composition*. New York: New York Academy of Sciences; 1963.

Dorn J, Hopkins B. *Thanatochemistry*. Reston, VA: Reston; 1985.

Fredrick JF. An alpha-glucan phosphorylase which requires adenosine-5-phosphate as coenzyme. *Phytochemistry* 1963;2:413–415.

Fredrick JF. *Embalming Problems Caused by Chemotherapeutic Agents*. Boston: Dodge Institute for Advanced Studies; 1968.

Gomori G. Microtechnical demonstration of phosphatase enzymes in tissue sections. *Proc Soc Exp Biol Med* 1939;42:23–26.

Goodman L, Gilman A, eds. *The Pharmacological Basis of Therapeutics*. 4th ed. New York: Macmillan; 1970.

Goth, A. *Medical Pharmacology*. 6th ed. St. Louis, MO: CV Mosby; 1972.

Julian RM. *A Primer of Drug Action*. San Francisco: Freeman; 1975.

Long YG. *Neuropharmacology and Behavior*. San Francisco: Freeman; 1972.

Merck, Sharpe, & Dohme. *Merck Index*. 10th ed. Rahway, NJ: Merck & Co.; 1983.

Physician's Desk Reference (PDR). Oradale, NJ: Medical Economics; 1984:No. 38.

Yessell ES, Braude MC. *Interaction of Drugs of Abuse*. New York: New York Academy of Sciences; 1976.

Windholz M, Budavari S. In: *Merck Index*. 10th ed. Rahway, NJ: Merck & Co.; 1983.

24

Selected Conditions

PURGE

Purge is defined as the postmortem evacuation of any substance from any external orifice of the body as a result of pressure. This condition can occur prior to, during, and after embalming. Purge is generally described by its source—stomach, lung, and so on. The pressure responsible for the purge can develop in several ways:

1. Gas: Gas in the abdominal cavity or in the hollow intestinal tract can create sufficient pressure on the stomach to force the contents of the stomach through the mouth or nose. This abdominal pressure can also push on the diaphragm with sufficient force to cause the contents of the lungs to purge through the mouth or nose. Gas can originate from early decomposition or from partial digestion of foods or may be true tissue gas formed by *Clostridium perfringens*.
2. Visceral expansion: When bodies have been dead for several hours and arterial solution is injected too fast, the hollow visceral organs (intestinal tract) tend to expand. As the abdomen is a closed cavity this expansion creates sufficient pressure to push on the stomach walls and create a stomach purge. The expansion also pushes on the diaphragm and squeezes on the lungs, possibly resulting in lung purge.

3. Arterial Solution:
   A. Injection of arterial solution at a fast rate of flow, especially in bodies dead for long periods, causes expansion of the viscera (see item 2).
   B. If an area of the stomach, upper bowel, or lung is ulcerated, the arterial solution can leak through the ulcerated vessels, fill the stomach, esophagus, or lung tissue, and the trachea, and develop into a purge.
   C. If esophageal varices break, sufficient blood and arterial solution can exit to create purge.
   D. Gastrointestinal bleeding accompanies a variety of diseases and the long-term use of many drugs. If a sufficient amount of arterial solution and blood leak from these tissues during injection, anal purge results.
   E. Purge can occur when leakage of arterial solution from an aneurysm in the thoracic or abdominal cavity develops sufficient pressure to push on the lungs or stomach.
   F. Sufficient injection pressure can cause leakage from recent surgical incisions. The arterial solution lost to the stomach or abdominal cavity builds up enough pressure to create purge.
4. Ascites and hydrothorax: When edema fills the thoracic or abdominal cavity prior to death, a great amount of pressure builds up and, on injection of arterial solution forces purge.

CONDITIONS PREDISPOSING TO PURGE

- Decomposition
- Long delay between death and embalming
- Drowning or asphyxia
- Recent abdominal, thoracic, or cranial surgery
- Tissue gas
- Hydrothorax or ascites
- Peritonitis or bloodstream infections
- Esophageal varices, ulcerations of the gastrointestinal tract, or internal hemorrhages

Protecting Skin Areas from Purge

When purge occurs prior to or during arterial injection from the nose or mouth, the surrounding tissues of the face should be protected by an application of massage cream. Stomach purge contains hydrochloric acid and can desiccate and discolor the skin. If arterial fluid is contained in the purge material, the dye from the fluid can stain the skin, making cosmetic application difficult. Cover the facial tissues and neck area with the massage cream. Only a light coating is needed. Be certain the inside of the lips is covered as well as the base of the nose. Tightly packing the throat, nostrils, and anus prior to embalming should greatly reduce the possibility of a purge during or after embalming.

General Preembalming and Embalming Treatments

When the abdomen is distended from gas or edema (ascites) prior to embalming, a trocar should be introduced into the upper area of the cavity. Piercing the transverse colon helps to relieve gas pressure. The stomach can also be punctured, as it can contain a great quanity of liquid. If ascites is present, removing some of the edema from the abdominal cavity will relieve the pressure that can cause purging during embalming. (The aspirating hose should be attached to the trocar.)

A nasal tube aspirator can be inserted into the nasal cavity and the throat to remove purge material.

Time Period Treatments

Two factors are necessary for purge to occur. First, there must be a substance to purge, such as stomach contents, blood, arterial fluid, and respiratory tract contents. Second, there must be pressure on an organ such as the stomach, rectum, or lung to evacuate the material.

Preembalming Purge

Stomach or Lung Purge. Preembalming purge generally consists of the stomach contents (Table 24–1). If esophageal varices have ruptured or if a stomach ulcer has eroded a blood vessel, blood can also be expected in the purge. As the stomach contains acid, this purge usually is brown. Stomach purge is often described as "coffee grounds" in appearance. Removal of this material at the beginning of

TABLE 24–1. POSTMORTEM PURGE

Source	Orifice	Description	Contents	Time
Stomach	Mouth/nose	Liquid/semisolid	Stomach contents	Preembalming
		"Coffee ground" appearance	Blood	Embalming
		Foul odor	Arterial solution	Postembalming
		Acid pH		
Lung	Mouth/nose	Frothy	Respiratory tract liquids	Preembalming
		Blood remains red	Residual air from lungs	Embalming
		Little odor	Blood	Postembalming
			Arterial solution	
Esophageal varices	Mouth/nose	Bloody liquid	Blood	Preembalming
			Arterial solution	Embalming
				Postembalming
Brain	Fracture in skull	White semisolid	Brain tissue	Preembalming
	Nose		Blood	Embalming
	Fractured ethmoid		Arterial solution	Postembalming
	Fractured ear			
	Temporal bone			
	Surgical opening			
Anus	Anal orifice	Semisolid/liquid	Fecal matter	Preembalming
			Blood	Embalming
			Arterial solution	Postembalming
Embalming solution	Mouth/nose	Color of arterial solution injected	Arterial solution	Embalming
	Anus/ear			
Cavity fluid	Mouth/nose	Color of cavity fluid	Cavity fluid	Postembalming
	Anal orifice	Blood present is brown in color		

embalming decreases the possibility of a postembalming purge. A nasal tube aspirator can be used to remove purge from the throat and nasal passages. Some embalmers prefer to disinfect the oral cavity and nose and tightly pack the passage with cotton. Others prefer to let the purge continue during embalming and make a final setting of the features after embalming. When restricted cervical injection is used the body can purge during injection. After arterial injection the body can be aspirated, the features set, nasal and throat passages tightly packed, and the head separately embalmed.

Anal Purge. Preembalming anal purge material should be forced from the body by applying firm pressure to the lower abdomen and flushed away with running water. It is recommended that this purge be allowed to continue during embalming. Quite often, fecal matter is difficult to aspirate from the body. The anal orifice can be tightly packed with cotton saturated with cavity fluid *after* cavity treatment.

Brain Purge. Preembalming brain purge results from a fracture of the skull, a surgical procedure in the cranial cavity, or a trauma such as a bullet penetrating the bone of the skull. It is possible for gas (a type of purge) to build up in the cranium and travel along the nerve routes to distend such tissues as the eyelids. Numerous foramina in the eye orbit communicate with the cranial cavity. Brain purge from the nose is rare and is usually the result of a fracture of the cribriform plate in the floor of the anterior cranial cavity. The ear can also be the site of brain purge, usually as a result of a fracture of the temporal bone. It is best to let these purges continue during the embalming procedure.

Embalming Purge

During arterial injection, the injected solution can expand the viscera. Pressure on the stomach or diaphragm results in expulsion of the contents of the stomach and/or the respiratory tract. Also during arterial injection, arterial solution can be lost to the respiratory tract, stomach, or esophagus as a result of ruptured capillaries, small arteries, or veins. Ulcerated or cancerous tissues easily rupture because of the pressure of the solution being injected.

Tuberculosis of the lungs, cancer, pneumonia, and bacterial infections of the lung can cause fluid loss through weakened capillaries. A second cause of lung purge during embalming is congestion in the right atrium of the heart, which easily occurs if disease has involved the valves of the heart. Assume that drainage is being taken from the right femoral vein but has been very difficult to establish. Blood continues to push into the right atrium but cannot be drained away. The pressure builds to the point where the blood flows into the right ventri-

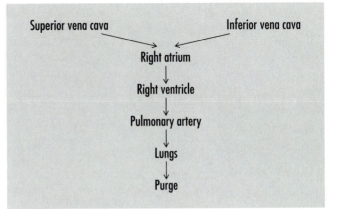

cle and into the pulmonary arteries, squeezing the lung tissues and forcing a purge. Rupture of small veins can also produce a bloody lung purge.

During embalming purge may simply be composed of the contents of the stomach, lung, or rectum or, as already explained, arterial solution. As a large amount of arterial solution is lost in the drainage and possibly as purge, be certain that a sufficient volume of arterial solution is injected to replace these losses. It is not always necessary to turn off the machine and begin a multipoint injection when purge contains arterial solution. When arterial solution is present in purge during arterial injection and *drainage is occurring,* inject a sufficient volume to satisfy the preservative demands of the body. When arterial solution is present in purge during arterial injection and *drainage has stopped,* a major fluid loss is occurring and distribution is not taking place. Evaluate the body and use sectional arterial injection where needed.

Rarely does anal purge contain arterial solution; however, long-term use of some drugs can cause gastrointestinal bleeding, rectal and colon cancers can erode tissues, and ulcerated colitis can destroy vessels. These conditions make possible a loss of arterial solution as well as blood drainage into the colon and rectum. If a sufficient amount of blood or arterial solution accumulates in the lower bowel, purge containing arterial solution can exit from the anal orifice.

It is usually during arterial injection that brain purge occurs. As already stated, for brain purge to occur, an opening must be present in the skull as a result of fracture, surgery, or trauma. Arterial solution escapes through small leaking arteries within the cranium, building up pressure that forces blood, arterial solution, and tissues of the brain through the openings.

Postembalming Purge

Purge that occurs prior to or during arterial injection can easily be controlled by the embalmer. It is the postembalming purge that should be of utmost concern to the embalmer. After cavity embalming, possibility of purge should be minimal. Many times, purge from the mouth, nose, or anal orifice after cavity embalming is simply cavity fluid that has been injected into these orifices. Tightly repack the nostrils with cotton, and replace moist cotton in the mouth with dry cotton.

Reaspirate prior to dressing whenever possible. If there appears to be a buildup of gas in the abdominal cavity, consider reinjection. Treat postembalming anal purge by forcing as much of the purge material from the body as possible. Then, pack the rectum with cotton saturated with a phenol solution, autopsy gel, or cavity fluid. Clothe the body in plastic pants or coveralls as added protection.

A purge that occurs from the mouth or nose after the body has been dressed and casketed may be temporarily stopped by removing the trocar button and passing a trocar through the viscera to relieve the pressure that has accumulated. The body should be reaspirated and reinjected.

Prevention of Postembalming Purge

1. Thoroughly aspirate the body cavities. Inject (in the adult body) at least 16 ounces (one bottle) of cavity fluid into the abdominal cavity, 16 ounces into the thoracic cavity, and, if possible, 16 ounces into the pelvic cavity.
2. Inject additional cavity fluid into obese bodies, bodies with ascites, bodies that have recently undergone abdominal surgery, and bodies which evidence decomposition.
3. If the abdominal trunk or buttock walls do not appear to have received sufficient fluid, hypodermically inject these areas with cavity fluids. Gases can form in unembalmed tissues and gradually move into the body cavities.
4. Reaspirate, especially those bodies that exhibit abdominal gas. This gas is easily detected when the trocar button is removed.
5. Reaspirate all bodies that have been shipped from another funeral home.
6. Pack the throat and nose with cotton. Nonabsorbent cotton should be used, because absorbent cotton may act as a "wick" to draw cavity fluid into the throat or upper nasal passages. Apply massage cream or autopsy gel to the nonabsorbent cotton before it is inserted into the nostrils or throat.
7. Remove moist cotton if purge has occurred during embalming. Be certain the mouth is completely dry.
8. When purge has been expelled from the skull as a result of fracture, decomposition, or surgical procedure (brain purge), the cranial cavity can be aspirated by passing an infant trocar or large hypodermic needle through the surgical opening, body fracture, or cribriform plate. To aspirate through the cribriform plate, insert the needle through the nostril. Direct the needle toward the anterior portion of the cranial cavity. The brain can be injected with a small amount of cavity fluid. This is best done with a large hypodermic needle and syringe.
9. A body that has had "tissue gas" in an extremity or cavity may need to be reaspirated and reinjected several times before dressing.
10. Inject a cavity fluid supplement (phenol solutions used for external bleaches) along with the cavity fluid into "problem" body cavities. (Labels of these products will indicate cavity injection.)
11. Tie off or sever the trachea and esophagus. This can be done through the incision used to raise the carotid artery.

GASES

Five types of gas may be found in the tissues of the dead human body: (1) subcutaneous emphysema, (2) air from the embalming apparatus, (3) gas gangrene, (4) tissue gas, and (5) decomposition gas (Table 24–2).

In the dead human body, gases move over time to the higher body areas. When the body is in the supine position with the head elevated, the gas will move into the unsupported tissues of the neck and face. The *source* of the gas can be in the *dependent* body areas. Gas can be detected in three ways in the body. It distends weak unsupported tissues such as the eyelids and the tissues surrounding the eye orbit, the temples, the neck, and the backs of the hands. In a firmly embalmed body, distension of veins is a possible sign that gas has formed. Pushing on the tissues where the gas is present may elicit a crackling sound that is both heard and felt. This is called **crepitation.** The area under the skin feels as if it is filled with cellophane.

Types of Gas Found in Tissues

Subcutaneous Emphysema. The most frequently encountered gas condition is caused by antemortem subcutaneous emphysema, brought about by a puncture or tear in the pleural sac or the lung tissue. As the individual gasps for air, more and more air is drawn into the tissues. Subcutaneous emphysema frequently follows compound fracture of a rib, tracheotomy, lung surgery, or projection of an object (such as bullet) into the pleural sac. A rib can be broken and the pleural sac or the lung itself torn if CPR is not administered with care, permitting a large amount of air to escape into the tissues.

TABLE 24–2. GASES THAT CAUSE DISTENSION

Type	Source	Characteristics	Treatment
Subcutaneous emphysema	Puncture of lung or pleural sac; seen after CPR; puncture wounds to thorax; rib fractures; tracheotomy	No odor; no skin-slip; no blebs; gas can reach distal points, even toes; can create intense swelling; rises to highest body areas	Gas escape through incisions; establishment of good arterial preservation; channeling of tissues after arterial injection to release gases.
"True" tissue gas	Anaerobic bacteria (gas gangrene) *Clostridium perfringens*	Very strong odor of decomposition; skin-slip; skin blebs; increase in intensity and amount of gas; possible transfer of spore-forming bacterium via cutting instruments to other bodies	Special "tissue gas" arterial solutions; localized hypodermic injection of cavity fluid; channeling of tissues to release gases
Gas gangrene	Anaerobic bacteria, *C. perfringens*	Foul odor, infection	Strong arterial solutions; local hypodermic injection of cavity chemical
Decomposition	Bacterial breakdown of body tissues; autolytic breakdown of body tissues	Possible odor; skin-slip in time; color changes; purging	Arterial injection of sufficient amount of the appropriate strong chemical; hypodermic and surface treatments; channeling to release gases
Air from embalming apparatus	Air injected by embalming machine (air pressure machines and hand pumps are in limited use today)	First evidence in eyelids; no odors; no skin-slip; amount depends on injection time	If distension is present, channeling after arterial injection to release gases

This condition is *not* caused by a microbe and does not continue to intensify after death. The gas, however, moves from dependent areas to the upper body areas such as the neck and face. No odor accompanies this condition; skin-slip or blebs do not form on the skin surface. In the male, the scrotum can distend to several times its normal size. It is best to remove the gas from the tissues *after* the body is embalmed.

COMMON CONDITIONS CAUSING ANTEMORTEM SUBCUTANEOUS EMPHYSEMA

- Rib fractures that puncture a lung
- Puncture wounds of the thorax
- Thoracic surgical procedures
- CPR compression causing a fractured rib or sternum to puncture a lung or pleural sac
- Tracheotomy surgery

Air from the Embalming Apparatus. The injection of air from the embalming machine is NOT a frequent problem today. Most machines automatically shut off when the tank has been emptied. This condition is most likely to occur when an air pressure machine or hand pump is used for injection. Air is forced into the closed container that contains the embalming solution. The pressure from the air forces the fluid into the body. The problem is of most concern if the face is being injected. The eyelids are one of the first areas to distend, even if a very small amount of air is accidentally injected.

Gas Gangrene. Gas gangrene is a fatal disease caused by contamination of a wound infection by a toxin-producing, spore-forming, anaerobic bacterium. This bacterium can be found in soil and the intestinal tract of humans and animals. *Clostridium perfringens* is the most common of the *Clostridium* bacteria responsible for this condition. The organisms grow in the tissue of the wound, especially muscle, releasing exotoxins and fermenting muscle sugars with such vigor that the pressure build up by the accumulated gas tears the tissues apart.

The gas causes swelling and death of tissues locally. The exotoxins break down red blood cells in the bloodstream and, thereby, damage various organs throughout the body. The bacteria enter the blood just before death (the incubation period is 1–5 days). Because of the destructive action of the exotoxins and enzymes produced, tissue involvement and spread are very rapid. Gas gangrene usually occurs after severe trauma, especially farm or automobile accidents and close-range shotgun discharges, where the wound may be contaminated with filth, manure, or surface soil. Gas gangrene is particularly likely after compound fractures; the bone splinters provide foreign bodies that enhance the infection as well as permit entrance of embedded debris or dirt.

The gangrenous process begins at the margins of the wound. The skin, dark red at first, turns green and then black, and there is considerable swelling that extends rapidly over the body. The tissues are filled with gas, sometimes to the point of bursting. The affected tissue decomposes, blisters and skin-slip form on the surface, and there is no line of demarcation. A very foul odor permeates the surroundings.

Gas causes the tissue to crackle when touched. The danger involved, as an embalming complication, lies in the fact that if death occurs shortly after injury, the gas gangrene may not be visible; it may be totally internal. If embalming treatment is not sufficient to control the spread of the organisms or their by-products, the symptoms of gas gangrene may show up several hours after embalming. In addition, if the postmortem examination is delayed, internal spread will be extensive and could create disastrous postembalming complications.

Tissue Gas. Tissue gas is caused primarily by *Clostridium perfringens*. It may begin prior to death as gas gangrene. After death, the condition may result from contamination of tissues by the gas bacillus, which has translocated from the intestinal tract. Contaminated hypodermic needles have also been known to transfer *C. perfringens* to tissues of the extremities. Contaminated autopsy instruments have spread this condition from one body to another. This condition may also be spread when embalming instruments (cutting instruments, i.e., scalpels, scissors, trocar, suture needles) are not thoroughly disinfected. These organisms are very resistant to most disinfectants. Thus, the condition can occur after the body has been embalmed if all the tissues of the body and the visceral organs have not been adequately sanitized and preserved (Fig. 24–1).

The gas is ordinarily formed more rapidly and with greater intensity in dependent tissues and organs. These areas are frequently congested with blood and later poorly saturated with arterial solution and, therefore, provide an ideal medium for bacterial growth. Being lighter than the liquids it displaces, the gas rises to the highest receptive parts of the body. In addition, the gas is larger in volume than the liquid it displaces and, thus, tears and distends the tissues.

Distension is usually greatest in soft tissue areas such as the eyelids, neck, and scrotum of the male. The gas spreads rather rapidly through the tissue, causing blebs to form on the surface. As the condition progresses, the blebs grow and burst, releasing the gas and putrefactive fluids and causing skin-slip.

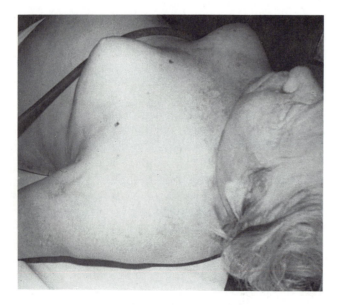

Figure 24–1. Body distended within 2 hours of death by tissue gas.

CONDITIONS PREDISPOSING TO TISSUE GAS

- Recent abdominal surgery
- Presence of gangrene at the time of death
- Intestinal ulcerations or perforations
- Contaminated skin wounds or punctures
- Intestinal obstruction or hemorrhage
- Unsatisfactory embalming
- Contact with contaminated instruments

Decomposition. In the dead human body two factors are responsible for decomposition: bacterial enzymes and autolytic enzymes. Gases are formed that accumulate in the visceral organs, body cavities, and the skeletal tissues. These gases are responsible for the odor of decomposition. As the gases accumulate in the body cavities, sufficient pressure is produced to cause purge. The gases produced by decomposition are not often as intense as tissue gas or gas gangrene. Likewise, decomposition cannot be spread from body to body by contaminated instruments. The generation of gas ceases when the tissues are properly embalmed. Gases can be removed by cavity aspiration and postembalming channeling of the tissues.

Embalming Protocol

Subcutaneous Emphysema. Because subcutaneous emphysema does not involve microbes, treatment involves merely removal of the gas from the tissues. There are no foul odors, blebbing, or skin-slip with this condition. During arterial injection, some of the gas in the tissues may relocate, most likely into the neck and facial tissues.

Restricted cervical injection should be used for the arterial injection. Fluid strength should be based on the postmortem and pathological conditions. A slightly stronger solution should be used to embalm the head, because if gas should relocate into the head after embalming (if the tissues are firm), sufficient resistance will be exerted to prevent distension. In restricted cervical injection, two incisions are made at the base of the neck. These incisions provide an exit for the gas in the tissues. The incisions can also be used as points from which to channel the neck so air can be pushed from the facial tissues.

Decomposition Gas, Gas Gangrene and "True" Tissue Gas. Decomposition gas, gas gangrene, and true tissue gas all have a bacterial origin. It is very important to saturate the tissues of the body with a very strong arterial solution. Restricted cervical injection should be used so large quantities of sufficient-strength arterial solution can be injected into the trunk. Chemicals specifically made for the treatment of decomposing bodies and tissue gas should be used, for example, special-purpose arterial fluids, coinjection chemicals, and cavity fluids that can be injected arterially.

If the gas appears to have originated in an extremity, sectional arterial embalming should be done. If the condition is well advanced, 100% chemical should be injected into the localized area. A coinjection chemical can be added for each ounce of arterial chemical. High pressure may be needed to inject the solution into the affected area. Often tissue gas is not noticeable at the time of death. As the organism responsible is anaerobic, after death the human body becomes an ideal medium.

Gases can form very rapidly after death. These postmortem changes can be devastating enough that a viewing of the body by family and the public would be impossible. It is imperative that the preparation be started as soon after death as possible. If the gas source is an extremity or an area such as the buttocks, a *barrier* can be made by hypodermic injection of undiluted cavity fluid in addition to sectional embalming.

Clinical Application

The source of the tissue gas appears to be a gangrenous condition of the left foot. The lower portion of the leg has turned a deep purple black. The leg is swollen and gas can be felt beneath the tissues. Injection is begun using a high-index special-purpose arterial fluid and employing restricted cervical injection as the primary injection point. Drainage is taken from the right internal jugular vein. The left femoral artery is then raised and the left leg arterially injected. Pulsation and high pressure are used to distribute the solution. A trocar is introduced from the medial side of the middle of the thigh. Cavity fluid is injected through the embalming machine throughout the area above the knee. In addition, the trocar is thrust into the deep tissues of the lower leg. Undiluted cavity fluid is injected. A barrier has now been formed with cavity fluid in an attempt to contain the *C. perfringens* and prevent it from migrating to other body areas.

In treatment of a body with true tissue gas, six-point injection can be employed with a strong arterial solution to ensure good preservation. The incisions for the arterial injection can remain open several hours, providing an exit for the gas.

Cavity treatment should be very thorough. Gas rises to the anterior portions of the viscera and cavity. Carefully aspirate the cavity, including the walls, to provide exits for the gas if it can be felt in the trunk walls. Inject a minimum of 16 ounces (or more) into each cavity. The trocar puncture can remain open to allow the escape of gases, later to be closed after reaspiration and reinjection.

Such bodies can be reaspirated and reinjected several times to ensure that bacterial activity has ceased. The treatment so far suggested are radical, but tissue gas is a very serious problem.

Tissue gas can form in bodies that have not been thoroughly embalmed. *C. perfringens* is a normal inhabitant of the gastrointestinal tract, which after death rapidly moves to other body areas.

Removal of Gas from Tissues

Regardless of the source of the gas, the method of removing it is the same. There is only one effective way to remove gas from distended tissues and that is to lance and channel the tissues and release the gas. Arterial injection and subsequent blood drainage may remove gases in the circulatory system, but do little to remove gas trapped in the subcutaneous tissue. The incision made to raise any vessels is an escape route for gas from the body.

Remember that in bodies with true tissue gas, release of the gas from the tissues does not stop its generation. The microbe causing the gas must be killed. Although gas accumulates in the superficial body tissues, the source of the gas may be located in a distal extremity or in dependent tissues.

Trunk Tissues. Gases in trunk tissues can be removed by trocar after arterial injection. During aspiration of the cavity, the trocar is channeled through the thoracic and abdominal walls. If the scrotum is affected, it too can be channeled by passing the trocar over the pubic bone.

Neck and Face. After arterial embalming, the trocar can be used to channel the neck to remove gas. Insert the trocar into the abdominal wall, after making certain the trocar can reach the neck tissues. Pass the trocar beneath the rib cage and under the clavicle to reach the neck. The trocar can also be inserted into the neck by passing under the clavicle. Make a large half-moon incision at the base of the neck lateral from the center of the right clavicle to a point lateral from the center of the left clavicle. Reflect this flap and, with an infant trocar or scalpel, channel the neck tissue. Squeeze the neck tissues. Force the gas toward the openings. The half-moon incision can also be used for restricted cervical injection. If restricted cervical injection is used, this incision prevents more gases from entering the neck and facial tissues. If possible, leave these incisions open several hours or until the body is to be dressed and casketed.

Eyelids and Orbital Areas. After embalming, the eyelids can be opened and slightly everted. Using a large suture needle, make punctures along the undersurface of the lids. Deep channels can also be made from this location to the surrounding orbital areas. By digital pressure move the gases from the most distal areas toward the punctures. A bistoury knife or large hypodermic needle can also be inserted from within the hairline of the temple area to remove gases in the orbital area and the temple. Cotton should be used for eye closure. It absorbs the small amount of liquid that may seep from the punctures. It may be best not to seal these punctures, for they are an escape route for any further gas that may accumulate in the orbital area. The closed eye can be glued after the gas is removed. In the autopsied body the orbital area can generally be channeled by carefully reflecting the scalp. A bistoury blade can be used to dissect into the orbital areas. All this can be done from beneath the skin surface through the tissues exposed by the cranial autopsy.

Facial Tissues. Gases present in the cheeks and facial tissues can easily be removed after arterial injection and cavity embalming (Fig. 24–2). Aspiration of the thoracic cavity and channeling of the neck tissues may help to remove some of the gas in the facial tissues. Open the mouth and insert a bistoury knife into the tissues of the face; run it deep to the facial bones to make channels for the gas to escape. This channeling provides escape routes for the gas. Digital pressure is needed to force the gas from the tissues to the exits. Begin at the distal points of the face and work the gas to the points where the bistoury knife or large hypodermic needle has been inserted. Any liquid leakage will drain into the mouth and throat areas. The lips can be glued. This is a radical treatment, but is the only way to provide an escape route for the gas. In the autopsied body, reflect the scalp with a bistoury knife or large hypodermic needle, and make channels into the facial tissues from the temple areas (Fig. 24–3). This may be sufficient to release the accumulated facial gases.

Instrument Disinfection

Tissue gas and gas gangrene involve a spore-forming bacillus, *C. perfringens,* which can easily be passed from one body to another via contaminated instruments. Great care should be taken in the disinfection of cutting instruments and suture needles. Wash instruments in cool

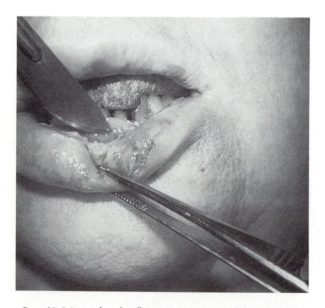

Figure 24–2. Lips are lanced to allow gas to escape (a postembalming treatment).

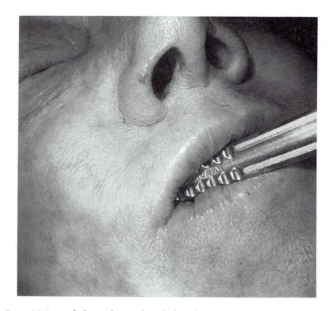

Figure 24–3. A scalpel is used to cut channels through which gas in the tissues can escape (postembalming treatment).

running water using a good disinfectant soap. Then, soak them in a very strong disinfectant solution for several hours. Be certain that the disinfectants used in the preparation room are active (most disinfectants have a specific shelf life). Place disposable scalpel blades in a sharps container. Care should be given to disinfection of the trocar and suture needles. Consult Chapter 3 for specific disinfectant recommendations.

BODIES WITH FACIAL TRAUMA

In the preparation of bodies with facial trauma, the embalmer's goal is maximum tissue preservation with a minimum amount of swelling. If good preservation can be established, the restorative and cosmetic procedures will be easier to perform and will provide satisfactory results.

Traumatic injuries vary greatly; however, facial trauma can be classified into two categories: injuries in which the skin is broken and injuries in which the skin is not broken.

Unbroken Skin	**Broken Skin**
Depressed fractures	Abrasion
Swollen tissues (hematoma)	Laceration
Ecchymosis	Incision
Simple fracture	Compound fracture

Traumatic injuries also vary with respect to their location on the head. A laceration of the cheek may be simple to restore; however, a lacerated upper eyelid may involve swelling and discoloration, as well as torn skin, resulting in a much more serious problem.

It is not within the scope of this text to detail the restorative treatments for each type of facial trauma and describe how treatment varies with location. It is the intent of this text to give a general outline of embalming protocol for traumatic facial injuries. Most of these injuries involve delay, for there usually is an inquiry by the coroner or medical examiner. Quite frequently, when an autopsy is performed, refrigeration may precede or follow the postmortem examination.

This discussion is concerned only with preparation of the head. If the body has been autopsied, the head is separately embalmed by injecting first the left common carotid artery and then the right common carotid. In the unautopsied body, restricted cervical injection can be used (right and left common carotid arteries are raised at the beginning of the embalming). Insert two arterial tubes into the right common carotid, one directed toward the trunk of the body and the other directed toward the right side of the head. Open the left common carotid artery, tie off the lower portion of the artery, and insert one tube into the artery directed toward the left side of the head. Leave both arterial tubes directed toward the head *open*. Inject the trunk first, then the left side of the head, and, finally, the right side. Drainage can be taken from the right internal jugular vein. Some embalmers prefer to drain from both the right and the left internal jugular veins when they inject the head.

General Considerations

Begin the preparation of these bodies by spraying the body with an effective topical disinfectant. Next, run cool water over the facial areas and hair to remove debris and blood. If glass was involved in the trauma, watch for small shards of glass that can easily rip gloves and cut the embalmer's fingers. Some glass can be flushed from the wounds with water, and forceps may be needed to pick glass pieces from broken tissues.

Align fractures. Incisions may have to be made prior to embalming to prop or align simple and depressed fractures. Next, align lacerated or incised skin areas. This is accomplished with a drop or two of super adhesive, or single (bridge) sutures of dental floss can be sewn with a small curved needle. Remove loose skin that cannot be embalmed by arterial means (this includes loose scabs). Apply surface preservative and bleaching compresses at this point or, if preferred, wait until the arterial injection is completed. Compresses of cavity fluid or phenol help to bleach, preserve, and dry the tissues. Phenol solutions work much faster than formaldehyde. Good tissue may be protected with a very small amount of massage cream.

Instant Tissue Fixation

Prepare a strong arterial solution. These solutions can vary depending on the arterial fluid chosen. Two examples are given here:

Solution 1 1 bottle (16 ounces) of 25- to 35-index arterial fluid
1 bottle (16 ounces) of coinjection chemical
Several drops of arterial fluid dye

Solution 2 1 bottle (16 ounces) of 25- to 35-index arterial fluid
$\frac{1}{4}$ gallon water
Several drops of arterial fluid dye

These solutions are very strong because the index of the fluid is high and there is little dilution.

Set the pressure gauge on the centrifugal injection machine at 20 psi (or higher) with the rate-of-flow valve closed.

After running some of the arterial solution through the machine to evacuate all air from the delivery hose, attach the delivery hose to the left common carotid artery. Now, open the rate-of-flow valve and allow the fluid to surge into the left side of the face. As soon as the fluid starts to flow, shut the valve off. Pause a few moments and repeat the process. The dye rises to the skin surface immediately so the embalmer is able to see what tissues are receiving fluid. In the autopsied body, the internal carotid artery may have to be clamped.

This method allows the embalmer maximum distribution, using a minimum amount of arterial solution. Keep in mind the strength of this solution. The dye helps to prevent postmortem graying of the tissues and also serves as a tracer for the fluid. Drainage is minimal and is not a concern. This method can also be used to inject the legs and arms when problems exist in the extremities.

In the unautopsied body, the trunk would generally be embalmed first and the facial area last. A suitable solution for preservation of the trunk and limbs can be used for injection. In the autopsied body the legs and arms are embalmed first, and the instant tissue fixation method is used to embalm the head.

BODIES THAT REQUIRE REEMBALMING

There are occasions when it may be necessary to reembalm a body:

- Fluid was not distributed to all areas.
- Too little solution was injected.
- The concentration of the fluid was too low to meet the preservative demands of the body.
- The injected solution was neutralized by the body chemistry (often seen in bodies dead from renal failure or edema).
- Rigor mortis was mistaken for embalming fluid tissue fixation.

Instant tissue fixation and waterless embalming techniques are good methods to use when a body must be reembalmed. Use multisite injection (if necessary) to inject the legs, arms, and head at high pressure but a pulsed rate of flow, as described for bodies with facial trauma.

In the unautopsied body cavity embalming will have been completed, so begin by aspiration before arterial injection. In this manner the drainage can be taken from the heart. It is not necessary to drain from each site of injection. As only a minimum amount of fluid is used in the instant tissue fixation process, drainage should not be a big concern. After injection, thoroughly aspirate and then inject a minimum of two or three bottles of concentrated cavity fluid into the cavities. It is always suggested that these bodies be reaspirated prior to dressing.

RENAL FAILURE

A more common complication associated with embalming today is due to kidney failure. Improvements in medicine and long-term drug therapy have increased the life span of persons with terminal diseases. The embalmer must check the death certificate carefully for references to renal failure or dysfunction. If the death certificate is not available, the embalmer should look for the signs of renal failure when making the preembalming analysis. Also, during and after embalming, if tissues fail to respond (by firming), the embalmer may suspect renal failure.

It has been estimated that six times more preservative chemical is needed to preserve tissues of bodies dead from the complications of renal failure. The embalmer can use some of the following signs to determine whether renal failure has affected a body:

- Sallow color to the skin as a result of urochrome buildup
- Uremic puritis (scratch marks on the extremities)
- Increase in the amount of urea, uric acid, ammonia, and creatine (urea and ammonia can be detected by their odor)
- Acidosis
- Edema (retention of sodium by the kidneys leads to increased retention of water)
- Anemia
- Gastrointestinal bleeding (blood in the gastrointestinal tract and purging)

As can be seen, a variety of signs indicate renal failure. The embalmer should realize that renal failure may be only a contributory cause of death, as it often accompanies other life-threatening diseases. Thus, the cancer or heart patient will display the bodily changes associated with these diseases, as well as the signs associated with kidney failure.

The importance of this disease to the embalmer lies in the fact that these bodies rapidly decompose. The acidity of the tissues leads to rupture of lysosomes, which contain the autolytic hydroenzymes that begin the de-

composition cycle. Edema present provides the moisture needed for the hydrolytic enzymes to act, blood in the intestinal tract provides an excellent medium for the growth of putrefactive microorganisms, and the abundant ammonia in the tissues readily neutralizes formaldehyde.

Embalming Protocol

Preparation of the body affected by renal failure calls for the use of strong arterial solutions. Preinjection fluid should be avoided, because if circulation is impaired, tissues can easily swell. Begin with at least a 2.0% formaldehyde-based arterial solution. The use of a 30- to 35-index fluid is advised. Many fluid manufacturers make high-index arterial fluid specifically for bodies dead from uremia. Follow the dilution instructions of the manufacturer. After surface blood discolorations have cleared and circulation is established, arterial solution in subsequent injections can be increased in strength. Use dye to indicate the distribution of arterial solution. If edema is extensive, inject a sufficient amount of fluid to dry some of the edema.

Some embalmers prefer to use an "average-strength arterial solution" made from a 20- to 30-index fluid. After surface blood discolorations are cleared and circulation is established, they add several ounces of a high-index formaldehyde-based arterial fluid to the arterial solution. This increases the strength of the solution being injected.

Two theories are held with respect to arterial solutions: (1) solution of one strength is used throughout the embalming procedure; (2) average solution is used at the beginning, and then strength is increased gradually until the desired tissue firmness is obtained.

When both edema and renal failure are present (in addition to side effects of drug therapy, effects of the immediate cause of death, and postmortem changes that have occurred if embalming was delayed), it is easy to understand why these bodies are so difficult to prepare and why fixation of the protein can be so difficult. It is most important to saturate these tissues with a strong preservative arterial solution. If this is not done the body will soften in a few hours, blebs can form, desquamation can develop, and the body can discolor and show signs of decomposition within a day or so.

To inject these strong solutions without overembalming the facial tissues, restricted cervical injection is advised. A large volume of very strong arterial solution can be injected into the trunk, and later a milder solution can be used to embalm the facial tissues.

The cavities should be thoroughly aspirated. Inject a minimum of one bottle of concentrated cavity fluid into each cavity. During arterial injection purge is possible from gastrointestinal ulcerations, so a large amount of blood and arterial solution may be present in the contents aspirated from the abdominal cavity. These bodies should be aspirated immediately after arterial injection.

It is also advised that these bodies be reaspirated and reinjected.

Some of the dependent areas press against the embalming table. These pressure point areas often do not receive sufficient arterial solution. These dependent areas are high in moisture, and so hydrolytic changes occur and the putrefactive bacteria flourish. Coveralls and possibly a unionall may be needed to prevent leakage if pitting edema is present. Preservative–deodorant powder should always be sprinkled inside the plastic goods.

ALCOHOLISM

The preparation of the body that has suffered from chronic alcoholism can present a number of problems for the embalmer.

Many of these bodies exhibit jaundice as a result of liver failure. The primary goal is good preservation. Liver failure can also cause edema in the skeletal tissues or the cavities (ascites, hydrothorax). In addition, hepatic failure depletes the blood of clotting factors; therefore, good drainage can be expected if the body is prepared a reasonable time after death. Both the common carotid artery and the femoral artery are good primary injection sites; however, if skeletal edema is extensive and a large volume of strong arterial solution must be injected, restricted cervical injection is recommended. Injection should proceed at a moderate rate of flow so the tissues can assimilate the arterial solution without swelling. A moderate rate of flow also helps to prevent purging and rupture of weakened esophageal veins.

Purge is often seen in these bodies. Bloody purge may exit the mouth or nose during arterial injection. Later, it turns into a fluid purge. A good sign that fluid is being distributed to the tissues is blood drainage. Inject a large volume of arterial solution to compensate for the fluid lost through purge. Arterial fluid dye is used to trace fluid distribution and to counterstain jaundice.

Because of the effect of long-term alcohol abuse on tissues, firming may be difficult to establish. These bodies should be injected with a moderate to strong preservative arterial solution. Do not use weak solutions even when the tissues may be emaciated or jaundiced. Add sufficient arterial fluid to firm the tissues.

Ecchymoses on the back of the hands can be treated by hypodermic injection of cavity fluid or phenol cautery solution after arterial injection. Before, during, and after arterial injection, compresses of cavity fluid, autopsy gel, or phenol solution may be applied to the skin surfaces to bleach and firm the ecchymotic areas.

Most of these bodies require tissue building after arterial injection. Tissues may be built up by injection of a restorative humectant in the last gallon of arterial solution.

At the beginning of the embalming, if ascites is present and the abdomen very distended, puncture and drain the abdomen of this serous fluid prior to or during arterial injection. By keeping the point of the trocar just beneath the surface of the anterior abdominal wall, no large vessels will be punctured. Cavity embalming should be thorough, and, of course, reaspiration is recommended.

OBESITY

Preparation of the obese body has been discussed elsewhere in this book. Some of the items discussed are reviewed here. The first concern is positioning. Just moving the heavy body on the preparation table can be difficult. Movement of a body is easier if it rests on a sheet or is clothed. Naked bodies are easier to move on a wet table.

Try to use a standard-size casket. Position the elbows close to the body. As the neck is usually quite short, keep the head straight and tie the feet together. Later, when the body is placed in the casket, tilt the shoulders and head slightly to the right.

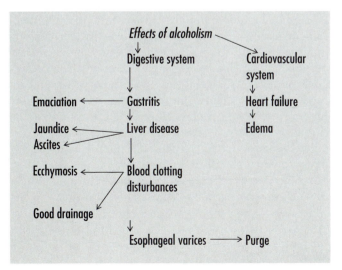

Atherosclerosis	→ Use of restricted cervical injection recommended
Varicose veins	→ Difficult drainage: Use right internal jugular vein
Diabetes	→ Poor peripheral circulation: Use dye for tracer
Weight	→ Drainage problems, increased preservative demand: avoid femoral arteries

The preceding scheme illustrates some of the complications associated with obesity.

Restricted cervical injection affords the use of the largest arteries, which should be free of arteriosclerosis. These vessels are not as deep as the femoral arteries. The right internal jugular vein can be used for drainage. It is the largest vein the embalmer can use in the unautopsied body.

Because of the short neck, drainage forceps are easier to use than a drain tube. The forceps can be inserted directly into the right atrium of the heart through the right internal jugular vein. If varicose veins are present, large clots may be observed in the drainage. The internal jugular vein allows passage of these clots out of the body.

If the obese person was also a diabetic, begin the embalming with the arms lowered over the sides of the table. Leave them in this position until the arterial solution reaches the tissues of the hands. Massaging the hands and radial and ulnar arteries promotes the flow of fluid into these peripheral areas.

This body will demand large volumes of solution. The solution can be an average dilution unless edema or other complications are present that call for stronger arterial solution mixtures. If restricted cervical injection is used, large volumes of solution can easily be injected without overembalming the facial tissues. Some embalmers prefer to increase the strength of the solution toward the conclusion of the embalming, before the head and face are injected. This increased solution strength helps to dry and firm tissues. A well-firmed body is much easier to dress and lift. Sufficient pressure should be used to overcome the resistance, particularly the resistance exerted against the large vessels by the weight of the viscera. Massage, manipulation, and intermittent drainage assist in fluid distribution.

If the legs do not receive sufficient arterial solution, try raising the external iliac artery at the level of the inguinal ligament. The vessels here are more superficial than the femoral artery. It is often observed that the arteries in obese bodies are quite small in size.

Purge is always a problem with obese bodies. Weight of the viscera pushing against the stomach can easily create sufficient pressure to cause a stomach purge. These bodies also retain heat for extended periods after death and gases easily form in the gastrointestinal tract. Again, restricted cervical injection allows the trunk to be embalmed first; then the cavities can be aspirated, the features set, and the head embalmed. Purge is thus easily dealt with. This order of embalming also eliminates the need to set features twice if the mouth becomes filled with purge material.

The shoulders of an obese body should be raised high off the table. The body should occupy three levels: the head is highest, then the chest, and, finally, the abdomen.

Keeping the head high facilitates raising of the vessels and helps to prevent purge. Keep the elbows as close to the body wall as possible. It may be necessary to tie the arms into position with cloth straps after embalming to keep the elbows high and as close as possible to the body.

When turning the body from side to side, place a sheet under it. It is much easier to move the body with this sheet. Some embalmers place undergarments on the large body, casket the body, and then dress the body in the casket. Others prefer to dress and then casket.

MYCOTIC INFECTIONS*

Mycotic infections are fungal infections that may have been present as an antemortem condition or occurred as the result of a postmortem invasion. Fungi may be saprophytic or parasitic; that is, they obtain their nourishment from dead organic material or from a living organism. Fungal infections are not rare in humans and frequently are serious. Often, skin and mucous membrane are affected by the fungal infection, as in athlete's foot and thrush. The more destructive parasitic fungi produce widespread chronic lesions.

In some fungal infections, the inflammatory response and tissue damage are the result of hypersensitivity to the fungal antigens. Fungi that are ordinarily saprophytic, such as *Aspergillus*, *Mucor*, and *Candida*, proliferate in patients receiving prolonged antibiotic, immunosuppressive, or steroid therapy and in those with predisposing diseases such as diabetes mellitus, leukemia, and AIDS. Although there are many types of fungal infections, discussion is limited to those specific to embalming.

Candidiasis (Moniliasis)

Candida species are commonly found in the mouth, intestinal tract, and vagina of healthy individuals. *Candida albicans* is the most common cause of candidiasis. A common form of the disease known as thrush affects the oral mucosa (tongue, gums, lips, and cheeks) and the pharynx and is seen most often in debilitated infants (especially premature) and children. The lesions, white patches on the mucosa, comprise an overgrowth of yeast cells and hyphae and a nonspecific acute or subacute inflammation of the underlying tissue. Similar lesions occur on the vulvovaginal mucosa, particularly in diabetic and pregnant women and women on birth control pills. The skin, especially moist skin (e.g., perineum, inframammary folds, and between the fingers), may be affected.

---

*This section on mycotic infections is taken from *Pathology of Human Disease* and *Synopsis of Pathology,* 10th ed. See the Bibliography at the end of the chapter.

Candida may produce lesions of the nails (onychia) and around the nails (paronychia), particularly in people whose hands are always in water (e.g., cooks). Occasionally, esophageal bronchopulmonary, and widely disseminated forms of candidiasis are observed. Invasiveness is promoted by the lowered resistance of the host, as may occur in various debilitating illnesses and with intensive antibiotic, immunosuppressive, or steroid therapy. Candidal endocarditis has been reported in drug addicts, as a result of the intravenous injection of narcotics, and in patients who have undergone cardiac surgery.

Oral candidiasis can occur at any age during the course of a debilitating disease. It can also occur under dentures and orthodontic appliances and can complicate other erosive mucosal diseases (e.g., pemphigus vulgaris). The moist folds at the corners of the mouth provide a friendly environment for a troublesome candidal infection.

Oropharyngeal candidiasis is a specific complication of AIDS, because individuals with AIDS are immunosuppressed. Mouth lesions can spread down the trachea and esophagus and produce extensive gastrointestinal infections.

Aspergillosis

Most species of the genus *Aspergillus* are saprophytic and nonpathogenic. Some are found as harmless invaders of the external auditory canal, nasal sinuses, and external genitalia and as secondary invaders in lung abscesses.

In involvement of the ear, the external auditory canal may be partially filled with foul moist material spotted with black granules. The lung appears to be the most common site of serious infection. Pulmonary lesions manifest as bronchopneumonia, abscesses, small infarcts (resulting from thrombosis caused by vascular invasion), or masses of *Aspergillus* mycelia ("fungus balls") in a newly formed cavity or a preexisting inflammatory (e.g., tuberculosis) or carcinomatous cavity. Chronic granulomatous reactions to the organisms in the lungs are also possible.

A primary fatal disseminated infection is relatively uncommon. Generalized aspergillosis is more frequent as a secondary complication and tends to occur in patients with debilitating diseases and in those who have received steroid, antibiotic, or immunosuppressive therapy. Aspergillosis occurs in various tissues and organs and is characterized by abscesses, necrotic and necrotizing lesions, and sometimes chronic granulomatous inflammation.

Phycomycosis

Phycomycosis is an infection of the lungs, ears, nervous system, and intestinal tract caused by a fungus commonly encountered as a saprophyte or contaminant. The lesions may display an intense necrotizing and suppurative inflammation process. Although this infection is commonly called mucormycosis, it may be caused by several members of the group Phycomycetes, including *Mucor, Rhizopus,* and *Absidia*. These fungi invade vessels and cause thrombosis and infarction. Phycomycosis is especially seen in patients with uncontrolled diabetes mellitus, leukemia, AIDS, and other debilitating diseases and in those receiving antibiotics, corticosteroids, chemotherapeutic agents, and irradiation. The resulting lesions are similar to those mentioned earlier.

Histoplasmosis (Reticuloendothelial Cytomycosis)

Histoplasmosis is caused by the oval, yeastlike organism *Histoplasma capsulatum*. Histoplasmosis occurs worldwide, although infection is particularly common in the Mississippi Valley of the United States. Positive diagnosis depends on identification of the organisms in cultures of sputum, blood, or bone marrow or in biopsied tissue from the lymph nodes. This infection may spread throughout the body.

Histoplasmosis is not generally spread between individuals. It appears to be contracted from soil contaminated with fecal material of chickens, pigeons, starlings, other birds, and bats. In South Africa, most of the recognized benign pulmonary infections seem to have been acquired from contaminated caves (cave disease). Histoplasmosis is endemic in many parts of the world, particularly near large rivers and in high-humidity warm-temperature regions. The lungs are believed to be the usual portal of entry of the organisms. Histoplasmosis can be classified into four forms: acute pulmonary, chronic pulmonary, acute disseminated, and chronic disseminated.

The acute pulmonary form may be asymptomatic or symptomatic. The basic reaction in the lungs and lymph nodes consists of foci of tuberculoid granulomas that tend to heal. Most cases of histoplasmosis are benign, asymptomatic pulmonary infections, with positive histoplasmin skin tests and healed calcified nodules in the lung and peribronchial lymph nodes, often resembling the healed primary complex of tuberculosis. The symptomatic pulmonary infections may be either mild and "flulike" or more severe, resembling atypical pneumonia. Usually the prognosis is good. Multiple pulmonary infiltrations, with or without hilar lymphadenopathy (involvement with the entrance to the glands), may be indicated in x-rays of the chest and, in the more prolonged cases, tend to calcify and simulate healed miliary tuberculosis. In some cases, a localized pulmonary tuberculoid granulomatous lesion with caseation necrosis, calcification, and fibrotic border (histoplasmoma) may occur, appearing in an x-ray of the chest as a "coin" lesion. This lesion is sometimes removed surgically because of the clinical suspicion of lung cancer.

The *chronic pulmonary* form is progressive, forming granulomatous inflammation with caseation necrosis and cavitation, and frequently is misdiagnosed as pulmonary tuberculosis, or it may occur as a secondary complication of tuberculosis. It is seen most commonly in otherwise healthy males over the age of 40. The prognosis is poor. Occasionally, either the acute primary complex of the chronic pulmonary type is disseminated, spreading through the blood to involve many organs. Involvement of the lymph system, liver, spleen, and bone marrow dominates the clinical picture. The organs involved are packed with macrophages stuffed with organisms, so the histologic picture resembles that of visceral leishmaniasis. Jaundice, fever, leukopenia, and anemia lead to a condition that mimics acute miliary tuberculosis.

The *acute disseminated* form may be either benign or progressive. The acute progressive form is rapidly fatal, and is usually encountered in young children or immunosuppressed (AIDS) adults. The spleen, lymph nodes, and liver are enlarged. There is a septic-type fever with anemia and leukopenia. Bone marrow smears may reveal the organisms or granulomas. Occasionally, the organisms may be found in mononuclear cells in blood smears.

The *chronic disseminated* form may occur in the elderly and otherwise healthy individuals and may be fatal. In the more protracted form, which occurs in otherwise healthy individuals, the clinical features vary according to the organ most severely involved. For instance, involvement of the heart valves leads to endocarditis, and involvement of the adrenal glands leads to Addison's disease. Other organs that can be affected are the gastrointestinal tract, spleen, liver, lymph nodes, lungs, bone marrow, and meninges. In some cases, infection and ulceration of the colon, tongue, larynx, pharynx, mouth, nose, and lips are initial manifestations.

Other Mycotic Infections

Several other mycotic infections may be encountered but are rare. These include dermatomycosis, cryptococcosis, North American blastomycosis, and protothecosis. More than 100,000 species of fungi are known, of which approximately 100 are human pathogens. For the most part, they occur as secondary complications of other diseases.

Significance of Mycotic Infections to Embalming

Mycotic infections are frequently encountered, especially in those with debilitating or immunosuppressive diseases and diabetes mellitus. The widespread use of immuno-suppressive drugs, combined with modern medical advances that keep patients alive but debilitated, has led to a considerable increase in the incidence of fungal infections. In the modern hospital, they are one of the most important and lethal examples of opportunistic infection.

The greatest danger presented is to the embalmer and to others who work directly with the dead human bodies. Many fungal infections produce superficial lesions on the skin and mucous membranes. As many of the fungi involved are saprophytic, they continue to multiply until they are effectively arrested. Other fungal infections involve the oral/nasal cavity, larynx, pharynx, esophagus, and lungs. These may also be saprophytic and continue to multiply in untreated or poorly embalmed dead human bodies.

In all fungal infections or unidentified lesions, careful handling of the remains is essential. When moving the remains, do not compress the abdominal or thoracic cavity. Such compression causes air and fungal organisms (including spores) to be expelled into the environment. The spores may lay dormant in the environment until conditions conducive to fungal growth arise. The spores and fungal organisms may also be inhaled by embalming personnel, establish colonies in the lungs and throat, and cause further infections.

Bodies with superficial lesions should never be handled with bare hands. A cut or break in the skin of the hands of embalming personnel represents a portal of entry for fungal and other organisms. Should the organisms enter the bloodstream, they can spread throughout the body and cause serious infections. In addition, the embalmer's clothing may harbor fungal organisms and spores, as well as other infectious organisms, which could be spread to other persons with whom the embalmer comes into contact.

Most, if not all, fungal organisms form spores. These spores may be resistant to weak disinfecting agents. Therefore, the spores may lay dormant in an improperly cleaned and disinfected preparation room and on improperly disinfected instruments. These spores could contaminate subsequent remains embalmed in that preparation room. The greater danger, however, lies in the possibility that unsuspecting embalming personnel might inhale airborne spores or contract them through cuts or breaks in the skin. Spores may enter the ventilation system and be spread to other areas.

Embalming personnel should wear protective garments in the preparation room (gloves, apron and/or impermeable disposable coveralls, oral/nasal mask, goggles, head and shoe coverings). Personal or bed clothing should be removed carefully and disposed of properly. The body should be thoroughly bathed with a proper disinfectant solution as soon as it is undressed. All superficial lesions should be treated immediately, and the mouth, nose, and eyes properly disinfected. All of these procedures must be accomplished before any embalming procedure is initiated (this would be true of all cases).

Once the external disinfection has been completed, embalming procedures may be carried out as prescribed by the preembalming analysis. Routine arterial injection of a solution of sufficient strength and thorough cavity treatment should control internal fungal infections. Oral, nasal, vaginal, and anal cavities may be packed with disinfectant-soaked cotton as an added precaution. For autopsied bodies, careful handling of drainage is recommended.

Students of funeral service education are taught that every body should be treated as though it were infectious, because it very well may be. This has been sound advice for many years and is especially important today in light of the fact that it is not always known what diseases the deceased may have had or may have come into contact with. Whether the body is a seemingly routine case or a victim of a severe infectious disease (e.g., hepatitis or AIDS), the protection of personal and public health rests solely in the procedures used by the embalming personnel.

KEY TERMS AND CONCEPTS FOR STUDY AND DISCUSSION

1. Define the following terms:
   crepitation
   esophageal varices
   instant tissue fixation
   lung purge
   mycotic infection
   postembalming purge
   preembalming purge
   purge
   renal failure
   stomach purge
   "true" tissue gas

2. Discuss the measures that can be taken to prevent postembalming purge.
3. Discuss the difference between subcutaneous emphysema and "true" tissue gas.
4. Outline the embalming of a body with tissue gas in the tissues of the right leg.
5. Discuss the problems encountered in embalming a body dead from chronic alcoholism.
6. List some mycotic infections encountered by the embalmer.
7. Discuss the problems encountered in preparation of the obese dead human body.
8. Discuss the complications encountered in embalming bodies dead from renal failure.

BIBLIOGRAPHY

Anderson WAD, Scotti M. *Synopsis of Pathology*. 10th ed. St. Louis, MO: CV Mosby; 1980.

Boehringer PR. Uremic poisoning. *ESCO Rev* 1964: second quarter.

Boehringer PR. *Controlled Embalming of the Head*. Westport, CT: ESCO Tech Notes: 1967;57.

Grant M. Selected embalming complications and their treatment. In: *Champion Expanding Encyclopedia*. Springfield, OH: Champion Chemical Co.; 1987:No. 573.

Mulvihill ML. *Human Diseases*. 2nd ed. Norwalk, CT: Appleton & Lange; 1987.

Robbins SL. *Pathology*. 3rd ed. Philadelphia: 1967.

Sheldon H. *Boyd's Introduction to the Study of Disease*. 9th ed. Philadelphia: Lea & Febiger; 1984.

Tissue gas cause and treatment. In: *Champion Expanding Encyclopedia*. Springfield, OH: Champion Chemical Co.; 1971:No. 420.

Walter JB. *Pathology of Human Disease*. Philadelphia: Lea & Febiger; 1989.

2

part

The Origin and History of Embalming
The History of Modern Restorative Art

Edward C. Johnson • *Gail R. Johnson* • *Melissa J. Williams*

The Origin and History of Embalming

Edward C. Johnson • Gail R. Johnson • Melissa J. Williams

A statement in 1875 by the N. Y. State Supreme Court is still relevant, concise, and conceptually complete:

> The decent burial of the dead is a matter in which the public have concern. It is against the Public Health if it does not take place at all and against a proper public sentiment should it not take place with decency.

Winston Churchill stated in his gifted style:

> Without a sense of history, no man can understand the problems of our time, the longer you can look back, the further you can look forward—the wider the span, the longer the continuity, the greater is the sense of duty in individual men and women, each contributing their brief life's work to the preservation and progress of the land in which they live, the society of which they are the servants.

Esmond R. Long, M.D., a medical historian, wrote:

> Nothing gives a better perspective of the subject than an appreciation of the steps by which it has reached its present state.
> *So it is with the subject of embalming. The authors of this chapter trust that this brief exposition of the origin and history of embalming will impart to the reader a sense of the tradition and technical advances achieved over the nearly 5000 years that the art and science of embalming have been practiced. There is a clear indication that both tradition and new technical advances will continue to be maintained in the future.*

Embalming, one of humankind's longest practiced arts, is a means of artificially preserving the dead human body.

I. **Natural means of preservation:** obtained without the deliberate intervention of humans
   1. Freezing: By this method bodies are preserved for centuries in the ice and snow of glaciers or snow-capped mountains.
   2. Dry cold: A morgue located on the top of St. Bernard Mountain in Switzerland was so constructed to permit free admission of the elements. True mummies were produced as a result of the passage of the cold, dry air current over the corpses.
   3. Dry heat: Natural mummies are produced in the extremely dry, warm areas of Egypt, southwestern America, and Peru.
   4. Nature of the soil at the place of interment: There are recorded instances of the discovery of bodies in a good state of preservation after long-term burial in a peat bog that had a high tannin content or in soils strongly impregnated with salts of aluminum or copper.

II. **Artificial means of preservation:** secured by the deliberate action of humans

1. Simple heat: Simple heat is the means employed to preserve bodies in the Capuchin Monastery near Palermo, on the island of Sicily. The Monastery is connected to a catacomb or underground burial vault composed of four separate chambers. Treatment of the bodies consists of slow drying in an oven that is heated by a mixture of slacked lime. The desiccated bodies, quite shrunken and light in weight, are placed in upright positions along the walls of the catacombs.
2. Powders: In powder methods, the body is placed on a bed of sawdust mixed with zinc sulfate or other preserving powder.
3. Evisceration and immersion (used by the Egyptians and others)
4. Evisceration and drying (the Guanche method)
5. Evisceration, local incision, and immersion (employed in Europe, particularly in France, during the period AD 650–1830)
6. Simple immersion (in alcohol, brine, or other liquid preservatives)
7. Arterial injection and evisceration (used by the Hunter brothers and others)
8. Cavity injection and immersion (method of Gabriel Clauderus)
9. Arterial injection (mode of treatment of Gannal, Sucquet, and many others)
10. Arterial injection and cavity treatment (method in daily use by all present-day embalmers; generally taught in schools and colleges of embalming today)
11. Artificial cold (by a system of refrigeration to reduce the body temperature to inhibit bacterial activity; in use in most hospitals and morgues today)

PERIODS OF EMBALMING HISTORY

Embalming originated in Egypt during the period of the first dynasty. It is estimated to have begun about 3200 BC and continued on until AD 650. The motive of Egyptian embalming was religious in that preservation of the human body (intact) was a necessary requirement for resurrection, their religious goal. During this nearly 4000-year period of embalming practice there obviously existed a number of variations of technique. Egyptian embalming began to decline with the advent of Christianity, as the early Christians rejected the practice, associating embalming with various "pagan religious rites." When the Arabs conquered Egypt they, too, rejected the practice of embalming.

The second period of embalming history extends from AD 650 to 1861 and its principal geographical area of practice and growth was Europe. This era is termed the *Period of the Anatomists,* as the motive was to advance the development of embalming techniques for the preservation of the dead to permit detailed anatomical dissection and study.

The third or modern period of embalming history extends from 1861 to the present day. It is during this period that embalming knowledge, which had been transferred from Europe to America during the previous period, finally reverted to its original use, principally for funeral purposes. Embalming again became available to all who requested it. Motives in this period are diverse, with sentiment probably predominant, as the average person desires to view the decedent free of evidence of the ravages of disease or injury. Public transportation is another reason to embalm, as the procedure prevents a dead body from becoming offensive during a protracted period of travel and is required by many public transport agencies.

Although the value of embalming to the public health is disputed and debated, it is most apparent that a decaying, unembalmed body is surely a health menace to those exposed to its effluvia. From earliest Egyptian times embalmers have been closely associated with the medical profession. In fact, most embalmers in the United States were doctors of medicine until the later portion of the 19th century.

ESTABLISHMENT OF EMBALMING SCHOOLS

The incentive for embalming in the period AD 650 to 1861 was the preservation of anatomical material to further the study of and research in anatomy. Those who made the early strides in embalming were the anatomists, but about the time of J.N. Gannal (early 19th-century France) and Thomas H. Holmes (late 19th-century United States), general public interest was aroused in the preservation of the dead. This interest and the later demand for preservation for funeral purposes of all human dead grew far beyond the means and desires of the few, trained embalmers in the medical profession. During the late 19th century in the United States, schools of embalming instruction were established by experienced embalmers. Many funeral directors and doctors attended the schools to study embalming and to seek employment. By the beginning of the 20th century in the United States, separation of the fields of embalming and medicine was complete. This brought about the advancement of both professions, particularly that of embalming, as it placed a complex art in the hands of specialists who are still striving to acquire more knowledge and skill in preserving the human dead.

How, then, and why did the practice of embalming develop?

EGYPTIAN PERIOD

During the early predynastic period, well before 3200 BC, the Egyptians had a very simple culture. When death occurred, the unembalmed body was placed in the fetal position (arms and legs folded), wrapped in cloth or straw mats, and placed in a shallow grave scooped out of the desert sand west of the Nile River. A few pieces of pottery and other artifacts were placed in the grave with the body, which was positioned on its side. The body was preserved by drying, from the contact with the arid, porous sand and the total absence of rainfall or other moisture. From time to time, desert winds uncovered the bodies in their shallow graves, and cemetary guards or relatives saw that the bodies were indeed preserved (Fig. 1).

As Egyptian civilization grew, towns and villages sprang up and commerce and industry created a substantial middle and upper class of landlords and other well-to-do persons, as well as a supreme class of tribal and area rulers. When members of this group died, the old practice of simple burial in the desert sands no longer sufficed. Graves were dug deeper and were lined with wooden boards or with stone slabs so that the body, still in the fetal position, remained untouched by the sand.

With these more prosperous or noble individuals were buried more valuable artifacts such as jewelry and furniture.

Then, as now, there existed members of society who were criminals, and some devoted themselves to grave robbing. When the cemetery custodians or family survivors of such elaborate burials noted the opening and desecration of burials, they also noted and were appalled that the corpse was no longer preserved, but had begun to decay. One attempt to forestall decomposition was the enclosure of the body within a solid stone coffin cut from a single mass of stone. The body of the coffin was without seams and the cover fit tightly. These burials were subsequently plundered and again the custodians or relatives contemplated the remains which, to their horror, had on many occasions completely decomposed to a skeletal status. Without a scientific knowledge of the process of putrefaction, they expressed the belief that the stone coffin ate the soft tissues. To this day, massive bronze and copper caskets are termed *sarcophagi* from the Greek *sarco* for "flesh" and *phagus* for "eater." The Egyptians, not wishing to revert to their simple burial-in-the-sands method, found it necessary to devise some system of preserving the human body—embalming.

It is not too difficult to understand how Egyptian embalming was first developed when it is kept in mind that Egypt has a basically warm climate. The culture was such that hunting and fishing provided some of the food requirements. Thus, a hunter or fisherman might have a successful catch and secure more birds, fish, or game than he or his family could consume immediately. Such animals, fish, or birds could, like the human body, quickly

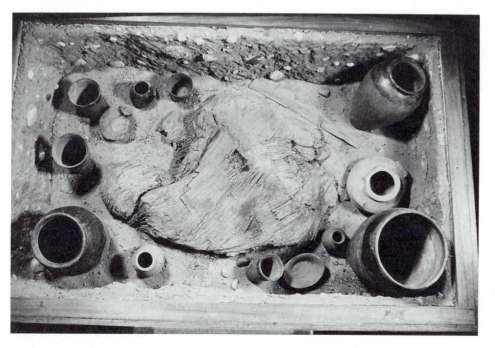

Figure 1. Predynastic (3200 BC) Egyptian burial site, west of the Nile. The unembalmed corpse is in the fetal position, wrapped in straw matting. *(Courtesy of the Royal Ontario Museum.)*

decay and become worthless for food. The hunter, however, knew how to prepare his catch and to preserve it. He eviscerated and bled his catch and then, by one or another method such as salting, sun drying, smoking, or cooking, preserved it for future consumption. *(This procedure for the preservation of food was common knowledge and it requires little imagination to recognize the ease with which the basic food preservation process could be adapted with refinements to the preservation of the dead human body.)*

Variation in Embalming Methods

The actual methods of embalming employed by the Egyptians varied from dynasty to dynasty according to custom and to the technique of the individual embalmer. History provides views of four contemporary writers on the subject who have frequently been quoted.

The earliest account is that of the Greek historian Herodotus, who lived about 484 BC:

> There are certain individuals appointed for the purpose [the embalming], and who profess the art; these persons, when any body is brought to them, show the bearers some wooden models of corpses; the most perfect they assert to be the representation of him whose name I take it impious to mention in this matter; they show a second, which is inferior to the first and cheaper; and a third which is cheapest of all. They then ask according to which of the models they will have the deceased prepared; having settled upon the price, the relations immediately depart, and the embalmers, remaining at home, thus proceed to perform the embalming in the most costly manner.
>
> In the first place, with a crooked piece of iron, they pull out the brain by the nostrils; a part of it they extract in this manner, the rest by means of pouring in certain drugs; in the next place, after making an incision in the flank with a sharp Ethiopian stone, they empty the whole of the inside; and after cleansing the cavity, and rinsing it with palm wine, scour it out with pounded aromatics. Then, having filled the belly with pure myrrh pounded, and cinnamon, and all other perfumes, frankincense excepted, they sew it up again; having so done, they "steep" the body in natrum, keeping it covered for 70 days, for it is not lawful to leave the body any longer.
>
> When the 70 days are gone by, they first wash the corpse, and then wrap up the whole body in bandages cut out of cotton cloth, which they smear with gum, a substance the Egyptians use instead of paste. The relations, having then received back the body, get a wooden case in the shape of a man to be made; and when completed, they place the body in the inside and then, shutting it up, keep it in a sepulchral repository, where they stand it upright against the wall. The above is the most costly manner in which they prepare the dead.
>
> For such who choose the middle mode, from a desire of avoiding expense, they prepare the body as follows: They first fill syringes with oil of cedar to inject into the belly of the deceased, without making any incision, or emptying the inside, but by sending it in by the anus. This they then cork, to hinder the injection from flowing backwards, and lay the body in salt for the specified number of days, on the last of which they release what they had previously injected, and such is the strength it possesses that it brings away with it the bowels and insides in a state of dissolution; on the other hand, the natrum dissolves the flesh so that, in fact, there remains nothing but the skin and bones. When they have done this they give the body back without any further operation upon it.
>
> The third mode of embalming, which is used for such as have but scanty means, is as follows: after washing the insides with syrmaea, they salt the body for the 70 days and return it to be taken back.

The second writer is Diodorus Siculus, who lived about 45 BC:

> When anyone among the Egyptians dies, all his relations and friends, putting dirt upon their heads, go lamenting about the city, till such time as the body shall be buried. In the mean time they abstain from baths and wine, and all kinds of delicate meats, neither do they during that time wear any costly apparel. The manner of their burials is three-fold: one very costly, a second sort less chargeable, and a third very mean. In the first, they say, there is spent a talent of silver ($1,200); in the second, 20 minae ($300); but in the last there is very little expense ($75). Those who have the care of ordering the body are such as have been taught that art by their ancestors. These, showing to the kindred of the deceased a bill of each kind of burial, ask them after which manner they will have the body prepared. When they have agreed upon the matter, they deliver the body to such as are usually appointed for this office. First, he who has the name scribe marks about the flank of the left side how much is to be cut away. Then he who is called the cutter or dissector, with an Ethiopian stone, cuts away as much of the flesh as the law commands, and presently runs away as fast as he can. Those who are present pursue him, cast stones at him, curse him, thereby turning all the execrations which they imagine due to his office upon him.
>
> For whosoever offers violence, wounds, or does any kind of injury to a body of the same nature with himself, they think him worthy of hatred; but those who are called embalmers are worthy of honor and respect; for they are familiar with their priests and go into the temples as holy men without any prohibition. So soon as they come to embalm the dissected body, one of them thrusts his hand through the wound into the abdomen and draws out all the viscera but the heart and kidneys, which another washes and cleanses with wine made of palms and aromatic odors.
>
> Lastly having washed the body, they anoint it with oil of cedar and other things for 30 days, and after-

wards with myrrh, cinnamon, and other such like matters, which have not only a powder to preserve it for a long time, but also give it a sweet smell; afterwards they deliver it to the kindred in such manner that every member remains whole and entire, and no part of it changed. The beauty and shape of the face seems just as it was before, and may be known, even the hairs of the eyebrows and eyelids remaining as they were at first. By this method many of the Egyptians, keeping the dead bodies of their ancestors in magnificent houses, so perfectly see the true visage and countenance of those that died many ages before they themselves were born that in viewing the proportions of every one of them, and the lineaments of their faces, they take as much delight as if they were still living among them.

The third account is given by Plutarch, who lived between AD 50 and 100:

The belly being opened, the bowels were removed and cast into the River Nile and the body exposed to the sun. The cavities of the chest and belly were then filled with the unguents and odorous substances.

The fourth description is by Perphry, who lived about AD 230 to 300:

When those who have care of the dead proceed to embalm the body of any person of respectable rank, they first take out the contents of the belly and place them in a separate vessel, addressing the sun, and utter on behalf of the deceased the following prayer, which Euphantus has translated from the original language into Greek: "O thou sun, our lord, and all ye gods who are the givers of life to men, accept me, and receive me into the mansions of the eternal gods; for I have worshiped piously, while I have lived in this world, those divinities whom my parents taught me to adore. I have ever honored those parents who gave origin to my body; and of other men I have neither killed any, nor robbed them of their treasure, nor inflicted upon them any grievous evil; but if I have done anything injurious to my soul, either by eating or drinking anything unlawfully, this offense has not been committed by me, but by what is contained in this chest." This refers to the intestines in the vessel, which is then cast into the River Nile. The body is afterwards regarded as pure, the apology having been made for its offenses, and the embalmer prepares it according to the appointed rites.

Differences in Translations

As may be observed, there were differences in embalming methods as described by the foregoing writers. This may be, in part, due to inaccuracies in copying and translating of the original manuscripts. Egyptologists generally dismiss the accounts of Plutarch and Porphyry as unreliable because the intestines either were removed and

placed in containers that were kept near the body or were replaced in the body. As to the accounts of Herodotus and Diodorus, they were given the seal of approval for their general verity. Scientific proof is lacking, however, with regard to the corrosiveness of oil of cedar, and it is believed that the covering of the corpse with natron took place before the filling of the trunk cavities with the spices and other substances.

Present-day translations of the *Book of the Dead,* a textbook guide for the Egyptian embalmer, do not agree on the 70-day period for the covering with natron. One of the chronologies of the most costly method states that the 1st to the 16th days were occupied with the evisceration, washing, and cleansing of the body; from the 16th to the 36th days, the body was kept under natron; from the 36th to the 68th days, the spicing and bandaging took place; and from the 68th to the 70th days, the body was coffined.

Steps in Egyptian Preparation

Step 1: Removal of the Brain.
The brain was generally removed by introducing a metal hook or spoon into the nostril and by forcing it through the ethmoid bone to the brain. As much as possible was scooped out in this way. In some mummies the brain was not removed. A few craniums had the brain removed through the eye socket. There is one case on record in which the evacuation of the cranium was accomplished through the foramen magnum, after excision of the atlas vertebra. After the body was removed from under natron, the cranium was usually repacked with linen bandages soaked in resin or bitumen. One writer tells of removing 27 feet of 3-inch linen bandage from the cranium of a mummy. Sometimes the cranium was filled with resin believed to have been introduced while molten with the aid of a funnel.

Step 2: Evisceration.
Many bodies were not eviscerated. The earliest incision was made vertically in the left side, extending from the lower margin of the ribs to the anterior superior spine (crest) of the ilium. This incision would measure between 5 and 6 inches in length. At a later period the incision became oblique, extending from a point near the left anterior spine (crest) of the ilium toward the pubis. A variant incision extended vertically from the symphysis pubis toward the umbilicus. In the very late 26th dynasty (665–527 BC) some bodies were eviscerated through the anus. The incision was usually made with a flint knife called Ethiopian stone because of its black color. All the viscera, with the exception of the kidneys and usually the heart, were removed, washed, and immersed in palm wine or packed in natron. (*Their disposition will be referred to later.*)

Step 3: Covering with Natron.
Natron is a salt obtained from the dry lakes of the desert and is composed of the chlo-

ride, carbonate, and sulfate of sodium and the nitrate of potassium and sodium. Because of its corrosive action on the body the embalmers had to affix the toes and fingernails to the body during the macerating period. This was accomplished by tying the nails on with thread or copper or gold wire. Alternatively, metal thimbles were fit over the ends of the fingers and toes for the same purpose. The body was then ready for the natron treatment. Early Egyptologists believed that the bodies were placed in a solution composed of natron dissolved in water, as described by Herodotus. Present-day authorities, in studying the original writing of Herodotus and other prime sources, detect a flaw in the translation of the text that is responsible for the misrepresentation. Present-day research, where the embalming process was recreated, indicates conclusively that only application of the concentrated dry salt over the body to some depth could dehydrate and preserve it. Experiments with different concentrations of the natron solution and immersion of specimens therein were largely unsuccessful in preventing decay.

Step 4: Removal from Natron. At the end of the 20th day of immersion in natron, the body was washed with water and dried in the sun.

Step 5: Wrapping and Spicing. The body was coated within and without by resin or a mixture of resin and fat. The skull was treated as in Step 1. The viscera, when removed from the body and not returned to the body, were placed in four canopic jars, the tops of which were surmounted by the images of the four children of Horus. Each jar held a specific portion of the viscera. The jar topped with the human head represented Imset and contained the liver. The jar covered with the jackal's head represented Duamutef and contained the stomach. The jar topped with the ape's head represented Hapy and held the lungs. The fourth jar, surmounted by a hawk's head, represented Qebeh-Snewef and contained the intestines. No mention is made of the disposition of the spleen, pancreas, or pelvic organs (Fig. 2).

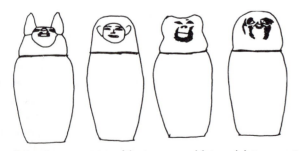

Figure 2. Canopic urns—containers of the viscera removed during embalming preparation and not returned to trunk of body. From left to right are the jackal's head, Duamutef (contained stomach); the human head, Imset (contained liver); the ape's head, Hapy (contained lungs); and the hawk's head, Qebeh-Snewef (contained intestines). *(Courtesy of Paula Johnson De Smet.)*

The canopic jars varied in size and material. They were from about 9 to 18 inches in height and 4 inches in diameter and were made of alabaster, limestone, basalt, clay, and other materials. The canopic jars were usually placed in a wooden box and kept near the body. When the viscera were placed in these jars, images in miniature of the jars were returned to the cavity, which was padded in straw, resin-soaked linen bandages, or lichen moss. On return to the body cavity, the viscera were usually wrapped in four separate parcels to which were attached specific images, as mentioned above. Originally, the incision was not sewn but merely had the edges drawn together. Sometimes the edges were stuck together by resin or wax; however, there are recorded instances in the 18th, 20th, and 21st dynasties (1700, 1250, and 1000 BC) of closure effected by sewing that closely resembles the familiar embalmer's stitch of today. The incision was covered, whether sewn or not, by a plate of wax or metal on which was engraved the eye of Osiris (Egyptian god of the dead).

Ancient Restorative Art

It was during this part of the preparation in the 20th dynasty (1288–1110 BC) that a little known process was performed. Most present-day embalmers feel that the restoration to normal of emaciated facial features of a corpse is of comparatively recent origin. On the contrary, the Egyptian embalmers performed this operation, but on a much more extensive scale. Not only were the facial features restored, but the entire bodily contours were subcutaneously padded to regain their normal shape. The methods and materials used varied.

The mouth was usually internally packed with sawdust to pad out the cheeks, while the eyelids were stuffed with linen pads. Then, working from the original abdominal incision by burrowing under the skin of the trunk in all directions, the packing material was forced into these channels. In places such as the back and arms that could not be reached from the original incision, additional local incisions were made through which to pass the padding material. In later periods, the cheeks and temples were padded with resin introduced through openings in front of the ears. This material, introduced while warm, could be molded to conform to the desired contour. The packing materials most commonly used were resin, linen bandages, mud, sand, sawdust, and butter mixed with soda. If was also during this stage of preparation that repair of bodily injuries took place. Broken limbs were splinted, and bed sores were packed with resin-soaked linen bandages and covered with thin strips of antelope hide.

There is a case of a crooked spine having been straightened. Eyes were sometimes replaced with ones of stone or, as in one instance, with small onions. The bodies that were to be gilded (covered with golden leaf) were then treated. Some were completely covered with a gold leaf; on others, only the face, fingernails, and toenails, or genitals were gilded, as there was much variation on this matter. After the complete covering of the body with a paste of resin and fat, the bandagers set to work. It is believed that there were individuals who specialized in wrapping certain parts of the body such as the fingers, arms, legs, and head. Each finger or toe was first separately swathed; then each limb. The body was first covered with a kind of tunic and the face covered with a large square bandage followed by the regular spiral bandages. Pads were placed between the bandages to aid in restoration and maintenance of the bodily contour. Lotus blossoms have been found between the layers of linen bandages. Some authorities claim that the living saved cloth all their lives to provide bandages for use as mummy wrappings. The bandages varied from 3 to 9 inches in width and up to 1200 yards in length and were inscribed at intervals with hieroglyphics indicating the identity of the enswathed person. Authorities believed that only one of ten mummies was prepared by the first method. The others were prepared by the cheaper methods, as described by the earlier writers. Another means of embalming used then was simple covering of the entire body with natron or molten resin. This latter process, while preserving the body, destroyed the hair and most of the facial features, fingers, and toes.

During the last 1000 years of Egyptian embalming practice, the emphasis gradually changed from producing a well-preserved body capable of withstanding decay for all eternity to creating an increasingly elaborate external appearance of the wrapped body. Wrapping patterns became quite elaborate and cartonage and plaster were employed to present a sometimes fanciful external recreation of the deceased. During the terminal centuries of Egyptian embalming, portraits on a flat surface were painted and placed over the head area, which more faithfully resembled the dead.

The Receptacles

The wrapped mummies were usually additionally encased and placed in boxes or coffins. An additional encasement, termed *cartonage,* was made of 20 or 30 sheets of linen cloth or papyrus saturated in resin, plaster of Paris, or gum acacia and placed over the wrapped body while wet. To ensure a tight fit, the material was drawn together in the back of the body by a kind of lacing not unlike present-day shoelacing. The cartonage, when dry, was as hard as wood and was covered with a thin coating of plaster, then painted with a representation of a human head and other designs. Two or more wood cases of cedar or sycamore might encase the cartonage and each other. These coffins or mummy cases were of different shape, depending on the period when they were made. The outer wooden case was, at times, rectangular in shape

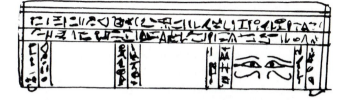

Figure 3. Wooden coffin. The body, placed inside, lies on its left side with the head at the end, where eyes are drawn facing eyes and thus looking outward *(Courtesy of Paula Johnson De Smet.)*

with a cover resembling the roof of a house. Early coffined embalmed bodies were placed within the coffins lying on their side. The exterior of the coffin contained the representation of a pair of eyes on one side near the head of the coffin (Fig. 3). This indicated the position of the body facing outward at this point. Coffins shaped like the human form were termed anthropoid or mummiform (Fig. 4). If the deceased was a member of a great family

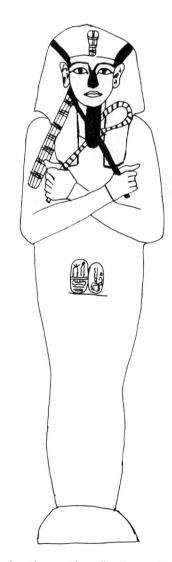

Figure 4. Wooden anthropoid or mummiform coffin. *(Courtesy of Paula Johnson De Smet.)*

he might be enclosed within a stone sarcophagus that was a stone coffin or vault fashioned of marble, limestone, granite, or slate.

Even in Egyptian times the tombs of the dead were plundered for their valuables. Many mummy cases were broken open and the mummies themselves were damaged. The embalmers were called on to repair the damaged mummies and to rewrap and recoffin them. This may explain, in part, the so-called faking of mummies. In the Field Museum of Natural History in Chicago there are numerous x-ray pictures of unopened mummy cases and unwrapped mummies. Some of these pictures show damage that may have occurred prior to or during the course of embalming. One x-ray photo of a young child displays the complete absence of the arms and bilateral fractures of the femurs at about their midpoint, with the lower broken portion entirely missing. Museum authorities advance the theory that this was done to fit the child into a smaller mummy case. Another x-ray photo reveals a wrapped mummy lacking arms and the trunk of the body. The head was connected to the legs by a board and the body had been represented by padding of straw or lichen moss.

Additional faking may be the result of a curious custom of the early middle ages of using bits of mummies as good luck pieces and as a drug for internal consumption. This demand created a brisk business for the Arabs of North Africa, and as the supply of natural mummies was difficult to maintain, the Arabs began to produce their own from the bodies of the lepers and criminal dead.

Animals were also embalmed, wrapped, and coffined in a manner similar to humans. The variety of animals so treated was large and included baboons, monkeys, full-grown bulls, gazelles, goats, sheep, antelopes, crocodiles, cats, dogs, mice, rats, shrews, hawks, geese, ibis, snakes, and lizards. X-ray examination of these wrapped packages discloses an occasional falsity. Some of these false mummies are composed of straw or rags wrapped in the form of the animal they were to represent. G. Elliot Smith, in his article on the Significance of Geographical Distribution of Practice of Mummification, states that knowledge of the Egyptian method of embalming was carried westward as far as the Canary Islands. He bases his decision on the similarity of the embalming procedures carried on in these areas of the world and the knowledge that the Egyptian method preceded those in all other known parts of the world.

THE PRACTICE OF BODY PRESERVATION OF VARIOUS ETHNIC GROUPS AND PLACES

Jews. The Jews did not embalm but simply washed and shaved the body and swathed it in sheets, between the folds of which were placed spices such as myrrh and aloes. The purpose of herbs and spices was to disguise the odor of decay of the body, not to preserve it.

Ancient Persians, Syrians, and Babylonians. Sometimes, the ancient Persians, Syrians, and Babylonians immersed their human dead in jars of honey or wax. Alexander the Great was said to have been so treated to preserve his body during the long journey from the place of death in Babylon in 323 BC (during a military campaign) to Egypt.

Ancient Ethiopians. The ancient Ethiopians eviscerated and desiccated their dead in a manner similar to the Egyptian method. The bodily contours were restored by applying plaster over the shrunken skin. The plaster-covered corpse was then painted with lifelike colors and given a coating of clear resinlike substance believed by some authorities to be a fossil salt and by others to be a type of amber, somehow rendered fluid at the time of application.

Canary Islands. (from at least 900 BC). In the Atlantic Ocean, about 4° south of the Madeira Islands, on the northwest coast of Africa, there is a cluster of 13 islands known as the Canary Islands. These islands were not subdued by any European nation until the Spaniards overran them in the late 15th century. The original inhabitants, known as Guanches, are thought to have been descendants of the lost continent of Atlantis. It is believed that only prominent and influential families had the dead embalmed. The Guanches' method of embalming their dead is very similar to the Egyptian method.

The Guanche embalmers were both men and women who performed the services for their own sex. These embalmers were well paid, although their touch was considered contaminating and they lived in seclusion in remote parts of the Islands. On the death of a person, the family bore the body to the embalmers and then retired. The embalmers placed the body on a stone table and an opening was made in the lower abdomen with a flint knife called *tabona*. The intestines were withdrawn, washed, cleaned, and later returned to the body. The entire body, inside and outside, was very thoroughly saturated with salt and the intestines were returned to the body along with numerous aromatic plants and herbs.

The body anointed with butter, powdered resin, brushwood, and pumice, was exposed to the sun, or, if the sun was not hot enough, the body was placed in a stove to dry. During the drying period the body was maintained in an extended position; the arms of men were placed along the sides of the body, while women's arms were placed across the abdomen.

The embalmers maintained a constant vigil over the body during this period to prevent it from being devoured by vultures. On the 15th or 16th day the drying process should be complete and the relatives would claim the body and sew it in goatskins. Kings and nobles were, in addition, placed in coffins of hollowed juniper logs. All bodies were deposited in caves in the hilly regions of the islands.

In another method of preparation described, a corrosive liquid believed to be juice of the spurge or euphorbia plant, was either introduced through the belly wall or poured down the throat; this was followed by the drying process described above. The mummies produced by these processes were called *xaxos* and the method of embalming was believed to have been introduced from Egypt about 900 BC. In T. J. Pettigrew's *History of Egyptian Mummies*, there is a description of a xaxos as found by a sea captain in 1764. The author points out the "flesh of the body is perfectly preserved, but it is dry, inflexible and hard as wood . . . nor is any part decayed. The body is no more shrunk than if the person had been dead only two or three days. Only the skin appears a little shriveled and of a deeply tanned, copper color." The xaxos were extremely light in weight, averaging about 6 to 9 pounds for bodies up to $5\frac{1}{2}$ feet in length.

Peru. Preservation of the body in Peru was practiced for at least a thousand years before the Spanish conquest in the early 16th century. It had for its motive a religious belief in the resurrection of the body. Most authorities agree that the Peruvians had no process of embalming, but that their mummies were a product of the extremely dry climate of the region. There are reports that the Incas or ruling classes were embalmed, and because only mummies of the common people have been discovered, this report may be true. The manner in which the Inca rulers are believed to have been prepared was by evisceration. The intestines were placed in gold vases, the cavity filled with an unspecified resin, and the body coated with bitumen. The bodies were said to have been seated on their thrones, clothed in their regal robes, hands clasped on the breast, and head inclined downward. There is mention of the use of gold to plate or replace the eyes.

The usual Peruvian mummy, of which there are many specimens in the Field Museum at Chicago, was often found buried with the face toward the west, together with provisions of corn and coca contained in earthen jars. The mummies themselves were wrapped in cloth and tied with a course rope. The outer covering was of matting and followed a roll of cotton which, in turn, enveloped a red or varied-color wool cloth wrapped about the body. The innermost wrapping was a white cotton sheet. The corpse was found in a squatting position, knees under chin, arm over breast, with the fists touching the jaws. The hands were usually fastened together, and on most mummies there was a rope passed three or four times around the neck. In the mouth there was usually a small copper, silver, or gold disk. The

greater part of the mummies was well preserved, but the flesh was shriveled and the features were disfigured. The hair was preserved, with the women's hair braided. Nearly all types of animals and birds have been found mummified, including parrots, dogs, cats, doves, hawks, heron, ducks, llamas, vicunas, and alpacas wrapped in the manner of human mummies.

Ecuador. The Jivaro Indians of the Marano River region of South America had a method of preserving heads by shrinking them. Technically, this process does not come under the heading of embalming, but a brief general description of the process is of interest.

The bones of the skull were first removed through long slits in the scalp. The skin of the head, with the hair attached, was boiled in water containing astringent herbs. On completion of this process, hot stones of gradually diminishing size were inserted into the space formerly occupied by the skull bones. When the shrinking process was completed, the stones were removed and the incisions were sutured as were the mouth and eyes. The finished shrunken head is about the size of a man's fist, with the features rather clear and retaining their proper proportions. It has been stated that this same process has been applied to an entire human body with equal success, although no such specimens have been found.

Mexico and Central America—Aztecs, Toltecs, and Mayans. On the basis of information received from Alfonso Caso, Mexico's outstanding anthropologist, there is no evidence of the employment of any artificial means of preservation of the body in the pre-Spanish era in these regions. There are accounts of finding mummies wrapped in matting and buried in the earth or in caves, but it is the opinion of Caso and others that such mummification was the result of the natural climate of the region.

North American Indians. Although no proof exists to substantiate claims that some of the Indian tribes embalmed their dead, there are quotes from two accounts of embalming means as recounted by H. C. Yarrow in his *Study of Mortuary Customs of North American Indians* from 1880, collected from earlier publications. On page 185 of the *History of Virginia* (by Beverly, 1722), this statement is found:

> The Indians are religious in preserving the corpses of their kings and rulers after death. First they neatly flay off the skin as entire as they can, slitting only the back; then they pick all the flesh off the bones as clean as possible, leaving the sinews fastened to the bones, that they may preserve the joints together. Then they dry the bones in the sun and put them into the skin again, which in the meantime has been kept from shrinking. When the bones are placed right in the skin, the attendants nicely fill up the vacuities with a very fine

white sand. After this they sew up the skin again, and the body looks as if the flesh had not been removed. They take care to keep the skin from shrinking by the help of a little oil or grease, which saves it from corruption. The skin being thus prepared, they lay it in an apartment for that purpose, upon a large shelf raised above the floor. This shelf is spread with mats for the corpse to rest easy on, and screened with the same to keep it from the dust. The flesh they lay upon hurdles in the sun to dry, and when it is thoroughly dried, it is sewed up in a basket and set at the feet of the corpse, to which it belongs.

Another account appeared in Volume XIII, page 39, of *Collection of Voyages* (Pinkerton, 1812), concerning the Werowance Indians:

> Their bodies are first bowelled, then dried upon hurdles til they be very dry, and so about most of their joints and neck they hang bracelets or chains of copper, pearl and such like, as they are used to wear. Their innards they stuff with copper beads, hatchets and such trash. Then they lap them very carefully in white skins and so roll them in mats for their winding-sheets.

The Indians are known to have wrapped their dead in cloth or leather and to have suspended the bodies in a horizontal manner in trees or buried them in the earth, in caves, or in the ground covered by rocks. This may have had a religious significance, but more likely it was done to prevent vultures or animals from devouring the dead.

Aleutian Islands and Kodiak Archipelago. It is believed that the inhabitants of the Aleutian Islands and Kodiak Archipelago practiced preservation of their dead from at least AD 1000, although the custom did not prevail on the mainland. The internal organs were removed through an incision in the pelvic region and the cavity was refilled with dry grass. The body was placed in a stream of cold running water, which was said to have removed the fatty tissues in a short time. The corpse was removed from the water and wrapped in the fetal posture, knees under the chin and arms compressed about the legs. This position was accomplished by use of force, breaking bones if necessary. In this posture the body was sun-dried and, as a final gesture, was wrapped in animal skins and matting.

PERIOD OF THE ANATOMISTS (AD 650–1861)

With the Arabic conquest of Egypt and the fall of the Roman Empire, European and Mediterranean civilizations declined virtually to the vanishing point. The old world of law and order as the Romans and others knew it was replaced by anarchy. Geographical areas were ruled by bands of armed men with little stability of con-

trol. The Dark Ages were to continue until the year 1000 when a gradual elimination of unstable leaders left a few more wise and capable individuals in charge of substantial geographical divisions of Europe. With a return to a more normal civilized existence came the establishment of schools and colleges in what is today Sicily, Italy, France, and England and later in Germany, Holland, Belgium, and Switzerland. The schools were, in part, the product of the Catholic Church, which throughout the Dark Ages had maintained and served as a sanctuary for work in the fields of medicine, nursing, teaching, copying of manuscripts, and establishment of orphanages and poorhouses.

The medical schools that were established used some texts originally written during the glory era of Egypt. In Alexandria, on the Mediterranean at the mouth of the Nile, there existed the greatest center for teaching that history had known. The Library, before its destruction, was said to have contained more than half a million manuscripts on subjects varying from astronomy to mathematics to engineering to medicine. It was here that a famous teacher and practitioner of medicine, Claudius Galen (130–200 AD), born in Pergamum, Asia Minor, taught and wrote on the subject of anatomy. His textbook on anatomy described human anatomy principally from dissections of animals such as the pig or monkey. It must be obvious today that there are substantial differences or variations between the anatomical structure of the pig or monkey and those of the human being. Galen and others were not encouraged to dissect the human body as it was considered a mutilation and a crime under Egyptian law. Nevertheless, Galen's teachings and writings on human anatomy were to be considered as the unchallengeable authority for the next 1000 to 1200 years.

With the emergence of Europe from the Dark Ages came a craving for learning that had to that time been suppressed. The medical schools lacked the authority to legally acquire dead human bodies for dissection and anatomical study until the 13th and early 14th centuries. Such authority was granted in 1242 by Frederick II, King of the two Sicilies, and again in 1302 for the delivery of two executed criminals to the medical school at Bologna, Italy, each year for dissection. Such dissections were public affairs, often conducted in open areas or amphitheaters always during the cold months of the year as the dissection subjects were not preserved. The dissection itself was rapid, frequently confined to a 4-day period. In the actual procedure, the anatomy professor, who was seated, read from Galen's text on anatomy while pointing out (with a wand) the body structures mentioned by Galen. An assistant, a barber–surgeon, did the actual dissection as the lecture progressed. Obviously, there were frequent contradictions between Galen's description of a body part and its actual appearance as disclosed by the dissection. These most evident discrepancies encouraged the more intelligent student and medical practitioner to steal bodies from cemeteries and gallows for personal study and research. Every part of such a purloined cadaver was probed speedily for knowledge of its structure or function until it became too loathsome to conceal and had to be disposed of. In many cases the soft tissues were thrown away and the bones boiled to secure the skeleton.

Military Religious Campaigns

During the period from 1095 to 1291 a series of military religious campaigns mounted by the Christian nations of Europe (termed *Crusades*) were conducted to recapture the Holy Land from the Moslems. The campaigns were successful early on, but with the passing of time the Christian occupation forces in the Holy Land became complacent and less martial and eventually were expelled from the entire conquered territory. Many prominent members of the nobility, including King Louis XIX of France, died far from home during the crusades. To allow the return to their homeland of their remains it was necessary to develop what became a gruesome procedure, as no certain means of embalming was available during the campaigns. The procedure consisted of disemboweling and disarticulating the body, cutting off all soft tissues, and then boiling the bones until they were free of all soft tissues. The bones were then dried and wrapped within bull hides and returned to their homeland by the couriers who maintained the communication lines.

In 1300 Pope Boniface VIII issued a Papal Bull (a directive) that prohibited the cutting up of the dead for the purpose of transport and burial under penalty of excommunication. For a brief period, this Papal Bull was interpreted by some members of the medical profession to ban anatomical dissection. For example, in 1345 Vigevano stated that dissection was prohibited, and Mondino (1270–1326) said sin was involved in boiling bones. In any case, such interpretations were rare and were seldom given any regard by the majority of anatomists.

As the years passed it became obvious that some system of preservation, even temporary, had to be contrived to permit a more careful and intensive study of body structure. Early efforts at preservation followed the ancient regimen of drying the parts, for moisture was and is the enemy of preservation. Preservation by drying of cadavers or their components was first sought by exposure to the natural heat of the sun. Later, use of controlled heat in ovens was employed to accomplish desiccation. Eventually, while probing the nature and extent of the hollow blood vessels, it was noted that warm air forced through the blood vessels removed blood and eventually dried out the tissue.

Reports of preservation attempts from the 15th century did not include injections of the blood vascular system. Such early injections into hollow structures of the body were made to trace the direction and continuity of blood vessels or to inflate hollow organs so as to reveal their size and shape or to make internal castings of areas under study. As early as 1326, Alessandra Giliani of Italy injected blood vessels with colored solutions that hardened; Jacobus Berengarius (1470–1550) employed a syringe and injected veins with warm water; Bartolomeo Eustaschio (1520–1574) used warm ink; Regnier De Graaf (1641–1673) invented a syringe and injected mercury; Jan Swammerdam (1637–1680) injected a waxlike material that later hardened. The great artist Leonardo Da Vinci (1452–1519), who is said to have dissected more than 30 corpses to produce hundreds of accurate anatomical illustrations, injected wax to secure castings of the ventricles of the brain and other internal areas.

Early Instruments for Injection

Early instruments for injection were crude and usually made in two parts: a container for the injection material and some form of cannula. The cannula was often contrived from a hollow straw, feather quill, hollow metal, or glass tube which was attached by ligature to an animal bladder (stomach or other intestine). The cannula was inserted into the hollow opening being studied and the bladder tied onto its free end. The bladder, in turn, was filled with a liquid and then tied to retain the bladder full. Entrance of the liquid material into the hollow area was secured by squeezing the bladder until it emptied.

As early as 1521 Berengarius wrote of using a forerunner of the modern syringe. Early syringes similar to the hypodermic syringes employed today were constructed. They were filled and then attached to a cannula in position within the opening to be injected. To refill the syringe the operator had to detach the syringe from the cannula, refill it, and then reattach it. Bartholin (1585–1629) developed the first continuous-flow syringe. It could be recharged during use without halting the injection process.

During the entire time from the end of the Egyptian embalming activity through the Dark Ages and into early medieval period, some members of the elite, clergy, nobles, tradesmen, and landowners were embalmed, a procedure ordinarily neither contemplated by nor available to the average European. The embalming procedure, not surprisingly, was virtually identical to the Egyptian technique described by Herodotus and others, with the exception that far less time was consumed in its execution.

One of the best accounts of nonanatomical embalming for burial purposes is related by the Dutch physician Peter Forestus (1522–1597), who wrote about embalming. His account, in German, is contained as an appendix in the 1605 edition of Peter Offenbach's treatise on *Wound Surgery*. Forestus specifically described the embalming process and the materials used in five named cases between 1410 and 1548, two of which he personally performed:

1410   Pope Alexander V of Bologna, Italy
1511   Lady Johanna of Burgundy, Holland
1537   Bishop Magoluetus of Bologna, Italy
1582   Countess of Hautekerken of The Hague, Holland
1584   Princess Auracius of Holland

As these cases are essentially similar, only one embalming report is cited in its entirety.

Most of the above embalmings were performed in the room of the residence where the death occurred, a practice rather commonly followed later (well into the 20th century) in many countries including the United States.

The following is the full description of the Forestus embalming of the Countess of Hautekerken. The others listed are quite similar with some individual variations such as opening the cranium and removing the brain and making long and deep incisions in the extremities to press out the blood, then filling the incisions with the powdered mixture.

> I personally was bidden to embalm the Countess of Hautekerken, who was a daughter of a nobleman of Egmont (Holland) and who died of childbirth on January 9, 1582 at The Hague (Holland) before Johannes Heurnius (1543–1604), my good friend, and professor at Leyden in Holland was asked. Preceding all things, before the embalment was begun, there was made the following preparation . . . I took $2\frac{1}{2}$ lbs. aloes; myrrh, $1\frac{1}{2}$ lbs.; ordinary wermut, seven handsfull; rosemary, four handsfull, pumice, $1\frac{1}{2}$ lbs.; majoran, 4 lbs.; storacis calamata, 2 loht; the zeltlinalipta muscata, $\frac{1}{2}$ loht. Mix all and reduce to a powder. Lay open the trunk of the body, remove all the viscera, afterwards take such sponges which were previously immersed in cold fresh water, afterwards dipped in aqua vita, and wash out the interior of the body by hand with the sponge. This having been done, fill the cavities (of the body) with a layer of cotton moistened in aqua vita; sprinkle over it a layer of the previously mentioned powders; place another layer of the moistened cotton and a layer of powder one over the other until the abdomen together with the chest is entirely full. Afterwards sew the above (abdominal walls) again together. Wrap around (the body) with waxed cloth and other things. Now having heard this you understand this embalment was performed by me, the aforementioned Heurnius and Arnold the Surgeon on January 10, 1562, in the dwelling of the wellborn Count and Countess Von Wassenaer in The Hague.

Ambroise Pare (1510–1590)

Born in France, Ambroise Pare was military barber–surgeon and eventually surgeon to French kings Henri II, Francois II, and Charles IX. He was famous for rediscovery and improvement of use of ligature to control bleeding after amputations, podalic version (changing the position of an unborn infant within the uterus) to facilitate delivery, and designing of artificial limbs. Pare, like many surgeons of the period, embalmed the bodies of prominent military leaders and noblemen killed during military campaigns as well as similarly prominent civilians dying of natural causes.

In one of his books written in 1585 and entitled *Apology and Account of His Journeys into Diverse Places*, Pare described embalming a follower of the Duke of Savoy, a Monsier de Martiques who died following a gunshot wound through the chest received in battle. The embalming was followed by coffining and transportation to the home of the deceased.

In his book *The Works of Ambroise Pare*, translated into English and published in London in 1634, he devotes a portion of the 28th chapter On the Manner Howe to Embalme the Dead:

> But the body which is to be embalmed with spices for very long continuance must first of all be embowelled, keeping the heart apart, that it may be embalmed and kept as the kinsfolkes shall thinke fit. Also the braine, the scull being divided with a saw, shall be taken out. Then shall you make deepe incisions along the armes, thighes, legges, backe, loynes, and buttockes, especially where the greater veines and arteries runne, first that by this means the blood may be pressed forth, which otherwise would putrifie and give occasion and beginning to putrefaction to the rest of the body; and then that there may be space to put in the aromaticke powders; and then the whole body shall be washed over with a spunge dipped in aqua vita and strong vinegar, wherein shall be boyled wormewood, aloes, coloquintida, common salt and alume. Then these incisions, and all the passages and open places of the body and the three bellyes shall be stuffed with the following spices grossely powdered. Rx pul rosar, chamomile, balsami, menthe, anethi, salvia, lavend, rorismar, marjoran, thymi, absinthi, cyperi, calami aromat, gentiana, ireosflorent, assacederata, caryophyll, nucis moschat, cinamoni, styracis, calamita, benjoini, myrrha, aloes, santel, omnium quod sut ficit. Let the incisions be sowed up and the open spaces that nothing fall out; then forthwith let the whole body be anointed with turpentine, dissolved oyle of roses and chamomile, adding if you shall thinke it fit, some chymicall oyles of spices, and then let it be againe strewed over with the forementioned powder; then wrap it in a linnen cloath, and then in cearecloathes. Lastly, let be put in a coffin of lead, sure soudred and filled up with dry sweete hearbes. But if

there be no plenty of the forementioned spices, as it usuall happens in besieged townes, the chirurgion shall be contented with the powder of quenched lime, common ashes made of oake wood.

The procedure described by Pare was the most prevalent in use from the end of the Egyptian system to well past the discovery of arterial injection.

Discovery of a New Technique

Anatomical dissection, nonpreservative injections, and study continued until inevitably the technique of arterial injection of some preservative substance into the blood vascular system to secure an embalmed subject was stumbled upon. Contrary to popular belief, three men, all Dutch and all friends, were involved and must be recognized for their contributions to the technique: Jan Swammerdam (1637–1680), the original inventor or discoverer; Frederick Ruysch (1638–1731), the great practitioner who refined the technique; and Stephen Blanchard (1650–1720), the person who openly published the method.

Swammerdam was educated in medicine but devoted the greatest part of his life to the study of insects and small animals. He perfected a system of injection to preserve even insects through tiny cannulas made of glass and manipulated by the aid of microscopes designed by Leeuwenhoek (the inventor of the microscope). His preservatives were said to have included various forms of alcohol, turpentine, wine, rum, spirits of wine (purer form of alcohol), and colored waxes. This injection technique was transmitted to Ruysch who applied it to human subjects, both entire bodies and portions thereof. His superb collections of anatomical specimens provided great teaching aids. His embalming of complete human remains included individuals such as British Admiral Sir William Berkley, who was killed during a sea battle off Holland in 1666, and whose body was recovered from the sea in a decomposing condition. Ruysch was requested by the Dutch government to embalm the body so that it might be returned to England for funeral and burial. It is said that the body was normal in appearance and color after his treatment.

In another episode the Russian Czar Peter the Great, during one of his visits to western Europe, visited the medical school of Leiden, Holland, and Ruysch's home, where his museum was situated. During the visit with Ruysch, it is related that some domestic problem required Ruysch's attention and he left Czar Peter alone for a few minutes. Czar Peter began to explore the various rooms and, in opening one door, discovered an infant apparently asleep. Tiptoeing into the room he contemplated the beautiful pink child, then bent down and kissed it, only to discover by its cold exterior that it was one of Ruysch's many preparations. Czar Peter purchased one

entire museum collection from Ruysch which some historians report was lost or destroyed. The truth is that it is still on exhibit in Leningrad today. Ruysch personally never did make a full disclosure of his technique or preservative. There are many who conjecture that his preservative was alcohol, turpentine, or even arsenic.

Blanchard, an anatomist of Leiden, published a book in 1688 entitled *A New Anatomy with Concise Directions for Dissection of the Human Body with a New Method of Embalming.* Pages 281 to 287 and several diagrams of syringes and instruments constitute the appendix describing his method of embalming. He mentions the use of spirits of wine and turpentine. In one of his embalming treatments, he began by flushing out the intestinal tract by first forcing water from the mouth to the anus. Then he repeated the flushing with spirits of wine and retained it in place by corking the rectum. He opened large veins and arteries and flushed out the blood with water, then injected the preservative spirits of wine. (**This technique described in the book appears to be the earliest mention of injection of the blood vessels for the specific purpose of embalming.**)

Ludwig De Bils (1624–1671)

Ludwig De Bils was a Flemish anatomist and resident of Leiden who was also an embalmer. As with Ruysch, he never divulged his embalming methods and is said to have gone to great lengths to prevent accidental discovery of his method by visitors to his museum. Gabriel Clauderus, while viewing De Bils' specimens, shrewdly moistened his forefinger and applied it to the skin of an embalmed body and, tasting the moistened finger, disclosed a salty flavor which led Clauderus to suspect that the principal ingredient in De Bils' fluid was salt. De Bils wrote several books on the subject of embalming but failed to disclose his methods.

Gabriel Clauderus (Late 17th Century)

Gabriel Clauderus, a physician from Altenburg, Germany, was a contemporary of De Bils. In 1695 he published a book, *Methodus Balsamundi Corpora Humani, Alique Majora Sine Evisceratione,* in which he described his method of embalming, which omitted evisceration. His fluid was made from 1 pound of ashes of tartar dissolved in 6 pounds of water, to which was added $\frac{1}{2}$ pound of sal ammoniac. After filtration it was ready for use and was denominated by Clauderus as his "balsamic spirit." He injected this fluid into the cavities of the body and then immersed the cadaver in the fluid for 6 to 8 weeks. The treatment was concluded by drying the corpse either in the sun or in a stove.

England's Customs and Achievements

Although the British Isles are geographically grouped with Europe, they developed different customs and their scientific achievements advanced at a pace different from that in continental Europe.

Some individuals regard the Company of Barber–Surgeons of London to be the first group licensed to embalm. A brief examination of the background of this organization reveals that from about 1300 to 1540 the Company of Barbers and the Guild of Surgeons were separate entities. In 1540 they received a charter from Henry VIII consolidating these two groups under the title of the Company of Barber–Surgeons and granting them the right to anatomize four executed criminals each year. In 1565 Queen Elizabeth I granted the same privilege to the College of Physicians. In 1745 the Surgeons and Barbers ended their joint relationship and again became two separate organizations. During the Barber–Surgeons period they were permitted to be the sole agency for embalming and for performing anatomical dissections in the city of London, although there is no record of any of the bodies for anatomy being embalmed.

This was never a well-respected or enforced monopoly. In their 200-year existence there were fewer than ten complaints, and in several of the cases cited in the College of Barber–Surgeons records, no fines or other punishment is noted. In several cases no conclusion of the case appears. Most complaints were lodged against members for performing private anatomical dissections not on the premises of the College. The more influential members such as William Cheselden and John Ramby simply ignored the rule and even withdrew from the organization as William Hunter did. (**The barber–surgeons made no progress in the development of licensing of embalmers as such and even today in the British Isles, no license or permit is needed from any governmental agency to perform embalming and never has been so required.**)

William Hunter, M.D.

William Hunter (1718–1783) was born in Scotland and studied medicine at the University of Glasgow and at Edinburgh. He finally settled in London where he specialized in the practice of obstetrics and taught anatomy. He became one of the great teachers of anatomy in English medical history and received many awards and appointments to honor societies, climaxed in 1764 by his appointment as Physician-Extraordinary to Queen Charlotte of England. He was the author of many brilliant treatises on medical subjects, perhaps the greatest being his *Anatomy of the Gravid Uterus*. His private collections of anatomical and pathological specimens, together with his lecture and dissecting rooms, occupied a portion of his home. All of this, plus a large sum of money, were donated to the University of Glasgow after his death.

Hunter was in the habit of delivering, at his private school at the close of the anatomical lectures, an account of the preparation of anatomical specimens and em-

balming of corpses. He injected the femoral artery with a solution composed of oil of turpentine, to which had been added Venice turpentine; oil of chamomile; and oil of lavender, to which had been added a portion of vermillion dye. This mixture was forced into the body until the skin exhibited a red appearance. After a few hours during which the body lay undisturbed, the thoracic and abdominal cavities were opened, the viscera were removed, and the fluid was squeezed out of them. The viscera were separately arterially injected and bathed in camphorated spirits of wine. The body was again injected from the aorta and the cavities were washed with camphorated spirits of wine. The viscera were returned to the body, intermixed with powder composed of camphor, resin, and niter, and placed in the eyes, ears, nostrils, and other cavities. The entire skin surface of the body was then rubbed with the "essential" oils of rosemary and lavender. The body was placed in a box on a bed of plaster of Paris for about 4 years. When the box was reopened, and if desiccation appeared imperfect, a bed of gypsum was added to complete the process.

One of Hunter's admonitions to his students, which is still applicable to attainment of the finest results, was to begin the embalming process within 8 hours of the death in the summer and within 24 hours in the winter.

Until the wartime aerial bombing of the Royal College of Surgeons Museum in 1941, the embalmed body of the wife of eccentric dentist Martin Van Butchell, a pupil of William Hunter, was on exhibition. There was a letter in Van Butchell's handwriting describing the embalming process. It is reproduced here verbatim:

12–Jan.–1775: At one half past two this morning my wife died. At eight this morning the statuary took off her face in plaster. At half past two this afternoon Mr. Cruikshank injected at the crural arteries five pints of oil of turpentine mixed with Venice turpentine and vermillion.

15–Jan.: At nine this morning Dr. Hunter and Mr. Cruikshank began to open and embalm my wife. Her diseases were a large empyema in the left lung (which would not receive any air), accompanied with pleuropneumony and much adhesion. The right lung was also beginning to decay and had some pus in it. The spleen was hard and much contracted; the liver diseased, called rata malphigi. The stomach was very sound. The kidneys, uterus, bladder and intestines were in good order. Injected at the large arteries oil of turpentine mixed with camphored spirits, i.e., ten ounces camphor to a quart of spirits, so as to make the whole vascular system turgid; put into the belly part six pounds of rosin powder, three pounds camphor and three pounds niter powder mixed rec. spirit.

17–Jan.: I opened the abdomen to put in the remainder of the powders and added four pounds of rosin, three pounds niter and one pound camphor. In all there were ten pounds rosin, six pounds niter and four pounds camphor, twenty pounds of powder mixed with spirits of wine.

18–Jan.: Dr. Hunter and Mr. Cruikshank came at nine this morning and put my wife into the box on and in 130 pounds of Paris plaster at eighteen d. a bag. I put between the thighs three arquebusade bottles, one full of camphored spirits, very rich of the gum, containing eight ounces of oil of rosemary, and in the other two ounces of lavender.

19–Jan.: I closed up the joints of the box lid and glasses with Paris plaster mixed with gum water and spirits wine.

25–Jan.: Dr. Hunter came with Sir Thos. Wynn and his lady.

7–Feb.: Dr. Hunter came with Sir John Pringle, Dr. Heberden, Dr. Watson and about twelve more fellows of The Royal Society.

11–Feb.: Dr. Hunter came with Dr. Solander, Dr. ——, Mr. Banks and another gentleman. I unlocked the glasses to clean the face and legs with spirits of wine and oil of lavender.

12–Feb.: Dr. Hunter came to look at the neck and shoulders.

13–Feb.: I put four ounces of camphored spirits into the box and on both sides of neck and six pounds of plaster.

16–Feb.: I put four ounces oil of lavender, an ounce of rosemary and $\frac{1}{2}$ ounces of oil of camomile flowers (the last cost four Sh.) on sides of the face and three ounces of very dry camomile flowers on the breast, neck, and shoulders.

(The body was said to resemble a Guanche or Peruvian mummy and was very dry and shrunken.)

John Hunter, M.D.

John Hunter (1728–1793) was born in Scotland, the younger brother of William Hunter, in whose anatomy classes he first proved so adept. After studying under the great surgeons of his time he was appointed to hospital staffs and lectured on anatomy. A region of the body he described was named in his honor: "Hunter's canal." He served as a surgeon in the British army during the campaign in Portugal (1761–1763) and, on his discharge from the service, settled in general practice in London. There he continued the collection and study of anatomical and natural subjects. He was a most brilliant and prolific writer on all phases of medicine and surgery and later founded his own private anatomy classes, which were unexcelled for the number of students who later distinguished themselves in medicine. Among these students were Jenner, Abernathy, Carlisle, Chevalier, Cline, Coleman, Astley Cooper, Home, Lynn, and Macartney.

In 1776 Hunter was honored by appointment as Surgeon-Extraordinary to the King of England. In 1782 he constructed a museum between his two homes in London to house his anatomical and natural history collections. These eventually contained nearly 14,000 items, and at his death were purchased by the British government for the Royal College of Surgeons. The main exhibit hall, measuring 52 by 28 feet, was lighted from above and had a gallery for visitors.

Many stories are told of body stealing for dissection and for securing specimens for collections. None would better illustrate this than John Hunter's acquisition in 1783 of the body of the Irish giant O'Brien, at a cost to him of about $2500.00. O'Brien, about 7 feet 7 inches in height and dreading dissection by Hunter had, shortly before his death, arranged with several of his friends that his corpse be conveyed by them to the sea and sunk in deep water. The undertaker, who it was said had entered into a pecuniary agreement with Hunter, managed that while the escort was drinking at a certain stage of the journey to the sea the coffin should be locked in a barn. Confederates, which the undertaker had concealed in the barn, speedily substituted an equivalent weight of stones for the body. At night, O'Brien's body was forwarded to Hunter who took it immediately to his museum, where it was dissected and boiled to procure the bones. The skeleton was on exhibit until May 1941, when three fourths of the museum of the Royal College of Surgeons, London, was destroyed by German bombers. Joshua Reynold's portrait of John Hunter displays the huge skeletal feet of O'Brien in the background.

Matthew Baillie

Baillie (1761–1823) was a nephew of William and John Hunter. He was educated by his uncles and became famous as a physician and writer on medical subjects. He modified the Hunterian method of embalming so as to provide as good preservation as ever in a shorter period. Using a solution of oil of turpentine, Venice turpentine, oil of chamomile, and oil of lavender (to which was added vermillion dye) he injected the femoral artery. He allowed several hours of elapse before he opened the body as in a postmortem examination and made a small incision in the bowel below the stomach, into which he inserted a small piece of pipe through which he introduced water to wash out the contents of the bowels. Then, ligating the rectum above the anus and the small bowel below the stomach, he filled the intestinal track with camphorated spirits of wine. The lungs were filled with camphorated spirits of wine via the trachea. The bladder was opened and emptied of its contents and a powder of camphor, resin, and niter was dusted over the viscera and the incision was closed. The eyeballs were pierced and emptied of their contents and repacked to normal with the powder mixture, as were the mouth and ears. The body was rubbed with oil of rosemary or lavender and placed on a bed of deep plaster.

Europe's Access to Cadavers

Continental European countries such as France, Germany, and Italy did not encounter the problems in supplying medical schools with cadavers as existed in Great Britain. Medical schools had access to bodies unclaimed for burial, a situation not present in the British Isles until after passage of the **Warburton Act in 1832.** The problem in continental Europe was different, consisting of securing a means to preserve cadavers for dissection with nonpoisonous chemicals. In France, for example, medical schools in the north had scheduled anatomical dissection classes during the cold months of the year as the cadavers were unembalmed.

By the late 18th and early 19th centuries, France and Italy had a number of different techniques and chemicals for embalming proposed by members of the medical or scientific communities.

Baron Leopold Cuvier (1769–1828) of France was a comparative anatomist whose classification of mammals and birds forms the groundwork for present-day systems. Cuvier advocated the use of pure alcohol as a preservative agent.

Francois Chaussier (1746–1828) of France recommended immersion of an eviscerated body in a solution of bichloride of mercury for preservation.[*]

Louis Jacques Thenard (1777–1857) of France was a brilliant teacher of and researcher in chemistry. He discovered the nature of hydrogen peroxide and made a study of human bile and the preservative action of bichloride of mercury. In 1834 he advocated introduction of an alcoholic solution of bichloride of mercury into the blood vessels to preserve cadavers for anatomical dissection.

G. Tranchina (also spelled Tranchini or Franchini) of early-19th-century Naples, Italy, openly advocated and successfully used arsenical solutions, arterially injected, to preserve bodies for both funeral and anatomical purposes. Tranchini's method of embalming varied, but the fluid was usually composed of 1 pound of arsenic dissolved in 5 pounds of alcoholic wine. He usually injected 2 gallons of this solution into the femoral artery without drainage of blood. At other times he injected the same amount into the right common carotid artery, sending the fluid first toward the head and then downward toward the body, allowing some drainage through the jugular vein. This was followed by incision of the abdomen, opening and emptying of the bowels, and moistening of the bowels with the injecting solution. The lungs were filled with the fluid via the trachea. A body prepared in this manner is said to have completely dried in 6 weeks.

J. P. Sucquet of France (mid-19th century) was one of the earliest proponents of the use of zinc chloride as a preservative agent. He injected about 5 quarts of a 20% solution of zinc chloride in water through the popliteal artery and also introduced some of this solution into the abdomen. One body prepared in this way was buried for 2 years, then disinterred and found to be in an excellent state of preservation. About 1845 an agent representing Sucquet sold the U.S. rights to his method and chemical to Chas. D. Brown and Joseph Alexander of New York City.

Jean Nicolas Gannal (1791–1852), a chemist in France (Fig. 5), began his life's work as an apothecary's assistant. From 1808 to 1812 he served in the medical department of the French Army, including the Russian campaign under Napoleon. After his discharge from the army he reentered the field of chemistry and was appointed assistant to the great French chemistry teacher Thenard. He later became interested in industrial chemistry and did research on methods of refining borax and improving the quality of glues and gelatins. In 1827 he was awarded the Montyon science prize for developing a method of treating catarrh and tuberculosis with chlorine gas. In 1831 he was asked to devote his time to de-

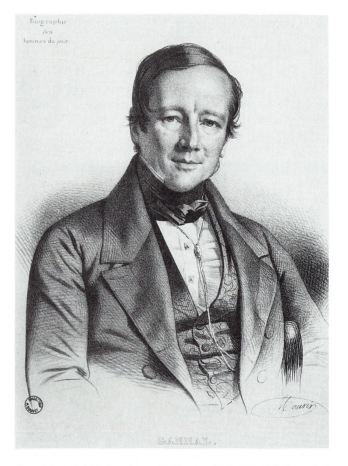

Figure 5. Portrait of J. N. Gannal at age 40. (*Courtesy of Ordre National de Pharmacien.*)

---

[*]**Bull. Hist. Med.** 1957; 30(5, Sept–Oct.): "Medicine in 16th Century New Spain," by Saul Jarcho, contains frequent mention of corrosive sublimate as a disinfectant for wounds.

vising an improved method of preserving cadavers for anatomical purposes. Close application to the problem resulted in success, which was recognized in 1836 by the award to Gannal of a second Montyon science prize.

His experiments included the use of solutions of acids (acetic–arsenous–nitric–hydrochloric), alkali salts (copper–mercury–alum), tannin–creosote–alcohol, and various combinations such as alum, sodium chloride, and nitrate of potash, and acetate of alumina and the chloride of alumina, the latter of which obliterated the lumen of blood vessels. His perfected method of embalming cadavers for anatomical purposes comprised the injection of about 6 quarts of a solution of acetate of alumina through the carotid artery without drainage of any blood. No evisceration or other treatment was used, although occasionally the bodies were immersed in the injecting solution until ready for dissection. Gannal used practically the same solution for embalming bodies for funeral purposes, although he did add a small quantity of arsenic and carmine to the solution. He injected about 2 gallons of this mixture, first upward and then downward in the carotid artery in less than one-half hour. No special treatment was given to the trunk viscera. In his book *History of Embalming*, he cited case histories of bodies he had embalmed and subsequently disinterred from 3 to 13 months after burial. Gannal states that in every such case the body was found in exactly the same state of preservation and appearance as when buried.

Gannal was involved in several precedent-making events. In mid-April 1840, a Paris newspaper published the following article:

> The young boy found murdered in a field near Villete not having been recognized and the process of decomposition having commenced, the Magistrates ordered it to be embalmed by M. Gannal's simple method of injection through the carotid arteries, so that this evidence of the crime may remain producible. This is the first operation of the kind performed by order of the Justices, and it was completed in a quarter of an hour.

In his translation of Gannal's *History of Embalming* (1840) (Fig. 6), Harlan mentions that the Paris police have access to Gannal's embalming process to preserve bodies in the Paris morgue where murder has been suspected.

Gannal was indirectly responsible for the passage of the first law prohibiting the use of arsenic in embalming solutions in 1846 (to which the use of bichloride of mercury was also prohibited in 1848).

There are several versions of the story. In one, Gannal had omitted stating that a portion of arsenic was added to his alumina salts embalming chemical, and when this solution was analyzed and arsenic found, the medical community was enraged and compelled the law to

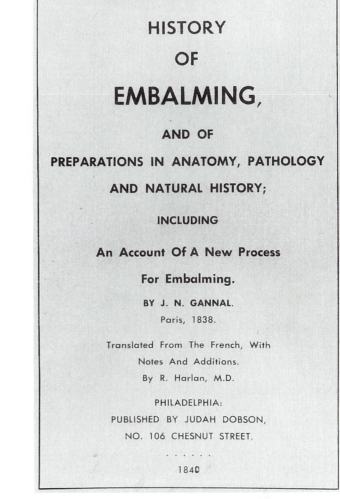

HISTORY
OF
EMBALMING,

AND OF

PREPARATIONS IN ANATOMY, PATHOLOGY

AND NATURAL HISTORY;

INCLUDING

An Account Of A New Process

For Embalming.

BY J. N. GANNAL.

Paris, 1838.

Translated From The French, With
Notes And Additions.
By R. Harlan, M.D.

PHILADELPHIA:
PUBLISHED BY JUDAH DOBSON,
NO. 106 CHESNUT STREET.

. . . . . .

1840

Figure 6. Title page of Harlan's translation of the *History of Embalming*.

be decreed. The other tale, never documented, relates that Gannal was retained to embalm the corpse of a member of the nobility who died suddenly. The members of the nobleman's family accused the decedent's mistress of poisoning him with arsenic. Under French law she was arrested and tried, the burden of her defense on her shoulders. Gannal followed the progress of the trial in the Paris newspapers and noted that the accused mistress was unable to prove her innocence. Finally, at the last possible moment, Gannal appeared at the trial and requested permission to testify in her behalf. He states that in his opinion the arsenic found in the body tissues of the deceased came there during the embalming with his embalming solution, as it contained arsenic . She was freed and the legal community petitioned for the abolition of arsenic in embalming solutions.

Gannal had two sons, Adolphe Antoine and Felix, who became physicians and continued the embalming practice after his death. They embalmed many famous people including De Lessups, who constructed the Suez Canal. The sons died in the early 1900s.

Richard Harlan (1796–1843) of Philadelphia, Pennsylvania, graduated from the Pennsylvania Medical College in 1818 and was placed in charge of Joseph Parrish's private anatomical dissection rooms in Philadelphia. After engaging in various projects in company with other Philadelphia physicians he became a member of the city health council. In 1838 he traveled to Europe and spent a portion of his time in Paris visiting various medical facilities and meeting local savants, among whom was J. N. Gannal. After being presented with a copy of Gannal's *History of Embalming,* he became so fascinated with it that he requested and received permission to publish an American edition translated into English. **The book, published in Philadelphia in 1840, became the first book devoted entirely to embalming procedures that was published in the United States in English** (Fig. 6).

Other Physicians and Anatomists

Girolamo Segato. A physician of Florence, Italy (17th century), Segato is known to have converted the human body to stone by infiltrating the bodily tissues with a solution of silicate of potash and succeeded this treatment by immersion of the body in a weak acid solution. The exact modus operandi is unknown.

Thomas Joseph Pettigrew. A London physician and surgeon, graduate of Guys Hospital, and fellow of the Royal College of Surgeons, Pettigrew (1791–1865) was one of the great historians of the science of embalming . His treatise *History of Egyptian Mummies,* published in London in 1834, is a masterpiece revealing Pettigrew's ability to accurately observe and minutely describe objects and processes of interest to students and practitioners of the art of embalming. This volume is to this day considered one of the fine works on Egyptian embalming methods and customs. In 1854 he withdrew from the practice of medicine and devoted his entire energy to the study of archaeology.

Dr. Falconry. A French physician of the mid-19th century, Falconry employed a means of preservation of cadavers for anatomical purposes that is of interest because of its simplicity. The corpse was placed on a bed of dry sawdust to which about a gallon of powdered zinc sulfate had been added. No injections, incisions, baths, or any additional treatment was used. The bodies so treated were said to have remained flexible for about 40 days, after which time they dried and assumed the appearance of mummies.

Thomas Marshall, M.D. Marshall was a London physician who published an account of a means of embalming in the *London Medical Gazette* in December 1839. His technique consisted of generously puncturing the body surface with needles or scissors and repeatedly brushing the body surface with strong acetic acid. A diluted acetic acid solution was introduced into the cavities of the body. The author claimed that the acetic acid would restore normal color even to gangrenous tissue.

Dr. John Morgan (Circa 1863). A professor of anatomy at the University of Dublin, Morgan made use of two principles that are widely recognized as necessary to achieve the best embalming results: (1) the use of the largest possible artery for injection and (2) the use of force or pressure to push the preserving fluid through the blood vessels. Also noted are his use of a preinjection solution (the earliest mention found) and his controlled technique of drainage. Morgan cut the sternum down its center, opened the pericardium to expose the heart, made an incision into the left ventricle or into the aorta, and inserted a piece of pipe about 8 inches long. This injecting pipe was connected by 15 feet of tubing to a fluid container that was maintained 12 feet above the corpse, thereby producing about 5 pounds of pressure (Fig. 7).

The tip of the right auricular appendage was clipped off to allow blood drainage. The first injection was composed of $\frac{1}{2}$ gallon of a saturated salt solution to which was added 4 ounces of niter. After this solution was allowed to "rush" through the circulatory system, a clamp was

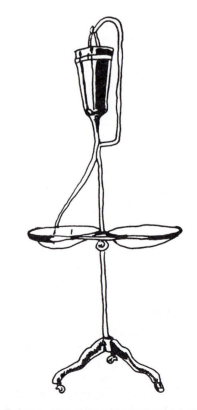

Figure 7. Gravity fluid injector. The jar filled with arterial chemical could be elevated several feet above the corpse, thus creating pressure for injection. *(Courtesy of Paula Johnson De Smet.)*

fastened over the auricular appendage when the drainage stopped. Several more gallons of a solution of common salt, niter, alum, and arsenate of potash was injected until the body was thoroughly saturated with the fluid. No special treatment of the internal organs or viscera was mentioned.

At this time there was virtually no embalming of the dead for funeral purposes available for the largest percentage of deaths. Many books were written regarding the dangers to the living of exposure to the dead buried or entombed (unembalmed) in churches or in city cemeteries. There was also concern for those who handled the dead.

Bernardino Ramazzini. The founder of occupational medicine, Ramazzini (1633–1714) wrote the *Diseases of Workers* in 1700, and an enlarged edition of that text was published in 1713. The latter edition contained a chapter on the Disease of Corpse Bearers.

Numerous publications varying in size from leaflets to bound books were printed inveighing against existing burial practices. A few relevant titles are *Considerations on the Indecent and Dangerous Custom of Burying in Churches and Churchyards etc.*, 1721, London, A. Batesworth; *Blame of Kirk Burial, Tending to Persuade Cemeterial Civility*, 1606 NP, Rev. William Birnie; *Gatherings from Graveyards, Particularly Those of London etc.*, 1830, G. A. Walker, surgeon, London; and *Sepulture, History, Methods and Sanitary Requisites*, 1884, Stephen Wickes, Philadelphia. The astonishing accounts contained in these or similar works should convince even the most skeptical opponent of embalming of the sanitary value of the embalming process.

From Europe to the Colonies

The transfer of embalming knowledge from Europe to the colonies in what today is the United States was accomplished by several means.

Anatomical study in the colonies as early as 1676 in Boston and again in 1750 recorded that "Drs. John Bard and Peter Middleton injected and dissected the body of an executed criminal for the instruction of young men engaged in the study of medicine." In 1752 the *N.Y. Weekly Postboy* carried an advertisement offering anatomy instruction by Dr. Thomas Wood. From 1754 to 1756, William Hunter, physician and student of the famed anatomy teacher Alexander Monroe I of Edinburgh, Scotland (and a relative of the Hunter Brothers), lectured on anatomy at Newport, Rhode Island. Doctors William Shippen and John Morgan of Philadelphia studied medicine in Europe and anatomy under British anatomists. On their return to the United States between 1762 and 1765 they became engaged in

teaching medical subjects, especially anatomy, in Philadelphia.

In 1840 the translation of Gannal's book *The History of Embalming* into English was to provide the first text in English printed in the United States devoted to embalming. In the mid-1840s the acquisition of Sucquet's embalming technique and chemicals as a franchise by Dr. Charles D. Brown and Dr. Joseph Alexander of New York City added to the increasing amount of embalming knowledge transferred to the United States.

MODERN PERIOD

By the year 1861 and the onset of the Civil War, the transfer of embalming knowledge from Europe to the United States was virtually concluded. A small group of medically trained embalmers existed together with printed information such as Harlan's translation of Gannal's textbook and various European embalming formulas and techniques that had been acquired.

Until the Civil War, however, little or no embalming was performed for funeral purposes. Most preservation, such as it was, for brief periods was provided by ice refrigeration when available.

With the outbreak of the Civil War in April 1861, there began the raising of troops by the North and South to prosecute the war. Little if any embalming was available to the Southerners during the war. Virtually all embalming was done by Northerners. As Washington, DC, was the capital city of the North, it became a center for troop concentration both to protect the city and to serve as a marshalling point for the armies moving against the south.

Northern troops composed of individual companies from small geographical areas and regiments from individual states as disparate as Vermont and Maine, Minnesota and Wisconsin, and Ohio, Pennsylvania, and New York crowded into the Washington, DC, area. Civilian embalmers Dr. Thomas Holmes, William J. Bunnell, Dr. Charles Da Costa Brown, Dr. Joseph B. Alexander, Dr. Richard Burr, Dr. Daniel H. Prunk, Frank A. Hutton, G. W. Scollay, C. B. Chamberlain, Henry P. Cattell, Dr. Benjamin Lyford, Samuel Rodgers, Dr. E. C. Lewis, W. P. Cornelius, and Prince Greer are known to have embalmed during the Civil War. There are others who, to this day, remain anonymous.

None of the embalming surgeons, as they were called, were ever employed in the military as embalmers. Some had been or would become military surgeons but did not perform embalming while in the military service.

Civil War Times

At the beginning of the Civil War, as in all previous wars fought by the United States, there was no provision for return of the dead to their homes. In the Seminole Indian Wars (during the 1830s), the Mexican War (1846–1848), and the campaigns against the Indians up to the outbreak of the Civil War, the military dead were buried in the field near where they fell in battle. It was possible for the relatives to have the remains returned to their home for local burial under certain conditions:

1. The next of kin was to request the disinterment and return of the body in a written request to the Quartermaster General.
2. On military authority confirmation that the burial place was known and disinterment could be effected, the family was advised to send a coffin capable of being hermetically sealed to a designated Quartermaster Officer nearest the place of burial.
3. Such Quartermaster Officer would provide a force of men to take the coffin to the grave, disinter the remains, and place them in the coffin and seal it. The coffined remains would then be returned to the place of ultimate reinterment.

During the early days of the Civil War and less frequently as the war dragged on, some family members of the deceased personally went to hospitals and battlefields to search for their dead and bring them home for burial. Civil War embalming was carried out with a variety of chemicals and techniques. Arterial embalming was applied when possible. An artery, usually the femoral or carotid, was raised and injected without any venous drainage in most cases. Usually, no cavity treatment was administered. When arterial embalming was believed impossible because of the nature of wounds or decomposition, other means of preparation of the body for transport were resorted to. In some cases the trunk was eviscerated and the cavity filled with sawdust or powdered charcoal or lime. The body was then placed in a coffin completely imbedded in sawdust or similar material. In other cases, the body was coffined as mentioned without evisceration.

Chemicals employed during the Civil War were totally self-manufactured by the embalmer and included, as basic preservatives, arsenicals, zinc chloride, bichloride of mercury, salts of alumina, sugar of lead, and a host of salts, alkalies and acids. An example of fluid manufacture of one of the most popular embalming chemicals, zinc chloride, was the immersion of sheets of zinc in hydrochloric acid until a saturated solution was obtained. The resulting zinc chloride solution was injected without further dilution. Many of the injection pumps employed were quite similar to what would be described as greatly enlarged hypodermic syringes. Many required filling of the syringe, attachment of a cannula, emptying of the syringe, unfastening of the syringe, and refilling. It was an extremely slow process! A few pumps were de-

signed to provide continuous flow, aspirating the embalming chemical continuously from a large source into the pump during the injection process. Others, such as the Holmes invention, were designed to fit over a bucket that could hold a gallon or more of liquid.

On May 24, 1861, 24-year-old Colonel Elmer Ellsworth, commander of the 11th N.Y. Volunteer Infantry, was shot to death in Alexandria, Virginia, as he seized a confederate flag displayed atop the Marshall House Hotel. He became the first prominent military figure killed in the war. His body was embalmed by Dr. Thomas Holmes, who had set up an embalming establishment in Washington, DC. Colonel Ellsworth had funeral services in the White House, in New York City, and in Albany, New York, with burial in his home town of Mechanicsburg, New York. His funeral set a pattern to be followed by prominent members of the military, culminating in President Lincoln's historic funeral services. Colonel Ellsworth's embalming and viewable appearance were widely and favorably commented on in the press and did much to familiarize the previously uninformed public with embalming.

The Army issued only two sets of orders relative to fatal casualties in the early stages of the war. On September 11, 1861, War Department General Order 75 directed the Quartermaster Department to supply all general and post hospitals with blank books and forms for the preservation of accurate death records and to provide material for headboards to be erected over soldiers' graves. On April 3, 1862, Section II of War Department General Order 33 stated:

> In order to secure as far as possible the decent interment of those who have fallen, or may fall in battle, it is made the duty of commanding generals to lay off lots of ground in some suitable spot near every battlefield, as soon as it may be in their power, and to cause the remains of those killed to be interred, with headboards to the graves bearing numbers, and when practicable the names of the persons buried in them. A register for each burial ground will be preserved, in which will be noted the marks corresponding with the headboards

This was the origin of what was to become the National Cemetery System.

Embalming Surgeons of the Civil War

Dr. Thomas Holmes (1817–1900). Holmes was born in New York City in 1817 and educated in local public schools and New York University Medical College, though the records of the period are incomplete and document only his attendance, not his graduation. He did practice medicine and was a coroner's physician in New York during the 1850s as numerous newspaper stories attest. He apparently moved to Williamsburg (now Brooklyn) and experimented with a variety of chemicals for embalming and techniques. When the Civil War broke out he opened an embalming office in Washington, DC, and Colonel Ellsworth became his first prominent client. Holmes subsequently embalmed Colonel E. D. Baker, a prominent politician and soldier killed in battle. This case brought more publicity both for Holmes and for embalming (Fig. 8).

Holmes ultimately prepared about 4000 bodies (including 8 generals), and patented many inventions relating to embalming during his lifetime. One in particular, a rubber-coated canvas removal bag, was far ahead of its time (Fig. 9).

When the war ended, Dr. Holmes returned home to Brooklyn and only occasionally practiced embalming. He operated a drugstore and manufactured a variety of products as diverse as embalming fluid and root beer! He invested heavily in a health resort and lost the investment. He wrote little about embalming, did not teach, and had no children. After a serious fall in his home he became periodically psychotic and occasionally required confinement. When he died in 1900 it was said that he wanted no embalming.

William J. Bunnell (1823–1891). Bunnell was born in New Jersey, moved to New York City, and in the 1850s be-

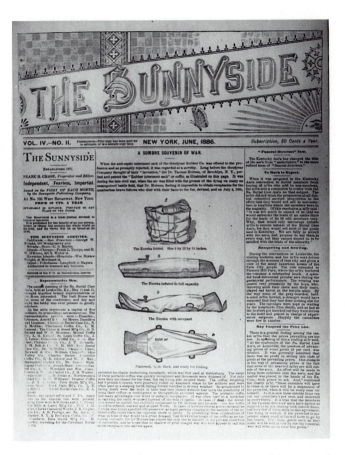

Figure 9. Front page of *The Sunnyside*, June 1886, featuring an article on Holmes's removal bag, citing its all-around utility as a sleeping bag and stretcher, its ability to be inflated as a raft, and, of course, its use as a corpse removal bag or coffin.

came acquainted with Dr. Holmes and married his sister. Dr. Holmes found him employment as an anatomy technician for some New York medical schools while teaching him embalming. When war broke out, Bunnell did not work directly with Dr. Holmes but formed his own Embalming Surgeon's organization with Dr. R. B. Heintzelman from Philadelphia as his active partner. Holmes and Bunnell did occasionally work together during the war at Gettysburg and at City Point, Virginia. After the war, it was reported that Bunnell was practicing medicine briefly in Omaha, Nebraska, and eventually opened an undertaking establishment in Jersey City, New Jersey. He became a marshall at the funeral of General Grant and became prominent in undertakers associations. His son, George Holmes Bunnell (1855–1932), followed his father in the business and was given assistance by his uncle, Dr. Holmes. George H. Bunnell had twin sons: Milton became a funeral director, and Chester became a physician.

Charles Da Costa Brown, Joseph B. Alexander, and Henry P. Cattell. Brown, Alexander, and Cattell were all active in the firm of Brown and Alexander, Embalming Surgeons. It is not

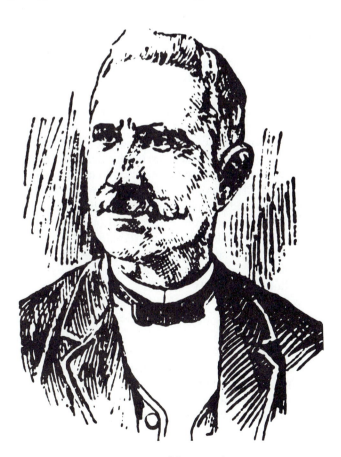

Figure 8. Portrait of Thomas H. Holmes.

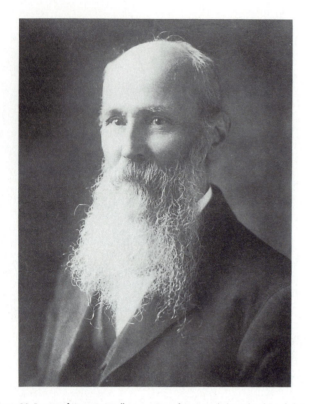

Figure 10. Portrait of Henry P. Cattell, an associate of Brown and Alexander, the embalming surgeons who embalmed Willie Lincoln in 1862 and President Lincoln in 1865.

known whether Brown and Alexander met in New York City in the late 1850s or in Washington, DC, in early wartime. Cattell (Fig. 10) is believed to have been the stepson of Dr. Charles Brown's brother, as his mother married a Brown in 1860. In any event, he entered the employment of the firm that embalmed Willie Lincoln, son of the President Abraham Lincoln, and later embalmed the President himself in 1865. After the war Dr. Brown abandoned embalming, returned to New York City, practiced dentistry, and became very active in the Masonic Lodge. He died in 1896 and is buried in Greenwood Cemetery in Brooklyn.

Alexander died in 1871 in Washington, DC. H. P. Cattell halted his embalming practice after the war, became a lithographer, and then entered the Washington, DC, police force. None of his family was ever aware that he had embalmed President Lincoln. He died in 1915 and is buried in Washington, DC.

Frank A. Hutton. Little is known of Hutton's personal biography. Born in or near Harrisburg, Pennsylvania, about 1835, he was a pharmacist by occupation. He had military service in the 110th Pennsylvania Volunteer Infantry ending in June 1862, was discharged in Washington, DC, and became a partner in the firm of Chamberlain and Hutton, Surgeons. This partnership did not last long and Hutton withdrew in February 1863. He

formed the firm of Hutton and Company with E. A. Williams, son of a Washington, DC, undertaker as his partner. Hutton advertised in the Washington City Directory, taking a full page space to extol his embalming expertise. He was also issued Patent 38,747 for an embalming fluid on June 1, 1863. The formula included alcohol, arsenic, bichloride of mercury, and zinc chloride.

During mid-April 1863, Hutton became embroiled in an argument with a client over charges for shipping his son's body to him. The client complained to Colonel L. C. Baker, provost marshall of the capitol, who, on April 20, 1863, arrested Hutton and seized the contents of his office as evidence. Hutton was confined in the Old Capitol Prison for about 10 days and then released. No details of his release or trial have been found. He subsequently relocated his quarters and continued in business with a much diminished clientele. Hutton is said to have returned to Harrisburg after the war ended and died there within a year.

Daniel H. Prunk (1829–1923). Born in Virginia in 1829, Prunk and his family migrated to Illinois where he attended college. After attending medical school in Cincinnati he began medical practice in Illinois and, in April 1861, moved to Indianapolis where he joined the 19th Indiana Volunteer Infantry as an assistant surgeon in September 1861. He was transferred to the 20th Indiana Volunteer Infantry in June 1862, and was arrested in November of that year and incarcerated in the Old Capitol Prison in Washington, DC, for about 3 months for conduct unbecoming an officer. He was then dismissed from the service. From July to October 1863 he was acting assistant surgeon at the 2nd Division Army Hospital at Nashville, Tennessee, and subsequently requested permission to provide embalming services in Nashville. The request was initially refused but finally granted late in 1863. He eventually had embalming establishments located not only in Nashville but also in Chattanooga nd Knoxville in Tennessee; at East Point, Atlanta, Dalton, and Marietta in Georgia; and at Huntsville in Alabama (Fig. 11).

In 1865 Dr. Prunk was licensed by the Army to practice embalming and undertaking. (He was also engaged in a wholesale grocery business, cotton trading, and money lending.) He made his own embalming fluid by dissolving sheets of zinc in muriatic acid (hydrochloric acid) until a saturated solution of zinc chloride was obtained to which a quantity of arsenious acid was added. The fluid obtained was injected quite warm without dilution or blood drainage.

Prunk sold all his embalming establishments in 1866 and returned to Indianapolis to practice medicine. It seems that he never engaged in embalming after his return to Indianapolis. He made one of the earliest written statements regarding the necessity of cavity treatment in

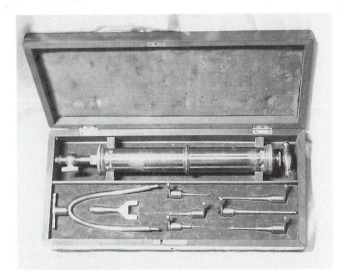

Figure 11. Injection syringe and cannulas of Daniel J. Prunk, Civil War embalming surgeon. *(Courtesy of the Illinois Funeral Directors' Foundation.)*

a letter written in 1872, to Dr. J. P. Buckesto of San Jose, California

> If I were going to ship a corpse from San Jose to New York City, we have advised for sometime the puncturing of the stomach to give vent to gases which accumulate at this time. In a subject with a large abdomen, where the bowels are discolored, the introduction of a couple of quarts into the peritoneal cavity by making a puncture near the umbilicus and throwing a thread of strong silk around it like a drawstring on a button cushion which can be readily closed after you are thru injecting.

Dr. Richard Burr. Although little biographical information other than his rumored origin in Philadelphia is available concerning Burr (who apparently practiced during the period 1862–1865), he has achieved immortality as the embalmer photographed by the Civil War photographer Brady in front of his embalming tent while injecting a subject (Fig. 12). W. J. Bunnell complained about Burr's unprofessional conduct, alleging that, among other things, he set Bunnell's embalming tent on fire! He was also one of the men against whom complaints had been

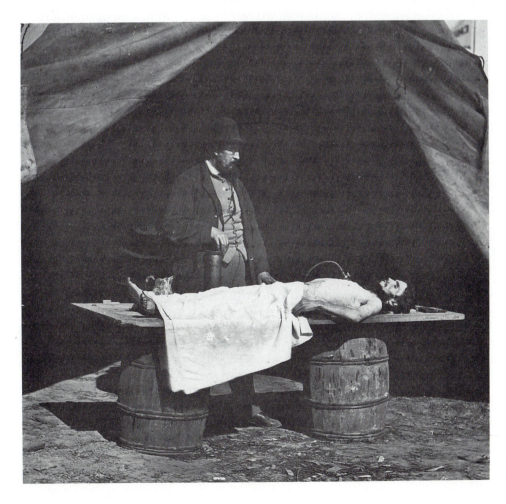

Figure 12. Richard Burr embalming near a battlefield during the Civil War. *(Courtesy of Library of Congress.)*

issued regarding inflated prices and poor services, which resulted in all embalmers' being excluded from military areas by order of General U.S. Grant in January 1865. **This resulted in establishment of the first set of rules and regulations for the licensing of embalmers and undertakers in the United States.**

The final Army order for embalmers contained some of the suggestions made by Dr. Barnes, chief of the Army Medical Service in December 1863, to the effect that a performance bond should be posted by any embalmer desiring to practice. In addition, the requirement stipulated by the Provost Marshall General ordered the embalmer to furnish a list of his prices as charged for work or merchandise to the Provost Marshall General, the medical director of the department, and the Post Provost Marshall.

U.S. Army General Order 39 concerning embalmers (March 15, 1865) read as follows:

1. Hereafter no persons will be permitted to embalm or remove the bodies of deceased officers or soldiers unless acting under the special license of the Provost Marshall of the Army, department, or district in which the bodies may be.
2. Provost marshalls will restrict disinterments to seasons when they can be made without endangering the health of the troops. They will grant licenses only to such persons as furnish proof of skill and ability as embalmers, and will require bonds for the faithful performance of the orders given them. They will also establish a scale of prices by which embalmers are to be governed, with such other regulations as will protect the interest of the friends and relatives of deceased soldiers.
3. Applicants for license will apply directly to the Provost Marshall of the Army or department in which they may desire to pursue their business, submitting in distinct terms the process adopted by them, materials, length of time its preservative effect can be relied on and such other information as may be necessary to establish their proficiency and success. Medical directors will give such assistance in the examination of these applications as may be required by the Provost Marshall.

In the Army of the Cumberland the following additional requirements were stipulated:

1. No disinterments will be permitted within the department between the 15th day of May and the 15th day of October.
2. The following scale of prices will be observed from and after this date: At Nashville and Memphis: for embalming bodies each at $15.00 to disinter, furnish metallic burial cases, well boxed, marked and delivered to the express office each at $75.00, zinc coffins and the above listed services each at $40.00. An additional charge of $5.00 may be made for embalming and also for either of the above styles of coffins at Murfreesboro, Chattanooga, Knoxville, and Huntsville, Alabama, or in the field.
3. No person will be permitted to operate as an embalmer under any license issued to him until he shall have filed a bond in this office in the penal sum of $1000 conditioned for the faithful observance of this order, and for the skillful performance of such works he shall undertake by virtue of his license. [Such licenses were not transferable from one individual to another.]

By 1864 the Armory Square Military Hospital in Washington, DC, had all its deceased patients routinely embalmed and the grave recorded so that the body could be disinterred and sent to family or friends when requested.

C. B. Chamberlain. Chamberlain is said to have Philadelphia as his origin. Although very little is known of the man, he definitely was an early partner of F. A. Hutton. He and Hutton apparently were not compatible, and he formed a new partnership with Ben Lyford. They both can be documented as practicing embalming surgeons on the scene at Gettysburg after the battle. Chamberlain is listed in the Washington, DC, City Directory as late as 1865 as a partner in Chamberlain and Waters Embalmers at 431 Pennsylvania Avenue. He is mentioned by F. C. Beinhauer, Pittsburgh undertaker, as being in the Pittsburgh area prior to and during the Civil War. Joseph H. Clarke also mentioned Chamberlain as a teacher of embalming in the post–Civil War period.

G. W. Scollay. Judging from the various patents issued to him, Scollay was apparently from St. Louis, Missouri. Very little personal information about him has been uncovered. He appeared to be an active embalming surgeon at the Gettysburg battlefield and in the area near Richmond. He has a listing in the 1865 Washington, DC, City Directory as a member of the firm of Scollay and Sands—Embalmers of the Dead. Frank T. Sands was a prominent undertaker in Washington, DC. Scollay patented two methods of embalming in the post–Civil War period, one in January 1867 and the other in October 1869. Both patents involved the use of gaseous compounds injected via the blood vascular system, one of the earliest recommendations for choice of gas rather than a liquid as a preservative introduced into the blood vascular system. In 1860, Scollay patented a two-piece cast glass coffin and, during the war, produced a number of different "sanitary" coffins.

Benjamin F. Lyford. Born in Vermont in 1841 and receiving public school education there, Lyford attended and graduated from Philadelphia University's 6-month course of medical studies. He first appears on the Civil War scene as a partner of C. B. Chamberlain, who provided embalming after the Battle of Gettysburg. Later he had altercations with Provost Marshall General Rudolf Patrick of the Army of the Potomac. This series of disagreements stimulated him to accept appointment on July 13, 1864, as assistant surgeon of the 68th Regiment of Infantry— U.S. Colored Troops. He reported to the unit in Missouri and subsequently served in Memphis. For a time he served as commanding officer of a small cavalry and artillery contingent in southern Alabama.

He returned to his regiment stationed near New Orleans, Louisiana, and went to leave in New Orleans. He was arrested inside a bordello in full uniform and faced court martial charges. Apparently found innocent of the charges, he was discharged from the Army on February 5, 1866, traveled to San Francisco, and opened an office for medical practice. One of his early patients was a wealthy widowed landowner who had an attractive daughter whom he fell in love with and married. The mother owned large tracts of land in Marin County across the bay north of San Francisco. Lyford built a health resort and dairy as well as his own home on this property and prospered.

In 1871 Lyford patented An Improvement in Embalming, which was a very complicated system consisting of the introduction through the blood vessels of specially distilled chemicals (including creosote, zinc chloride, potassium nitrate, and alcohol) while the body was enclosed in a sealed container. The container, to have the air within it alternatively evacuated to create a vacuum and reversed to create pressure. Finally, the body was eviscerated and the trunk cavity filled with an arsenical powder. His final recommendation was the use of cosmetics to color the features; he was one of the first to make this recommendation. In 1870, a local newspaper carried a story describing a body he had successfully embalmed. Lyford died in 1906 without issue and had a large well-attended funeral.

Dr. E. C. Lewis, W. P. Cornelius, and Prince Greer. This most interesting account of the Civil War embalming surgeons relates the method of the transmission of embalming technique from a medically trained practitioner to an undertaker, who, in turn, trained a layman in the skill. Dr. E. C. Lewis was a former U.S. Army surgeon, W. P. Cornelius (1824–1910) was a successful undertaker in Nashville, Tennessee, and Prince Greer was a former orderly, body servant, and slave of a Colonel Greer of a Texas cavalry regiment who died in the fighting in Tennessee.

Thomas Holmes wrote:

In the forepart of the war a young ex-Army doctor named E. C. Lewis called at my headquarters in Washington and wished me to instruct him in the embalming profession and sell him an outfit to go to the western Army and locate at Nashville. He offered as security a property holding in Georgetown, DC for any amount of fluid I would trust him for. I made a bargain with him and he used many barrels of fluid. I was often surprised at his large orders. (*Note:* Dr. Lewis' headquarters were at Mr. Cornelius' undertaking establishment in Nashville.)

Cornelius stated:

It was during the year 1862 that one Dr. E. C. Lewis came to me from the employ of Dr. Holmes and proposed to embalm bodies. It was new to me but I at once put him to work with the Holmes fluid and Holmes injector. He was quite an expert, but like many men could not stand prosperity and soon wanted to get into some other kind of business, which he did. When Lewis the embalmer quit, I then undertook the embalming myself with a colored assistant named Prince Greer.

Cornelius explained that Prince Greer had earlier brought the body of Colonel Greer of a Texas cavalry regiment to Cornelius for shipment back to Texas. After shipping back the body Prince Greer remained at Cornelius' premises and was asked what he wanted to do to earn his room and board. Prince Greer indicated he would do anything.

Cornelius continued:

Prince Greer appeared to enjoy embalming so much that he himself became an expert, kept on at work embalming during the balance of the war, and was very successful at it. It was but a short time before he could raise an artery as quickly as anyone and was always careful, always of course coming to me in a difficult case. He remained with me until I quit the business in 1871.

Prince Greer is the first documented black embalmer in U.S. history.

Public and Professional Acceptance

With the ending of the war and the assassination of President Lincoln, the Civil War's last major casualty, the public had been familiarized with the term *embalming* and obtained personal knowledge of the appearance of an embalmed body. This knowledge was acquired by the hundreds of thousands who viewed not only President Lincoln but other prominent military and civilian figures as well as the ordinary soldiers embalmed and shipped to their homes.

Despite the end of the war and the establishment of peace there was no wide adoption of embalming by civilian undertakers of the United States. There were many reasons for this apparent reluctance to adopt a worthwhile new practice. Undertakers in the United States at the end of the Civil War were an unorganized, largely rural group of individuals lacking a professional body of knowledge and skills. Specifically, they lacked textbooks of instruction on embalming, instructors and schools of embalming, professional journals, and professional associations. Until these necessities became available embalming would not flourish.

The first step taken was to attempt the sale of embalming fluid to undertakers. Some Civil War embalming surgeons, such as Dr. Thomas Holmes, engaged in this endeavor on returning home. Holmes had a large local market (metropolitan New York City) for his preservative chemical, which he had named *Innominata*, and he promoted it well. Holmes, like other embalming chemical salesmen, realized quickly that the undertakers were interested in the preservative qualities of such chemicals but the clients were without knowledge of embalming techniques. Holmes therefore promoted the use of his Innominata as an external application, to wash the body and to saturate cloths to place over the face. His fluid was also poured into the mouth and nose to reach the lungs and stomach. Holmes' early practices were duplicated by other purveyors of embalming chemicals.

In these early post–Civil War years some instruction of undertakers in arterial embalming was imparted by the occasional knowledgeable traveling salesman who sold embalming chemicals. C. B. Chamberlain is reported to have done this in the late 1860s and early 1870s.

Examples of chemical embalming fluid patents include one issued to C. H. Crane of Burr Oak, Michigan, in September 1868. It was a powdered mixture of alum salt, ammonium chloride, arsenic, bichloride of mercury, camphor, and zinc chloride. It could be used as a dry powder or dissolved in water or alcohol to form an arterial solution and was named Crane's electrodynamic mummifier. In 1876 he sold the patent rights to this or a similar formulation to a Professor George M. Rhodes of Michigan. Another early embalming chemical manufacturer in 1877 was the Mills and Lacey Manufacturing Company of Grand Rapids, Michigan, whose embalming fluid featured arsenic as its preservative.

Instruments and chemicals available in the post–Civil War period included rubber gloves at $2 per pair (1877); anatomical syringes and three cannulas in a case for $20 to $22; surgical instruments in cases for $4 to

$5; Rulon's wax eyecaps and mouth closers at $1 each; and Segestor embalming fluid for $4.50 per dozen pint bottles (1873). Professor George M. Rhodes was said to have sold 100,00 bottles of his dynamic Electro Balm in 1876 with more than 3000 undertakers using the product. Egyptian Embalmer Fluid (1877) sold for $6.50 per dozen pint bottles and was also available in 5- and 10-gallon kegs as well as $\frac{1}{2}$ and 1-gallon carboys at $3.00 per gallon.

Until the first quarter of the 20th century, embalming was most frequently carried out in the home of the deceased or, in some communities, in the hospital where death occurred. There were early attempts in some funeral homes in the 1870s to provide both a preparation room and chapel space for the wake and services. In issues as early as 1876 of both *The Casket* and *The Sunnyside,*[*] there were accounts of the installation of preparation rooms. For example:

> Maynard Funeral Home, Syracuse, N.Y., had a morgue fitted with marble slabs and running water for storing bodies.
> Hubbard and Searles Undertaking establishment at Auburn, N.Y., could provide seating for 100 persons at a service and had a cooling room with cement floor and marble slabs (2 × 8 feet) and running water connection.
> Knowles Undertaking establishment at Providence, R.I., had a preserver room and a corpse room where surgical procedures and postmortems were made.
> The Douglas Undertaking Co. of Utica, N.Y., had a room for funeral services and a cooling vault in the cellar which had walls three feet thick and also contained shelves for body storage.

Dr. Auguste Renouard. In 1876, Dr. Renouard (1839–1912) became a regular contributor to *The Casket* of articles on all phases of embalming knowledge, which greatly implemented interest in embalming. He was born on a plantation in Point Coupee Parish, Louisiana, and received his early schooling locally. He is said to have attended the McDowell Medical School in St. Louis, Missouri, and, at the outbreak of the Civil War, to have returned to Louisiana to enlist in the Confederate Army. Despite his claim to military service in the confederate forces, no documented evidence has been found in some 50 years of searching. In the postwar period he secured employment as a pharmacist in various cities such as New York, Memphis, and Chicago, where he was married. His son, Charles A., was born shortly before the Chicago fire of

---

[*]The most significant impetus to spreading embalming knowledge was the founding of the professional journals *The Sunnyside* in 1871 and *The Casket* in 1876. Both, from their inception, carried advertisements for various embalming chemicals.

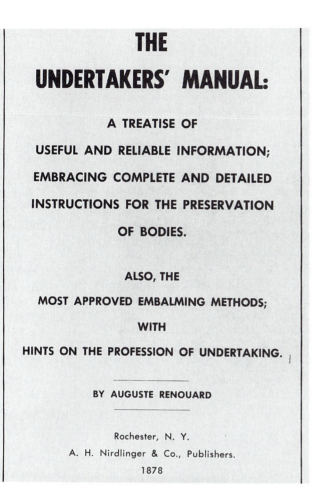

THE UNDERTAKERS' MANUAL:

A TREATISE OF

USEFUL AND RELIABLE INFORMATION;

EMBRACING COMPLETE AND DETAILED

INSTRUCTIONS FOR THE PRESERVATION

OF BODIES.

ALSO, THE

MOST APPROVED EMBALMING METHODS;

WITH

HINTS ON THE PROFESSION OF UNDERTAKING.

BY AUGUSTE RENOUARD

Rochester, N. Y.

A. H. Nirdlinger & Co., Publishers.

1878

Figure 13. Title page of Auguste Renouard's first edition of *The Undertaker's Manual.*

1871. Losing everything in the fire, Renouard traveled to Denver, Colorado, and secured employment as a bookkeeper for a combination furniture store and undertaking establishment. Because of its altitude, Denver at this time was regarded as a health resort for treatment of lung diseases.

The undertaking section of the firm returned many bodies to the east and south for hometown burial, and Renouard became interested in the procedures employed at his firm for shipment of the bodies. After studying the existing rudimentary system he suggested to his employer that he be permitted to prepare the bodies for shipment by arterial embalming. This consent was given and it almost immediately produced a volume of letters from the receiving undertakers inquiring about the procedure used to create such beautiful corpses, which resembled a person asleep. Renouard graciously replied, explaining his chemicals and technique to the extent that it assumed the proportions of a correspondence course. Additionally, there were a number of individual undertakers who traveled to Denver to receive personal instruction in embalming from Renouard.

The publisher of *The Casket* urged Dr. Renouard to write a textbook on embalming and undertaking for use by undertakers. In 1878 he published *The Undertaker's Manual*, which contained 230 pages of detailed instruction on anatomy, chemistry, embalming procedures, instruments, and details of undertaking practice (Fig. 13). **This was the first book published specifically as an embalming textbook in the United States and would be followed by a horde of others.** In 1879, notices appeared in *The Casket* that undertakers in states such as Connecticut and Pennsylvania were agents for the sale of Auguste Renouard's chemical formulas and techniques (Fig. 14).

In 1881 the doctor was requested to open a school of embalming in Rochester, New York, but, for a variety of reasons, this did not become a reality until early 1883.

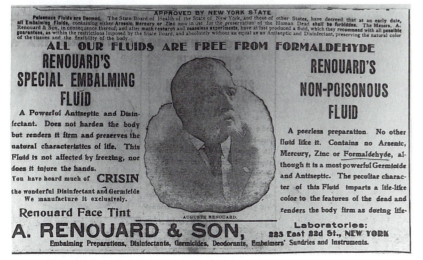

Figure 14. Auguste Renouard's advertisement for embalming fluid.

In 1880 the state of Michigan was the first to form an undertakers' association, which, in 1881, changed its name to Funeral Directors Association. Other states quickly followed the Michigan lead and organized state associations. **The various state associations met in 1882 in Rochester and organized the National Funeral Directors Association, another important step toward professionalism.** Renouard provided demonstrations of embalming in Rochester at the first national convention of the Association. This set a pattern for many years of an obligatory embalming demonstration at state and national conventions. During the 1882 gathering, agents of an English firm (Dotridge Brothers, Funeral Supply Firm) offered Renouard a 5-year contract to teach embalming in London at $5000 per year, which he rejected.

The Rochester School of Embalming headed by Dr. Renouard under the auspices of the Egyptian Chemical Company opened in 1883 and he continued his affiliation with this school until December 1884. He then entered into an agreement with Hallett and Company Undertakers in Kansas City, Missouri, to locate his school, the School of Embalming and Organic Chemistry, on the company's premises. By mid-1886 he terminated his school in Kansas City and returned to Denver. He then began to travel to distant points such as Ft. Worth, Texas, and Toronto and Montreal, Canada, providing embalming instruction for periods ranging from 3 days to 2 weeks.

In 1894 Dr. Renouard made his final move to New York City and established the U.S. College of Embalming. The school had no fixed term classes and the student remained until he was able to embalm. In 1889 the doctor's son, Charles A., was reported to be a shipping clerk with the firm of Dolge and Huncke—Embalming Chemical Manufacturers. Early in 1899 Charles opened the Renouard Training School for Embalmers in New York City and, in February 1900, Auguste Renouard closed the U.S. College of Embalming and joined Charles at his school. Charles provided several months of embalming instruction in London, England, on behalf of the O. K. Buckhout Chemical Company of Grand Rapids, Michigan. In 1906 Auguste traveled to England and continental Europe where he was most graciously received and entertained.

Auguste Renouard died in his home in 1912. A monument paid for by voluntary subscription of his former students was an example of the esteem in which he was held by those he instructed. **He can, without question, be regarded as the first major figure to provide embalming instruction for undertakers in the United States.** His son Charles continued the Renouard Training School for Embalmers until his death in 1950.

Joseph Henry Clarke. Born in Connersville, Indiana, Joseph Henry Clarke (1840–1916) received his early education in pharmacy and enrolled as a student in a medical col-

lege in Keokuk, Iowa. His studies, however, were interrupted by the Civil War. He volunteered for service with the Union Army but was rejected because of physical defects. He was permitted to serve as a civilian and later held the position of assistant hospital steward in the 5th Iowa Infantry. After the death of his father, he returned home before the end of the war to support his family. He married and secured employment as a casket salesman. During the course of his travels he became acquainted with a fluid manufacturer and became sufficiently interested in embalming to sell embalming fluids as a sideline. His interest in embalming grew as he realized the need to demonstrate the method of use of the fluid he hoped to sell to his patrons. This, in turn, led to his study of and experimentation with embalming chemicals to solve problems relating to preservation of the dead. He enrolled in an anatomy course conducted by Dr. C. M. Lukens of the Pulte Medical College in Cincinnati, Ohio, which broadened into a lifetime friendship and professional partnership in the founding of the Clarke School of Embalming at Cincinnati in 1882 (Fig. 15).

The school lacked permanence because Mr. Clarke traveled most of the year giving courses of instruction, each course varying in length from 2 to 7 days. His second course of instruction away from Cincinnati was presented in New York City. One class member was Felix A. Sullivan, who would later become a well-known teacher and writer in the embalming field. Sullivan and Clarke became rivals and bitter enemies. One major clash occurred when General and ex-President Ulysses S. Grant

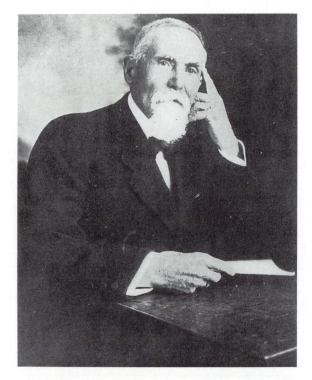

Figure 15. Portrait of Joseph Henry Clarke, founder of the Cincinnati College of Embalming.

died on July 23, 1885, at Mt. McGregor, New York. Clarke had been advised by the Holmes Undertaking Company (no relation to Thomas Holmes) of Saratoga, New York, that the company would be retained to handle the funeral of General Grant and that they wanted Clarke to do the embalming. Clarke was in Baltimore on the day of Grant's death, but he became ill and went to his Springfield, Ohio, home where he was bedridden for 3 to 4 weeks. The embalming was accordingly performed by one member of the Holmes Undertaking Company family and a Dr. McEwen using Clarke's proprietary embalming chemical (Fig. 16).

After the body had been embalmed Rev. Stephen Merritt, clergyman and undertaker of New York City and also General Grant's religious adviser, arrived together with Felix A. Sullivan and announced that they were to take charge. The Holmes personnel withdrew from the premises and Sullivan proceeded to reembalm the body. He claimed he withdrew all previously injected arterial fluid and replaced it with the chemical made by the company he represented. Clarke rebuffed these claims in the professional journals. A reporter from the *New York Times* wrote that Mr. Holmes (of Saratoga, New York) was too drunk to carry out the necessary preparation of the body. *The New York Times* was subsequently sued for libel and lost the case, and Mr. Holmes was awarded several thousand dollars in damages.

The name of the embalming school was changed in 1899 to the Cincinnati College of Embalming and was established on a permanent basis. Mr. Clarke conducted only occasional lecture tours at that time. He was ably assisted in the management of the school by his son, C. Horace Clarke. In 1907 Charles O. Dhonau became associated with him and later took over operation of the school. Mr. Clarke was a capable teacher, lecturer, and author of several texts on embalming, and he held several patents in the embalming field. He retired in 1909 to San Diego, California, where he died in 1916.

Felix Aloysius Sullivan (1843–1931). Sullivan was born in Toronto, Ontario, Canada, in 1843, the son of a Scotch immigrant undertaker and an Irish mother. He unquestionably had the most interesting, controversial, riotous, and successful career as a practitioner, writer, teacher, and lecturer of embalming and related subjects. His career was so full of incidents that it would be impossible to recount all but a few highlights.

After the usual parochial school education and some experience working with his father, Sullivan, together with several other friends, crossed the border into the United States and enlisted in a New York cavalry regiment during the Civil War. Military records verify his service but reveal he deserted the service near the end of the war. He claims to have assisted in embalming while in the service, but the claim can neither be affirmed nor denied as it lacks proof.

After the Civil War he followed various occupations and traveled. He eventually drifted to New York City where he secured employment with various casket companies and finally became a funeral director for hire. He studied anatomy and other medical sciences and, by 1881, became an embalmer of some local repute. He was hired to go to Cleveland, Ohio, to reembalm President Garfield, who died from an assassin's bullet, and seems to have been successful in this venture. Sullivan attended Clarke's embalming class in New York City in 1882 to learn how such a class of instruction was conducted. Sullivan, together with W. G. Robinson, opened the New York School of Embalming in 1884 and a year later was again involved in the embalming of a president, this time President Ulysses Grant (see previous information on Clarke's career). He then entered and left a long list of employers. In 1887 he was in Chicago when the anarchists who bombed the police in 1886, killing and wounding police and civilians, were condemned to die. One ex-

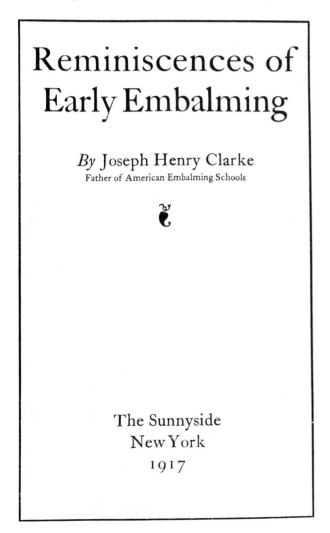

Reminiscences of Early Embalming

By Joseph Henry Clarke

Father of American Embalming Schools

The Sunnyside
New York
1917

Figure 16. Title page of an article by Joseph Henry Clarke for *The Sunnyside.*

ploded a dynamite cap in his mouth in jail and the others were hung. He prepared all bodies and was praised for his plastic surgery on the "mad bomber."

Sullivan continued his erratic employment or work habits, working for one firm, quitting, and then working for another. By 1891 he was again a lecturer/demonstrator, this time for the Egyptian Chemical Company. By 1892 he reached the height of his career as a lecturer, speaking and teaching in more cities to larger classes than anyone previously had. He was expelled from the State Funeral Directors convention in 1893 in St. Louis, Missouri, and a resolution was passed to forbid ever inviting his return. Sullivan settled in Chicago and opened a school of embalming. Local papers relate his arrest there together with a female companion (not his wife) on charges of adultery and wife and child desertion. When he finally settled the charges he underwent a cure for alcoholism and resumed teaching in a succession of short-lived appointments at various schools.

In 1900, the O. K. Buckhout Company of Michigan, a manufacturer of embalming chemicals, had Charles A. Renouard under contract to lecture, and sent him to London, England, to present a 3-week course of instruction that was very well received. Renouard returned home to attend similar engagements in the United States. The Buckhout Company had to find someone to continue the successful course of instruction in England, and the position was offered to Sullivan, who immediately accepted. Sullivan began teaching in London on October 8, 1900, a career that would extend to 1903. He lectured throughout the British Isles and helped to organize the British Embalmers Society as well as a journal entitled the *British Embalmer*.

He related that when Queen Victoria died in 1901 he was consulted about the possibility of embalming her. He recommended against it since it was impossible to guarantee perfect results. When he returned to the United States, he purchased an embalming school in St. Louis, Missouri, but the venture proved unprofitable. He then moved to Denver and Salt Lake City and eventually back to St. Louis, where he died. Sullivan wrote hundreds of articles plus eight books, taught thousands to embalm, and probably received more gifts from his classes than any other teacher before or since his time.

Increase in Embalming Schools

Some early "graduates" of embalming courses of instruction gave up regular employment at an undertaking establishment to provide embalming service to a number of undertakers who had no staff member trained to embalm. **This is how the terms *embalmer to the trade* or *trade embalmer* originated.**

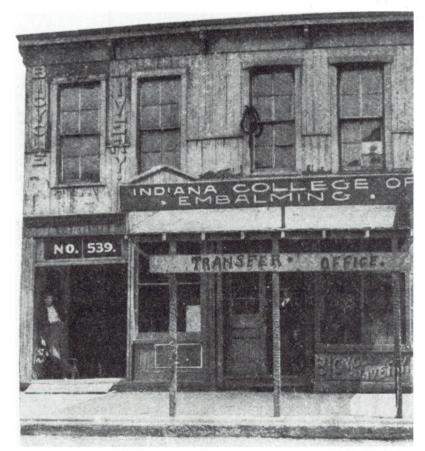

Figure 17. Old Indianapolis College of Embalming, Indianapolis, Indiana.

Many undertakers and/or their assistants were eager to learn to embalm but were unable to absent themselves from their business or employment to take advantage of such training. Some, however, managed to attend the 3 to 5-day schools, sponsored by the embalming chemical companies, in their city where they were taught the basic skills by the itinerant instructors. Others augmented their meager knowledge by enrolling in home study courses offered by many of the established schools of embalming.

Schools of instruction in embalming increased in number and activity by the beginning of the 20th century. Many manufacturers of embalming chemicals entered into the business of teaching embalming to maintain and increase the market for their products. Although the repair of injuries to the dead caused by disease or trauma had been dealt with since Egyptian times, it was not until 1912 that a systematic treatment for such cases was developed by a New York City embalmer, Joel E. Crandall (1878–1942). From this time on the schools of embalming slowly began to adopt instruction in this special phase of embalming treatment. Today, the subject area is commonly referred to as **restorative art**. It would be impossible to list in this text every personality who became an embalming professor or every school that was established, but a few should be mentioned.

Carl Lewis Barnes. Born into a family that operated an undertaking establishment in Connellsville, Pennsylvania, Barnes (1872–1927) studied medicine in Indiana, opened an embalming school there (Fig. 17), and moved it to Chicago. He manufactured embalming chemicals, wrote many books and articles on the subject, and had the largest chain of fixed-location schools in history in New York, Chicago, Boston, Minneapolis, and Dallas. While serving overseas as a medical colonel in the U.S. Army in World War I, his business failed. He never reopened the schools, continuing the practice of medicine until his death (Fig 18).

Albert H. Worsham. Worsham (1868–1939) attended Barnes' school and was on the faculty from 1903 to 1911 when he opened his own school in Chicago, with his wife Laura and brother Robert as faculty members. He lectured widely and was noted principally for contributing to the early foundation of postmortem plastic surgery.

Howard S. Eckels. Eckels (1865–1937) was a manufacturer of embalming chemicals and the founder of Eckels College of Embalming in Philadelphia, Pennsylvania. *(The school and chemical plant were in the same building, which was not an uncommon arrangement.)* Eckels wrote many articles and books, was successfully sued for plagiarism, and was not adverse to engaging in prolonged debates in the press. After his death his son John managed the school well into the post–World War II period

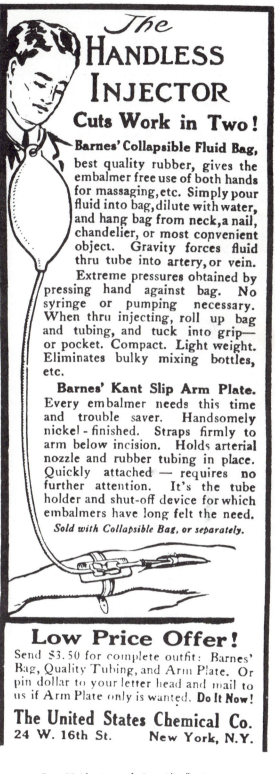

Figure 18. Advertisement for Barnes' handless injector.

when it closed after a period of affiliation with Temple University.

William Peter Hohenschuh. Born in Iowa City, Iowa, the son of an undertaker, Hohenschuh (1858–1920) took over the family business on the death of his father and began to teach embalming, which he had learned by correspondence from Auguste Renouard in the mid-1870s. Hohenschuh was active in the Iowa State Association and was elected president to the National Funeral Directors Association. He operated an embalming school in Chicago and, in 1900, in partnership with Dr. William S. Carpenter (1871–1944), opened the Hohenschuh–Carpenter School of Embalming in Des Moines, Iowa. He also operated a funeral home. In 1930 Dr. Carpenter moved the school to St. Louis and merged it with the Moribund American College of Embalming owned by F. A. Sullivan. After Dr. Carpenter's death his daughter Helene Craig an her son Golden Craig operated the school as well as the American Academy in New York City. This continued well into the post–World War II period.

Clarence G. Strub. Born in Iowa March 1, 1906, Strub attended the University of Iowa in Iowa City, Washington University in St. Louis, Missouri, and the Hohenschuh–Carpenter College of Embalming in Des Moines, Iowa. He became an instructor at Hohenschuh in 1929. In 1930, the school was moved to St. Louis where it merged with the, American College of Embalming and operated under the name of the St. Louis College of Mortuary Science. In 1934 he became a member of the staff of the Undertaker's Supply Company of Chicago and conducted clinics and demonstrations throughout the United States and Canada. He taught embalming and funeral management at the University of Minnesota and the Wisconsin Institute of Mortuary Science and was the director of research for the Royal Bond Chemical Company for many years (Fig. 19).

His greatest contributions to embalming lie in his ability to write clearly and simply, explaining embalming theory and practices. During his career he published well over 1000 articles, as well as many teaching outlines and quiz compendia. His little text, *The Principles of Restorative Art,* was the true prototype of all present-day texts on the subject. He also authored the monumental textbook *Principles and Practice of Embalming,* published by L. G. "Darko" Fredericks, which became the standard embalming text used by most colleges of mortuary science. Strub also wrote several technical movies such as the *Conquest of Jaundice* and *The Eye Bank Story,* as well as many purely children's stories and movies. He was the architect of the Eye Bank System in Iowa, which set the national pattern, as well as the curator of the state of Iowa's anatomical donation program. He died in Iowa City, Iowa, on August 6, 1974.

Women Embalmers. Women as well as men were trained as embalmers and not only practiced embalming but

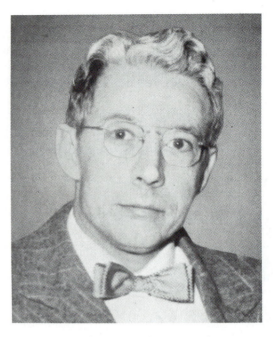

Figure 19. Photograph of Clarence G. Strub.

founded schools of instruction. Among these women were **Mrs. E. G. Bernard** of Newark, New Jersey, who founded the Bernhard School of Embalming; **Mme. Linda Odou,** who founded the Odou Embalming Institute in New York City (Fig. 20); and **Lena R. Simmons,** who founded and operated the Simmons School of Embalming in Syracuse, New York, until her son Baxter took over the management.

MORTUARY EDUCATION

Mortuary colleges, as known today, are relatively recent in origin. The development of mortuary education has followed the general pattern common to all professional fields. It emerged slowly from a period in which knowledge was transmitted from preceptor to student by means of observation and informal discussion to its present academic status.

A system for national accreditation of mortuary schools was first introduced in 1927 by the Conference to Funeral Service Examining Boards, a national association of state licensing boards. Higher standards governing qualifications of faculty, the curriculum, and teaching facilities were established and enforced.

The first teachers' institute was held in Cincinnati in the spring of 1946. On November 8 and 9, 1947, the second teachers' institute was held at the Pittsburgh Institute of Mortuary Science, at which time the first curriculum in embalming was adopted (Fig. 21). The committee chairman was Professor Ronald F. Hannum of the Cleveland College of Mortuary Science. A basic course content in anatomy was also adopted. This committee

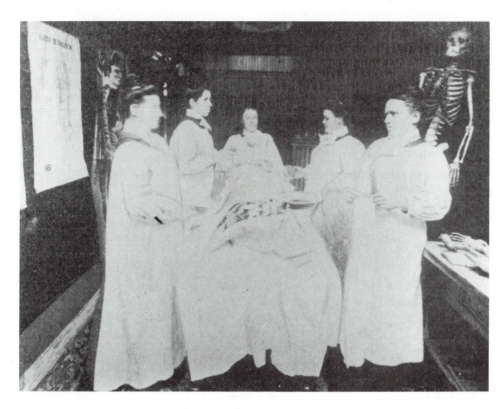

Figure 20. Anatomy class at Odou Institute of Embalming, New York, circa 1900 (Professor Odou at center of group).

was chaired by Dr. Emory S. James of the Pittsburgh Institute of Mortuary Science. On November 10, in Pittsburgh, the National Association of Colleges of Mortuary Science met and adopted what became the Morticians' Oath, still administered today to graduates of mortuary science.

CONCERN FOR TREATMENT

Early embalming reports concerning arterial injection indicated some concern for special treatment of the trunk viscera. Most such treatments consisted of removal, treatment, and replacement of viscera in the trunk cavity

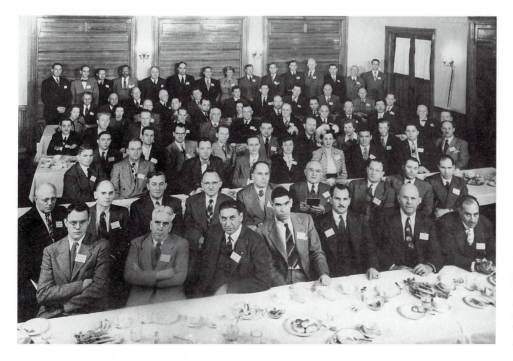

Figure 21. Educators from across the United States gathered for the Second Teachers Institute held in Pittsburgh, Pennsylvania, November 8 and 9, 1947. At this meeting the first curriculum in anatomy and embalming was established and the Mortician's Oath was adopted. (Courtesy of the Pittsburgh Institute of Mortuary Science, Pittsburgh, Pennsylvania.)

together with some preservative material, either powdered or liquid. Other reports, such as those of the Gannal–Sucquet era, indicate dependence for total preservation solely on the arterial injection unaccompanied by any special treatment for the trunk cavities. Gabriel Clauderus had advocated preservation based on introduction of his preservative chemical into the trunk cavity followed by immersion of the entire body in the preservative.

It was not until the mid-1870s that a "modern" system of treatment for the cavities was designed. The inventor of the trocar, Samuel Rodgers (listing Los Angeles, New York City, and San Francisco as his residence) secured two patents for the trocar, one in 1878 and the second in 1880. The `1878 patent described the trocar much as it exists today. The 1880 patent was issued for a system of embalming that consisted of introduction of his trocar, thrust through a single point in the navel into all the organs of the trunk to distribute a preservative fluid throughout the trunk viscera. The simplicity of this treatment and its modest success made it appealing to men who, for whatever reason, did not adopt arterial embalming, which required greater knowledge of anatomy and surgical skill. The inevitable result was a confrontation between "belly punchers" (cavity treatment advocates) and "throat cutters" (arterial embalmers) concerning the merits of their respective means of preservation.

It slowly became evident that neither system was always completely successful and that combination of the two systems, arterial injection followed by cavity treatment, offered the greatest promise of embalming success. Although Rodgers did not mention aspiration prior to injection of preservative chemicals in his process, Auguste Renouard did specifically recommend this in his *Undertaker's Manual*. Rodgers' method of a single-entrance opening into the trunk cavity was a brilliant concept not followed by all his contemporary "authorities." Espy's and Taylor's books of embalming instruction, for example, advocated multiple (three to four) points of insertion through the trunk wall for the trocar. Rodgers formulated an embalming preservative chemical named *Alekton*, which was believed to have phenol as its principal preservative. He also recommended cavity treatment followed by hypodermic injections using his trocar, inserted into the limbs of the corpse.

Since the introduction of arterial injection of the blood vessels in the late 17th century no other system of corpse preservation explored had ever been even seriously used. In 1884 a British physician, Dr. B. W. Richardson, devised what he termed **needle embalming**. The process consisted of inserting a trocar (the needle), such as Rodgers' invention, at the medial corner of the eye socket and forcing it into the brain area, where the injection process was repeated. After removal of the trocar from

the brain area, cavity treatment, aspiration, and injection were carried out. This process was most often referred to as the **eye process**. Rodgers in his early patent had proposed insertion of his trocar through the nose to inject preservative chemicals into the brain area, but did not suggest that this process would preserve the entire body as Richardson contended. It eventually was to be called the **nasal process**. Professor Sullivan, ever alert for any new procedure to interest his students, adopted Richardson's eye process and exploited its simplicity to the maximum.

Carl Barnes offered a variation of the procedure by inserting the trocar through the neck and into the brain via the foramen magnum. T. B. Barnes, his brother and school instructor associate, inserted the trocar between dorsal vertebrae into the spinal canal. In this method, Dr. Eliab Meyers drilled a hole through the center of the vertex of the skull, permitting direct access for a small trocar into the superior sagittal sinus. The process, regardless of point of access, is said to have delivered the preservative chemical eventually into blood vessels within the cranium and then to the rest of the body.

A dramatic test demonstration of the process is both described and illustrated in Barnes' textbook, *The Art and Science of Embalming*. A severed head of a dissection room subject had trocars inserted into the brain area through the eye socket route. Rubber tubes connected the carotid arteries and jugular veins with collecting bottles. As fluid was injected through the trocars into the brain area, fluid flowed into the collecting bottles via the carotid arteries and jugular veins. The process achieved moderate popularity until about 1905 when it became extinct. Not all teachers of embalming were advocates of it, and J. H. Clarke was a vigorous critic.

A variation of the process was the short-lived attempt to insert the trocar into the left ventricle of the heart and inject the arterial system. The great difficulty encountered in positively locating the left ventricle quickly discouraged this procedure. The intentional application of an electric current directly to a corpse for the intended purpose of simulating the effect of lightning or accidental electrocution on the blood—destruction of blood coagulation—has been attempted many times without any appreciable success.

One early experimenter was Charles T. Schade of McAlester, Oklahoma, who as early as 1909 conceived the idea of applying an electric current, powered by dry cell batteries, to the body surface, in the belief that this would cause small muscles to contract and hence force blood out of the areas of discoloration. No effect was noted concerning the ability of an electric current applied externally to a corpse to prevent normal postmortem blood coagulation or promote dissolution of any existing intravascular clots. Similar attempts to accomplish this desirable effect have been attempted through the years down to the present both in the United States and England without success. Those who have experimented have concluded that the dead human body does not conduct an electrical current well enough to accomplish the intended purpose.

PROFESSIONALISM IN EMBALMING

Toward the end of the 19th century and on into the 20th century a number of events were to occur that would accelerate embalming toward the level of professionalism. A convergence of two movements became apparent about 1897, with the appearance of advertisements by embalming fluid companies stating that their fluid contained formalin. For some years there had been arguments to eliminate arsenic and other poisons from inclusion in embalming fluid formulas for the same medicolegal reason that the French prohibited arsenic in 1846 and bichloride of mercury in 1848. Now that a powerful disinfectant, **formalin,** was available and reasonably priced, the opportunity to eliminate poisonous chemicals was at hand. The state of Michigan led the way in 1901 and was followed by other states.

The second movement was to require regulations for both licensing and governing those who practiced embalming, and in 1893–1894 the state of Virginia became the first state to do so. Formalin content fluids were not a total blessing and were not as favorably received as might have been expected. Embalmers of the period were unaccustomed to the very different characteristics of the new preservative. For example, bodies embalmed with arsenic were said to have been relatively supple, making dressing and positioning relatively easy. Many of the poisonous chemicals had bleaching qualities and left the body quite white. Only a few left any undesirable coloration, such as those reported to contain copper, which tended to produce a bluish color in the skin. Then too, little or no problem was reportedly encountered to the penetration of all the body tissues, with or without blood drainage. There was also the proven ability of such poisonous chemicals to preserve the body tissues. There were, of course, some negatives such as the possible absorption of poisonous chemicals through the embalmer's unprotected skin, various skin irritations, and thickened and cracked fingernails.

Embalmers beginning to experiment with the formalin-based embalming fluids had to learn that they must remove the blood in all cases and began to use low-formalin-content or nonformalin fluids to wash the blood out before injection of the preservative formalin-based solutions. They also learned that they had to position the body properly before injection and the hardening effected by formalin or they would encounter serious problems later in trying to properly position hands together. To their astonishment, embalmers also discovered that formalin reacted with the bile pigments present in the skin of jaundiced bodies to produce an unsightly green-colored skin.

The opponents of formalin fluids were highly critical of the formaldehyde fumes, which irritated mucous membranes, claiming these effects were more dangerous to health than the poisonous chemicals. Reason and science prevailed and the embalming fluid formulas were improved to overcome most of the early problems. With the eventual transfer of the site of embalming from the family home bedroom to the funeral home preparation room, proper ventilation tended to eliminate most of the irritation problem. Chemicals became more diverse. For example, different formulas were developed for specific uses, such as arterial and cavity, preinjection, coinjection, and for special purposes as in decomposing cases. The delivery of embalming fluids in concentrated form, to be added to water to create the desired dilution strength, was a distinct contrast to the former embalming chemical packaging which was delivered in containers already combined with water ready to inject. Thus, the embalmer had to become more experienced and intelligent in the mixing of the formalin embalming solution than he had formerly.

UTILIZATION OF NEW DEVICES

Over the years of embalming in bedrooms of the home of the deceased, little in the way of improvements was instituted in injection pumps or aspirating devices. With the transfer of the majority of embalming preparations to the funeral home, however, new devices could be used. In the last quarter of the 19th century most embalming pumps or injectors were based on the gravity bowl, the hand pump, or the rubber bulb syringe. The gravity bowl was simply a container suspended above the body and connected to the arterial tube by a length of rubber tubing. The height of the bowl above the body determined the pressure. Its main advantage was that it did not require the constant pumping by the embalmer and, therefore, left hands free to perform other tasks. The hand pump could produce either pressure or vacuum for injection or aspiration into or from a glass container.

When the preparation of the body was moved to the funeral home, water pressure was used to create suction to aspirate. Special aspirators, such as the Penberthy, Worsham, and Slaughter, generated suction by water pressure and were made to attach to preparation room sink faucets, connected by rubber tubing to the trocar. Later in the 1950s special electric motor-driven aspirators were devised and were found to overcome the aggravation encountered by low water pressure during high-water-use periods. *Most communities today have requirements relating to the need for preventing suction of aspirated material into the water system.*

At a New York state convention in 1914, a battery-powered electric pump, the Falcon Electric Embalmer for injecting embalming chemicals, was demonstrated but was not widely adopted. Some new instruments devised to simplify or improve certain embalming procedures were developed in the 1920s and 1930s. A new method of jaw closure was devised involving "barbed tacks" driven into the mandible and maxillae by a spring-propelled hammer. Wires attached to the "tacks" were then twisted together to secure the desired degree of jaw closure. A plastic, threaded, screwlike device called the **trocar button** became the most useful waterproof seal for trocar punctures, bullet wounds, and even for intravenous needle punctures (when surgically enlarged). A metal dispensing device that was attached directly to any standard 16-ounce bottle of cavity fluid (by screwing it into the bottle opening in place of the cap) simplified cavity fluid injection. The dispenser was connected to the trocar by a length of rubber hose and injection was accomplished by gravity after the cavity fluid bottle was elevated and inverted.

It was not until the mid-1930s that electric-powered injection machines were available and in use. Some were simply electric motors with fittings to produce pressure or vacuum-connected to suitable containers by rubber tubing. One of the first "self-contained" embalming fluid injection machines put on the market in the 1930s was the Snyder/Westberg device. It was originally designed to hold $\frac{1}{2}$ gallon of embalming fluid. The machine was compact, durable, and trouble free, and was originally designed with motor and the fluid container side by side. Model II was designed so that the fluid container was placed above the injection motor; thus, the fluid was "gravity fed" to the pump. This arrangement has become standard on all self-contained units. In 1937 the Slaughter Company developed an all-metal fluid injection tank equipped with a pressure gauge; in 1938 the Flowmaster electric-powered injection machine was announced; in 1939 the Frigid Fluid Company developed a pressure injector consisting of a metal container for holding embalming fluid complete with exit connection with shut-off and a carbon dioxide gas cylinder to create the necessary pressure to inject the fluid. **In mid-1939 the Turner Company announced the availability of the Porti Boy, which was to become the all-time most popular injection machine.** Several improvements over the years included a pulsator device, a larger fluid tank, and the ability to produce extreme high-pressure injections. By the 1960s, extreme high-pressure injection machines such as the Sawyer were available and in use.

AVAILABILITY OF MORE MATERIALS

With the end of World War II, metal and other materials became available to produce various new embalming devices. The concept of using externally generated agitation to assist in blood removal became popular. Some embalming tables had such pulsating devices built in as an integral part of the structure. Other pulsating devices were devised to be attached to existing operating tables or were handheld devices to be applied to the body over the course of the major blood vessels. Disillusionment with this development came after a short period of use. The vibrations produced by such devices made it impossible to keep instruments, and even the body itself, from sliding downward toward the foot of the table.

Another innovation was the development of a conventional embalming fluid by the Switzer Corporation of Cleveland that contained a large quantity of fluorescent dye. The dye was to act as a tracer or indicator of the degree of circulation or penetration of the embalming fluid when viewed under an ultraviolet light illuminator furnished with the embalming fluid. Although the system did indeed disclose the extent of the distribution of the embalming chemical and its fluorescent dye, it never was proof positive that areas of the body beneath the skin were thoroughly embalmed.

In the wake of Hiroshima and Nagasaki and other major disasters such as airline crashes, earthquakes, mudslides, and building collapses, a search was instituted for some new means of quickly processing (preserving) huge numbers of dead. Over the years, different means of processing (preserving) the victims of such tragedies were devised, tested, and found unsuitable for a variety of reasons. Experiments were conducted with processes using ultrasound, radiation, atomic bombardment, and ultracold. No process tried seemed to be capable of preserving a tremendous number of bodies in a brief period. The search continues!

Indisputably the greatest change in embalming procedures began in the 1980s by the intervention of federal government agencies. The Federal Trade Commission (FTC) adopted rules concerning the necessity for embalming and the securing of consent for same. The Occupational Safety and Health Administration (OSHA) adopted rules relating to embalming procedures, funeral home personnel protection, and similar public health and hygienic measures. The Environmental Protection Agency (EPA) issued rules concerning the use and control of formaldehyde and chemicals used by embalmers.

Although it has been generally conceded that formaldehyde-based fluids performed well as preserving and fixing agents for the embalming process, chemical research for an improvement in embalming chemicals has always been active.

During the 1930s, Hilton Ira Jones of the Hizone Company performed extensive research on glyoxal, a chemical that seemed to display much promise for use in an embalming formula. World War II, however, reduced the available supply and thus the research in this direction.

Another chemical, glutaraldehyde, was thoroughly researched and developed into an embalming formula by the Champion Company.

At the time of publication of this textbook edition, an announcement had been made by as many as three embalming fluid companies of formulations that replace formaldehyde in embalming solutions.

Since the intervention of OSHA in embalming procedures, the search has intensified to find a substitute for formaldehyde and thus eliminate the vexatious problems of monitoring formaldehyde fume levels and wearing filter masks as required by OSHA regulations.

It is astonishing what has been achieved in the embalming field in nearly 5000 years of growth of knowledge, skill, and experience. Naturally, what the future holds is unknown, but those working in the field feel it will be as exciting and rewarding as the past millenia.

KEY TERMS AND CONCEPTS FOR STUDY AND DISCUSSION

1. List and describe the natural means of preservation.
2. List and describe the artificial means of preservation.
3. Describe the three periods of embalming history.
4. Describe the procedures employed in each of the five steps used by the Egyptians in the preparation of mummies.
5. Explain the contributions made to the development of embalming by each of the following:
   A. William Harvey
   B. Marcello Malpighi
   C. Jean Nicholas Gannal
   D. Gabriel Clauderus
   E. John Hunter
   F. Richard Harlan
   G. John Morgan
   H. Thomas Holmes
   I. Frederick Ruysch
   J. Joseph Henry Clark
6. Explain the following terms:
   anthropoid (mummy) form coffin
   Canopic jars
   cartonage
   evisceration
   natron
   needle embalming

preinjection fluid
sarcophagus
trade embalmer
trocar

BIBLIOGRAPHY

Beverly R. *History of Virginia.* 1922:185.

McClelland EH. *Bibliography on Embalming* (mimeo copy). New York: National Association of Mortuary Science (limited to 100 copies); 1949.

McCurdy CW. *Embalming and Embalming Fluids—With Bibliography of Embalming.* Wooster, OH: Hearld Printing; 1896

Oatfield H. *Literature of the Chemical Periphery—Embalming.* Advances in Chemistry Series No. 16 (a key to pharmaceutical and medicinal chemistry literature). Washington, DC: American Chemical Society.

Pinkerton J. *Collection of Voyages.* (Vol. 13), 1812.

Surgeon General's Catalogue. Washington, DC: U.S. Army; 1883–1884.

Townshend J. *Grave Literature* (a catalogue of some books relating to the disposal of bodies and perpetuating the memories of the dead). New York (private collection); 1887.

Egypt

Aliki. *Mummies Made in Egypt.* New York: Thomas J. Crowell; 1979.

Arcieri GP. *Note E Ricordi—Sulla Preservatione Del Corppo Umano.* Rivista Di Storia Delle Scienze Medicine E Naturoli, No. 1. Florence; 1956.

Bardeen CR. Anatomy in America. *Bulletin of University of Wisconsin,* No. 115. September 1905.

Budge EAW. *The Mummy.* Cambridge: University Press; 1893.

Choulant L. *History and Bibliography of Anatomical Illustration.* New York: 1962 (reprint).

David AR, ed. *Manchester Museum Mummy Project.* Manchester, England: Maney and Sons; 1979.

Harris JE, Weeks KR. *X-Raying the Pharaohs.* New York: Charles Scribner's Sons; 1973.

Hemneter E. *Embalming in Ancient Egypt.* Ciba Symposia, Vol. 1, No. 10, Summit, NJ: Ciba Pharmaceuticals; January 1940.

Herodotus. *History* (translated by George Rawlinson). New York: Dial and Tudor Presses; 1928.

Liebling R, et al. *Time Line of Culture in the Nile Valley and Its Relationship to Other Countries.* New York: Metropolitan Museum of Art; 1978.

Martin RA. *Mummies.* Anthropology Leaflet No. 36. Chicago, IL: Chicago Natural History Museum Press; 1945.

Mendelsohn S. *Embalming*. Ciba Symposia, Vol. VI, No. 2. Summit, NJ: Ciba Pharmaceuticals; May 1944.

Moodie RL. *Anthropology Memoirs*. Vol. III: *Roentgenologic Studies of Egyptian and Peruvian Mummies*. Chicago, IL: Field Museum Press; 1931.

Pettigrew TJ. *History of Egyptian Mummies*. London: Longman, Rees; 1834.

Pons A. *Les Origines de L'Embaument et L'Egypte Predynastique*. Montpelier, France: Inprimerie Grollier; 1910.

Smith GE, Dawson WR. *Egyptian Mummies*. New York: Dial Press; 1924.

Steuer RO, Saunders JB de CM. *Ancient Egyptian and Cnidian Medicine*. Berkeley/Los Angeles: University of California Press; 1959.

Peru[*]

Garcillaso de la Vega. *Royal Commentaries of Peru*. (translated by Paul Rycant). London; 1688.

Prescott WH. *History of the Conquest of Peru*. (2 vols.). Philadelphia: JB Lippincott; 1882.

Rivero ME, Von Tschudi JJ. *Peruvian Antiquities*. (translated by Francis L. Hawks), New York: George Putnam; 1853.

Von Hagen VW. *Realm of the Incas*. New York: New American Library of World Literature; 1957.

Alaska and Aleutian Islands

Quimby GI. *Aleutian Islanders*. Anthropology Leaflet, No. 35. Chicago: Natural History Museum; 1944.

North American Indians

Yarrow HC. *Study of Mortuary Customs Among the North American Indians*. Washington, DC: U.S. Government Printing Office; 1880.

Equador—Jivaro Indians

Cottlow LN. *Amazon Head Hunters*. New York: Signet Book/Henry Holt; 1953.

Flornoy B. *Jivaro*. New York: Library Publishers; 1954

Canary Islands

De Espinosa A. *The Guanches of Tenerife*. London: Hakluyt Society; 1907.

Hooton EA. *The Ancient Inhabitants of the Canary Islands*. Harvard African Studies, Vol. II. Cambridge, MA: Harvard University Press; 1925.

Europe (Early Period)

Bradford CA. *Heart Burial*. London: Allen & Unwin;1933.

Castiglioni A, Robinson V. *The Anatomical Theater*. Ciba Symposia, Vol. III, No. 4. Summit, NJ: Ciba Pharmaceuticals; May 1941.

Clauderus G. *Methodus Balsamundi Corpora Humane Aliaque Majora sine Evisceratione et Sectione Hucusque Solita*. Altenberg, Germany: G. Richterum; 1679.

De Villihardouin G, DeJoinville J. *Memoirs of the Crusades*. New York: EP Dutton; 1938.

Dionis M. *Cours D'Operations de Chirurqie*. Paris: d'Houry; 1746.

Garrison FH. *Introduction to the History of Medicine*. Philadelphia: 1929.

Greenhill T. *Nekrokadeia—Or the Art of Embalming*. London: printed for the author; 1705.

Guichard C. *Des Funerailles et diverses Manieres*. Lyon, France: D'ensevelir; 1582.

Guichard C. *Funerailles*. Lyon, Grance: Jean de Tovrnes; 1581.

Guybert P. The charitable physitian showing the manner to embalm a dead corpse. In: *The Charitable Physitian*. London: Thomas Harper Printer; 1639.

Pare A. *How to Make Reports and to Embalm the Dead*. (translated). London: Cotes & Young; 1634.

Pilcher LS. The Mondino myth (reprint). *Med Library Hist J*. 1906; 4(4, Dec.).

The Art and Science of Embalming Dead Bodies (taken from the 29th book of Peter Forestus and translated from the Latin into German), contained in *A New Medical Treatise* by Petrum Offenbach, M.D. Frankfort: Zacharian Palthenium; 1605.

Treece H. *The Crusades*. New York: Random House; 1962.

Walsh JJ. *The Popes and Science*. New York: Fordham University Press; 1908.

Walsh JJ. *The 13th—Greatest of Centuries*. New York: Catholic Summer School Press; 1907.

Wellcome HS. *The Evolution of Antiseptic Surgery*. London: Burroughs Wellcome; 1910.

Young S. *The Annals of the Barber Surgeons of London*. London: Blades East & Blades; 1890.

Europe (Late Period)

Bailey JB. *The Diary of a Resurrectionist 1811–1812*. London: Swan-Sonnenschein; 1896.

Ball JM. *The Sack em Up Men*. London: Oliver & Boyd; 1928.

Bayle DC. *L'Embaumement*. Paris: Adrien Delahaye; 1873.

Blanchard S. *Anatomia Reformata—Balsamatione*,

[*]Also see Moodie in list under Egypt.

Novus Methodus. Leiden: Boutesteyn & Lughtmans: 1687.

Cole FJ. *A History of Comparative Anatomy*. London: MacMillan: 1944.

Coliez A. *Conservation Artificielle des Corps*. Paris: Amedee Legrand; 1927.

Cope Z. *The History of the Royal College of Surgeons*. Springfield, IL: Charles C Thomas; 1959.

Dawson WR. Life and times of Thomas J. Pettigrew. *Med Life*. (3 issues) 1931;38 (1–3, Jan./Feb./March).

DeLint JG. *Atlas of the History of Medicine*, Vol. I. London: HK Lewis; 1926.

Eriksson R, ed, translator, *Andreas Vesalius 1st Public Anatomy at Bologna—1540*. Uppsala: Almquist & Wikselle; 1959.

Gannal JN. *Histoire des Embaumements*. Paris: Ferra Librairie; 1838.

Gannal JN (as translated by R. Harlan): *History of Embalming*. Philadelphia: Judah Dobson; 1840.

Gerlt-Wernich-Hirsch. *Biographisches Lexikon Der Herrvorragenden Arzte Aller Zeiten und Volker*. Berlin: Urban & Schwarzenberg; 1932.

Laskowski S. *L'Embaumement, la conservatione des Sujets et les Preparations Anatomiques*. Geneva: H. Georg; 1886.

Mann G. The anatomical collections of Fredrick Ruysch at Leningrad. *Bull Cleve Med Library*. 1964;11 (No. 1, Jan.).

Nordenskiold E. *The History of Biology*. New York: Tudor; 1928.

Paget S. *John Hunter*. London: T. Fisher University; 1898.

Peachy GC. *The Homes of Hunter in London*. London: Bailliere, Tindall & Cox; 1928.

Pettigrew JT. Fredrick Ruysch. In: *Pettigrew's Medical Portrait Gallery*. London: Whitaker; 1840.

Ramazzini B. *De Morbio Artificum* (ed 2, 1713). *Diseases of Workers* (translated by WC Wright). New York: Hafner; 1964.

Richardson BW. *The Art of Embalming*. In *Wood's Medical and Surgical Monographs*. Vol. III. New York: 1889.

Sigerist HE. *The Great Doctors*. Garden City, NY: Doubleday; 1958.

Singer C. *Studies in the History and Method of Science*. (2 vols.). Oxford, England: Clarendon Press; Vol I.—1917, Vol II.—1921.

Sucquet JP. *De L'embaumement et des Conservation pour l'etude de l'anatomie*. Paris: Adrien Delahaye; 1872.

Sucquet JP. *Traits du Visage Dans L'embaumement*. Paris: Adrien Delahaye; 1862.

United States

Barnes CL. *The Art and Science of Embalming*. Chicago, IL: Trade Periodical; 1905.

Clarke CH. *Practical Embalming*. Cincinnati, OH: C. H. Clarke; 1917.

Clarke JH. Reminiscences of early embalming. *The Sunnyside*, 1917.

Crane EH. *Manual of Instructions to Undertakers*. 8th ed. Kalamazoo, MI: Kalamazoo; 1888.

Dodge AJ. *The Practical Embalmer*. Boston: A. Johnson Dodge; 1908.

Eckels HS. *Practical Embalmer*. Philadelphia: H.S. Eckels Co.; 1903.

Espy JB. *Espy's Embalmer*. Springfield, OH: Espy Fluid Co.; 1895.

Gallagher T. The body snatchers. *Am Heritage*, June 1967.

Johnson EC. Civil war embalming. *Funeral Directors Rev*, June/July/August; 1965.

Johnson EC, Johnson GR. A Civil War embalming surgeon—The story of Dr. Daniel H. Prunk. *The Director* (NFDA publication), January 1970.

Johnson EC, Johnson GR. *Alone in His Glory*. Unpublished manuscript, Civil War Mortuary Practices.

Johnson EC, Johnson GR. *Prince Greer—America's First Negro Embalmer*. Liaison Bulletin, International Federation of Thanatopractic Association, Paris, April 1973.

Johnson EC, Johnson GR. The undertakers manual. *Canadian Funeral News*, Calgary, July 1980.

Johnson EC, Johnson M. D.H. Rhodes—Conscientious caretaker of Arlington National Cemetery. *Am Funeral Director*; January 1984.

Johnson EC, Johnson GR, Johnson Williams M. Dr. Renouard's role in embalming history. *Am Funeral Director* 1987. August 1987.

Johnson EC, Johnson GR, Johnson M. Dr. Thomas Holmes—Pioneer embalmer. *Am Funeral Director* July/August 1984.

Johnson EC, Johnson GR, Johnson Williams M. History of modern restorative art. *Am Funeral Director* January–April 1988.

Johnson EC, Johnson GR, Johnson Williams M. The trial, execution and embalming of two Civil War soldiers. *Am Funeral Director* December 1986.

Johnson M. *A historic precedent to the FTC rules of 1977 (Civil War licensing for embalmer requirements)*. NFDA Bulletin, 1979.

Johnson M. Lena R. Simmons—The grand dame of early embalmers. *Am Funeral Director* January 1977.

Johnson M. *Lina Odou—Embalmer*. July 1977.

Keen WW. *Addresses and Other Papers*. Philadelphia: Saunders; 1905.

Mendelsohn S. *Embalming Fluids*. New York: Chemical Publishing; 1940.

Mills and Lacey Mfg. Co. (no author stated). *Practical*

Directions for Embalming the Dead. Grand Rapids, MI: Stevens, Cornell and Dean; 1881.

Myers E. *Champion Textbook on Embalming*. Springfield, OH: Champion Chemical Co.; 1908.

Renouard A. *Undertakers Manual*. Rochester, NY: A. Nirdlinger; 1878.

Renouard CA, ed. *Taylor's Art of Embalming*. New York: H. E. Taylor; 1903

Samson H, Crane ON, Perrigo AB, Hatfield MD. *Pharmaceutical, Anatomical and Chemical Lexicon* (the NFDA official textbook). Chicago, IL: Donohue & Henneberry; 1886.

Strub CA, Frederick LG. *The Principles and Practice of Embalming*. 4th ed. Dallas, TX: L.G. Frederick; 1986.

Sullivan FA. *Practical Embalming*. Boston: Egyptian Chemical Co.; 1887.

The Faculty of the Cincinnati School for Embalming, Lukens CM and Clarke JH. *Textbook on Embalming*. Springfield, OH: Limbocker; 1883.

War Department. General Order 33, April 3, 1862.

War Department. General Order 39, March 15, 1865.

War Department. General Order 75, September 11, 1861.

Wightman SK. In search of my son (Civil War). *Am Heritage*, February, 1963.

The History of Modern Restorative Art

Edward C. Johnson • *Gail R. Johnson* • *Melissa J. Williams*

The reader is advised to reread the section on Egyptian embalming procedures entitled Ancient Restorative Art found in the preceeding section of this text.

To date, no record of a restorative art procedure applied during the anatomical or middle period of embalming history has been found. Virtually all documented reports of embalming in this period include the practice of enclosing the preserved body within a metal-lined, hermetically sealed coffin, which precluded viewing. To satisfy some medieval customs relating to funeral practices and chivalry, an imago or effigy of the decedent was created by preparing a death mask as the basis for the head. The features were painted to closely resemble the normal lifelike appearance, and effigies were often adorned with a wig. The completed head was attached to a torso, complete with arms and legs, proportional to the life size of the decedent. The effigy was dressed in the clothing or armor of the decedent and placed on the coffin containing the corpse, where it remained during the entire period preceding actual interment (Fig. 22).

A few examples of effigies still remain in storage at Westminster Abbey, London, England.

During the U.S. Civil War a few, a very few, documents indicate that some effort was made to repair traumatic injuries. One such document in the Frank Hutton collection is a letter from the family of a Union Army soldier who was embalmed and sent home for burial. The family wrote in their letter to Hutton, that the corpse "looked pretty good for being dragged by mules."

By and large, however, it can be stated without fear of contradiction that very little of what is referred to today as restorative art was practiced until the second decade of the 20th century. There were exceptions occasionally, such as the treatment of the anarchist bomber's suicide in Chicago briefly described in the section on Felix Aloysius Sullivan (see the preceeding section). Joseph H. Clarke briefly mentions the treatment of a tumor case in his book *Reminiscences of Early Embalming*.

What is termed restorative art today represents the greatest remaining challenge to the skill, the ability to improvise, and the courage of the practicing embalmer. It is the last frontier and poses problems to test those who choose to grapple with its manifest difficulties. Formerly known most commonly by several popular terms such as plastic surgery, demisurgery, and dermasurgery, it is today most commonly referred to as restorative art.

The term *restorative art*, not adopted until the early 1930s, is in reality a poorly contrived label for specialized postmortem treatment accorded those dying of trauma or debilitating disease, the practice of which is most often believed to have originated entirely in the United States in recent years. Such a premise is false inasmuch as the practice of restorative art is dependent on and inseparable from the embalming procedure. Thus,

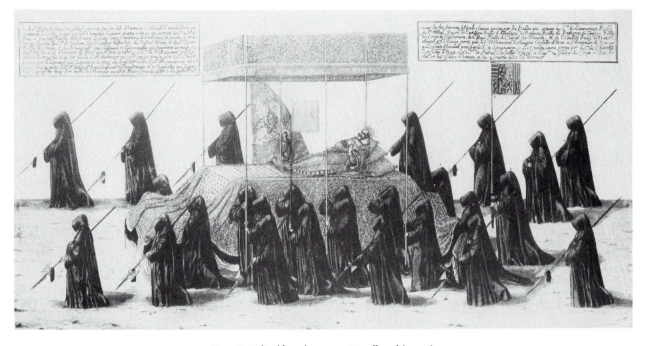

Figure 22. Medieval funeral procession. Note effigy of deceased.

one realizes that restorative art has been practiced from the origin of embalming in Egypt and so it was (Fig. 23).

The year 1912 marks the establishment of the modern era of what is today known as restorative art. The first articles appeared in the April 19, 1912, issue of *The Sunnyside. Demisurgery,* as it was to be termed by its founder, was "the art of building or creating parts of the body which have been destroyed by accident, disease, decomposition or discoloration, and making the body perfectly natural and lifelike."

The science of restorative art as known today was founded by one man, Joel E. Crandall, then an embalmer in New York City. Although many others made impor-

tant contributions to this science through the years, no other one person can claim the honor of stimulating the interest of fellow embalmers in this most difficult technical subject area.

An editorial in the April 19, 1912 issue of *The Sunnyside* stated that "the photographs of before and after appearance of a mutilated body show what can and should be done. The originator of the new art of demisurgery is Joel E. Crandall of New York City and his first article on the new technique appears in the pages of this issue of *The Sunnyside*" (Fig. 24).

An early acknowledgment of Crandall's primacy in the field was made by Howard S. Eckels in a letter pub-

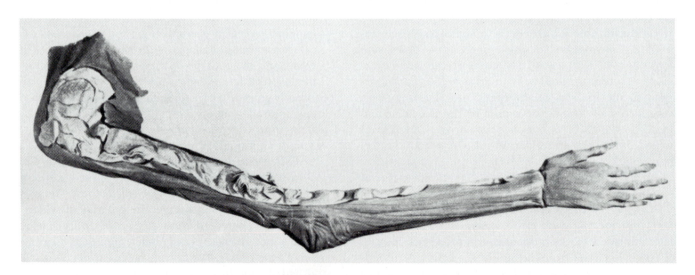

Figure 23. Arm of a mummy of the XXIst Dynasty, showing the packing material.

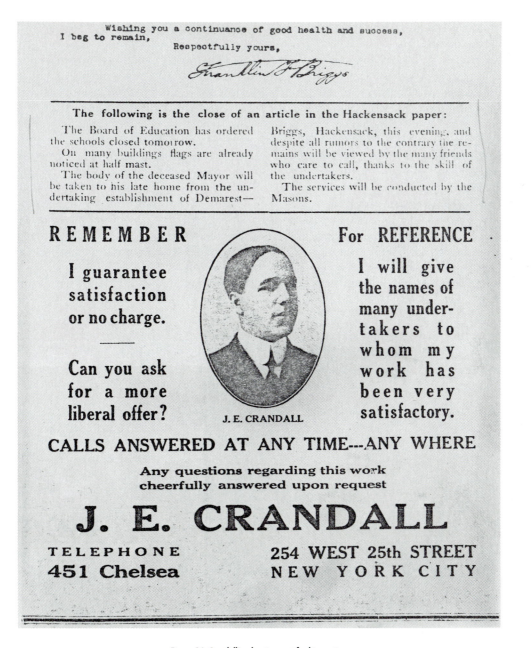

Figure 24. Crandall's advertisement for his services.

lished in the May 14, 1914, issue of *The Sunnyside*, stating that the science of demisurgery was indeed founded by Joel E. Crandall.

A. Johnson Dodge quoted in the June 1, 1917, issue of *The Casket*,

How to care for mutilated or postmortem cases, or bodies which from any cause have become unsightly and make them presentable, should constitute a part of the education of the embalmer. Thorough instruction in this difficult part of the art should be given by the instructors in our schools. But this part of the work requires special experience and some study either to

practice or teach it successfully. It was first taught as a specialty by Mr. Joel E. Crandall of New York City, and to him belongs the credit of introducing it. We think Mr. Crandall is the only person who has attained any great degree of success in the practice of this art, and would recommend the student who wishes to attain a high degree of proficiency in this part of his profession to apply to Mr. Crandall for instruction, as he appears to be the only known person really competent to teach it.

Joel E. Crandall (1878–1942) was born on September 16, 1878, in Whitesville, New York, the son of Norris Crandall and Caroline Andrews Crandall.

Following the customary education available at the time, he worked at a variety of jobs. At about 20 years of age he began working for a New York City undertaker. Deeply interested in embalming and becoming increasingly skillful, his services were much in demand and he was employed by both the Frank E. Campbell and Stephen Merritt undertaking establishments as well as the National Casket Company.

Writing in 1912 about his efforts to repair mutilated cases, he stated that he had studied the problems over a period of 10 years. His early efforts to use conventional materials such as plaster of Paris were abandoned for any use except as an interior deep filler in contact with bone. He formulated covering cosmetics and a waxlike putty to fill in missing or damaged areas.

His earliest experiments were on severely mutilated bodies that neither the family nor the undertaker believed could be restored to viewability. Little by little over the years, by trial and error, he developed a successful system for treatment of mutilated cases that eventually embodied most present-day principles or techniques.

Among the requirements Crandall advocated were a recent photograph of the decedent as a reference for the restoration, hardening of the soft tissues of the face as a prerequisite to demisurgery, and enough working time to carry out the entire treatment. Crandall also made the earliest mention of the use of "concealed stitches" to close lacerations and "corrective surgery" to remove remnants of features or tissue impossible to incorporate into the restoration. For his early research he made use of plaster life-size heads that he mutilated and repaired: a procedure that was eventually adopted in one form or another by most embalming schools for laboratory practice and is generally used to this day.

Crandall began his career in demisurgery by offering his services anywhere within a 400-mile radius of

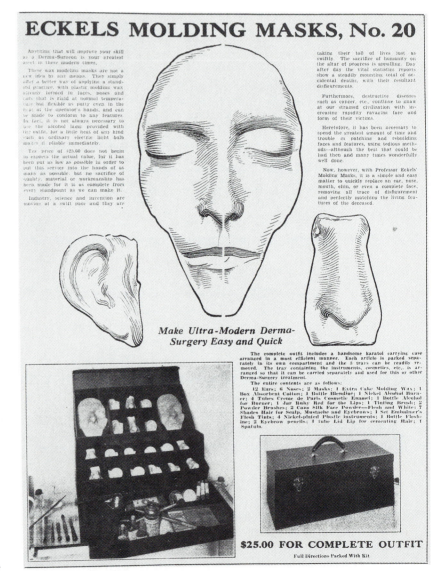

Figure 25. Advertisement for Eckels molding masks.

New York City. Gradually, by demand, he was compelled to offer instruction in demisurgery. Each class was limited to 25 students for a 1-month period of instruction.

About the same time he manufactured and sold the first demisurgical grip containing all required instruments, cosmetics, brushes, prefabricated mustaches and eyelashes, and preformed facial features of wax.

The use of prefabricated features as a base for individual modification of the decedent's facial topography enabled the unskilled or untrained embalmer to perform a reasonable restoration otherwise impossible. Crandall's brilliant concept was to be duplicated by others a number of times over the ensuing years.

A report of a restoration in 1924 mentions the use of prefabricated eyes and nose. The manufacturer of the parts, William Collier of New York City, advertised a kit containing prefabricated features in 1929 and patented the same in 1931. The Eckels Company of Philadelphia offered a similar kit in October of 1930 (Fig. 25), as did the Paasche Air Brush Company of Chicago in 1936. An interesting improvement on prefabricated features was developed by a dental plastic surgeon named C. J. Speas, who taught restorative art at Gupton–Jones College of Mortuary Science in Nashville, Tennessee, in the late 1940s. The basic concept was the "family resemblance theory," that is, members of the same family frequently resemble one another very closely. Thus, for example,

when a nose is destroyed, a mold is made of the nose of a family member most closely resembling the decedent, cast in wax, and fitted into the decedent's face. Thus, a custom-made prefabrication is created.

Crandall purchased the Clerihew Undertaking Company located at 133 Broadway, Paterson, New Jersey, in 1913, and continued to maintain premises in New York City for his demisurgical supply company and school. Crandall must have written at some length on the subject of demisurgery, as *The Funeral Director's Encyclopedia,* a proposed three-volume work, each volume supposed to contain about 600 pages, was described in *The Sunnyside* in 1916 as having 100 pages on the art of demisurgery by Joel E. Crandall. No copies of this three-volume encyclopedia are known to exist and it is suspected that it was never published. The 100 pages on demisurgery referred to were most likely the basic lectures used by Crandall in the resident course of instruction at the Demisurgical Institute of New York and as a teaching text in his correspondence course in 1918 (Fig. 26). (The writers have never seen this material and would be most grateful to any member of our profession having a copy of same, making it available for inspection and study.)

The greatest impact of Crandall's influence on the embalmers of America resulted from his published photographs of mutilated cases taken before and after treat-

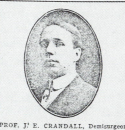

Figure 26. Copy of the first ad for demisurgery in 1918.

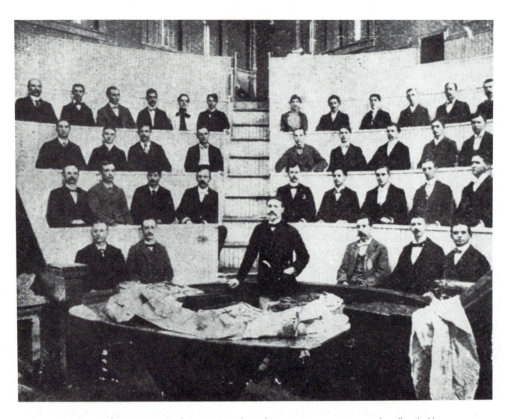

Figure 27. Carl L. Barnes giving a demonstration in the Cook County Morgue, contiguous to the college building.

ment, most of which were extremely difficult to restore even by today's standards. His work was exceptionally well done and was an inspiration to embalmers who desired to improve their skills, for he showed and proved that difficult cases could be restored to a viewable condition.

The effect of Crandall's announcement of the founding of the art of demisurgery on the embalming schools of the country varied. Some heads of schools such as Robbins of Boston, C. O. Dhonau of Cincinnati, and Thorton Barnes of New York were rather vocal in their protest concerning Crandall's claim to founding the science (Fig. 27). All three claimed that their schools had taught the subject for years, though in truth no mention of the matter in advertising nor listing of the subject matter in the school curricula is noted prior to April 1912. Barnes' Schools began to advertise the teaching of Der-Mort-Ology, and the Cincinnati School added a course in demisurgery, whereas Robbins stated that his school taught artistic embalming, decoloration, and postmortem surgery. C. A. Renouard stated that he neither taught nor recommended the use of cosmetics and, further, that much of demisurgery was unnecessary and unwelcome. Before his death, in 1953, Renouard was to reverse his opinion to the extent of even providing special short-term courses in restorative art.

Dhonau additionally accused Crandall of publish-

ing retouched photographs of his restored cases. This so incensed Crandall that he secured affidavits from everyone concerned—the undertaker, the photographer, lawyers, and family representatives, who attested to the authenticity of his work as represented by the case photographs.

Lena Simmons composed a satirical account of a fictional Lemuel, the young embalmer at Burrywell & Company who "fixed him up." She skillfully concocted a case report using quotations from published articles on demisurgical procedures by Robbins and others, but curiously enough did not include any by Crandall.

The interest in the new art of demisurgery was immediate and has continued to the present day. The professional journals increasingly carried both photographs and case reports of successful treatment of mutilated cases, while advertisements multiplied for cosmetics, instruments, and demisurgical materials.

Crandall's career blossomed as he lectured on demisurgery at the New York State Embalmers Convention in the fall of 1912 and continued a busy demisurgical practice.

Among the cases Crandall treated was the famous Colonel Jacob Astor, who in 1912 as a passenger on the Titanic died at sea. His body, like hundreds of others, was taken from the sea near the site of the sinking and transported to Halifax, Nova Scotia, and from there returned to New York City for burial. Crandall was called by the New York undertaker in charge to treat Astor's badly discolored face. By means of Crandall's cosmetic skill, the casket was open for viewing of the body as it lay in state at the Astor estate near Rhinebeck, New York.

The February 1917 issue of *The Sunnyside* carried a notice that Crandall had motion pictures taken of a number of his demisurgical cases and that the films would be available for teaching purposes and presentation at conventions. Historically, this is the first known recording of any restorative procedures in motion pictures.

Crandall continued to be in demand to lecture before large crowds at state conventions on this new and intriguing subject, appearing on several state programs in New England in 1917. By 1918 the effect of World War I on the funeral profession was becoming evident and Crandall was interviewed by *The Sunnyside* for his views on the application of demisurgery to U.S. war casualties. He was most forthright in his conviction that all our war dead should be embalmed shortly after death and restored later at a convenient time and place (Fig. 27).

Crandall's illustrated demisurgical case reports continued to be seen in professional journals through 1922. From 1923 on, however, Crandall fades in national note, though continuing to operate his Paterson, New Jersey, funeral home until death on July 19, 1942.

Joel E. Crandall demonstrated that any case, no matter how badly mutilated, could be restored to viewability. Further, he devised not only the materials for his newly created science of demisurgery, but the technical instructions to accomplish this new skill.

All practicing embalmers owe a debt of gratitude to Joel E. Crandall, demisurgeon and founder of demisurgery, known today as restorative art.

The sudden and unforeseen arrival of Joel E. Crandall on the educational scene as the founder of the new art of demisurgery created the problem of partial loss of educational leadership for the American embalming schools. Recovering quickly from this threat, most schools began to teach the subject, although some, out of pride or vanity, refused to give the new art Crandall's title: demisurgery.

The immediate exception was Cincinnati College, which called the subject demisurgery but insisted that the subject had been taught there for years. Eckels College used the term *demisurgery* and acknowledged Crandall as its founder. Boston College called the course *postmortem surgery and the art of decoloration,* and the Barnes School dubbed it *Der-Mort-Ology and dermasurgery.* An article describing Albert Worsham's demonstration of demisurgery calls it *plastic work.* The terms *dermasurgery* and *plastic surgery* also were noted as descriptive titles for the art, although one of the most original titles was used in 1917 by the New York School of Embalming (formerly Barnes School), which advertised derma sculpture taught by a sculptor and demisurgery taught by an embalmer. An advertisement for Dermatol Cosmetics in 1913 stated that it was not necessary to go to school to learn demisurgery or cosmetic application as everything one needed to know was in the pamphlet wrapped around each jar of cosmetics.

From 1912 onward the pages of our professional journals disclose early contributions to the science of what today is termed restorative art. More and more advertisements are seen for cosmetics, demisurgery kits, and equipment (Fig. 28). Before-and-after case photos, pioneered by Crandall, appeared with some frequency in product advertisements as well as in articles. Demonstration of demisurgery at meetings and conventions became every bit as popular and as well attended as embalming demonstrations had been 30 years earlier.

Many prominent teachers and heads of embalming colleges wrote about the "new art." Some made first mention of standard basic procedures or techniques still employed today. Others advanced practices that were proven later to have little real value; for example, Robbins, in 1912, advocated the grafting of skin from one area of the body to replace damaged skin on the head. Such procedures were seldom very successful.

Robbins together with Lena Simmons, in 1912, mentions invisible or blind stitching (subcutaneous sutures), and C. O. Dhonau in the same year recommended baseball stitching with wax covering and concealing the sutured area, a rather unsatisfactory technique. Razorless shaving cream (a depilatory) made a brief but unsuccessful appearance in 1914, as it has a number of times since then.

Basic principles of demisurgery practice, such as using very concentrated fluid to produce firm tissue as ideal for final restoration and performing basic restoration to a near-normal anatomical relationship prior to arterial injection, were reiterated by C. O. Dhonau, Robbins, Worsham, Lena Simmons, and others. Some recommended removal of tumors and other surgical procedures prior to embalming, but Worsham and most modern authorities recommended that this be done after arterial injection. Most early authorities agreed that it was necessary to wait between completion of the arterial treatment and final application of wax and cosmetics. Most recommended a minimum of 6 to 10 hours' timelapse to ensure drying and halting of leakage from torn tissues.

In 1915 Worsham mentions using cotton and Collodion as a cavity filler to within one-sixteenth of an inch of the normal surface, then covering this surface with wax. He also used the cotton and Collodion to form such basic features as lips, ears, nose, and eyelids.

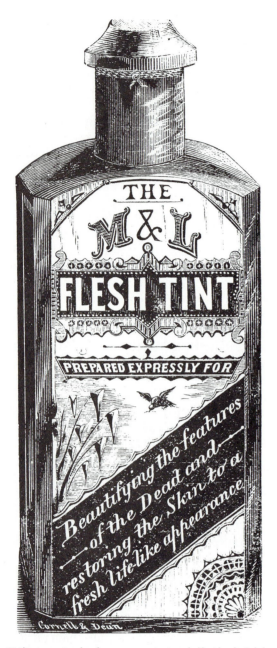

Figure 28. This preparation, though not a preservative is a valuable aid to the Embalmer's art.

Dhonau, writing at some length on demisurgery in 1915, called attention to the individuality of the human face, differences in the lateral halves, as well as cosmetic skin variations. His suggestion, noted for the first time, to do the "work in the same light as that in which the body will rest until its final disposition," is still heeded today. In 1915 he demonstrated modeling of the facial features on a plaster skull, a technique that is today fairly standard throughout the schools for the teaching of restorative art.

One of the more dramatic demisurgical cases of the era was that treated by Worsham in Chicago in mid-

1917. A lion tamer was attacked, mangled, and killed while performing in the lions' cage. A Chicago undertaker, Lafayette C. Ball, who was present at the attack, ran to his nearby funeral home, secured several bottles of formalin-based cavity fluid, returned to the circus cage, and poured the contents of the bottles over the dead lion tamer's torn body. This ingenious technique stopped the lions from further mangling the body, and permitted the circus personnel to retrieve it. Worsham, called on to prepare the body, was confronted with the need to replace both ears, much of the face, and both arms, and to close the torn open abdomen from which some viscera had been devoured. Before and after photos disclose a reasonable restoration.

Practicing embalmers were stimulated to try to repair difficult cases, too. *The Sunnyside* issue of September 15, 1914, published a story and before-and-after photos of two cases, a murder and suicide by shotgun. In both, the skulls had been shattered by the 16-gauge shot. Mr. and Mrs. G. A. Rousevell of Lead, South Dakota, restored the bodies to a virtually normal appearance.

During the period 1910–1920 there was much preoccupation with the problem of jaundice. Every fluid manufacturer who made, as most did, a formalin-based arterial fluid received complaints about the change in color of a jaundiced body from yellow to green after embalming. Despite the manufacture of numerous new formulas by many companies through the intervening years, this problem remains not completely solved to the present day.

During 1924 J. H. De Normandie of New York City developed a treatment for jaundice. He injected a solvent (not specified) into the carotid artery without drainage and allowed it to remain for 20 minutes, during which time a special ointment was applied to the face and the face covered with hot moist towels. This was followed by the injection of about 3 gallons of arterial fluid and drainage from the jugular vein. The system was declared successful but chemical components were never fully disclosed.

Other individual embalmers experimented with the use of various bleaching solutions such as phenol, chlorine (laundry bleach), and hydrogen peroxide, none of which produced any measure of uniform results.

In 1917 C. O. Dhonau announced a new technique for treating swollen, blackened eyes. He incised the underside of the affected lid or lids, pressed out the accumulated blood and serum, and then applied 50% phenol solution to shrink and bleach the area.

At this time the schools, which conducted courses of instruction of quite varying lengths averaging 3 months' duration at most, allotted some instruction time to demisurgery. Some schools scheduled regular periods in the laboratory for learning to form facial features in wax or clay on a plaster skull. Unique among these courses was that taught by Worsham, whose class in demisurgery was most often given at the end of the entire course of instruction. By the 1930s it amounted to 25 to 40 total hours of laboratory work. The actual practice was carried out on mutilated human heads left over from the anatomy dissection classes. The heads were stored in preservative fluid between class sessions and were, of course, rather wet, distorted, and chemically malodorous. The actual practice, however, was realistic, as all suturing, cavity filling, feature forming, and cosmetizing were practiced just as on an actual case.

In 1948 at the Postgraduate Institute of Restorative Art of Chicago, the laboratory teaching system was modified by the recreation of dozens of mutilated heads in plastic and rubber, which permitted suturing, waxing, and cosmetizing. The school was headed by Dean Edward C. Johnson.

Before-and-after photos of a case handled by the faculty and students of the Simmons School in 1921 indicate good results. In 1924 Cincinnati College featured its postmortem plastic surgery laboratory in an advertisement for the first time. In 1926 Dhonau criticized fluid manufacturers for issuing diplomas in demisurgery to those in attendance at their free clinics. This was a throwback to 35 years earlier when fluid manufacturers were criticized for issuing diplomas to those attending their embalming clinics.

Virtually every issue of *Casket and Sunnyside* during the 1920s carried at least one feature article about demisurgery, whether a case history, before-and-after photos, new products for the demisurgeon, or editorial praise and commendation for the procedure. In 1925 an advertisement appeared announcing that Clyde E. Richardson of Paterson, New Jersey, was available for dermasurgical cases. It is believed he was trained by Joel E. Crandall. The April 1, 1925, issue of *Casket and Sunnyside* had a four-page insert by the Eckels Chemical Company of Philadelphia on dermasurgery. The copy was a combination of a sales pitch for the Eckels Company's cosmetics, instruments, and other materials and technical advice on case treatment.

Some American folk heroes were the subjects of restorative treatment. One of the earliest was Floyd Collins, who in 1925 was trapped in Sand Cave, Kentucky, where he died. Eighty-three days later, his body was recovered and removed to Bowling Green, Kentucky, where it was embalmed and the destroyed facial features (eyes, nose, and mouth) were replaced. His mother expressed satisfaction with his appearance in the casket.

Three notorious criminals—John Dillinger, Bonnie Parker, and Clyde Barrow—died at the hands of law enforcement agents in July 1934. Dillinger, dead from bullet wounds in a Chicago Alley, was taken to the Cook County morgue, where a Worsham College of Mortuary Science instructor, Don Asheworth, was requested to make a death mask of Dillinger for the FBI. Asheworth related to the writers that he was visited by the FBI at 2 AM and that he was persuaded to hand over the extra mask.

Bonnie and Clyde were slain near Arcadia, Louisiana, and taken to a mortuary there. Both were embalmed in Louisiana, but Clyde was taken to the Sparkman–Holly–Brand Mortuary in Dallas, while Bonnie was taken to McKamy–Campbell Funeral Home, also in Dallas. Clyde, his head shattered, received more than 100 bullet or shotgun pellet wounds; Bonnie received more than 50 bullet wounds. Both bodies were restored and viewed in their respective caskets by an estimated 50,000 people.

In 1936 the convicted kidnapper and murderer of Charles A. Lindbergh's baby, Bruno Hauptmann, was executed by electrocution. Reports of his preparation state that restorative art procedures were required to repair burns on his face and head. Services were private, however, and followed by cremation.

In the December 1926 issue of *Casket and Sunnyside* appeared the first advertisement for the electric-heated spatula, manufactured by the Montez Manufacturing Company, of Addison, Michigan (Fig. 29). This device, highly touted when first developed as an excellent spatula to smoothe and model wax as well as to reduce swollen areas, was less effective than anticipated. The heat of the iron had a tendency to melt wax and leave an unnaturally shiny surface. When used to reduce swelling, the device produced only a very minor evident reduction after much effort. Perhaps its best use was to "iron" tissue.

In August 1927 during the Minnesota 37th State Convention at St. Paul, the term *restorative art* was first used. The Worsham College advertisement of December 1927 used the term *restorative art* but later reverted to the term *dermasurgery*. In 1929, the McAllister School listed Robert C. Harper as professor of restorative art. In November 1928 William G. Collier, Collier School, New York City, stated in an address, "Any man can be taught the principles of this restorative art." It was to take some years, however, before the term *restorative art* was adopted and uniformly applied to the subject area first termed demisurgery by Joel E. Crandall in 1912.

By the mid-1920s, articles by teachers and practitioners of embalming on restorative art appeared with frequency in most professional journals and house organs of chemical manufacturers and supply companies. One such writer and practitioner was William G. Collier, a trade embalmer of New York City who became a prolific author of articles on restorative art. Collier, scion of a well-established funeral service family, first appeared in print in *Casket and Sunnyside* in 1925 with an article on jaundice treatment. From that moment on he was a

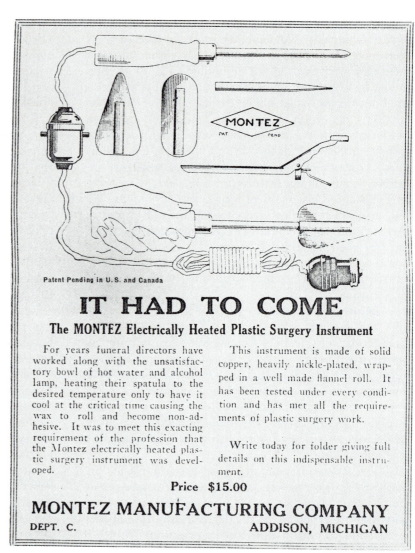

Figure 29. Early heated spatula used to smooth wax and reduce swollen facial tissues, circa 1926.

more or less regular contributor of articles dealing with treatment of facial cancer, decapitation, general demisurgical procedures, and cosmetics.

Collier founded both a school of embalming instruction and a shipping service in New York City, and was the holder of several patents for restorative wound fillers and preformed facial features. Collier is remembered as a patient teacher, excellent speaker, and excruciating writer.

The Champion Company in March 1929 introduced the subject area to the readers of its house organ, *Champion Expanding Encyclopedia of Mortuary Practice,* with an article entitled The Art of Plastic Surgery. Such written articles by the supervising chemist, A. O. Spriggs, on a variety of subjects (e.g., treatment of gunshot cases, subcutaneous suture, hypodermic injection of tissue filler cream) were assembled into a textbook in 1934 that is still available today under the title *Champion Restorative Art.*

As early as 1927, C. F. Callaway was lecturing, demonstrating, and writing on the subject of restorative art. Callaway became a special representative of the Undertaker's Supply Company of Chicago, and wrote many articles on plastic surgery for its house organ, as well as trade publications. Ten years later he was joined in these activities by Ralph Hensen, who later taught mortuary science subjects at the College of Mortuary Science at St. Louis, and by Clarence G. Strub (Fig. 30), whose last years in a long and distinguished professional career in funeral service were spent with the University of Iowa as curator of the Anatomy Department of the Iowa Medical College eye enucleation training program. Strub's early contribution to restorative art was his publication in 1932 of a small textbook of 32 pages entitled *The Principles of Restorative Art As the Embalmer Should Know Them* (Fig. 31). The little text was extremely well written in a simple and direct style with emphasis on the practical application of technique, though

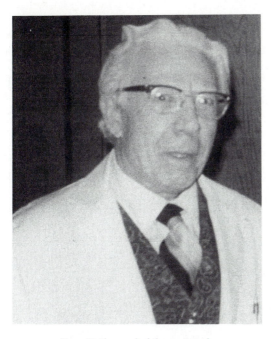

Figure 30. Photograph of Clarence G. Strub.

Stallard and Slocum produced pamphlets of instruction on the subject of embalming and restorative art, which were much sought after and highly prized by practicing embalmers.

In 1945 *Casket and Sunnyside* inaugurated a monthly feature, Restoration Clinic by E. C. Johnson. Each monthly article described treatment for a particular type of case and was illustrated by before-and-after photographs of each case. The series continued monthly for more than 14 years.

The spring of 1931 was marked by the untimely death of one of the early full-time embalming college teachers of restorative art, Ivan P. Bowsher. Bowsher, dying at age 33, was a World War I veteran who had graduated from Cincinnati College in the class of 1921. While a student at the college he was recognized as a gifted artist and was invited to join the faculty, on graduation, as a teacher of restorative art. For 10 brief years he gave the students of Cincinnati College one of the best courses of instruction in restorative art available. On his death, the college instituted the Ivan P. Bowsher Medal for outstanding achievement in restorative art to be awarded to one member of each graduating class. Cincinnati College had another outstanding teacher of restorative art, G. Joseph Prager, who with Dean C. O. Dhonau wrote an excellent textbook entitled *Manual of Restorative Art*, published in 1934. Prager continued and expanded the restorative art curriculum inaugurated by Bowsher and in 1955 published another textbook entitled *Post Mortem Restorative Art*.

The post-World War II era witnessed the publication of a number of textbooks on restorative art, ranging in quality from poor to classic. An example is the *Technique of Restorative Art* by Maude Adams Adair

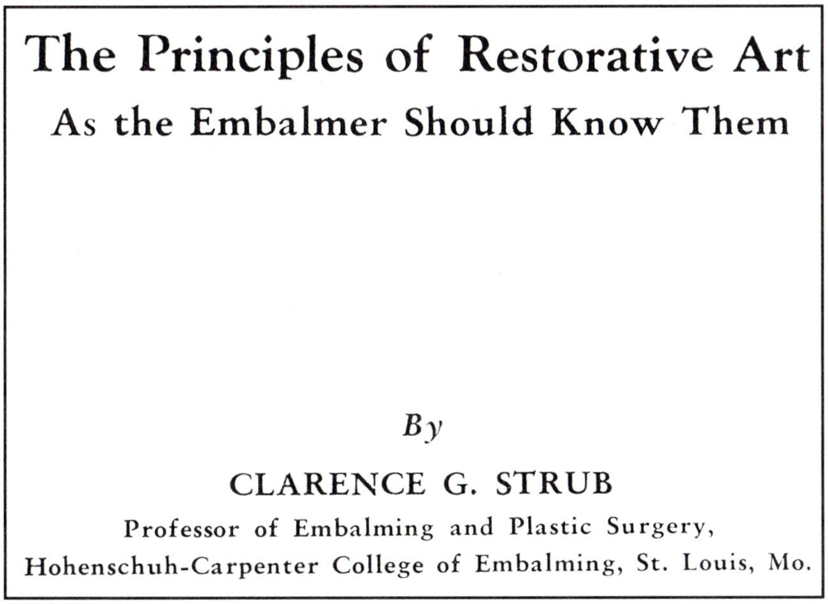

it did embody some elements of theory. Taken as a whole, the book can be recognized as the true prototype of the best contemporary restorative art textbook.

The Dodge Chemical Company, during this period, also had a team of talented writers, lecturers, and demonstrators in the persons of Frank Stallard, a voluminous writer whose articles appeared for years in trade publications and the Dodge Chemical Company house organ, and Ray Slocum, a most popular embalming and restorative art demonstrator on the Dodge "faculty." Both

The Principles of Restorative Art
As the Embalmer Should Know Them

By

CLARENCE G. STRUB

Professor of Embalming and Plastic Surgery,
Hohenschuh-Carpenter College of Embalming, St. Louis, Mo.

Figure 31. Title page of Clarence G. Strub's book.

published in 1948. The text is superficial, and has a conglomeration of nonrelevant subject matter ranging from flower arrangement, to hairdressing, to the National Funeral Directors Association's code of ethics, to committal services.

An excellent book that deals with a very limited area of the field of restorative art, written by Gladys P. Cury of Boston in 1947, is titled *A Textbook of Facial Reconstruction*. Gladys Curry was an internationally recognized authority on the identification of the dead, and her expertise was often requested in disasters such as the infamous Coconut Grove nightclub fire, which claimed more than 500 victims, and the recovery of decomposing bodies of the crew members of the submarine Sqaulus lost in U.S. waters in 1939.

Her book is well illustrated with photographs depicting the step-by-step reconstruction or replacement on the bare skull of the soft tissues of the face and neck to the individual's normal appearance. The task is carried out logically and methodically by replacing the muscles in their normal position as to origin and insertion and finally sculpting the features and skin surface and adding the hair. The Curry system has been successfully employed by a number of embalmers who have assisted various law enforcement agencies in the identification of skeletal remains.

The Curry text is devoted solely to instruction in reconstruction of the soft tissues of the head and neck with clay or wax, and is devoid of any instruction on or concern with the ordinary restorative problems or embalming of such cases. This text is highly recommended as an invaluable addition to an embalmer's library for reference on modeling and identification techniques.

The contemporary standard textbook on restorative art was written by the late Sheridan Mayer (Fig. 32), pub-

lished as a lengthy treatise in 1940 and as a fully hardbound textbook in 1943 entitled simply *Restorative Art*. This work has gone through many revisions and is now used in most mortuary science college programs. Mayer also wrote the treatises *Workbook on Color* published in 1947 and *Mortuary Cosmetology* published in 1948. In 1973 he published the textbook *Color and Cosmetics*, which is in use in mortuary science college programs.

Mayer was born in a Philadelphia suburb in 1908 and was educated in primary schools in the area. He attended the University of Pennsylvania and a number of private schools where he enrolled in courses largely in the field of art, sculpture, and public speaking. His allied interests included the theater; he acted on stage and studied, taught, and was employed as a theatrical cosmetician and makeup specialist in the Philadelphia and New York City areas.

It is noteworthy and to his great credit that Mayer overcame the handicap of not being a practicing embalmer and yet was able to impart instruction intelligently. Mayer is one of the very few, if not the only, truly successful teachers who had never been a practicing embalmer.

His introduction to the teaching of restorative art was at a clinic at the Eckels College of Mortuary Science in Philadelphia, September 6–8, 1939, where he appeared on the program with the famed Covermark cosmetic formulator Lydia O'Leary. His dynamic and informative presentation was so well received by all in attendance that he was offered a position on the faculty, which he accepted and retained until 1947.

During 1943 to 1945 Mayer volunteered for duty in the U.S. Maritime Service and was assigned to the harbor antisubmarine net division. In 1947 he joined the faculty of the Pittsburgh Institute of Mortuary Science, where he met Otto S. Margolis and formed an admiration for him. In 1951 when Margolis assumed control of the American Academy of Mortuary Science in New York City, Mayer accompanied him there to strengthen the faculty. The American Academy merged with the McAllister Institute in 1964.

Mayer has written extensively on the subject of cosmetics and restorative art and has written articles for many professional journals. His greatest contribution to the subject of restorative art, however, has been his influence and steady guidance of mortuary colleges toward the development and acceptance of a uniform course of instruction, as well as the adoption of uniform standards of facilities for such instruction and relevant examination questions. He has been the chairman of the restorative art course content committee of mortuary science schools and colleges for many years, where he accomplished monumental tasks in curriculum studies and syllabus preparation and screening of a bank of examination questions on the subject of restorative art. Mayer

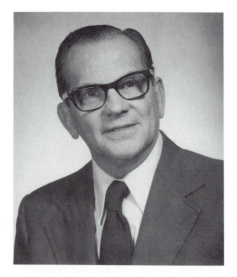

Figure 32. Photograph of J. Sheridan Mayer.

taught until 1975. In December of 1993, he died in Cincinnatti, Ohio, where he had retired.

Unfortunately, not all who have taught restorative art were as dedicated or qualified as Mayer. Some were individuals with basic training in art or sculpture, who had little interest or understanding of the problems involved in restorative art. Some examples come to mind. In one case an instructor had his students practice modeling each feature in supersize; ears, for example, were a foot long. Another instructor was most insistent that the students practice sculpturing of the eyes and mouth open! Surely such practices lack any semblance of relevance to normal professional procedures. The writers personally believe very strongly that the teaching of embalming and restorative art requires not only a background of practical experience in such areas, but, equally important, a continuing experience of practice while teaching.

The present-day requirement of the possession of a college degree to become a faculty member at colleges of mortuary science sharply limits the employment of many capable potential teachers with genuine expertise in embalming and restorative art. The words of A. Johnson Dodge, as so well stated in 1917, are still valid today: "How to care for mutilated bodies and make them presentable should constitute a part of the education of the embalmer. Thorough instruction in this difficult art should be given by instructors in our schools. But this part of the work required *special experience* and some study either to practice or teach it successfully."

One area of instruction in restorative art that has been recognized increasingly as a valuable practical working asset is the study of physical anthropology. Physical anthropology has been defined as a science that deals with the physical likenesses and differences of the races and sexes as well as the changes wrought by age and disease of humans. Such study has been most helpful in the practice of restorative art. It has been particularly invaluable in identification and reconstruction of skeletal remains. Study of skeletal remains can reveal sex, race, age, general height range, as well as individual characteristics such as right or left handedness, old trauma, (e.g., healed fractures), and diseases. Perhaps the most interesting use of such knowledge is the reconstruction of the face on a fleshless skull.

The technique used today by experts such as Betty Catliff, assistant to Clyde Snow, physical anthropologist, retired Chief of the Federal Aviation Authority, Physical Anthropology Unit, at Norman, Oklahoma, is virtually identical to the original system devised by Wilhelm His of Leipzig University in Germany.

In brief in 1895, His was compelled to devise a method of identifying a skull as to whether or not it and its associated bones were the remains of the renowned composer Johann Sebastian Bach. The bones had been disinterred from the church cemetery during enlargement of the church of St. John and a new more elaborate grave and monument for the remains, if indeed they were his, were planned. Proof of the identity was imperative.

His studied the bones in his anatomy laboratory and recognized the key to the solution. The bones of the face support the soft tissues, muscles, fat, and skin. The soft tissues vary in thickness at various points, for example, thin over the forehead, nose, and prominences of the temples, cheeks, lips, and chin. He also deduced that tissue thickness was fairly uniform at about 15 key points over the anterior and lateral skull surface of individuals of like sex, name, and age.

His began assembling measurements of the key points from the numerous undissected cadavers in his laboratory. He recorded each point thickness for each corpse, then averaged these measurements to secure a single working measurement for each such point. He had small metal markers constructed that were labeled A, B, and so on, to correspond with the tissue thickness at that point.

He secured the services of a well-known sculptor who agreed to undertake the project of reconstruction of the skull using the His technique. The metal markers were put in position on the skull, embedded in clay. When they were all correctly placed, strips of clay were applied connecting the points, and these in turn were interconnected. Finally the vacant spaces were filled in and the features formed. The reconstructed skull appearance obtained closely resembled contemporary portraits and sculptures of Bach and the committee for construction of the new tomb and monument was satisfied.

This technique has been updated from time to time by creating new tables, as His did, of females and other races. The technique has produced good results even by those using the procedure for the first time.

While the schools of mortuary science steadily increased the hours allotted to the teaching of restorative art, they recognized the fact that many practicing embalmers felt a distinct lack of ability in this field. Consequently, from time to time virtually all schools of mortuary science offered practicing embalmers special short courses varying in length from 1 to 7 days. Some featured actual demonstrations on mutilated bodies, whereas others offered only practice modeling of features.

Through the years special schools were founded to teach cosmetic application and restorative art. An example of such a school, unaffiliated with an existing school of mortuary science, was the Embalmers Graduate College formed in Chicago in 1937 by L. Roy Davenport and Honora D. Mannix, which offered 30 hours of instruction and practice in both cosmetology and restorative art.

In 1948 the Post Graduate Institute of Restorative

Art was organized in Chicago. The curriculum included a short 2-week course and the standard 7-month course that offered 25 hours per week of instruction. When the school was merged into Worsham College in 1955, the course had been taken by 16 mortuary college restorative art instructors or their assistants.

Education of embalmers at all levels of skill in restorative art has been enhanced by the production of photographic records of actual restorative procedures. Some of these productions were in black and white, some in full color, some in motion, and others in still pictures. Most are silent and very few have either sound or voice accompaniment.

The earliest still photographs of restorative art cases taken before, during, and after restoration were, of course, those of cases treated by demisurgeon Joel E. Crandall dating no later than 1912. Crandall also bears the distinction of producing the first black and white motion pictures of restorative procedures made in the year 1917 (See Fig. 24).

Other great early teachers such as C. A. Renouard and Albert Worsham made films prior to 1920 not only on the subject of restorative art but also on embalming technique and anatomical dissections.

The truly classic motion picture on restorative procedures was produced in color in the early 1930s by the

late Earle K. Angstadt (Fig. 33) of the Auman Funeral Home of Reading, Pennsylvania, who also performed all the actual restorative art techniques displayed in the film. The silent film has subtitles and is expertly photographed. It depicts classic technique, flawlessly performed, during the restoration of a surgically removed mandible, reduction of facial swelling, hypodermic tissue filling of face and hand, and replacement of eyelids and eyelashes damaged beyond salvage by an infection. This film, still available from either National Selected Morticians or National Funeral Directors Association headquarters, will never be improved on.

Another much longer film recording many more cases of severe trauma was produced in the late 1930s by the late R. Victor Landig, founder of the Landig College of Mortuary Science at Houston. The photography of the 10 or 12 cases recorded on the film varies widely from poor to good, with respect to color fidelity, focus, and technique, whereas restorative skill is uniformly good except for the handling of hair restorations.

The Los Angeles College of Mortuary Science produced a fine color motion picture complete with sound and voice in the late 1940s. The film depicts no actual cases but does show how to produce plaster practice masks and provides excellent modeling instruction for producing the individual facial features. The Champion Company of Ohio has a motion picture in color made in the 1940s by A. O. Spriggs, featuring his technique in treating a small group of actual restorative cases. E. C. Johnson has slides recording the treatment of several hundred cases, including virtually every conceivable problem requiring restorative art treatment.

Our profession desperately needs more visual aids such as the foregoing to provide wider exposure of our practitioners to successful techniques at conventions, meetings, seminars, and workshops.

While textbooks, films, and teachers were providing more instruction and training for every level of embalmer competence, skill, and capability, the chemical and embalming supply manufacturers were also active in providing better tools and materials for the embalmer to complete restorations more skillfully.

In 1933 the Hydrol Chemical Company made a most significant announcement in the trade journals concerning the patenting of liquid tissue builder that coagulated or jelled on being hypodermically introduced into the body tissue. This, of course, was a vast improvement over ordinary liquids such as glycerin, then in use for this purpose, as such liquids, remaining liquid, tended to settle away from the high point in response to the law of gravity. This failure of the hypodermically deposited material to maintain its position obviously ultimately destroyed the effect of such treatment.

Another equally vexatious problem resulting from the use of such permanent-liquid-state tissue builders was

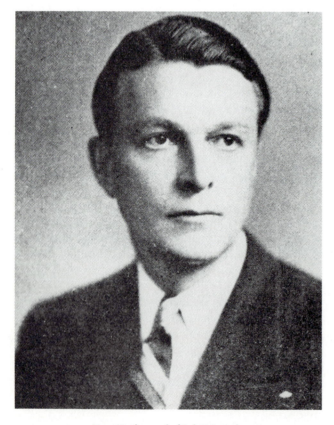

Figure 33. Photograph of Earle K. Angstadt.

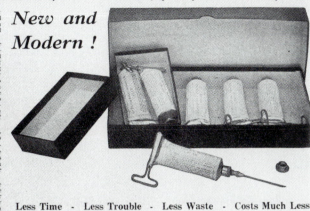

Hypo-Derma Molding Cream

➤ For Filling In the Emaciated Face, Neck and Hands, Quickly and Efficiently ◄

New and Modern !

Emaciated cases from tuberculosis, chronic anemia, or long illness can be greatly improved in appearance by injecting Eckels' Hypo-Derma Cream into the tissues of hollow cheeks and temples.

There are quite a number of ways, all more or less helpful, for the improvement of this condition. In the past, hand-heated wax has answered the purpose and still does with quite a few, but it is a more or less laborious way of doing it; whereas, the modern injection of an especially compounded cream is much quicker, easier to handle and to control. Our new Hypo-Derma Cream, especially made to inject, as it is, in the tissue by merely attaching the needle directly to the tube, does not even require filling the hypodermic syringe. The cream is injected into the tissue simply by turning the key on the end of the tube.

The body should first be thoroughly embalmed, particularly the parts in which this cream is to be injected and the tissues should be fairly firm.

The operator should insert the needle in the hairline to inject the hollow places in the temples and inside of the nose or corner of the mouth for the purpose of filling out the cheeks in order not to leave the marks of the needle to view.

The needle itself should be injected into the tissue first and then the tube attached. The point of the needle should be inserted to the far end of the hollow spot and worked back slowly over the entire area in order that sufficient cream be forced into the tissue, so that it may be properly distributed throughout the depressed area. After this is done and you have injected the cream the needle may gradually be withdrawn with the entire depression filled.

Should it be found that there is an uneven distribution of cream this may be overcome and smoothed out by the use of a hot towel.

Less Time - Less Trouble - Less Waste - Costs Much Less

Also prevents contracting and drying of the skin, particularly the lips and nose.

This new package containing 6 tubes, attachment and needle, sells complete for $3.00. Included in this outfit is a smaller case holding two tubes which can be readily slipped into your pocket or grip.

Figure 34. Tissue filler using cream, circa 1930.

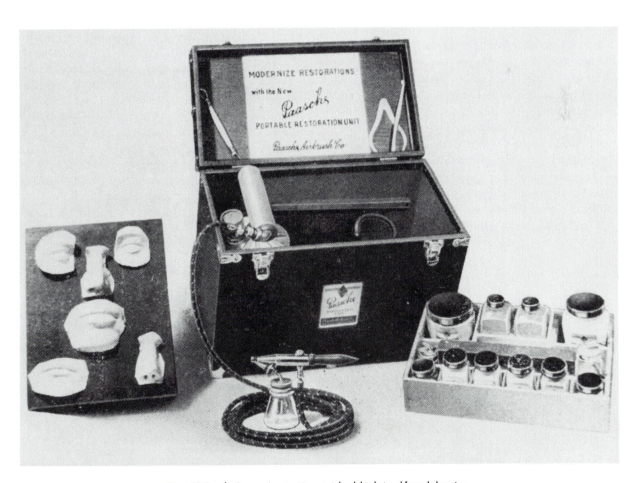

Figure 35. Paasche Company's restorative art air brush kit designed for embalmers' use.

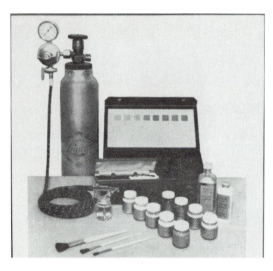

Figure 36. Master Nuance Aire-Tynt Unit.

the most disturbing occurrence of seepage from the point of insertion of the hypodermic needle. Both of these problems were corrected by the new jelling tissue builder as it would neither seep or shift its position due to the change in its structure from liquid to semisolid to solid.

An alternative material such as hand cream or petroleum jelly had been used, but the technique for successful use required that both the filled syringe and the large-diameter needle be kept warm to permit a free flow of the semisolid material. Special hypodermic syringes with screw-threaded plungers were devised to make the ejection of thick creams easier, but they never did become very popular, and after introduction of coagulable liquid filler, they virtually disappeared from the market (Fig. 34).

In 1935 the Dodge Chemical Company introduced De-Ce-Co needle injector and needles as an improved means of securing mouth closure, and in 1937 offered a complete set of eight specially designed restorative art instruments. In addition the company, like many others,

offered a complete range of cosmetics, waxes, and restorative art chemicals.

Methods of cosmetic application, but primarily application of highlight or accent cosmetics over waxed areas, had always required improvement. The difficulty in applying accent cosmetics evenly and naturally on waxed surfaces is a problem familiar to all experienced embalmers. The best solution is to apply the cosmetics with an air brush or power sprayer. By these means the cosmetics are literally floated into position, and disturbance of either the underlying base cosmetics or the wax surface is completely avoided.

As far back as 1911, spray applicators, powered by carbon dioxide cylinders, were available to the embalmer for cosmetic application, but it was not until the 1930s that the need and desire for sprayer-applied cosmetics became popular.

In 1934 the Undertaker's Supply Company announced the availability of the E-Z Way manually operated spray cosmetic applicator and a compatible cosmetic. The device was well received as it was most efficient and was generally conceded to be the best of the non-power-operated sprayers, many of which are still in use today.

In 1936 the Paasche Company of Chicago, a manufacturer of industrial and artistic air brush equipment, offered a restorative art air brush kit designed for embalmers' use (Fig. 35). The kit contained an electric-powered air compressor, an air brush applicator of high quality, restorative art wax, cosmetic instruments, preformed features such as ears, nose, and lips, and an instruction pamphlet. The Nuance Aire-Tynt cosmetic applicator was advertised in 1937 by J. Horace Griggs of Amarillo, Texas (Fig. 36). The air brush applicator could be adapted to apply cosmetics, whether powered by a manually operated pump, an electric-powered air compressor, or a carbonic gas cylinder.

Today many embalmers have been using, when the need arises, inexpensive easily available handheld model

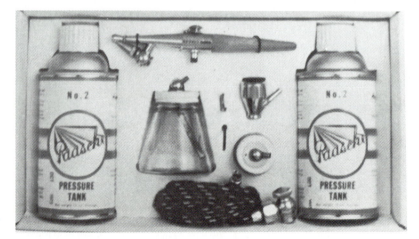

Figure 37. Hand-held model paint sprayer powered by small replaceable containers of freon gas.

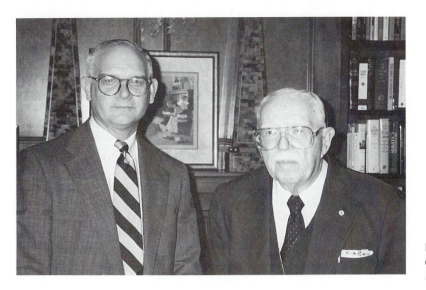

Figure 38. Robert G. Mayer (left) and Edward C. Johnson are instructors of embalming and restorative art. They are the primary authors of *Embalming: History, Theory, and Practice.*

paint sprayers that are powered by small replaceable containers of freon gas. These units, readily available in hobby shops, hardware stores, or paint stores, serve the purpose equally as well as the more expensive air compressor-powered sprayers (Fig. 37).

Restorative art was considered of sufficient importance in 1945 to have Richard G. Reichle, registrar of Worsham College, address the National Funeral Directors Association convention in Chicago on the continuing value and need for these procedures. The National Funeral Directors Association has recognized the importance of restorative art at several of its professional conferences in the past years.

American advances in restorative art over the years has been significant. We have ample supplies of materials and equipment, fine school laboratory teaching facilities, and dedicated teachers, yet the most important need of all remains unchanged. Now, as in the origin of the art, it is necessary for the individual embalmer, in charge of the case, to initiate the restoration of that case and to bring it to a successful conclusion. No amount of material, equipment, or training can substitute for the individual will and determination to overcome a most distressing case. The individual, now as always, is the key to success. The will to succeed and the ability to improvise are more often of value than any other asset.

Today, while you are reading this, the American way of funeral service is under attack by a variety of critics. It is therefore necessary that we in funeral service rededicate ourselves to the fulfillment, to the very best of our ability, of the American way—the funeral with the body present and viewable (Fig. 38).

BIBLIOGRAPHY

Benkard E. *Undying Faces* (a collection of death masks from the 15th century to the present). London: Hogurth Press; 1929.

Clarke CH. *Practical Embalming.* Cincinnati, OH: C. H. Clarke; 1917.

Crane EH. *Manual of Instruction to Undertakers,* 8th ed. Kalamazoo, MI: Kalamazoo; 1888.

Curry GP. *Facial Reconstruction.* Boston; 1947.

Dhonau CO, Prager GJ. *Manual of Restorative Art.* Cincinnati, OH: Embalming Book Co; 1932

Dodge AJ. *The Practical Embalmer.* Boston: A. Johnson Dodge; 1908.

Dutra FR. Identification of person and determination of cause of death. *Archives of Pathology* 1944;38: 339.

Eckles HS. *Derma Surgery.* Philadelphia: H. S. Eckles;

Espy JB. *Espy's Embalmer.* Springfield, OH: Espy's Fluid Co.; 1895.

Gerasimov MM. *The Face Finder.* Philadelphia/New York: Lippincott; 1971.

Gradwohl RBH. *Legal Medicine.* St. Louis, MO: CV Mosby; 1954.

His W. *Anatomische Forschungen über Johann Sebastian Bach's Gegeine und Antlitz Nebst Bermerkungen über dessin Bilder.* Leipzig: S. Hirzel; 1895.

Hooten EA. *Up from the Ape.* New York; Macmillan; 1946.

Johnson EC. *Restorative Art.* Chicago: Worsham College; 1948.

Krogman W. *A Guide to the Identification of Human Skeletal Material.* Washington, DC: FBI Law Enforcement Bulletin.

Krogman W. *The Human Skeleton in Forensic Medicine.* Springfield, IL: C C Thomas; 1962.

Mayer JS. *Workbook on Color.* 1947.

Mayer JS. *Mortuary Cosmetology.* 1948.

Mayer JS. *Color and Cosmetics.* Bergenfield, NJ: Paul Publishing; 1973.

Mayer JS. *Restorative Art.* Dallas, TX: Professional Training Schools; 1993.

Michel G. *Scientific Embalmer.* Cleveland, OH; 1922.

Quiring DP. *Skeletal Identification.* Address to Ohio State Coroners Association; May 23, 1951.

Reichle RG. *Practical Problems in Restorative Art.* Chicago: Lecture - NFDA 63rd Convention; 1945.

Smith E, Dawson WR. *Egyptian Mummies.* New York; Dial Press; 1924.

Spriggs AO. *Plastic Surgery.* 4th ed. Springfield, OH: Champion Chemical; 1946.

Stewart TD. *Essentials of Forensic Anthropology.* Springfield, IL: Charles C Thomas; 1979.

Strub CG. The principles of restorative art. *Embalmer's Monthly.* 1932.

Wentworth B, Wilder HH. *Personal Identification.* Chicago: T. G. Cooke Fingerprint; 1932.

3

part

Glossary*

*1995 Glossary of Terms for the Course Content in Embalming. Prepared by the American Board of Funeral Service Education.

Abdominal anatomical regions. (1) Nine regions of the abdomen as demarcated by four imaginary planes, two of which are horizontal (indicated by lines drawn across the right and left tenth ribs and across the right and left anterior superior iliac spines) and two sagittal (indicated by lines drawn from the midpoint of inguinal ligament to the nipples on the chest, right and left sides). Upper row: right hypochondriac, epigastric, left hypochondriac. Middle row: right lateral, umbilical, left lateral. Lower row: right inguinal, pubic, left inguinal. (2) Four regions of the abdomen as demarcated by two imaginary planes, one horizontal and the other midsagittal: upper right quadrant, upper left quadrant, lower right quadrant, lower left quadrant.

Abrasion. Antemortem injuries resulting from friction of the skin against a firm object and causing removal of the epidermis.

Abut. To touch or contact, as with the tarsal plates of the closed eyelids.

Accessory Chemicals. Chemicals used in addition to vascular (arterial) and cavity embalming fluids. Include but are not limited to hardening compounds, preservative powders, sealing agents, mold-preventive agents, and compress application agents.

Acquired immunodeficiency syndrome (AIDS). Specific group of diseases or conditions that are indicative of severe immunosuppression related to infection with the human immunodeficiency virus (HIV). Persons who died with AIDS may exhibit conditions such as wasting syndrome, extrapulmonary tuberculosis, and Kaposi's sarcoma.

Action level (AL). Exposure limit usually one half of the Occupational Health and Safety Administration (OSHA) legal limit for a regulated substance. This level is established to ensure adequate protection of employees at exposures below the OSHA limits, but to minimize the compliance burdens for employers whose employees have exposures below the 8-hour permissible exposure limit (PEL). The AL for formaldehyde is 0.5 ppm.

Actual pressure. See Pressure.

Adipocere/Grave Wax. Soft, whitish, crumbly or greasy material that forms on postmortem hydrolysis and hydrogenation of body fats.

Adsorption. Assimilation of gas, vapor, or dissolved matter by the surface of a solid or liquid.

Aerobic. In the presence of free oxygen.

Aerosolization. Dispersal as an aerosol. Minute particles of blood and water become atomized and suspended in air when water under pressure meets the blood drainage or when flushing an uncovered flush sink.

Agglutination. Intravascular: increase in viscosity of blood brought about by the clumping of particulate formed elements in the blood vessels.

Agonal algor. Decrease in body temperature immediately before death.

Agonal coagulation. In reference to blood, a change from a fluid into a thickened mass.

Agonal dehydration. Loss of moisture from the living body during the agonal state.

Agonal edema. Escape of blood serum from an intravascular to an extravascular location immediately before death.

Agonal fever. Increase in body temperature immediately before death.

Agonal period. Period immediately before somatic death.

Agonal Translocation. See Translocation.

Algor Mortis. Postmortem cooling of the body to the surrounding temperature.

Alternate drainage. Method of injection–drainage in which embalming solution is injected and then injection is stopped while drainage is open.

Amino acids. Building blocks of which proteins are constructed, and the end products of protein digestion or hydrolysis. The basic formula is NH_2–CHR–COOH–amino group, an alpha carbon, any aliphatic or aromatic radical, and a carboxyl group.

Anaerobic. In the absence of free oxygen.

Anasarca. Severe generalized edema.

Anatomical guide. Method of locating structures by reference to an adjacent known or prominent structure.

Anatomical limits. Points of origin and points of termination in relation to adjacent structures. Used to designate the boundaries of arteries.

Anatomical position. The body is erect, feet together, palms facing forward, and thumbs pointed away from the body.

Aneurysm. Localized abnormal dilation or outpocketing of a blood vessel resulting from a congenital defect or a weakness of the vessel wall.

Aneurysm hook. An embalming instrument that is used for blunt dissection and in raising vessels.

Aneurysm needle. An embalming instrument used for

blunt dissection and in raising vessels that has an eye in the hook portion of the instrument for placing ligatures around the vessels.

Angular spring forceps. Embalming instrument used as a drainage instrument.

Anomaly. Deviation from the normal.

Antecubital. In front of the elbow/in the bend of the elbow.

Antemortem. Before death.

Anterior. Toward the front.

Anterior superior iliac spine. A bony protuberance that can be palpated topographically, found on the ilium, the superior broad portion of the hip bone; the origin of the inguinal ligament and the sartorius muscle.

Anticoagulant fluid. Ingredient of embalming fluids that retards the natural postmortem tendency of blood to become more viscous or prevents adverse reactions between blood and other embalming chemicals.

Apparent death. Condition in which the manifestations of life are feebly maintained.

Arterial (vascular) fluid. Concentrated, preservative, embalming chemical that is diluted with water to form the arterial solution for injection into the arterial system during vascular embalming. Its purpose is to inactivate saprophytic bacteria and render the body tissues less susceptible to decomposition.

Arterial solution. Mixture of arterial (vascular) fluid and water used for the arterial injection. May include supplemental fluids.

Arterial tube. Tube used to inject embalming solution into the blood vascular system.

Arteriosclerosis. Term applied to a number of pathological conditions causing a thickening, hardening, and loss of elasticity of the walls of the arteries.

Articulation. Place of union between two or more bones.

Ascites. Accumulation of serous fluids in the peritoneal cavity.

Asepsis. Freedom from infection and from any form of life. Sterility.

Asphyxia. Insufficient intake of oxygen. Numerous causes.

Aspiration. Withdrawal of gas, fluids, and semisolids from body cavities and hollow viscera by means of suction with an aspirator and a trocar.

Atheroma. Fatty degeneration or thickening of the walls of the larger arteries occurring in atherosclerosis.

Autoclave. Apparatus used for sterilization by steam pressure, usually at 250°F (121°C) for a specific time.

Autolysis. Self-destruction of cells. Decomposition of all tissues by enzymes that form without microbial assistance.

Autopsy. Postmortem examination of the organs and tissues of a body to determine cause of death or pathological condition. Necropsy.

Bactericidal agent. Agent that destroys bacteria.

Bacteriostatic agent. Agent that has the ability to inhibit or retard bacterial growth. No destruction of viability is implied.

Balsamic substance. Resin combined with oil. A fragrant, resinous, oily exudate from various trees and plants.

Base of the axillary space. Armpit.

- **Anterior boundary.** Established by drawing a line along the fold of skin that envelops the lateral border of the pectoralis major muscle.
- **Posterior boundary.** Established by drawing a line along the fold of skin that envelops the lateral border of the latissimus dorsi muscle.
- **Medial boundary.** Established by drawing a line that connects the two points where the pectoralis major and latissimus dorsi muscles blend into the chest wall.
- **Lateral boundary.** Established by drawing a line that connects the two points where the pectoralis major and latissimus dorsi muscles blend into the arm.

Biohazard. Biological agent or condition that constitutes a hazard to humans.

Biological Death. Irreversible somatic death.

Bischloromethyl ether (BCME). A carcinogen potentially produced when formaldehyde and sodium hypochlorite come into contact with each other. Normally occurs only in a controlled laboratory setting and requires a catalyst.

Bleaching agent. A chemical that lightens a skin discoloration.

Blood. Cell-containing fluid that circulates through the blood vascular system and is composed of approximately 22% solids and 78% water.

Bloodborne pathogens. See Bloodborne Pathogen Rule.

Bloodborne pathogen rule. Occupational Health and Safety Administration (OSHA) regulation concerning exposure of employees to blood and other body fluids. The following are OSHA definitions.

- **Blood.** Human blood, human blood components, and products made from human blood.
- **Bloodborne pathogens.** Pathogenic microorganisms that are present in human blood and can cause disease in humans. These pathogens include, but are not limited to, hepatitis B virus (HBV) and human immunodeficiency virus (HIV).
- **Contaminated.** Marked by the presence or reasonably anticipated presence of blood or other potentially infectious materials on an item or surface.
- **Contaminated laundry.** Laundry that has been soiled with blood or other potentially infectious materials or may contain sharps.
- **Contaminated sharps.** Any contaminated object that can penetrate the skin including, but not limited to, needles, scalpels, broken glass, and exposed ends of wires.
- **Engineering controls.** Controls (e.g., sharps disposal container, self-sheathing needles) that isolate or remove the bloodborne pathogen hazard from the workplace.
- **Exposure incident.** Specific eye, mouth, other mucous membrane, nonintact skin, or parenteral contact with blood or other potentially infectious materials that results from the performance of an employee's duties.
- **Occupational exposure.** Reasonably anticipated skin, eye, mucous membrane, or parenteral contact with blood or other potentially infectious materials that may result from the performance of an employee's duties.
- **Parenteral.** Introduced into the body by way of piercing the mucous membranes or the skin barrier, for example, by needlesticks, human bites, cuts, and abrasions.
- **Personal protective equipment (PPE).** Specialized clothing or equipment worn by an employee for protection against a hazard.
- **Universal precautions.** An approach to infection control in which all human blood and certain human body fluids are treated as if they are contaminated with HIV, HBV, and other bloodborne pathogens.
- **Work practice controls.** Controls that reduce the likelihood of exposure by altering the manner in which a task is performed (e.g., prohibiting recapping of needles, not allowing blood splatter or aerosolization of blood while draining during the embalming process).

Blood discoloration. Discoloration resulting from changes in blood composition, content, or location, either intravascularly or extravascularly.

Blood pressure. Pressure exerted by the blood on the arterial wall in the living body and measured in millimeters of mercury.

Blood vascular system. Circulatory network composed of the heart, arteries, arterioles, capillaries, venules, and veins.

Blunt dissection. Separation and pushing aside of the superficial fascia leading to blood vessels and then the deep fascia surrounding blood vessels, using manual techniques or round-ended instruments that separate rather than cut the protective tissues.

Boil. Acute, deep-seated inflammation in the skin. Usually begins as a subcutaneous swelling in a hair follicle.

Bridge suture (temporary interrupted suture). Individual stitch knotted at the tissue edge. May be applied prior to embalming to align tissues.

Buccal cavity. Vestibule of the oral cavity. Space between the lips, gums, and teeth.

Buffer. Embalming chemical that effects the stabilization of acid–base balance within embalming solutions and in embalmed tissues.

Bulb syringe. Self-contained, soft rubber manual pump designed to create pressure to deliver fluid as it passes through oneway valves located within the bulb. It is used only to deliver fluids; it cannot be used for aspiration.

Cadaver. Dead human body used for medical purposes, including transplantation, anatomical dissection, and study.

Cadaveric lividity. Postmortem intravascular red–blue discoloration resulting from hypostasis of blood.

Cadaveric spasm. Prolongation of the last violent contraction of the muscles into the rigidity of death.

Calvarium. Domelike superior portion of the cranium. That portion removed during cranial autopsy.

Calvarium clamp. Device used to fasten the calvarium to the cranium after a cranial autopsy.

Canalization. Formation of new channels in a tissue.

Capillaries. Minute blood vessels, the walls of which comprise a single layer of endothelial cells. Capillaries connect the smallest arteries (arteriole) with the smallest veins (venule) and are where pressure filtration occurs.

Capillary permeability. Ability of substances to diffuse through capillary walls into the tissue spaces.

Carbohydrate. Compound containing hydrogen, carbon, and oxygen. Sugars, starches, and glycogen.

Carbuncle. Circumscribed inflammation of the skin and deeper tissues that ends in suppuration and is accompanied by systemic symptoms, such as fever and leukocytosis.

Carcinogen. Cancer-causing chemical or material.

Cavitation. Formation of cavities in an organ or tissue. Frequently seen in some forms of tuberculosis.

Cavity embalming. See Embalming.

Cavity fluid. Embalming chemical that is injected into a body cavity following aspiration in cavity embalming. Cavity fluid can also be used as the chemical in hypodermic and surface embalming.

Cellular death. Death of the individual cells of the body.

Center of fluid distribution. Ascending aorta and/or arch of the aorta.

Center of venous drainage. Right atrium of the heart.

Centers for Disease Control and Prevention (CDCP, CDC). Major agency of the Department of Health and Human Services, with headquarters in Atlanta, Georgia, concerned with all phases of control of communicable, vectorborne, and occupational diseases.

Centrifual force machine. Embalming machine that uses motorized force, pulsating and nonpulsating type.

Chelate. Substances that bind metallic ions. Ethylenediaminetetracetic acid (EDTA) is used as an anticoagulant in embalming solutions.

Chemical postmortem change. Change in the body's chemical composition that occurs after death, for example, release of heme leading to postmortem staining.

Chemotherapy. Application of chemical reagents in the treatment of disease in humans. May causes a elevated preservation demand.

Chin rest. One of several methods used for mouth closure (antiquated).

Clinical death. Phase of somatic death lasting from 5 to 6 minutes in which life may be restored.

Clostridium perfringens. Anaerobic, saphrophytic, spore-forming bacterium, responsible for tissue gas. Referred to as a gas bacillus.

Coagulating agents. Chemical and physical agents that bring about coagulation.

Coagulation. Process of converting soluble protein into insoluble protein by heating or contact with a chemical such as an alcohol or an aldehyde. Solidification of a sol into a gelatinous mass. Agglutination is a specific form of coagulation.

Coinjection fluid. Fluid used primarily to supplement and enhance the action of vascular (arterial) solutions.

Coma. Irreversible cessation of brain activity and loss of consciousness. Death beginning at the brain.

Communicable disease. Disease that may be transmitted either directly or indirectly between individuals by an infectious agent.

Concurrent disinfection. Disinfection practices carried out during the embalming process.

Concurrent drainage. Method of drainage in which drainage occurs continuously during vascular (arterial) injection.

Condyle. Rounded articular process on a bone.

Congealing. See Coagulation and Agglutination.

Conjunctiva. Mucous membrane that lines the eyelid and covers the white portion of the eye.

Contagious disease. Disease that may be transmitted between individuals, with reference to the organism that causes a disease.

Contaminated. See Bloodborne Pathogen Rule.

Cornea. Transparent part of the tunic of the eyeball that covers the iris and pupil and admits light into the interior.

Corneal sclera button. That portion of the cornea recovered for transplantation in situ.

Coroner. Official of a local community who holds inquests concerning sudden, violent, and unexplained deaths.

Corpulence. Obesity.

Cosmetic fluid. Embalming fluid that contains active dyes and coloring agents intended to restore a more natural skin tone through the embalming process.

Counterstaining compound. Dye that helps to cover jaundice.

Coverall. Plastic garment designed to cover the body from the chest down to the upper thigh.

Cranial embalming. Method used to embalm the contents of the cranial cavity through aspiration and injection of the cranial chamber by passage of a trocar through the cribriform plate.

Cremated remains. Those elements remaining after cremation of a dead human body.

Crepitation. Crackling sensation produced when gases trapped in tissues are palpated, as in subcutaneous emphysema or tissue gas.

Creutzfeldt–Jakob disease. Disease of the central nervous system with unknown etiology, assumed to be a slow virus. Because etiology is unknown, caregivers using invasive procedures use extreme caution.

Cribriform plate. Thin, medial portion of the ethmoid bone of the skull.

Death. Irreversible cessation of all vital functions—non-legal definition.

Death rattle. Noise made by a moribund person caused by air passing through a residue of mucus in the trachea and posterior oral cavity.

Death struggle. Semiconvulsive twitches that often occur before death.

Decay. Decomposition of proteins by enzymes of aerobic bacteria.

Decomposition. Separation of compounds into simpler substances by the action of microbial and/or autolytic enzymes.

Dehydration. Loss of moisture from body tissue that may occur antemortem or postmortem (antemortem: febrile disease, diarrhea, or emesis; postmortem: injection of embalming solution or through absorption by the air).

Denatured protein. Protein whose structure has been changed by physical or chemical agents.

Dental tie. Antiquated method of mouth closure.

Desiccation. Process of drying out.

Desquamation (skin-slip). Sloughing off of the epidermis, wherein there is a separation of the epidermis from the underlying dermis.

Dialysis. Separation of substances in solution by the difference in their rates of diffusion through a semipermeable membrane.

Differential pressure. See Pressure.

Diffusion. Movement of molecules or other particles in solution from an area of greater concentration to an area of lesser concentration until a uniform concentration is reached.

Diffusion (fluid). Passage of some components of the injected embalming solution from an intravascular to an extravascular location. Movement of the embalming solutions from the capillaries into the interstitial fluids.

Digits. Fingers and toes. The thumb is the No. 1 digit for each hand and the large toe is No. 1 digit for each foot.

Discoloration. Any abnormal color in or on the human body.

Disease. Any deviation from or interruption of the normal structure or function of a body part, organ, or system.

Disinfectant. An agent, usually chemical, applied to inanimate objects/surfaces to destroy disease-causing microbial agents, but usually not bacterial spores.

Disinfection. Destruction and/or inhibition of most pathogenic organisms and their products in or on the body.

Distribution (fluid). Movement of embalming solutions from the point of injection throughout the arterial system and into the capillaries.

Drain tube. Embalming instrument used to aid the drainage of venous blood from the body.

Drainage. Discharge or withdrawal of blood, interstitial fluid, and embalming fluids from the body during vascular embalming, usually through a vein.

Drench shower. Occupational Safety and Health Administration-required safety device for release of a copious amount of water in a short time.

Dry gangrene. See Gangrene.

Dye (coloring agent). Substances that, on being dissolved, imparts a definite color to the embalming solution. Dyes are classified as to their capacity to permanently impart color to the tissue of the body into which they are injected.

Ecchymosis. Extravasation of blood into a tissue. A bruise.

Edema. Abnormal accumulation of fluids in tissue or body cavities.

Electric aspirator. Device that uses a motor to create a suction for the purpose of aspiration.

Electric spatula. Electrically heated blade that may be used to dry moist tissue, reduce swollen tissue, and restore contour.

Electrocardiogram (ECG, EKG). Record of the electrical activity of the heart.

Electroencephalogram (EEG). Record of the electrical activity of the brain.

Embalming. Process of chemically treating the dead human body to reduce the presence and growth of microorganisms, to retard organic decomposition, and to restore an acceptable physical appearance. There are four types of embalming:

- **Cavity embalming.** Direct treatment other than vascular (arterial) embalming of the contents of the body cavities and the lumina of the hollow viscera. Usually accomplished by aspiration and then injection of chemicals using a trocar.
- **Hypodermic embalming.** Injection of embalming chemicals directly into the tissues through the use of a syringe and needle or a trocar.
- **Surface embalming.** Direct contact of body tissues with embalming chemicals.
- **Vascular (arterial) embalming.** Use of the blood vascular system of the body for temporary preservation, disinfection, and restoration. Usually accomplished through injection of embalming solutions into the arteries and drainage from the veins.

Embalming analysis (case analysis). That consideration given to the dead body prior to, during, and after the embalming procedure is completed. Documentation is recommended.

Engineering controls. See Bloodborne Pathogen Rule.

Environment. Surroundings, conditions, or influences that affect an organism or the cells within an organism.

Environmental Protection Agency (EPA). Governmental agency with environmental protection regulatory and enforcement authority.

Enzyme. Organic catalyst produced by living cells and capable of autolytic decomposition.

Excision. Removal as by cutting out. The area from which something has been cut out.

Expert tests of death. Any procedure used to prove a sign of death, usually performed by physicians.

Exposure incident. See Bloodborne Pathogen Rule.

Extravascular. Outside the blood vascular system.

Extravascular blood discoloration. Discoloration of the body outside the blood vascular system, for example, ecchymosis, petechia, hematoma, and postmortem stain.

Extrinsic. From outside the body.

Eye enucleation. Removal of the eye for tissue transplantation, research, and education.

Eye enucleation discoloration. Extravasation of blood as a result of eye enucleation.

Eyecap. Method used to close the eyes in which a thin, plastic, dome-shaped disk is placed just beneath the eyelids.

Eyelid overlap. Method of eye closure in which the upper lid is placed on top of the lower lid.

Eyewash station. Occupational Safety and Health Administration-required emergency safety device providing a steady stream of water for flushing the eye.

Fat. Organic compound containing carbon, hydrogen, and oxygen. Chemically, fat is a triglyceride ester composed of glycerol and fatty acids.

Fatty acids. Product of decomposition of fats.

Febrile. Characterized by a high fever, causing dehydration of the body.

Fermentation. Bacterial decomposition of carbohydrates.

Fever blisters. Lesions of the mucous membrane of the lip or mouth caused by herpes simplex type I or II virus or by dehydration of the mucous membrane in a febrile disease.

Firming. Rigidity of tissue due to chemical reaction.

Fixation. Act of making tissue rigid. Solidification of a compound.

Fixative. Agent employed in the preparation of tissues, for the purpose of maintaining the existing form and structure. A large number of agents are used, the most important one being formalin.

Flush (flushing). Intravascular blood discoloration that occurs when arterial solution enters an area (such as the face), but due to blockage, blood and embalming solution are unable to drain from the area.

Formaldehyde (HCHO). Colorless, strong-smelling gas that when used in solution is a powerful preservative and disinfectant. Potential occupational carcinogen.

Formaldehyde gray. Gray discoloration of the body caused by the reaction of formaldehyde from the embalming process with hemoglobin to form methylhemoglobin.

Formaldehyde rule. Occupational Safety and Health Administration regulation limiting the amount of occupational exposure to formaldehyde gas.

Furuncle. See Boil.

Gangrene. Necrosis, death, of tissues of part of the body usually due to deficient or absent blood supply.

- **Dry gangrene.** Condition that results when the body part that dies had little blood and remains aseptic. The arteries but not the veins are obstructed.

- **Gas gangrene.** Necrosis in a wound infected by an anaerobic gas-forming bacillus, the most common etiologic agent being *Clostridium perfringens*.
- **Moist (wet) gangrene.** Necrotic tissue that is wet as a result of inadequate venous drainage. May be accompanied by bacterial infection.

Germicide. Agent, usually chemical, applied either to inanimate objects/surfaces or to living tissues to destroy disease-causing microbial agents, but usually not bacterial spores.

Gooseneck. Rubber stopper containing two tubes, one to create vacuum or pressure and the other to deliver fluid or achieve aspiration. Possibly used in conjunction with a hand pump.

Grave wax. See Adipocere.

Gravity filtration. Extravascular settling of fluids by gravitational force to the dependent areas of the body.

Gravity injector. Apparatus used to inject arterial fluid during the vascular (arterial) phase of the embalming process. Relies on gravity to create the pressure required to deliver the fluid (0.43 pounds of pressure per 1 foot of elevation.)

Groove director. Instrument used to guide vein tubes into vessels.

Hand pump. Historical instrument resembling a large hypodermic syringe attached to a bottle apparatus. Used to create either pressure for injection or vacuum for aspiration.

Hard water. Water containing large amounts of mineral salts. These mineral salts must be removed from or sequestered in water (vehicle) to be used in mixing vascular embalming solutions.

Hardening compound. Chemical in powder form that has the ability to absorb and to disinfect. Often used in cavity treatment of autopsied cases.

Hazard Communication Standard (Rule). Occupational Safety and Health Administration regulation that deals with limiting exposure to occupational hazards.

Hazardous material. Agent or material exposing one to risk.

Headrest. Piece of equipment used to maintain the head in the proper position during the embalming process.

Hematemesis. Blood present in vomitus. Vomiting of blood.

Hematoma. A swelling or mass of clotted blood caused by a ruptured blood vessel and confined to an organ or space.

Heme. Nonprotein portion of hemoglobin. Red pigment.

Hemoglobin. Red respiratory portion of the red blood cells. Iron-containing pigment of red blood cells functioning to carry oxygen to the cells.

Hemolysis. Destruction of red blood cells that liberates hemoglobin.

Hepatitis. Inflammation of the liver that may be caused by a variety of agents, including viral infections, bacterial invasion, and physical or chemical agents. It is usually accompanied by fever, jaundice, and an enlarged liver.

Hepatitis B virus (HBV). Severe infectious bloodborne virus.

Herpes. Inflammatory skin disease marked by small vesicles in clusters, usually restricted to diseases caused by herpesvirus.

High-index fluids. Special vascular (arterial) fluid with a formaldehyde content of 25 to 36%.

Household bleach. Five percent sodium hypochlorite solution. Mixing 12 ounces of household bleach with 116 ounces of water yields 1 gallon of a 10% household bleach solution (5000 ppm sodium hypochlorite).

Human immunodeficiency Virus (HIV). Retrovirus that causes acquired immunodeficiency syndrome (AIDS).

Human remains. Body of a deceased person, including cremated remains.

Humectant. Chemical that increases the ability of embalmed tissue to retain moisture.

Hydroaspirator. Apparatus that is connected to the water supply. When the water is turned on, a suction is developed and is used to aspirate the contents of the body's cavities.

Hydrocele. Abnormal accumulation of fluids in a saclike structure, especially the scrotal sac.

Hydrocephalus. Abnormal accumulation of cerebrospinal fluids in the ventricles of the brain.

Hydrolysis. Reaction in which water is one of the reactants and compounds are often broken down. In the hydrolysis of proteins, the addition of water accompanied by the action of enzymes results in the breakdown of protein into amino acids.

Hydropericardium. Abnormal accumulation of fluid within the pericardial sac.

Hydrothorax. Abnormal accumulation of fluid in the thoracic cavity.

Hygroscopic. Absorbing moisture readily.

Hypertonic solution. Solution having a greater concentration of dissolved solute than the solution with which it is compared.

Hypodermic embalming. See Embalming.

Hypostasis. Settling of blood and/or other fluids to dependent portions of the body.

Hypotonic solution. Solution having a lesser concentration of dissolved solute than the solution with which it is compared.

Imbibition. Absorption of the fluid portion of blood by the tissues after death, resulting in postmortem edema.

Incision. A clean cut made with a sharp instrument. In embalming, a cut made with a scalpel to raise arteries and veins.

Index. Strength of an embalming fluid, indicated by the number of grams of pure formaldehyde gas dissolved in 100 mL of water. Index usually refers to a percentage; an embalming fluid with an index of 25 usually contains 25% formaldehyde gas.

Infant. Child less than 1 year of age.

Infectious disease. Disease caused by the growth of a pathogenic microorganism in the body.

Infectious waste. See Biohazard.

Inferior. From a given reference toward the feet.

Inguinal ligament. Anatomical structure forming the base of the femoral triangle; Extends from the anterior superior iliac spine to the pubic tubercle.

Injection. Act or instance of forcing a fluid into the vascular system or directly into tissues.

Injection pressure. See Pressure.

Instant tissue fixation. Embalming technique that employs a very strong arterial solution (often waterless). The solution is injected under high pressure in spurts into a body area. Very little solution is used.

Instantaneous rigor mortis. Instantaneous stiffening of the muscles of a dead human body.

Intercellular. Between the cells of a structure.

Intercellular fluid. Fluid inside cells of the body (constituting about one half of the body weight).

Intercostal space. Space between the ribs.

Intermittent drainage (restricted drainage). Method of drainage in which the drainage is stopped at intervals while the injection continues.

Interstitial fluid. Fluid in the supporting connective tissues surrounding body cells (about one fifth the body weight).

Intravascular. Within the blood vascular system.

Intravascular blood discoloration. Discoloration of the body within the blood vascular system, for example, hypostasis, carbon monoxide, and capillary congestion.

Intravascular fluid. Fluid contained within vascular channels (about one twentieth of the body weight).

Intrinsic. From within the body.

Isotonic solution. A solution having a concentration of dissolved solute equal to that of a standard of reference.

Jaundice. Conditions characterized by an excessive concentration of bilirubin in the skin and tissues and deposition of excessive bile pigment in the skin, cornea, body fluids, and mucous membranes with the resulting yellow appearance of the patient.

Jaundice fluid. Arterial fluid with special bleaching and coloring qualities for use on bodies with jaundice. Usually, formaldehyde content is low.

Jugular drain tube. Tubular instrument of varying diameter and shape, preferably with a plunger, that is inserted into the jugular vein to aid in drainage.

Laceration. Wound characterized by irregular tearing of tissue.

Larvicide. Substance used to kill insect larvae.

Lateral. Away from the midline.

Legionnaires' disease. Severe, often fatal bacterial disease characterized by pneumonia, dry cough, and sometimes gastrointestinal symptoms (Legionella pneumophilia).

Lesion. Any change in structure produced during the course of a disease or injury.

Ligate. To tie off, as in ligating an artery and vein on completion of embalming or ligating the colon in autopsied bodies.

Linear guide. Line drawn or visualized on the surface of the skin to represent the approximate location of some deeper lying structure.

Lipolysis. Decomposition of fats.

Livor mortis. See Cadaveric Lividity.

Lumen. Cavity of a vein, artery, or intestine.

Lysin. Specific antibody acting destructively on cells and tissues.

Lysosome. Organelle that exists within a cell, but separate from the cell. Contains hydrolytic enzymes that break down proteins and certain carbohydrates.

Maggot. Larva of an insect, especially a flying insect.

Mandibular suture. Method of mouth closure in which a suture is passed through the septum of the nose and around the mandible.

Masking agent. See Perfuming Agents.

Massage. Manipulation of tissue in the course of preparation of the body.

Material safety data sheet (MSDS). Form that must accompany a hazardous product. Requirement of the Department of Labor and Occupational Safety and Health Administration under the Hazard Communication Standard.

Medial. Toward the midline.

Medical examiner. Official elected or appointed to investigate suspicious or unnatural deaths.

Meningitis. Inflammation of the meninges.

Microbe (microorganism). Minute one-celled form of life not distinguishable as to vegetable or animal nature.

Midaxillary Line. Vertical line drawn from the center of the medial border of the base of the axillary space.

Millicurie (mCi). That amount of radioactive material in which 37 million atoms disintegrate each second.

Modifying agents. Chemicals for which there may be greatly varying demands predicated on the type of embalming, the environment, and the embalming fluid to be used.

Mold-preventive agents. Agents that prohibit the growth of mold.

Moribund. In a dying state. In the agonal period.

Mouth former. Device used in the mouth to shape the contour of the lips.

Multiple-site (Multipoint) injection. Vascular injection from two or more arteries. A minimum of two sites are prescribed in the suggested Minimum Standard for Embalming.

Musculature suture. Method of mouth closure in which a suture is passed through the septum of the nose and through the mentalis muscle of the chin.

Nasal cavity. Space between the roof of the mouth and the floor of the cranial cavity.

Nasal tube aspirator. Embalming instrument used to aspirate the throat by means of the nostrils.

Necrobiosis. Antemortem, physiological death of the cells of the body followed by their replacement.

Necropsy. See Autopsy.

Necrosis. Pathological death of a tissue still a part of the living organism.

Needle injector. Mechanical device used to impel specially designed metal pins into bone.

Nephritis. Inflammation of the kidneys.

Nitrogenous waste. Metabolic by-products that contain nitrogen, such as urea and uric acid. These compounds have a high affinity for formaldehyde and tend to neutralize embalming chemicals.

Noncosmetic fluid. Type of arterial fluid that contains inactive dyes that will not impart a color change on the body tissues of the deceased.

Obese. Having an abnormal amount of fat on the body. Corpulent.

Occupational exposure. See Bloodborne Pathogen Rule.

Occupational Safety and Health Administration (OSHA). A Governmental agency with the responsibility for regulation and enforcement of safety and health matters for most U.S. employees. An individual state OSHA agency may supercede the U.S. Department of Labor OSHA regulations.

One-point injection. Injection and drainage from one location.

Opaque cosmetic. A cosmetic medium able to cover or hide skin discolorations.

Operative corrections. Any and all techniques to treat a problem area, for example, excision, incision, and wicking.

Ophthalmoscope. Optical instrument with an accompanying light that makes it possible to examine the retina and to explore for blood circulation.

Optimum. Most favorable condition for functioning.

Oral cavity. Mouth and vestibule, or the opening to the throat.

Osmosis. Passage of solvent from a solution of lesser to one of greater solute concentration when the two solutions are separated by a semipermeable membrane.

Packing forceps. Embalming instrument used in closing the external orifices of the body.

Palpate. To examine by touch.

Parallel incision. Incision on the surface of the skin to raise the common carotid arteries. It is made along the posterior border of the inferior one third of the sternocleidomastoid muscle.

Parenteral. See Bloodborne Pathogen Rule.

Parts per million (ppm). In contaminated air, the parts of vapor or gas (formaldehyde) per million parts of air by volume. In solution, the parts of chemical per million parts of solution.

Passive transport system. Method by which solutes and/or solvents cross through a membrane with no energy provided by the cells of the membrane. In embalming, examples include pressure filtration, dialysis, diffusion, and osmosis.

Pathological discoloration. Antemortem discoloration that occurs during the course of certain diseases such as gangrene and jaundice.

Pediculicide. Substance able to destroy lice.

Percutaneous. Effected through unbroken skin.

Perfuming agents (masking agents). Chemicals found in embalming arterial formulations having the capability of displacing an unpleasant odor or of altering an unpleasant odor so that it is converted to a more pleasant one.

Perfusion. To force a fluid through (an organ or tissue), especially by way of the blood vessels. Injection during vascular (arterial) embalming.

Peritonitis. Inflammation of the peritoneum, the membranous coat lining the abdominal cavity and investing the viscera.

Permissible exposure limit (PEL). Maximum legal limit established by the Occupational Safety and Health Administration for a regulated substance. These are based on employee exposure and are time-weighted over an 8-hour work shift. When these limits are exceeded, employers must take proper steps to reduce employee exposure. For formaldehyde, the PEL is 0.75 ppm.

Personal protective equipment (PPE). See Bloodborne Pathogen Rule.

Petechia. Antemortem, pinpoint, extravascular blood discoloration visible as purplish hemorrhages of the skin.

Pharmaceutical. Drug or medicine.

Pitting edema. Condition in which interstitial spaces contain such excessive amounts of fluid that the skin remains depressed after palpation.

Pneumonia. Acute infection or inflammation of the alveoli. The alveolar sacs fill up with fluid and dead white blood cells. Causes include bacteria, fungi, and viruses.

Positioning devices. Preparation room equipment for properly positioning bodies prior to, during, and after vascular embalming.

Posterior. Toward the back.

Postmortem. Period that begins after somatic death.

Postmortem caloricity. Rise in temperature after death due to continued cellular oxidation.

Postmortem examination. See autopsy.

Postmortem physical change. Change in the form or state of matter without any change in chemical composition.

Postmortem stain. Extravascular color change that occurs when heme, released by hemolysis of red blood cells, seeps through the vessel walls and into the body tissues.

Potential of hydrogen (pH). Degree of acidity or alkalinity. The scale ranges from 0 to 14—0 being completely acid, 14 completely basic, and 7 neutral. Blood has a pH of 7.35 to 7.45.

Potential pressure. See pressure.

Precipitant. Substance bringing about precipitation. The oxilates formerly used in water conditioning chemicals are now illegal because of their poisonous nature.

Preinjection fluid. Fluid injected primarily to prepare the vascular system and body tissues for the injection of the preservative vascular (arterial) solution. This solution is injected before the preservative vascular solution is injected.

Preparation room. That area or facility wherein embalming, dressing, cosmetizing, or other body preparation is effected.

Preservation. See Temporary Preservation.

Preservative demand. Amount of preservative (formaldehyde) required to effectively preserve and disinfect remains. Depends on the condition of the tissues as determined in the embalming analysis.

Preservative powder. Chemical in powder form, typically used for surface embalming of the remains.

Pressure. Action of a force against an opposing force (a force applied or acting against resistance).

- **Actual pressure.** That pressure indicated by the injector gauge needle when the arterial tube is open and the arterial solution is flowing into the body.
- **Blood pressure.** Pressure exerted by the blood on the vessel walls measured in millimeters of mercury.
- **Differential pressure.** Difference between potential and actual pressures.
- **Injection pressure.** Amount of pressure produced by an injection device to overcome initial resistance within (intravascular) or on (extravascular) the vascular system (arterial or venous).
- **Intravascular pressure.** Pressure developed as the flow of embalming solution is established and the elastic arterial walls expand and then contract, resulting in filling of the capillary beds and development of pressure filtration.
- **Potential pressure.** Pressure indicated by the injector gauge needle when the injector motor is running and the arterial tubing is clamped off.

Pressure filtration. Passage of embalming solution through the capillary wall to diffuse with the interstitial fluids by application of positive intravascular pressure. Embalming solution passes from an intravascular to an extravascular position.

Primary dilution. Dilution attained as the embalming solution is mixed in the embalming machine.

Primary disinfection. Disinfection carried out prior to the embalming process.

Procurement. Recovery of organs or tissues from a cadaver for transplantation.

Prognathism. Projection of the jaw or jaws that may cause problems with mouth closure and alignment of the teeth.

Protein. Organic compound found in plants and animals that can be broken down into amino acids.

Proteolysis. Decomposition of proteins.

Ptomaine. Any one of a group of nitrogenous organic compounds formed by the action of putrefactive bacteria on proteins, for example, indole, skatole, cadaverine, and putrescine.

Pubic symphysis. Fibrocartilage that joins the two pubic bones in the median plane.

Purge. Postmortem evacuation of any substance from an external orifice of the body as a result of pressure.

Pursestring suture. Suture used to close small punctures or holes. A series of small stitches are made through the skin around the circumference of the opening. The ends of the thread are then knotted.

Pus. Liquid product of inflammation containing various proteins and leukocytes.

Pustular lesion. Characteristic pus-filled wound of a disease, such as smallpox, syphilis, and acne.

Putrefaction. Decomposition of proteins by the action of enzymes from anaerobic bacteria.

Radiation protection officer. Supervisor, in an institution licensed to use radionuclides, who has the responsibility to establish procedures and make recommendations in the use of all radioactive matter.

Radionuclide. Chemical element that is similar in chemical properties to another element, but differs in atomic weight and electric charge and emits radiation. An atom that disintegrates by emission of electromagnetic radiation.

Rate of flow. Speed at which fluid is injected, measured in ounces per minute.

Razor burn (razor abrasion). Mark of desiccation.

Reaspiration. Repeated aspiration of a cavity.

Reducing agent. Substance that easily loses electrons and thereby causes other substances to be reduced. Formaldehyde is a strong reducing agent.

Resinous substance. Amorphous, nonvolatile solid or soft side substance, a natural exudation from plants. Any of a class of solid or soft organic compounds of natural or synthetic origin.

Restoration. Treatment of the deceased in the attempt to recreate natural form and color.

Restorative fluid (humectant). Supplemental fluid, used with the regular arterial solution, whose purpose is to retain body moisture and retard dehydration.

Restricted cervical injection. Method of injection wherein both common carotid arteries are raised.

Restricted drainage. See Intermittent Drainage and Alternate Drainage.

Right atrium. Chamber on the right side of the heart seen as the center of drainage. Used as a site of drainage via instruments from the right internal jugular vein and direct via the trocar or through the thoracic wall.

Rigor mortis. Postmortem stiffening of the body muscles by natural body processes.

Saccharolysis. Decomposition of sugars.

Sanitation. Process to promote and establish conditions that minimize or eliminate biohazards.

Saponification. Process of soap formation. As related to decomposition, the conversion of fatty tissues of the body into a soapy waxy substance called adipocere or grave wax.

Saprophytic bacteria. Bacteria that derive their nutrition from dead organic matter.

Scalpel. Two-piece embalming instrument consisting of a handle and a blade used to make incisions and excisions.

Sealing agents. Agents that provide a barrier or seal against any leakage of fluid or blood.

Secondary dilution. Dilution of the embalming fluid by the fluids in the body, both vascular and interstitial.

Sepsis. Pathologic state resulting from the presence of microorganisms or their products in the blood or other tissues.

Septicemia. Condition characterized by the multiplication of bacteria in blood.

Sequestering agent. Chemical agent that can "fence off" or "tie up" metal ions so they cannot react with other chemicals.

Serrated. Notched on the edge like a saw, as seen with forceps.

Sharps. Hypodermic needles, suture needles, injector needles, scalpel blades, razor blades, pins, and other items sharp enough to cause percutaneous injury, penetration of unbroken skin. May include other items normally not disposed of following use such as scissors, teeth, fingernails, and ribs.

Sharps container. Occupational Safety and Health Administration-required receptacle for proper disposal of sharps.

Short-term exposure limit (STEL). Legal limits established by the Occupational Health and Safety Administration to which workers can be exposed continuously for a short period without damage or injury. Exposures at the STEL should not be longer than 15 minutes and not repeated more than four times per workday.

Sign of death. Manifestation of death in the body.

Sodium hypochlorite. Unstable salt usually produced in an aqueous solution and used as a bleaching and disinfecting agent. (See Household bleach).

Solute. Substance that is dissolved in a solution.

Solution. Liquid containing dissolved substance.

Solvent. Liquid holding another substance in solution.

Somatic death. Death of the organism as a whole.

Split injection. Injection from one site and drainage from a separate site.

Sterilizers. Oven or appliance for sterilizing. An autoclave that sterilizes by steam under pressure at temperatures above 100°C.

Sterilization. Process that renders a substance free of all microorganisms.

Stethoscope. Delicate instrument used to detect almost inaudible sounds produced in the body.

Stillborn. Dead at birth. A product of conception either expelled or extracted dead.

Subcutaneous. Situated or occurring beneath the skin.

Subcutaneous emphysema. Distension of the tissues beneath the skin by gas or air. An antemortem condition brought about by a surgical procedure or trauma.

Superficial. Toward the surface.

Superior. Anatomically toward the head.

Supplemental fluid. Fluid injected for purposes other than preservation and disinfection. Supplemental fluids generally fall into one of three categories: preinjection, coinjection, and humectants or restorative fluids.

Surface compress. An absorbent material (pack) saturated with an embalming chemical and placed in direct contact with the tissue.

Surface discoloration. Discoloration due to the deposit of matter on the skin surface. These discolorations may occur antemortem or during or after embalming of the body. Examples are adhesive tape, ink, iodine, paint, and tobacco stains.

Surface embalming. See Embalming.

Surfactant (surface tension reducer; wetting, penetrating, or surface-active agent). Chemical that reduces the molecular cohesion of a liquid so it can flow through smaller apertures.

Temporary preservation. Science of treating the body chemically so as to temporarily inhibit decomposition.

Terminal disinfection. Institution of disinfection and decontamination measures after preparation of the remains.

Test of death. Any procedure used to prove a sign of death.

Thanatology. Study of death.

Third-degree burns. Burns that result in destruction of

cutaneous and subcutaneous tissues (seared, charred, or roasted tissue).

Time-weighted average (TWA). Exposure that is time-weighted over an established period. It allows the exposure levels to be averaged generally over an 8-hour period.

Tissue coagulation. See Coagulation.

Tissue gas. Postmortem accumulation of gas in tissues or cavities brought about by an anaerobic gas-forming bacillus, *Clostridium perfringens*.

Tobacco tar. Yellow/brown discoloration of the fingernails and fingers from excessive use of cigarettes.

Topical disinfection. Disinfection of the surface of the body or an object.

Translocation. Agonal or postmortem redistribution of host microflora on a hostwide basis.

Transplantation. Grafting of living tissue from its normal position to another site or of an organ or tissue from one person to another.

Transverse. Lying at right angles to the long axis of the body.

Trauma. Physical injury or wound caused by external force or violence.

Trocar. Sharply pointed surgical instrument used in cavity embalming to aspirate the cavities and inject cavity fluid. The trocar may also be used for supplemental hypodermic embalming.

Trocar button. Plastic, threaded screwlike device for sealing punctures and small round trocar openings.

Trocar guide. Line drawn or visualized on the surface of the body or a prominent anatomic structure used to locate internal structures during cavity embalming, from a point of reference 2 inches to the left of and 2 inches superior to the umbilicus.

Unionall. Plastic garment designed to cover the entire body from the neck down to and including the feet.

Universal precautions. See Bloodborne Pathogen Rule.

Vacuum breaker. Apparatus that prevents the back-siphoning of contaminated liquids into potable water supply lines or plumbing cross-connections within the preparation room.

Vascular (arterial) embalming. See Embalming.

Vehicle. Liquid that serves as a solvent for the numerous ingredients incorporated into embalming fluids.

Viral hepatitis. Inflammation of the liver caused by a virus (possibly as many as seven in number) capable of causing acute or chronic hepatitis illness. The transmission can be oral-fecal, parenteral, or sexual.

Viscosity. Resistance to the flow of a liquid. Thickness of a liquid.

Water conditioner. Complexing agent used to remove chemical constituents from municipal water supplies that could interfere with arterial formulations.

Water hardness. Quality of water containing certain substances, especially soluble salts of calcium and magnesium.

Waterless embalming. Arterial injection of an embalming solution composed of arterial fluid, humectant, and co-injection fluid. No water is added to the solution.

Waterlogged. Condition resulting from the use of an embalming solution containing an insufficient amount of preservative to meet the preservative demand of the tissues. The interstitial spaces are overly filled, engorged with water.

Wet gangrene. See Gangrene.

Wetting agent. See Surfactant.

Work practice controls. See Bloodborne Pathogen Rule.

ACRONYMS

ACGIH	American Congress of Governmental Industrial Hygienists
AIDS	Acquired immunodeficiency syndrome
AL	Action level
BCME	Bischloromethyl ether
CDCP	Centers for Disease Control and Prevention
ECG	Electrocardiogram (also EKG)
EEG	Electroencephalogram
EPA	Environmental Protection Agency
FTC	Federal Trade Commission
HBV	Hepatitis B virus
HIV	Human immunodeficiency virus
mCi	Millicurie
MSDS	Material Safety Data Sheet
NIOSH	National Institute for Occupational Safety and Health
OSHA	Occupational Safety and Health Administration
PEL	Permissible exposure limit
pH	Potential of hydrogen
PPE	Personal protective equipment

ppm	Parts per million
STEL	Short-term exposure limit
TLV	Threshold limit value
TWA	Time-weighted average

REFERENCES

Benenson AS. *Control of Communicable Diseases in Man.* 15th ed. Baltimore: Victor Graphics; 1990.

Embalming Course Content Syllabus. American Board of Funeral Service Education; 1991.

Frederick LG, Strub CG. *The Principles and Practices of Embalming.* 5th ed. Dallas: Professional Training Schools; 1989.

Mayer RG. *Embalming: Theory, Practices, and History,* Norwalk, CT: Appleton & Lange; 1990.

Merriam Webster's Collegiate Dictionary. 10th ed. Springfield, MA: Merriam-Webster; 1993.

Thomas CL. *Taber's Cyclopedic Medical Dictionary.* 17th ed. Philadelphia: F.A. Davis; 1993.

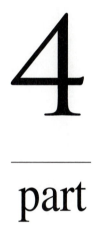

part

Selected Readings

The following articles have been reprinted for extra research and information:

1. *The Mathematics of Embalming Chemistry: Part I. A Critical Evaluation of "One-Bottle" Embalming Chemical Claims*, by Jerome F. Fredrick (1968)

2. *Final Report on Literature Search on the Infectious Nature of Dead Bodies for the Embalming Chemical Manufacturers Association*, September 1, 1968, by Maude R. Hinson (1968)

3. *Multiple Death Disaster Response Handbook*, by Robert D. Carpenter, James M. Dorn, Barbara M. Hopkins, and Todd W. Van Beck (1989)

4. *Occupational Exposure to Formaldehyde in Mortuaries*, by L. Lamont Moore and Eugene C. Ogrodnik (1986)

5. *Formaldehyde Vapor Emission Study in Embalming Rooms*, by Edward J. Kerfoot (1975)

6. *Reported Studies on Effects of Formaldehyde Exposure*, by Leandro Rendon (1983)

7. *Dangers of Infection*, by Leandro Rendon (1980)

8. *In-Use Evaluation of Glutaraldehyde as a Preservative–Disinfectant in Embalming*, by Robert N. Hockett, Leandro Rendon, and Gordon W. Rose (1973)

9. *The Antimicrobial Activity of Embalming Chemicals and Topical Disinfectants on the Microbial Flora of Human Remains*, by Peter A. Burke and A. L. Sheffner (1976)

10. *The Microbiologic Evaluation and Enumeration of Postmortem Specimens from Human Remains*, by Gordon W. Rose and Robert N. Hockett (1970)

11. *Recommendations for Prevention of HIV Transmission in Health-Care Settings* (1987)

12. *CDC's Universal Precautions in the Context of Medical Waste Management*, by Michael P. Kiley (1989)

13. *Can Magnesium Sulfate Be Safely Used to Rid the Body of Fluid in the Lower Extremities?* by Murray Shor (July, 1965)

The Mathematics of Embalming Chemistry*: Part I. A Critical Evaluation of "One-Bottle" Embalming Chemical Claims

Jerome F. Frederick, Ph.D.
Director of Chemical Research, Dodge Chemical Company

Few concepts can be more misleading and destructive to the professional future of the modern embalmer than the belief that "one-bottle embalming" is technically possible or even ethically admissible. The faulty reasoning behind this kind of wishful thinking is predicated on the premise that one single 16-ounce bottle of embalming chemical can be made to contain *all* of the essential chemical components required for the complete embalming of the "average" case, regardless of the condition-variables present in such a case.

Certain unscrupulous "fluid merchants," who are actually not bonafide embalming chemical manufacturers at all, have good reason to foster this misleading and unrealistic view. They do so with an obvious ulterior motive in mind. To put it plainly, they hope to win favor in the profession on the strength of a sensational economy appeal by claiming that embalming can be accomplished far more inexpensively with just one bottle of their super-duper elixir. Nothing could be further from the truth. To those who really understand the science of tissue preservation, such a claim smacks strongly of the chicanery and flim-flam of the old-time "medicine men" who in earlier days ranged the frontiers in their flashy horse-drawn vans and sold cure-alls "good for man or beast" to the trusting pioneer folk in the far-flung outposts of expanding America. Times have changed, but credulity, it seems, remains a dominant factor of human nature even in this enlightened day and age. Although stemming more from trustfulness than ignorance, unquestioning belief in the impossible and impractical still threatens the success of the misguided individual, but even more important, tends to undermine the very foundation of funeral service itself.

Misleading, illogical, and technically faulty, the "one-bottle" concept must be explored in depth before its pitfalls can be made clear to all ethical embalming practitioners, for if allowed to gain momentum unopposed, such a trend can only give the critics and detractors of funeral service valid evidence to win public support for their destructive efforts.

---

*Reprinted from the *De-Ce-Co Magazine* 1968;60(5).

In order to guide our readers toward a true and realistic evaluation of the hazards inherent in the "one-bottle" concept, we will divide discussion of the subject into two parts. In the first portion we will center our analysis upon a hypothetically "perfect case"—one in which no type of chemotherapy had been administered prior to death and where no problems other than those met within the normal course of tissue preservation face the embalmer. We must realize, of course, that no such case actually exists. But it gives us the unbiased starting point needed to expose the fallacies of the "one-bottle" embalming chemical concept and so reveal its hidden threat to the profession.

In cases where modern chemotherapy has been brought into play prior to death—and this encompasses some 90% of the cases treated by embalmers nowadays—the calculations for the analysis and critical evaluation must be revised. For here the hazards of "one-bottle embalming" take a sharp upward turn—and its inadequacy becomes greatly intensified.

We know, for instance, that cases in which the new antibiotic *kanamycin* has been used for some time prior to death require a much greater concentration of the arterial chemical than that indicated for cases which have not been treated with this drug. Expressed in its simplest terms, this requirement stems from the fact that the antibiotic causes changes in the kidneys. In consequence, the kidney tissues accumulate large concentrations of nitrogenous and ammoniacal wastes. And, as every embalmer knows, there is no more effective way to neutralize formaldehyde than reacting it with ammonia.

This part of our discussion, however, we shall take up at a later date and for the present confine ourselves to an analysis of the "perfect case," keeping in mind that it is purely hypothetical—for nowhere in our present chemotherapeutic era will the professional embalmer ever encounter such a case! Remember also that in any discussion concerning a topic such as this one, it is necessary to establish and accept certain basic scientific assumptions. While these may not apply directly to 100% of our cases in actual practice—"perfect" or otherwise—they do take into consideration the most common variables and so hypothesize a truly realistic and typical "specimen" case. For example, an *average* adult cadaver weighing 65.3 *kilograms* (or 65,300 grams) has been shown to contain a *total protein* content of 10.7 kilograms (or 10,700 grams of protein), by Brozek et al. (*Ann NY Acad Sci* 1963;110:123).

When formaldehyde reacts with protein, and *only* protein—and here again, we simplify the discussion by deliberately overlooking the fact that formaldehyde will also react with *other* components of the human body besides protein—it requires about 4.0 to 4.8 grams (or 4.4 *grams* average) of formaldehyde to totally react with and fix exactly *100 grams of a soluble protein.* Nonsoluble proteins require even more preservative.

Now, as pointed out by J. F. Walker in his treatise (*Formaldehyde,* 2nd ed., New York: Rheinhold; 1953:315), the 4.4 grams of formaldehyde are required to totally fix and preserve, for "all times," the 100 grams of soluble protein.

The average cadaver has about 10,700 grams of protein. To totally and "forever" preserve *all* the protein present in this average cadaver, we would need

$$10,700/100 \times 4.4 = 470.8 \ grams \ of \ formaldehyde$$

Let us consider, then, an average 16-ounce bottle of arterial fluid. If it contains only 30% formaldehyde (most modern arterials contain other preservatives in addition to formaldehyde) it would be technically defined as a "firming" or "high-index" fluid. Its formaldehyde content is computed as follows:

1 U.S. fluid ounce = 29.6 ml

16 fl oz = 473.6 ml of fluid, of which 30% is formaldehyde,

hence $0.03 \times 473.6 = 142.08 \ grams \ of \ formaldehyde.$

If we require 470.8 grams of formaldehyde to totally preserve all the protein in an average body, then that amount of this chemical in a 30% fluid will contain only enough formaldehyde to preserve

$$142.08/470.8 = 0.3 \ or \ 30\% \ of \ all \ the \ protein \ in$$
$$that \ average \ cadaver.$$

These calculations, as we pointed out earlier in this article, are necessarily predicated upon assumptions which must be accepted in order to establish a basis for computation. But even allowing the most liberal margin of error, it can be readily seen that *no single 16-ounce bottle of fluid* could possibly deliver the minimal acceptable degree of preservation—even in a "high-index" formulation! And this, remember, is calculated on the conditions of an *average* case!

Yet, as theoretical figures, these must not be construed as applicable to every like instance. There are many truly capable and excellent embalmers whose professional standards demand the most critical technical perfection who can point to instances where they have achieved adequate preservation with as little as $1\frac{1}{2}$ or 2 bottles of arterial fluid.

But none among them would rightfully claim that he uses *only one* bottle of arterial per case as *standard operating procedure,* for to do so would reflect unfavorably upon his professional judgment. Even the most ingenious and careful practitioners must admit that they are compelled to vary the concentrations of arterial chemical to meet the exigencies and special conditions present in each specific case. Most conscientious embalmers, in fact, use the full complement of "adjunct" chemical when the need for them is indicated—restorative humectants when there's evidence of emaciation or dehydration, water conditioners to neutralize chemical conflict in their solutions, modifiers, preinjections, coinjections, and vascular conditioning expedients. It is their familiarity with these "tools of the trade" which sets them apart as an elite professional class, where attitude and course of action are closely patterned on that of the medical man who employs every pharmaceutical and surgical expedient available to him as the need becomes apparent and modifies his treatment according to the conditional factors present in the case at hand. Imagine, if you can, a doctor who would be content to use the *same drug* in the *same concentration* on every case he treats! The analogy is very close to "one-bottle embalming."

But even if it were possible to produce a reasonably acceptable, if not perfect, embalming result with the "one-bottle" tactic, the embalmer who chose to place such paltry economy above the true objectives of his profession would indeed be asking for trouble. For the value of his reputation can scarcely be counted in fluid ounces of arterial chemical. Sensibly enough, few are ready to risk so much for so little in return—and the profession can well spare those who fall by the wayside with "one-bottle embalming."

Now, back to the hard facts of embalming chemistry:

Even if it were technically possible to increase the amount of formaldehyde in a 16-ounce bottle of arterial chemical to an absolute 100%, we'd have barely enough to "fix" the total protein present in the "average perfect case." This, of course, is not feasible because of the intrinsic chemical–physical nature of formaldehyde. But mere "fixation" or stabilization of the body proteins does not constitute total embalming. The result of using such an arterial would be a rock-hard, ghastly gray cadaver—a far cry indeed from the lofty standards of modern embalming! And where would we put our diffusion-stimulating constituents in a 100% formaldehyde fluid? Our cosmetic modifiers, blood solvents, and vascular conditioning components? Without these, could this super-duper 100% formaldehyde arterial do the job we want it to do? Could it penetrate and preserve *all* the proteins in our hypothetical "average" case? Could it get past the "average" number of circulatory obstacles we'd be almost certain to encounter in such a case? Lacking its normal complement of supporting constituents, it's hardly likely that this 100% formaldehyde fluid would win any applause from experienced professionals.

It should be plainly apparent at this point in our discussion that the "one-bottle" technique offers more danger to embalming results and professional reputation than the earnest, ethical embalmer is willing to risk. But

our analysis and evaluation would not be quite complete if we did not take a moment to quiet the suspicion that "one-bottle" embalming might become valid through technical advances in injection equipment. We refer specifically to the use of high-pressure embalming. Although embalming under such pressures may *appear* to use only one bottle of arterial chemical to achieve preservation, the technique merits the most critical scientific scrutiny. There is now evidence that high-pressure embalming actually causes the preservation to be "blown" to the superficial areas of the body. The result is a "taut skin" appearance which gives the *impression* of true preservative firming, but actually fails to embalm the deep underlying tissues, creating a condition which can obviously cause the embalmer a great deal of trouble.

In any event—no matter which technique is employed—we must face the incontrovertible mathematical truths of embalming. Knowing the way proteins react with preservatives leaves no illusions that one-bottle embalming will ever become a practical reality. Claims to the contrary should be viewed with cautious skepticism, for there is every indication that they will prove wholly false and unworthy of acceptance by the ethical professional.

Final Report on Literature Search on the Infectious Nature of Dead Bodies for the Embalming Chemical Manufacturers Association, September 1, 1968*

Maude R. Hinson
Medical Research Librarian, Downers Grove, Illinois

INTRODUCTION

In recent years, critics of American funeral practices and customs have charged that embalming is an economic waste and that it serves no useful purpose in protecting the public health. This claim is based on the theory that "the germ dies with the host." Therefore, it is argued, the unembalmed dead human body is harmless and not a source of possible infection and disease. Although such

*Literature search conducted by Maude R. Hinson, Medical Research Librarian, Bibliographic Service, 4912 Wallbank Avenue, Downers Grove, IL 60515.

statements have sometimes been credited to men who would be expected to be knowledgeable in the field (in one notable instance, a pathologist), no scientific, documented facts have been offered to substantiate the statements.

To disprove this theory, or to prove that the dead human body does harbor infectious organisms, that it can be a public hazard, and that modern embalming lessens that hazard, the Embalming Chemical Manufacturers Association (ECMA) sponsored this literature research project. The principle guidelines for the search were to avoid any literature published by an embalming chemical manufacturer, a college of embalming, or any related "interest." The search was to be centered in literature in the fields of medicine, pathology, biology, and related sciences.

THE SEARCH

The search began with a review of *Index Medicus* for the years 1963, 1964, 1965, and part of 1966, from which 265 references were selected. Eighty-eight book references were taken from the 1966 *Subject Guide to Books in Print,* published by R. R. Bowker. These lists were submitted to a committee of ECMA to select the articles to be photocopied at the National Library of Medicine in Bethesda, Maryland, and the books to be purchased. Photocopies were not ordered of all 265 reference articles, nor were all 88 books purchased. Some were passed over because they seemed too general to have direct bearing on the subject under investigation; others were passed because they appeared too similar to others already ordered. Twenty-one foreign language articles were translated to English. Not all of the articles photocopied will be cited in this report, again because of similarities among several of the articles. To include them would serve only to lengthen the report, without substantially increasing the weight of documentation.

DISCUSSION

To reasonably maintain the proposition that embalming has a real public health value, two questions must be answered. The first question concerns the validity of the claim that an infectious organism will invariably die when its host organism dies. If this theory has basis in fact, it must be conceded that the dead human body is harmless and does not present a public health hazard. If, on the other hand, we find this theory in error, we are led to another question. Can these organisms endanger public health?

Since the second question is somewhat rhetorical, perhaps it can be dealt with most simply. Establishing the reality of contact infection is an integral part of the proof that dead bodies can support living organisms. Establishing the validity of airborne infection may be even more pertinent, since it would be a hazard only to a small circle of mourners, funeral home personnel, pathologists, medical students, etc.

In "Airborne Infection: How Important for Public Health?" Alexander Langmuir maintains the reality and danger of airborne infection based upon systematic epidemiological studies, supported by extensive laboratory studies in experimental animals and human subjects. He lists psittacosis, Q fever, histoplasmosis, coccidioidomycosis, anthrax, brucellosis, primary tuberculosis, and primary mycosis as only a few diseases which are "intrinsically and exclusively airborne infections."[1]

Having broken order to eliminate a fairly straightforward question, we now turn back to question number one, which is perhaps the crux of this investigation. Do infectious organisms live on in a dead human body? There may be differing opinions on this question among laymen, but little variance of opinion can be found at the scientific level. In his article Virulence of Some Organisms in Cadavers, Giuseppe Fiorito says "Obviously, not all bacteria die in a cadaver."[2] He points out that even the process of putrefaction itself "is largely bacterial." He continues, "The high and rapid toxicity of cultures from cadavers indicates that restraining influences in living humans cease with death."[2] Fiorito injected one group of guinea pigs with *E. coli* from cadavers. The bacteria were 100% lethal in 9 to 55 hours. In a second group inoculated with *E. coli* from living humans, some guinea pigs survived completely and none lived less than 9 days. As is most often the case in recent articles, the article by Carpenter and Wilkins, Autopsy Bacteriology: Review of 2,033 Cases,[3] takes for granted the proposition that bacteria live in cadaver. If infectious organisms die with the host, the phrase "autopsy bacteriology" would have no meaning. In this article, the researchers show that length of postmortem and number of bacteriological organisms were positively correlated. That is, the longer the dead body is untreated, the higher the bacteria count.

In a study by J. Putnoky,[4] it was discovered that 68.5% of a sample of 400 cadavers "had bacteria in their internal organs." An article entitled Growth Conditions for Pathogenic Organisms in Dead Tissues[5] lists dermatomycetes, trichophyton fungi, *Anchorion quinckeana*, staphylococci, and *B. anthracis* as a few of the many organisms that linger on after death of the host. Vincenzo Mario Palmieri[6] has determined the life span of many organisms in dead, untreated tissue. For example, tetanus lives 234 days and typhus, 90 days. The supply of such articles is unending. Five others[7–11] are listed in the References.

Up to this point, we have mentioned only articles documenting the life of infectious organisms, in general, after the death of the host. There is an abundance of scientific literature which deals with specific infectious organisms and demonstrates their ability to survive in dead tissue. Perhaps the greatest number of articles have been written on tuberculosis. In The Dissemination of Tubercle Bacilli from Fresh Autopsy Material,[12] Ruell A. Sloan concludes: "First, methods of examination which make use of a compression technique contaminate the atmosphere in the vicinity of the autopsy. Second, within the limitations of this study, fresh tuberculosis lungs are decidedly dangerous and are a potent source of atmospheric contamination against which methods of proper protection should be devised."

A statement from a paper by Hans Popper and colleagues[13] is rather convincing: "Blood from living tuberculosis patients gave no conclusive results in culturing tuberculosis bacilli. That is, the tests failed to prove the existence of bacillemia. Yet 85–90% of blood samples, arterial and venous, from tubercular cadavers yielded viable cultures after miliary or pulmonary tuberculosis." We have found a great number of additional papers dealing with tuberculosis in dead tissue.[14–21]

Studies of tuberculosis, while numerous, are by no means the only such studies of disease existing in a dead host. A. Tjoschkoff and others, in Further Studies of the Causes of Easy Infection During the Postmortem Examinations of Septic Cadavers,[22] concentrate on the problem caused by staph and strep in these circumstances. We learn, "staphylococci multiply 10–100 times and even more in the blood and tissues of corpses kept at room temperatures." They maintain that the danger is compounded by the fact that after death "there is an increase not only in the number of microbe cells," but also "of their virulence (infectious potency) and to an exceptionally high degree." In a paper by Erich Hoffman[23] we find, "the dangerous teaching that syphilis cannot be transmitted from cadavers to autopsy workers is refuted." Among 38 previous case histories, such transmission was proved in 20 and was probable in 14. In cases involving animal cadavers known to be infected with B. anthracis, P. Begnescu[24] has found, "Burial in animal cemeteries and throwing into dry wells do not suffice." Rather than fill this report with quotation, after quotation other articles on this subject will simply be listed in the References.[25–28]

SUMMARY

In the light of several references cited here, it seems that there is no sound, scientific basis for the "germ dies with the host" theory. Secondly, we have established the fact that these infectious organisms can be spread by physical contact or may be airborne. Laboratory studies indicate that compounds such as aldehydes, phenols, alcohols, etc., are effective disinfectants and preservatives.

Since these compounds and similar ones are incorporated in modern embalming formulations, it can be predicted that such chemicals, when injected and used according to present-day embalming techniques, will also be effective in killing and reducing bacterial flora.

REFERENCES

1. Langmuir AD. Airborne infection: How important for public health? *Am J Public Health* 1964; 54(10):1666–1668.
2. Fiorito G. Virulence of some organisms in cadavers. *Riforma Med* 1924;40:270–273.
3. Carpenter HM, Wilkins RM. Autopsy bacteriology: Review of 2,033 cases. *Arch Pathol* 1964;77:73–81.
4. Putnoky J. Bacteriological test results from 400 autopsies. *Zentralbl Bakteriol Parasitenkunde Infectionskrankheiten Hyg* 1932;126:248–252.
5. Truffi G. Growth conditions for pathogenic organisms in dead tissues. *G. Ital Dermatol Sifilol* 1932; 73:839–857.
6. Palmieri YM. Resistance of pathogenic organisms to putrefaction and biological reactions in cadavers. *Rasseqna Int Clin Ter* 1930;11:648–653.
7. Wood WH, Oldstone M, Schultz RB. A re-evaluation of blood culture as an autopsy procedure. *Am J Clin Pathol* 1965;43(43):241–247.
8. Branch A, Lo M. Occurrence of bacteremia in one hundred consecutive autopsy cases. *Med Services J Canada* 1964;20:232–234.
9. Sulkin ES, Pike RM. Survey of laboratory acquired infections. *Am J Public Health* 1951;41(7):769–781.
10. Hunt HF, et al. A bacteriologic study of 567 postmortem examinations. *J Lab Clin Med* 1929; 14(10):907–912.
11. Epstein EZ, Kugel MA. The significance of postmortem examination. *J Infect Dis* 1929;44: 327–334.
12. Sloan RA. The dissemination of tubercle bacilli from fresh autopsy material. *NY State J Med* 1942;42: 133–134.
13. Popper H, et al. Culturing tuberculosis bacilli from cadaver blood. *Virchow's Arch Pathol Anat Physiol Klin Med* 1932;285:789–802.
14. Reid DD. Incidence of tuberculosis among workers in medical laboratories. *Br Med J* 1957;July: 10–14.
15. Morris SI. Tuberculosis as an occupational hazard during medical training. *Am Rev Tuberculosis* 1946;54:140–158.
16. Woringer F. Dissection tuberculosis in an autopsy orderly, a case of pulmonary bacillosis. *Bull Soc Fr Dermatol Syphilogr* 1933;40:204–206.
17. Hein J. Tubercles in cadavers and autopsy lesions

followed by general tubercular infection. *Beitrage Klin Tuberkulose* 1933;82:682–696.

18. Neuhaus C. Culturing tubercle bacilli from cadavers. *Zentralbl Allg Pathol Pathol Anat* 1928; 42:337–344.
19. Purrman W. Tuberculosis as an occupational disease. *Dtsch Gesundheit* 1964;19:2389–2390.
20. Hedvall E. The incidence of tuberculosis among students at Lund University. *Am Rev Tuberculosis* 1940;41:770–780.
21. Alderson HE. Tuberculosis from direct inoculation with autopsy knife. *Arch Dermatol Syphilol* 1931;24:98–100.
22. Tjoschkoff A, et al. Further studies of the causes of easy infection during the postmortem examinations of septic cadavers. *Dokl Bolq Akad Nauk Tome* 1965;18(2):179–181.
23. Hoffman E. Occupational syphilitic infection from cadavers. *Dermatol Wochenschr* 1929;88:284–286.
24. Begnescu P. Local excharizing in combating zoonoses microbiologia. *Parazitol Epidemiol* 1964;9(1):73.
25. Weilbaecher JO, Moss ES. Tularemia following injury while performing postmortem examination on human case. *J Lab Clin Med* 1938;24:34–38.
26. Zurhelle E, Stempil R. Studies on viability & virulence retention in *Spirochaeta pallida* in dead tissue. *Arch Dermatol Syphilis* 1927;153:219–266.
27. Mgaloblischwili P. Syphilis infection from cadavers. *Dermatol Z* 1927;51:167–189.
28. Balbi E. Development of pathogenic bacteria in dead tissue. *Pathologica* 1931;23:351–354.

Multiple Death Disaster Response Handbook*

Robert D. Carpenter • James M. Dorn • Barbara M. Hopkins, Ph.D. • and Todd W. Van Beck
Funeral Service Educators, Cincinnati College of Mortuary Science, Cincinnati, Ohio

GENERAL GUIDANCE

Our purpose is to establish means and methods for the most reasonable and proper care and handling of the dead in multideath disaster situations.

*Published by the National Funeral Directors Association, Milwaukee, WI (1989).

The Mortuary Team is responsible for aiding your county or area coroner/medical examiner in the recovery, evacuation, identification, sanitation, and preservation (such as embalming, if necessary), notification of the next of kin, and facilitating the release of the identified dead to the next of kin or their agent. Your coroner/medical examiner is by law in charge of the dead at all times. We are working as a support group when requested.

This information booklet is to give you better direction and information about where to receive proper professional advice, or a team of trained mortuary coordinators if requested. You are not in the disaster alone. NFDA [National Funeral Directors Association] at this time has over 2500 trained qualified professionals and 100 certified disaster mortuary coordinators. They are as close as your telephone.

A very important area to cover is the stress of the disaster worker. A high percentage of workers change jobs or quit within a year following a disaster unless they have been exposed to a psychological first-aid program (group debriefing, by a professional counselor) within 24 to 48 hours following the disaster.

This program is not and cannot be all things to all people, but by following the information and requesting proper help I am sure it will assist you toward being professional when the country is looking.

THE DISASTER WORKER AND DEATH

One of the problems that arises following a multideath disaster is the relationship between those people who are called upon to be disaster workers and the nature of the work they must do. Since funeral directors deal with death on a routine basis, it is often believed that they should be able to handle the disaster/death situation without much difficulty. This is not necessarily the case since funeral directors are accustomed to dealing with only one or a few deaths at the same time in familiar surroundings.

DO:

- Be familiar with the problems, both emotional and situational, that are inherent in emergency disaster work.
- Be familiar with the ways in which disaster workers prepare themselves for work in multiple death disasters.
- Understand the symptoms of disaster work burnout and the risks of being exposed to death overload.
- Know the strategies for helping other disaster workers cope with their own personal psychosocial needs during and after extensive disaster involvement.

DON'T:

- Don't compete in a disaster situation. It is a community challenge and working together with the community is the most effective way to meet the challenge.
- Don't be afraid to share your own dismay over the disaster. Your strength will be in how you perform your help, not by being the rock of strength.
- Don't forget that disaster work is unique and difficult for even the most seasoned person to cope with. If you experience difficulty following a disaster yourself—seek help.
- Don't underestimate death overload. Each of us has our own special point of tolerance. Be respectful and aware of your own tolerance in a disaster situation.

DEALING WITH THE MEDIA IN TIME OF EMERGENCY

During a disaster, communication with a number of different groups—the immediate survivors, the coroners, the police, the firefighters, the mass media, and the disaster workers themselves—occurs. This section deals with one of these groups—the mass media—so it is about communicating with the communicators.

DO:

- Designate one person to deal with the press. This person should be cool under fire, articulate, respected by officials, credible to reporters, low key, accessible.
- Inform the press corps of the designated person.
- Tell everyone working at the scene the identity of the designated representative to the press.
- Caution all to refer questions to the press liaison person.
- If you are the press liaison person or asked by him/her to speak with the press, be prepared with the information they need and be certain it is correct. Only comment in your area of expertise.

DON'T:

- Don't give ill-informed, spur-of-the-moment interviews at the scene.
- Don't feel compelled to answer every question asked of you by the press. Do not speculate. Do not lie.
- Don't play favorites among the reporters except for giving information to the wire services.
- Don't go before a camera or talk to a reporter without first giving careful thought to what you will say and how you will say it.

COMMUNICATIONS WITH IMMEDIATE SURVIVORS

Since funeral directors will have contact with the survivors of the victims of a disaster soon after the event has occurred, they shoud help the survivors to begin the grief process.

DO:

- Have a good working knowledge of the dynamics of the grief process.
- Recognize that a disaster presents unique dimensions of grief.
- Understand that survivors of disaster victims experience problems relating to short- and long-term grief reactions.
- Be familiar with the sequence and relationships of the tasks the bereaved will need to go through in their grief work.

DON'T:

- Don't be too verbal. Actions speak louder than words in a disaster crisis.
- Don't attempt to tell the bereaved how he or she feels. This is a time for support, not analysis.

DEVELOPING AND EQUIPPING A MORGUE SITE

The focal point of activity for the caring of the dead is the morgue, where remains are received, processed for identification, and prepared for final disposition. In this building, interviews also are held with the next of kin and other authorized persons. Great care should be exercised in the selection of the temporary morgue facility (Fig. 1).

DO:

- Get to know the coroner/medical examiner in your area in preparation for working under his/her jurisdiction during a disaster.
- Be aware of possible locations in your area that could be used as morgue sites.
- Be sure that morgue sites have adequate space, running water, adequate ventilation, good lighting, sufficient electrical outlets, multiple drains.
- Recognize that the morgue site will need to accommodate a variety of personnel.
- Develop a list of resources from whom perishable materials can be obtained.
- Stockpile nonperishable items.

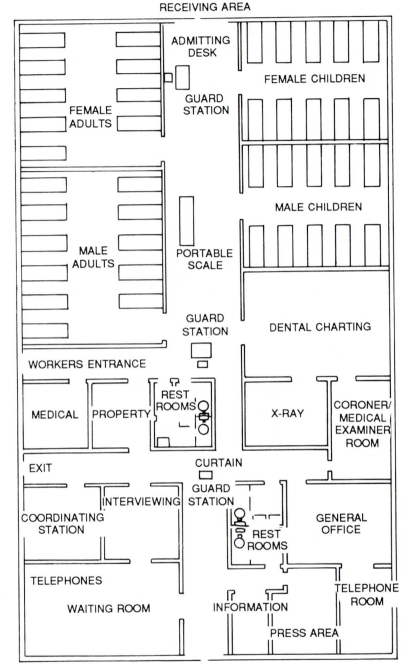

Figure 1. Suggested disaster temporary morgue.

DON'T:

- Don't attempt to take charge of the morgue site. The coroner/medical examiner has legal jurisdiction over the dead.
- Don't plan only one morgue site in a given area. Have multiple options.
- Don't stockpile perishable items.

THE HANDLING AND DECONTAMINATION OF RADIATION FATALITIES

In order to safely handle and properly decontaminate radiation fatalities, the disaster worker needs to be familiar with a certain amount of technical information. From a practical viewpoint, a body that is contaminated with radiation can be likened to one that has been contaminated with an infectious agent. In both cases, the object of decontamination procedures is to remove the source of contamination as much as possible from the body and, while doing this, to use protective measures to minimize one's own exposure to the contaminant and to prevent contamination of the work area.

DO:

- Become familiar with the three types of radiation emitted by radionuclides, the concept of half-life and activity, and the devices used to measure radioactivity, before a disaster involving radiation occurs.
- Set up an area separate from that for other types of disaster victims for receiving and decontaminating radiation accident victims.
- Consult a radiation protection specialist or health physicist, if possible, for guidance.
- Wear dosimeters in order to monitor personal exposure to radiation.
- Try to identify the radionuclide and its activity present in or on a body.
- Make use of the protective measures of time, distance, and shielding. Minimize the amount of time of contact with a radioactive source; maintain distance from a radioactive source if possible; wear protective clothing, including plastic aprons, long-sleeved scrub suits, and two pairs of rubber gloves.

DON'T:

- Don't be afraid to handle a radioactive case. With proper training, and by following certain commonsense practices, your risk of being harmed by radiation is low.
- Don't touch any source of radioactivity with your bare hands. Sealed sources, splinters of wood, glass, and metal that are radioactive should only be removed with a long (8 inches) forceps.
- Don't spend unnecessary time in close contact with a body contaminated with radiation.
- Don't stand near a source of radiation unless necessary for performance of your duties.
- Don't leave the area where decontamination is occurring until you have been monitored for contamination.

GUIDELINES AND DISASTER RESPONSE PROTOCOL FOR A MAJOR TRANSPORTATION ACCIDENT

A funeral director may be called on to perform certain procedures before the remains are shipped to a receiving funeral director who is acting at the request of the fam-

ily of the deceased. The following guidelines must be followed by the shipping funeral director.

REMOVAL FROM TEMPORARY MORGUE

- Use only licensed personnel to make removals.
- Receive clearance to enter the temporary morgue in advance.
- Use only a professional hearse for removals and/or any transportation.

PREPARATION

- Remove the deceased from the original disaster pouch or place the entire pouch in a new heavy-duty opaque pouch.
- Use the best chemical process available for treating the remains.
- Wrap the deceased in absorbent material, if possible.
- Place the deceased in a fresh heavy-duty opaque pouch.
- Casket the deceased.
- Place identification tape with number and name on the casket at the foot.
- Place casket in a shipping tray.
- Mark identification name and number on the outside of the air tray.

DELIVERY

- Recheck all data gathering, vital statistics, and documents including permits and foreign shipping papers. Make sure all is included in the shipping envelope.
- Use only a professional hearse for the delivery to the receiving funeral director or common carrier. Do not use a van or station wagon.

Follow the office setup guidelines below to ensure thorough and correct procedures are employed:

- Staff the office with funeral directors.
- Select a proper facility to have the office. The room must be large enough for wall charts with the following information:

1. Names, when identified
2. Method of shipping (i.e., carrier, time, etc.)
3. Name, address, phone, and receiving funeral home
4. Funeral home doing the preparation and shipping

- Provide ample telephones so that the office staff may be in frequent contact with the casualties' families.
- Standardize all paperwork including:

1. Work sheets including all paper work relative to

the identification: dental charts, fingerprints, photos, jewelry, tattoos, scars
2. Death certificates
3. Release forms from the temporary morgue and cremation authorization
4. Also need: receiving funeral home; common carrier including flight, time, destination (airport); records of who worked on particular case, stake numbers, method of embalming

Please note: The above protocol is suggested by the insurance adjustors (as a working guideline). Since they are in charge and making payment for services rendered, their wishes must be followed.

LEGAL AND FINANCIAL CONSIDERATIONS IN MULTIPLE DEATH DISASTERS

In a discussion of multiple death disasters, it is important to be aware of sources of financial assistance. These include both governmental and nongovernmental agencies.

DO:

■ Before a disaster be aware of local, state, and federal laws regarding financial assistance.
■ Before a disaster occurs be aware that for victims of natural disasters certain private organizations such as the Red Cross, the Salvation Army, and religious groups may provide financial assistance.
■ Recognize that in human-caused disasters monies to cover the costs of your services will come through insurance companies.
■ Know if your state funeral directors association has set aside funds for the use of the funeral directors who work with local government officials in response to multideath disasters.

DON'T:

■ Don't assume that state or federal funds are available to disaster victims unless the disaster has been officially declared.
■ Don't assume that government agencies will cover all costs incurred by disaster-related deaths.

COORDINATING POSTDEATH ACTIVITIES

As funeral directors are called upon to serve in disasters, they must not lose sight of the fact that regardless of the numbers of persons killed, each one had an individual relationship to those who survive. Those survivors should be served in a manner that meets their individual needs.

DO:

■ Recognize that it is extremely important for a family or someone representing them to identify the deceased in order to begin their grief work.
■ Be aware of the value of ceremonial and ritualistic elements in a funeral with the immediate survivors of a multiple death disaster.
■ Know the different ways to solve the wide range of disaster problems of final disposition of multiple disaster victims.
■ Tell the families of disaster victims that there will be coordination of all activities between the funeral director on location and the funeral director at the point of final disposition.

DON'T:

■ Don't try to do everything. Attend to the matters that concern you (embalming, coordination of remains, bereavement care, etc.).
■ Don't forget the value of ritual in a disaster aftermath. Funerals help to bring a sense of order and structure. This is a need of disaster survivors.
■ Don't be afraid to follow your own instincts during a disaster. You possess skills and knowledge which are of extreme value in a disaster. Take the necessary training, and put it to use.

HUMAN BEHAVIOR IN DISASTER

A disaster is a sudden unexpected event that overtaxes both the resources of a social unit and its ability to respond. It involves groups of people and the aftermath generally requires aid and assistance from other social units. Human behavior is altered by a disaster situation. An understanding of the nature of such behavior and the potential outcomes should be helpful for the funeral director in dealing with disasters.

DO:

■ Be able to distinguish disasters from accidents.
■ Be aware that people will react differently to a natural disaster than to a human-caused disaster.
■ Become familiar with the four levels of disaster response that exist in a developed social system: societal, community, organizational, and individual.
■ Recognize that after a disaster the organizational structure in a community may shift considerably and may be difficult to understand.

DON'T:

■ Don't be surprised if great anger, hostility, and

other-directed behavior are present in human-responsible disasters.

- Don't ignore its informal structure as an influence on how a community responds to a disaster.
- Don't be surprised if the norms that govern people's sense of right and wrong are significantly altered in response to a disaster.

Occupational Exposure to Formaldehyde in Mortuaries*

L. Lamont Moore, CIH, CSP
Safety Sciences Department, Indiana University of
Pennsylvania, Indiana, Pennsylvania

Eugene C. Ogrodnik, MS
Dean, Pittsburgh Institute of Mortuary Science,
Pittsburgh, Pennsylvania

A short-term project was conducted to evaluate occupational exposure to formaldehyde in mortuaries. The study group consisted of 23 mortuaries located in Allegheny County, Pennsylvania. These establishments had business volumes ranging from 35 to 500 embalmings per year. On-site surveys were conducted at each location to examine ventilation systems and review work practices. Breathing zone and room air samples were subsequently collected during actual embalming procedures in a number of the smaller facilities with less well designed ventilation systems. One of the primary objectives of the project was to educate participating mortuary directors about the potential health hazards associated with occupational exposure to formaldehyde. An extensive literature review was completed to summarize related epidemiological and environmental studies for participants. Additionally, the monitoring data were compared to previous observations and exposure estimates. Results of this study did not reveal employee exposures which approached existing limits established by the Occupational Safety and Health Administration (OSHA).

Formaldehyde is a colorless, pungent, irritant gas that is water soluble and most frequently marketed as 37–56% aqueous solutions, commonly known as formalin. Formaldehyde vapor is very irritating to the respiratory tract, eyes, and exposed surfaces of the skin. Inhalation of high concentrations can cause laryngitis, bronchitis, and bronchopneumonia. Liquid formaldehyde solutions may cause severe burns on contact with the eye. Formaldehyde will act as a primary skin irritant, causing an erythematous or eczematous dermatitis reaction.

Formaldehyde solutions do not have a high degree of systemic toxicity, and acute and chronic exposures generally result in vaying degrees of irritation which are usually localized. Symptoms commonly experienced by the general population are nonspecific, transient, exposure dependent, and usually mild. In some cases, however, formaldehyde may act as an allergic (immunologically mediated) skin sensitizer, and it may also exacerbate respiratory distress in individuals with preexisting or formaldehyde-induced bronchial hyperreactivity. It may not be feasible for sensitized persons to work in an area where there is any possibility of exposure, even at very low levels.

Formaldehyde has an odor threshold far below 1 part per million (ppm). Stern[1] reported the lower limit for odor detection to be 0.05 ppm with throat irritation first occurring at 0.5 ppm. Bourne and Seferman[2] established the threshold for eye irritation at 0.13 to 0.45 ppm. The experience of numerous investigators has been that rapid inurement to such concentrations develops and there is a general absence of complaints from most workers exposed below 2 or 3 ppm.[3] According to existing OSHA regulations, the permissible limit for 8-hour time-weighted average exposure to formaldehyde is 3 ppm. The acceptable ceiling concentration is 5 ppm and the acceptable maximum peak is 10 ppm for 30 minutes. This standard was adopted in the mid-70s based on the irritant properties of formaldehyde.

The American Conference of Governmental Industrial Hygienists[3] has listed formaldehyde as a substance suspect of carcinogenic potential for man. In 1983 they proposed an 8-hour time-weighted average exposure limit of 1 ppm with a short-term exposure limit of 2 ppm for a maximum of 15 minutes. They point out that these concentrations may not be sufficient to prevent sensitized persons from suffering irritation but should be adequate to avoid development of persistent adverse effects.

In 1976 the National Institute for Occupational Safety and Health[4] recommended to OSHA that occupational exposure to formaldehyde be limited so that no employee is exposed at concentrations which exceed 1 ppm during any 30-minute period. This recommendation presumably was designed to protect the health of employees over their working lifetime, but may not be adequate to protect sensitized or hypersensitive individuals.

Plunkett and Barbela[5] completed a mail survey of 57 embalmers in 20 California funeral homes during

---

*Reprinted from the J Environ Health 1986;49(1), with permission.

1976. Nine had symptoms compatible with acute bronchitis, and 17 were considered to have chronic bronchitis. No data on formaldehyde exposure levels, work practices, ventilation, or frequency of exposure was gathered. Nevertheless, there was enough evidence to suggest that more in-depth studies of this profession should be considered.

Levine et al[6] studied nearly 100 West Virginia morticians who were attending an educational program during 1978. Standardized respiratory disease questioninaires and pulmonary function tests were administered to the group. The pulmonary function of morticians compared favorably with that of residential populations in Oregon and Michigan. Among the study group, those who had presumably embalmed the largest number of bodies did not demonstrate a higher than expected incidence of chronic bronchitis or pulmonary function deficits. The authors concluded that long-term intermittent exposure to low levels of formaldehyde had exerted no meaningful chronic effect on respiratory health. No actual data on formaldehyde exposures, ventilation, or work practices were gathered as part of this study.

Williams et al[7] recently published the results of exposure studies conducted in seven West Virginia funeral homes. Area and personal samples were used to evaluate the embalmers' exposure to formaldehyde, phenol, and 23 organic solvents and particulates. Twenty-five personal samples revealed time-weighted average formaldehyde concentrations which ranged from 0.1 to 0.4 ppm during the embalming of intact bodies, and ranging between 0.5 and 1.2 ppm during preparation of autopsied cases. The overall average exposures were 0.3 ppm and 0.9 ppm, respectively. Concentrations of other airborne chemicals and of particulates were negligible. Time-weighted averages were calculated over the length of time actually required for the embalming. Embalming technique and condition of the body appeared to be the major determinants of formaldehyde exposure in preparing autopsied bodies. The importance of room air exchange rate could not be determined from this study. Overall, exhaust ventilation appeared to reduce formaldehyde concentrations in general room air but had little effect on the embalmer's personal exposure.

Kerfoot and Mooney[8] completed an extensive study of six funeral homes in the Detroit area, collecting 187 air samples under a variety of conditions. The vapor concentrations encompassed a range between 0.09 and 5.26 ppm. The average formaldehyde concentrations ranged between 0.25 and 1.30 ppm under normal working conditions with an overall average of 0.74 ppm.

It was not clear whether personal or area samples were obtained. Ventilation systems were evaluated in terms of air changes per hour and compared with average concentrations of formaldehyde found in each facility. The largest number of air changes did not always cor-

respond to the lowest concentration of vapors. The authors concluded that the location of the fan and size of the room were also significant factors. They also pointed out that all six establishments were above average facilities and inferred that formaldehyde concentrations in smaller, less well designed funeral homes might be markedly higher.

In 1979, NIOSH[9] conducted a health hazard evaluation of the embalming laboratory at the Cincinnati College of Mortuary Science. The request had been prompted by the early disability retirement of an embalming instructor who had developed asthmatic bronchitis after 5 years of laboratory exposure. Air samples were collected via general area and personal breathing zone sampling during actual work conditions and simulated accidents involving spillage of embalming fluids. Formaldehyde concentrations exceeded the proposed ACGIH threshold limit value of 1 ppm in 7 of 13 samples collected. All of the excessive concentrations were detected during simulated (worst case) situations, or during one afternoon when the ventilation system was inoperable.

A study of mortality among undertakers licensed in Ontario, Canada, was completed by R. J. Levine[10] in late 1982. He selected a cohort of 1477 embalmers licensed between 1928 and 1957 and examined the cause of death in 337 men who had died prior to 1978. The ratio of observed to expected deaths from each cause was expressed as a percentage or standard mortality ratio. No significant increase in mortality was detected for any form of cancer. Deaths from cancers at sites of potential contact with formaldehyde—skin, nose, oropharynx, larynx, and esophagus—were less than expected, as were deaths from cancer of the lung.

Walrath and Fraumeni[11] of the National Cancer Institute published a study in 1983 which investigated whether embalmers in New York State, compared with the general population, had a greater proportion of cancer deaths that might be associated with exposure to formaldehyde. The study group consisted of approximately 1132 deceased embalmers who had been licensed to practice in New York State between 1902 and 1979. The difference between observed and expected numbers of deaths from malignant neoplasms was elevated, but not significantly. Skin cancer mortality was significantly elevated, primarily among those licensed for more than 35 years. Mortality was slightly elevated for kidney cancer, leukemia, and brain cancer. No excess mortality was observed for cancers of the respiratory tract and no deaths ascribed to nasal cancer.

Walrath and Fraumeni[12] published the results of a similar study of California embalmers in 1984. The authors examined the death certificates of 1007 embalmers and calculated proportionate mortality ratios for the major causes of death. Mortality was significantly elevated for total cancer, arteriosclerotic heart disease, leukemia, as well as cancers of the colon, brain, and prostate. There were no deaths from nasal cancer and the pattern of lung cancer mortality was unremarkable. One of the inherent weaknesses of both the California and New York studies is that sample sizes were of insufficient size to detect rare conditions such as nasal cancer. Although the respiratory tract would presumably be the prime target site for formaldehyde carcinogenicity, the authors conclude that available epidemiological evidence suggests attention should be given to possible cancer risks at other sites, including the brain, bone marrow, and colon. It may be of significance to note that the Ontario study[10] did not indicate an elevated risk of cancer based on a study of 300+ death certificates. However, larger studies performed in New York[11] and California[12] both showed excess deaths from leukemia and brain cancer.

Patty's text[13] suggests that aldehydes cannot be regarded as potent carcinogens. The irritant properties of the compounds preclude substantial worker exposure under normal conditions. The extreme reactivity of formaldehyde, acrolein, and chloroacetaldehyde, for example, produces reactions at epithelial surfaces which tend to limit their absorption into the body. The rapid metabolic conversion to innocuous materials also may limit those critical reactions necessary to initiate systemic tumorigenesis. However, formaldehyde-induced tissue irritation may promote tumor formation initiated by another compound. Therefore, caution is warranted, and certainly further epidemiologic studies must be performed to define any hazard that may exist.

Since 1979, there have been several research reports linking formaldehyde exposure to cancer. These studies were based on exposure of rats and mice to concentrations of 2, 6, and 15 ppm for 30 hours per week over a period exceeding 2 years.[14] Based on these findings, NIOSH recommended in 1981 that as a prudent measure, occupational exposure be reduced to the lowest feasible limit.

MATERIALS AND METHODS

On-site surveys were conducted at each facility to interview the funeral director about work procedures, evaluate the overall floor plan, calculate room volume, and record air flow measurements where appropriate. Subsequently, air sampling was conducted in a number of the funeral homes with poorly designed ventilation systems. Where feasible, samples were collected from the breathing zone of the embalmer during the entire period required for the embalming, usually 45–75 minutes.

Air was drawn through a liquid sampling medium using MSA Model G pumps set at a flow rate of 500 cubic centimeters per minute. Calibration was accomplished prior to the surveys using a primary standard (soap-bubble meter) as suggested by the manufacturer. Pumps were adjusted as necessary to maintain the desired flow rate throughout the sampling period. A midget impinger with fitted glass bubbler containing 15 ml of a 10% aqueous methanol solution was used to collect air samples to be analyzed for formaldehyde. At the conclusion of the sampling period, samples were transferred to polyethylene bottles, sealed, labeled, and shipped to an approved industrial hygiene laboratory.

At the laboratory, samples are reacted with hydrazine reagent to form a hydrazone derivative, then analyzed by differential pulses polarography. This sampling and analytical technique (ID-102) was developed at OSHA's Analytical Laboratory in Salt Lake City, Utah. The coefficient of variation (CY_T) for the total sampling and analytical technique is 0.08. This value corresponds to a standard deviation of 1 mg/m^3 at the OSHA permissible exposure limit of 3 ppm.

RESULTS AND DISCUSSION

The embalming rooms examined as part of this study varied significantly in terms of their size, layout, and the effectiveness of the ventilation system. Preparation rooms were equipped with ventilation systems which produced from 0 to 20 air changes per hour with a mean of 7.6 air changes per hour. Three facilities had exhaust systems which produced no measurable air movement at all. Only 17% of these rooms had an exhaust grate or fan which was positioned to prevent fumes from being drawn through the breathing zone of the employee.

The size of embalming rooms ranged from 735 to 5000 ft^3 with a mean of 1950 ft^3. Less than 10% of the establishments had any provisions for the introduction of makeup air into the work area. The only source of makeup air would have been leakage around doors or windows throughout the structure.

Eight personal samples were collected from the breathing zone of funeral directors during separate embalming procedures in six different funeral homes. None of these establishments had ventilation systems which would be considered above the norm described above. Exposure concentrations summarized in Table 1 show a range of 0.03 to 3.15 ppm with an overall average of 1.1 ppm during the period required for the embalming. Embalming procedures typically last 45–75 minutes depending on the condition of the subject. When we assumed zero exposure during the unsampled portion of the shift, 8-hour time-weighted average exposures ranged from 0.01 to 0.49 ppm, with an overall mean of 0.16 ppm.

The data summarized in Table 2 provide a comparison of our limited data with that of more extensive stud-

TABLE 1.   SUMMARY OF FORMALDEHYDE EXPOSURE MEASUREMENTS BASED ON PERSONAL SAMPLING

	Low	High	Average
Time-weighted average exposure during the period required for the embalming procedure	0.03 ppm	3.15 ppm	1.1 ppm
Exposure estimate for the full workshift, an 8-hour time-weighted average	0.01 ppm	0.49 ppm	0.16 ppm

Note: Calculation of 8-hour time-weighted averages was completed making the assumption that exposure would have been zero during the unsampled portion of the workshift.

TABLE 3.   COMPARISON OF FORMALDEHYDE CONCENTRATIONS DETECTED IN WORKROOM AIR DURING EMBALMING PROCEDURES—AREA VS PERSONAL SAMPLING

	Low	High	Average
Area samples taken in proximity to preparation tables	N.D.[a]	0.84 ppm	0.45 ppm
Personal samples collected from the breathing zone of embalmers	0.03 ppm	3.15 ppm	1.1 ppm

[a]N.D. signifies "not detected."

ies by Kerfoot and Mooney[8] and Williams et al.[7] Allegheny County exposure estimates reflect slightly higher formaldehyde concentrations which may be associated with the smaller, poorly designed preparation rooms where sampling was conducted. Plans for a longer term study were abandoned when our initial monitoring revealed 8-hour time-weighted average exposures to be well below the OSHA permissible exposure limit of 3 ppm.

Six area samples were also collected from general workroom air in proximity to preparation tables, usually in conjunction with personal sampling. Results summarized in Table 3 suggest that area sampling is not representative of the embalmers' actual exposure. Where concurrent sampling was carried out, concentrations found in the employee's breathing zone were up to twice as high as measurements taken from general workroom air several feet away.

There are a number of conclusions to be drawn from this study, despite its limited scope. First, the authors found many funeral directors to be largely unaware or poorly informed about the continuing controversy over the carcinogenic potential of long-term exposure to formaldehyde. Second, it was clear that most funeral homes in this study had ventilation systems or floor plans which were largely ineffective in controlling exposure during embalming procedures. The position of the exhaust grate commonly draws contaminants through the embalmer's breathing zone. Third, the authors' data sug-

gest that personal, breathing zone samples are likely to provide the most accurate indicator of employee exposure in the embalming room.

Occupational exposure to formaldehyde in funeral homes should rarely exceed permissible exposure limits established by OSHA. These limits were adopted in the early 1970s to protect employees against the irritant properties of formaldehyde, and may not be sufficiently stringent in view of the chemical's suspected carcinogenic potential. It is reasonable to assume, however, that there are regular occasions where embalmers' exposures exceed the short-term exposure limits of 2 ppm during any 15-minute period recommended by ACGIH in 1983 and the NIOSH recommendation of 1981 which suggests exposure be kept at the lowest feasible limit.

More extensive epidemiological and laboratory studies will be carried out before the issue of formaldehyde carcinogenicity is resolved. Funeral directors or embalmers represent a profession which should be of continuing interest to epidemiological researchers studying the long-term exposure to formaldehyde. Should more definitive evidence be developed with regard to the carcinogenic effects of formaldehyde, large-scale education efforts and installation of improved engineering controls will become priority within the funeral home industry.

TABLE 2.   COMPARISON OF ALLEGHENY COUNTY EXPOSURE DATA WITH PREVIOUS STUDIES

	Estimated Formaldehyde Exposure During Embalming (in ppm)		
	Low	High	Average
Kerfoot/Mooney (1975)[8]	0.25 ppm	1.39 ppm	0.74 ppm
Williams/Levine/Blunden (1984)[7]			
Intact cases	0.10 ppm	0.40 ppm	0.30 ppm
Autopsied cases	0.50 ppm	1.20 ppm	0.90 ppm
Allegheny County (1984)	0.03 ppm	3.15 ppm	1.10 ppm

REFERENCES

1. Stern AC. *Air Pollution*. New York: Academic Press; 1968;Vol. 1, p. 484.
2. Bourne HG, Seferman S. Wrinkle proofed clothing may liberate toxic quantities of formaldehyde. *Ind Med Surg* 1959;28:232.
3. American Conference of Governmental Industrial Hygienists. *Documentation of the Threshold Limit Values*. Cincinnati, OH: ACGIH; 1983: 197.1.
4. National Institute of Occupational Safety and Health. *Criteria for a Recommended Standard. . . . Occupational Exposure to Formaldehyde*. Baltimore, MD: NIOSH; 1976:P.B. 76-273805.
5. Plunkett ER, Barbela T. Are embalmers at risk? *Am Ind Hyg Assoc J* 1977;38:61-62.
6. Levine RJ, DalCorso RD, Blunder PB, Battigelli MC.

The effects of occupational exposure on the respiratory health of West Virginia morticians. *J Occup Med* 1984;26:91–98.

7. Williams TM, Levine RJ, Blunden RB. Exposure of embalmers to formaldehyde and other chemicals. *Am Ind Hyg Assoc J* 1984;45:172–176.

8. Kerfoot EJ, Mooney TF. Formaldehyde and paraformaldehyde study in funeral homes. *Am Ind Hyg Assoc J* 1975;36:533–537.

9. National Institute of Occupational Safety and Health. *Health Hazard Evaluation.* Cincinnati: College of Mortuary Science Embalming Laboratory; 1980:HHE 79-146-670, NTIS Pub. PB80-192099.

10. Levine RJ. Mortality of Ontario undertakers. In: *C.I.I.T. Activites.* Research Triangle Park, NC: Chemical Industry Institute of Toxicology; 1982.

11. Walrath J, Fraumeni JF. Mortality patterns among New York embalmers. *Int J Cancer* 1983;31:407–411.

12. Walrath J, Fraumeni JF. Cancer and other causes of death among California embalmers. *Cancer Res* 1984;44:4638–4641.

13. Clayton GD, Clayton FE (Eds). *Patty's Industrial Hygiene and Toxicology.* 3rd ed. New York: John Wiley & Sons; 1981:Vol 2A.

14. National Institute of Occupational Safety and Health. *Intelligence Bulletin 34: Formaldehyde: Evidence of Carcinogenicity.* Baltimore, MD: NIOSH; 1981.

Formaldehyde Vapor Emission Study in Embalming Rooms

Edward J. Kerfoot, Ph.D. Applicant
Department of Physiology, Department of Occupational and Environmental Health, College of Medicine, Wayne State University (Graduate of Department of Mortuary Science, Wayne State University), Detroit, Michigan

Most funeral service licensees are familiar with the physical properties and uses of formaldehyde, but few are fully aware of its toxic properties. Industries that use formaldehyde, as permanent-press fabric and paper processing, show concern about this gas and its effect on their workers. Investigation revealed that no experimentation had ever been done to determine the concentrations of formaldehyde to which funeral licensees are exposed.

It seemed that some study in this area was needed—not only to determine if the concentrations of formalde-hyde during embalming were within accepted "safe" levels, but also to evaluate the effectiveness of controls on the formaldehyde concentrations and to consider some possible adverse effects of this gas.

It may be worthwhile here to describe some of the properties of formaldehyde that are important to this particular study. Formaldehyde is a toxic gas and classified as an upper respiratory irritant because it has a high solubility in water and is held by the moisture covering the upper respiratory tract. Gases that dissolve more slowly in water travel more deeply into the respiratory tract before they are dissolved. So, under ordinary circumstances, formaldehyde, though toxic, does't cause any damage. Formaldehyde possesses distinctive physiological properties causing symptoms very familiar to all funeral licensees such as burning of the eyes, lacrimation, and irritation of the upper respiratory passages. These symptoms allow formaldehyde to act as its own warning agent as other gases like ammonia do.

The main purpose of this research was to determine the concentration of formaldehyde vapors that embalmers inhale while embalming. In six Detroit area funeral home preparation rooms the formaldehyde content during embalming procedures was determined chemically. These establishments were not representative of a general cross section of all funeral homes but were actually better than average. The concentration of formaldehyde vapors for the total 187 samples taken ranged from 0.09 to 5.26 ppm (parts per million). At the higher levels of this range, the fumes caused such severe upper respiratory distress that the licensees and sampler were unable to remain in the room.

Ventilation systems in the preparation rooms were evaluated in two ways. First, samples of formaldehyde concentrations were taken with the fan off (with an average of 1.34 ppm), then with the fan on (with an average of 0.74 ppm), indicating that use of a fan reduces the vapors by about half. Secondly, the fans were evaluated in terms of air changes per hour. The larger number of air changes did not always correspond to the lower concentration of formaldehyde vapors, indicating the probability that other factors, specifically the location of the fan and size of the room, were also significant in the efficiency of the ventilation systems.

At one funeral home, still another factor was evaluated. A surgical cloth mask was placed in the sample holder and the concentration of formaldehyde after being filtered through the mask again determined. Here the samples showed average values of 2.50 ppm with no ventilation or mask, 1.21 ppm with ventilation but without a mask, and 0.78 ppm using both the ventilation system and mask. This indicated that as the use of the fan reduced the formaldehyde concentrations by half, the further use of a mask reduced the concentrations by nearly half again. Masks are not commonly used during embalming but concerned licensees should be aware of the efficiency of a mask in reducing the amount of formaldehyde vapors inhaled.

Air samples containing embalming powders and hardening compounds were taken with a thermal precipitator and then sized microscopically; the mean particle size was found to be 1.6 microns. This finding was of definite importance because particles between 1 and 2 microns are respirable, deposited, and, most importantly, retained in the lung depths. Larger particles could not penetrate as deeply and smaller particles, which could penetrate deeply, are too small to be retained but would be exhaled. Also, the particles of paraformaldehyde powders have the ability to absorb formaldehyde vapors in the air, so that not only the particles of paraformaldehyde but the attached formaldehyde vapors (which normally affect only the upper respiratory tract) may be carried into the lower repiratory tract of the licensee.

A small-scale toxicity survey was done among the licensees at these funeral homes; they filled out questionnaires concerning the known toxic effects of formaldehyde. This study clearly demonstrated that formaldehyde is mainly an upper respiratory irritant causing eye and nose burns, sneezing, coughing, and headaches: It is interesting that 3 out of 7 men suffered from asthma or sinus problems, which is a somewhat higher proporiton than in the general population.

The workers who were bothered more by the irritant action of formaldehyde were exposed to the higher concentrations and those who spent more of their work time embalming also experienced more severe symptoms. Keep in mind that these symptoms were experienced by workers who spend only part of their work day exposed to formaldehyde and at concentrations well below the present limit.

The study, then, showed several facts of importance. For one thing, it found the formaldehyde vapor concentrations to which licensees who embalm are exposed to be within the levels of the present TLV (threshold limit value). This means that if the concentrations exceed 5 ppm they pose a possible health hazard to the worker but under this level the worker is "safe." It must be mentioned here that the current TLV of 5 ppm is being challenged and proposals have been made (by OSHA) to lower it to 2 ppm. If this happens it would mean that some licensees would be working in concentrations of formaldehyde far above the accepted "safe" limit.

The results of the toxicity survey verified the fact that formaldehyde is mainly an upper respiratory irritant because all involved experienced, to some degree, the symptoms of upper respiratory irritation. The possibility that more serious damage could occur, however, was evident with the determination of paraformaldehyde particle size. Because it's known that these powders can absorb formaldehyde, the fact that their size makes them able to be carried deep into the lungs and retained there becomes a finding of much importance. It means that these powders and compounds, as well as the attached formaldehyde vapors, can reach an area where they may cause serious lung damage.

This research also showed that ventilation systems reduce the vapor concentration roughly by half and also showed that great variations in the effectiveness of ventilation systems existed. The importance of several factors, namely the size of the fan, the size of the room, and the location of the fan, in influencing the effectiveness of a good ventilation system was shown. Further, it showed that these concentrations can be reduced by almost half again by the use of a mask.

From these results some conclusions may be drawn:

There definitely is a need for further study in this area, particularly concerning the paraformaldehyde powders and their ability to penetrate the lung depths.

The need for lowering the TLV to 2 ppm (as has been proposed) seems quite evident. As previously mentioned, when the formaldehyde concentrations approached the present TLV of 5 ppm, the licensee and sampler were too distressed to remain in the embalming room, and the irritating effects experienced by those involved in the toxicity survey at much lower levels seem to back this up.

There certainly is good reason for licensees to be well educated in the known and even possible effects of formaldehyde as well as in the effectiveness of the controls available to them. This knowledge might make more licensees responsible in protecting themselves as well as they can, even to employing the annoyance of a mask, especially when the embalming powders and hardening compounds are used.

Finally, there is a real need for setting up definite standards regarding formaldehyde exposure. Definite regulations should be set up regarding size of embalming rooms, size of fans, and their locations in the embalming rooms to insure good ventilation systems. Perhaps even the number of hours that one embalmer could be exposed in a given amount of time should be limited. Whether such standards will be determined will depend, in large part, on the interest of funeral service licensees themselves.

Reported Studies on Effects of Formaldehyde Exposure*

Leandro Rendon
Director of Research and Educational Programs,
Champion Chemical Company, Springfield, Ohio

The general effects related to human exposure to formaldehyde appear to include many different symp-

*Reprinted from the *Expanding Encyclopedia*, No. 542, Springfield, OH: Champion Chemical Co.; 1983, with permission.

toms and conditions. Perhaps, the most frequently mentioned effects are those associated with the pungent, irritating properties of formaldehyde involving the eyes, nose, and throat. The degree of response will vary depending upon the amount of formaldehyde present and from individual to individual.

It has long been known that high concentrations of formaldehyde are irritating to man and that it can cause skin sensitization. Because of formaldehyde's importance, the Chemical Industry Institute of Toxicology (CIIT) sponsored a conference in November 1980, in which current research on formaldehyde was presented. The event brought scientists and government regulators together to hear and discuss the wide variety of then-current research.

Issue no. 517, May 1981, of the *Expanding Encyclopedia* discussed some of the available data regarding "Health Risk From Formaldehyde." Since then, more information has become available and it is the purpose of this discussion to update what is known regarding effects of formaldehyde exposure.

In his presentation at the November 1980 conference, Richard J. Levine et al[1] distinguished two important categories of embalming practice in relation to exposure: the embalming of "normal" (nonautopsied) and of autopsied remains. In their studies, the group found time-weighted-average formaldehyde concentrations to be 0.3 ppm during the embalming of nonautopsied cases and 0.9 ppm for autopsied remains. The highest concentrations were 0.4 ppm and 2.1 ppm, respectively. The investigator commented that while exposures found in embalming autopsied bodies are more intense, autopsied bodies usually comprise only a minority of total bodies embalmed. He further stated:

In a summary, pulmonary function of West Virginia (where the study was performed) morticians compared favorably to that of residential populations in Oregon and Michigan. Among morticians, high exposure was linked neither to chronic bronchitis nor to pulmonary function deficits. The results suggest that intermittent exposure to low levels of formaldehyde gas over the long term exerts no meaningful chronic effect on respiratory health.

At the same CIIT conference on November 1980, Walrath et al[2] presented a preliminary study that investigated whether embalmers, compared with the general population, have a greater proportion of cancer deaths that might be associated with exposure to formaldehyde. The study group consisted of deceased embalmers licensed to practice embalming in New York State between 1902 and 1979. The death certificates revealed data indicating that the embalmers in that group experienced a slightly elevated mortality from cancer, a significant excess of arteriosclerotic heart disease, and a very low incidence of pneumonia deaths. Skin cancer mortality was significantly elevated as well as kidney and brain cancers. On the other hand, there was no excess mortality from cancer of the respiratory tract, including the nasal passages. The investigators point out, however, "that embalming fluids contain a mixture of other chemicals that are partly intended to offset the adverse reactions of formaldehyde."

It should be pointed out that commercially available fluids from 1902 to approximately the late 1930s tended to be rather harsh and astringent compositions. The embalmer did not often use or wear gloves when working with embalming compositions as happens today. It is possible to assume that prolonged contact of the embalming fluids with the skin could produce adverse effects. Also, it is possible that adequate ventilation and exhaust systems were not available in preparation rooms in the "early" days.

On November 3, 1982, the Formaldehyde Institute sponsored a formaldehyde toxicology conference as a means of continuing the open dialogue between interested parties that was initiated at the November 1980 meeting. Another important paper was presented at that meeting by Dr. Richard J. Levine et al.[3]

The investigators made a study of the mortality of Ontario undertakers during the period between 1928 and 1957. As was the purpose in the study among West Virginia funeral licensees, Dr. Levine was interested in learning more about possible effects of formaldehyde among groups of workers who are known to work with the compound possibly to a greater extent than others and over a longer period of time.

The sites felt to be of particular interest as being of a special risk for cancer from exposure to formaldehyde were skin, nasal passages, buccal cavity, pharynx, and larnyx. Among the Canadian funeral licensees no deaths due to nasal cancer were observed. Mortality attributed to cancers of the buccal cavity, pharynx, and respiratory system exclusive of trachea, bronchus, and lung was less than expected.

Cirrhosis of the liver was the only cause of death found to be significantly in excess. The investigators felt that perhaps this might be due to a higher consumption of alcoholic beverages by this group than the general population. They believed this might account for the increases in mortality from liver cancer, disease of the circulatory system, and acute respiratory diseases, which are characteristically elevated among alcoholics. The preliminary conclusion is that formaldehyde exposure among Ontario's funeral licensees has had no effect on cancer mortality.

A new British epidemiology study released in August 1983 contains some interesting information. Dr. E. A. Acheson, Director of the British Medical Research

Council's Environmental Epidemiology Unit, Southampton General Hospital, in the United Kingdom, presented a report based on a study of more than 7700 chemical workers from six factories among the country's chemical industry where formaldehyde has been manufactured or used for more than 15 years. The study sought to find an increase in the incidence of cancer types among long-term employees exposed to formaldehyde. The levels workers were exposed to over the period studied were as much as three times higher than those allowed under present regulations.

Results of the Acheson study show no excessive risk for formaldehyde workers of contracting nasal, lung, prostrate, brain, skin, kidney, or bladder cancers. The report, according to the Formaldehyde Institute, brings the total number of epidemiology studies performed to 12, all revealing no excess cancer types in persons exposed to formaldehyde. In this country, the major manufacturers of formaldehyde have accomplished similar studies among their workers and report data similar to those of Acheson.

In Iowa, a study was accomplished jointly by the Iowa State Department of Health and the University Hygienic Laboratory. The study was carried out with the endorsement of the Board of Mortuary Science Examiners and the Iowa Funeral Directors Association. The first phase of the two-part study determined formaldehyde exposure during embalmings. The second part examined cancer death rates among funeral directors as compared to the general population.

During the study, personnel from the Iowa State Department of Health visited 44 funeral homes that had been randomly selected throughout the state. At each place, two samples of formaldehyde gas were collected during embalming procedures—one at the operator's breathing zone and one ambient room air sample. According to the Iowa State Department of Health, the following determinations were found as a result of the study, June 1983;

Formaldehyde concentrations measured in breathing zone samples ranged from nondetectable to 3.5 ppm. The *average* detectable level of formaldehyde in the breathing zone was 0.84 ppm. Ambient room sample concentrations ranged from nondetectable to 1.99 ppm, with an *average* reading of 0.23 ppm determined.

The Iowa State Department of Health reported its findings to the Iowa Funeral Directors Association and listed the following measures that should be followed to reduce exposure whenever practicable *although none of the reported levels were in excess of federal standards:*

1. Local exhaust ventilation should be used whenever persons are working in the preparation room, particularly during embalming procedures. Significantly higher concentrations of formaldehyde would be expected when no local exhaust ventilation is used during embalming procedures. Ventilation systems should be properly designed with consideration for room volume, embalming workload, and avoidance of dead air spaces.
2. During embalming procedures, personnel should avoid working in locations between the exhaust vent and sources of formaldehyde (for example, embalming tank, mixing tank, etc.)
3. Situations in which formaldehyde is exposed to room air (for example, spills, open tanks, open bottles, etc.) should be minimized. In situations where opportunities for volatilizing formaldehyde into the room air cannot be avoided, the length of exposure should be maintained at as short an interval as is practicable.
4. Direct skin contact with formaldehyde should be avoided. Use of protective equipment, such as rubber gloves and aprons, will reduce the chances of skin exposure. In this study, at least one instance of contact dermatitis was reported to occur from embalming fluid.

ACKNOWLEDGMENT

Acknowledgment is hereby extended to the Iowa Funeral Directors Association for making available the preceding information which should be of immense interest to all funeral licensees.

REFERENCES

1. Levine RJ, et al. The effects of occupational exposure on the respiratory health of West Virginia morticians. In: *Formaldehyde Toxicity.* New York: Hemisphere Pub. Corp.; 1983:212–226.
2. Walrath J, et al. Proportionate mortality among New York embalmers. In: *Formaldehyde Toxicity.* New York: Hemisphere Pub. Corp.; 1983:227–236.
3. Levine RJ, et al. Mortality of Ontario undertakers: A first report. In: *Formaldehyde Toxicology–Epidemiology–Mechanisms.* New York: Marcel Dekker; 1983:127–140.

Dangers of Infection*

Leandro Rendon
Director of Research and Educational Programs, Champion Chemical Company, Springfield, Ohio

The possibility of acquiring disease as the result of handling and caring for human remains is very real and is of

*Reprinted from the *Expanding Encyclopedia,* No. 508. Springfield, OH: Champion Chemical Co.; 1980, with permission.

concern to funeral licensees. Unfortunately, there are those who do not seem to be aware of the potential risks involved or who do not seem to believe such danger exists or that it is even possible. Such individuals, in and out of funeral service, seem to minimize the existence of disease-producing organisms in dead human remains.

At the Continuing Education program sponsored April 18, 1980, by the faculty of San Antonio College, San Antonio, Texas, Dr. Kendall O. Smith, Professor of Microbiology, University of Texas Health Science Center at San Antonio, was one of the participants. He presented information about some of the biological hazards that should be of concern to the funeral licensee. The following discussion is based on some of the information presented by Dr. Smith. It is hoped this discussion serves to further stress the potential dangers of infection that the licensee does encounter in his or her work and the need, therefore, to follow prescribed hygienic practices and certain procedures of disinfection and decontamination to protect himself or herself against infection.

The most often reported infections associated with handling of human remains are tuberculosis and infectious hepatitis. In the survey among funeral licensees made by this Department some time ago, of those who sustained one or more infections, about 14% said they had contracted tuberculosis and 12.7%, infectious hepatitis. The medical literature makes reference to similar and other incidences of infection (*Proc Roy Soc Med* 1973:66-25).

Causes of death in cancer patients for the year 1970 were studied in New York (*J Med* 1975;6:61) at a hospital on the basis of clinical and pathology reports of 506 cases. The single major causes of death was infection (36%), which also was a contributory factor in an additional 68% of the cases. The organisms causing the infection were mostly gram-negative, antibiotic-resistant bacteria. Other important causes of death were hemorrhagic and thromboembolic phenomena (18%) which also were contributory factors in an additional 43%.

In a study performed by personnel of the M. D. Anderson Hospital and Tumor Institute, Houston, Texas (*Am J Med Sci* 1974;268:97), the causes of death in patients with malignant lymphoma were reviewed. The records of some 206 patients over an 8-year period were used for the report. The commonest cause of death in those patients was infection which accounted for 51% of the deaths. These infections were primarily caused by gram-negative bacilli.

Toxoplasmosis is a disease caused by infection with the protozoan *Toxoplasma*. In infants and children, the disease usually is characterized by an encephalomyelitis. In adults, a form clinically resembling a spotted fever has been reported.

Five patients with lethal disseminated toxoplasmosis were seen within a 2-year period at the Swedish Hospital Medical Center and the University of Washington Hospital (*Arch Intern Med* 1974;134:1059). In all patients, there was a severe underlying disease treated with various chemotherapeutic agents, corticosteroids, splenectomy, or irradiation. Although the clinical symptoms were variable and masked by the underlying illness, therapeutic measures, or concomitant infectious processes, or both, the autopsy findings were strikingly uniform in that the brain, myocardium, and lungs were invariably affected. Reports in the literature and the experience of the investigators indicate that disseminated toxoplasmosis in compromised hosts is being recognized with increasing frequency.

One episode has been repoted (*JAMA* 1967; 202:284) in which toxoplasmosis was transmitted during postmortem examination. The occurrence of lymphadenitis in human toxoplasmosis is well recorded. However, the mode of transmission and time course of the disease remain far from clear.

Most of the knowledge of acquired toxoplasmosis is based on infections in laboratory workers and on occasional cases of accidental inoculation. A case is recorded where a pathologist became acutely ill with toxoplasmosis 2 *months* after the autopsy of a patient who died with Hodgkins's disease and toxoplasmic ventriculitis.

Personnel from the National Institute of Neurological Diseases and Stroke, National Institutes of Health, call attention to another type of potential infection (*J Neurosurg* 1974;41:394). Precautions are mentioned in conducting biopsies and autopsies on patients with presenile dementia.

The report mentions that such patients may have Creutzfeldt–Jakob disease, a disease transmissible by a virus likely to be extremely resistant to inactivation. It is recommended:

1. That instruments used in any surgical or autopsy procedures on patients with presenile dementia be autoclaved for at least 30 minutes
2. That all organs, including those fixed in formalin, be treated as infectious materials
3. That floors and other surfaces in contact with tissues from such patients be decontaminated with a solution known to inactivate the scrapie agent, for instance, 0.5% NaOC1 solution. The fact that the agent is susceptible to sodium hypochlorite but not to the well-known disinfectants tells us something about the newly emerging pathogens that seemingly are highly resistant to the commonly used chemical sterilants.

The literature references many instances of cross-infections among patients in hospitals. The May 1980 issue (No. 507) of this *Encyclopedia* alludes to infections of this type among hospitalized populations. A typical situation found in the literature is the following case. Serological evidence of cross-infection in a dialysis unit hepatitis B epidemic has been reported (*Kidney Int* 1974;6:118).

It is of interest to call this report to the attention of the reader because it points to the ease with which personnel can acquire infections. If this can happen in a hospital, consider the possibility of such occurrence in the preparation room while handling the remains of individuals who have been in a dialysis unit. There were 74 patients and staff who developed HB-Ag-positive hepatitis during a 28-month surveillance period. Twenty-six (26) of these cases were intimately related to the dialysis unit (21 dialysis/transplant patients and 5 hospital staff) and 48 were not. Representative sera from each group of cases were further tested for HB-Ag subtype specificity. Thirteen (13) of fourteen (14) dialysis/transplant patients had subtype *ay* whereas 10 of 15 general hospital patients had the alternate pheonotype *ad*.

All four staff individuals who had probably acquired their infection from dialysis/transplant patients were *ay* subtype. Eight of the dialysis/transplant patients had never received blood. Transfusion rate in the infected dialysis patients was one third that of leukemic patients but the hepatitis rate was higher. The bacteriological procedures are mentioned in detail simply to illustrate the thoroughness of establishing proof of cross-contamination. There is little doubt as to the source of the infection.

An interesting incident is found in the literature (*Am J Clin Pathol* 1969;51:260) that should be of pertinent interest to funeral licensees—tubercular infection. Inoculation tuberculosis of the skin, occuring in physicians and medical students engaged in performing postmortem examinations, has been referred to by a variety of names among which "prosector's wart" appears to be a particularly appropriate term. A medical student–prosector developed typical primary cutaneous tuberculosis of the hand despite having practiced most currently accepted precautionary methods in performing an autopsy on a patient who had harbored active turberculosis. The nature of the infection was established by culture as well as by demonstration of acid-fast bacilli in the surgically excised lesion of the hand.

In a study to establish the incidence of tuberculosis among workers in medical laboratories, an investigator (*Br Med J* 1957;5035:10–14) at the London School of Hygiene and Tropical Medicine made a survey among personnel of the National Health Service and the Public Health Laboratory Service. There was a larger number of incidences of infection among individuals employed in laboratory and mortuary tasks which exposed them to the risk of contact with infected pathological material. The incidence was highest in the second and third years of such employment.

Tuberculosis as an occupational disease among workers in pathology institutes is the subject of a report from West Germany (*Dtsch Gesundheit* 1964;19:2389–2390). Incidence of tuberculosis among pathologists was found to be 20-fold greater in one study, and 25-fold greater in another, than in the general population.

Investigators in Europe (*Dokl Bolg Akad Nauk* 1965;18:179–181) have shown that streptococci and staphylococci multiply 10–100 times and even more in the blood and tissues of corpses kept at room temperatures. Additional investigations have also shown that there is an increase not only of the number of septicemic agents (Pasteurellae, the erysipelosis, and *Bact. pyocyaneum*), but also in their virulence. The virulence of the strains isolated from dead remains held at room temperatures rises immediately after death and reaches maximum at the 5th to the 7th hours for the streptococci and the 10th to the 12th hours for the staphylococci after which it may gradually decrease.

The newly emerging pathogens that are frequently arriving on the scene seem to be "unconventional" types. They are difficult to isolate in some cases and present problems in classification. Some seem to be able to change their structure, i. e., mutate, and thereby become resistant to commonly used drugs.

Often, infections are acquired and the host is unaware of the infection. The organisms may not indicate their presence for days, weeks, months, and even years. As can be seen from the very brief overview of the literature, there is ample scientific evidence for the need to practice effective measures in the preparation room to reduce, as much as possible, the risk factor of such environment.

In-Use Evaluation of Glutaraldehyde as a Preservative–Disinfectant in Embalming*

Robert N. Hockett, M.S.
Research Associate, School of Dentistry, University of Michigan, Ann Arbor, Michigan

Leandro Rendon, M.S.
Director of Research and Educational Programs, Champion Chemical Company, Springfield, Ohio

*Reprinted from abstracts of the annual meeting of the American Public Health Association, Session 449. Contributed papers: Microbiology–Immunology, November 1973.

Gordon W. Rose, Ph.D.
Associate Director, Department of Mortuary Science,
Wayne State University, Detroit, Michigan

INTRODUCTION

The use of formaldehyde as a disinfectant has been described by Walker,[1] Lawrence and Block,[2] and Spaulding.[3] Walker states that its commercial importance as a fungicide is probably greater than as a bactericide, and that a 4.0% solution will destroy all vegetative and many spore-forming bacteria "in less than 30 minutes."

The three "high-level" germicides described by Spaulding are 3 to 8% formaldehyde (7.5–20% formalin), 2.0% alkalinized glutaraldehyde, and gaseous ethylene oxide. He reports that in order for formaldehyde to exert a "high level of disinfection" or destruction of large numbers of bacterial and fungal spores, tubercle bacilli, and enteric viruses, including the hepatitis viruses, it should be used in a concentration of 8.0% (20% formalin). The indicated exposure time for formaldehyde (8.0%) plus alcohol (60–70%) was 12 hours in situations calling for high-demand disinfection.

The concentration of formaldehyde solution used as a preservative-disinfectant in funeral service and other areas of biologic preservation seldom exceeds 2.0% (5.0% formalin).[4] Inasmuch as 2.0% alkalinized glutaraldehyde possesses "high-level" disinfection properties equal to or surpassing those of 8.0% formaldehyde, it was decided that an in-use evaluation of glutaraldehyde as a preservative–disinfectant in the embalming of human remains should be conducted. Further, this study and similar unpublished investigations were suggested by earlier reports from pathologists that several etiologic agents of infection are recoverable from human remains embalmed with conventional formaldehyde-base chemicals. *Klebsiella pneumoniae, Hemophilus influenzae, Mycobacterium tuberculosis, Nocardia asteroides, Histoplasma capsulatum,* and other recognized pathogens were recovered from human remains embalmed for extended periods of time.[5–7]

Rubbo et al,[8] Pepper and Lieberman,[9] and Stonehill et al[10] reported that buffered aqueous solutions of glutaraldehyde may be employed without loss of effectiveness for up to 3 weeks. The consensus from available reports indicates that the most effective use-concentration of glutaraldehyde for rapid sporicidal effect, with or without alcohol, is 2.0% by weight and buffered to a pH of 7.4–8.5. Concentrations as low as 0.05% are equally effective against some vegetative bacteria. The use of 2.0% alkalinized glutaraldehyde for the sterilization of urological instruments[11] and anesthesia equipment[12] in the

medical care area fulfilled many of the criteria of an "ideal" cold sterilizing agent. Also of particular interest were the reports of low toxicity for the user. No toxicity or tissue irritation were reported after extensive use. Buffered glutaraldehyde was so highly regarded as a broad-spectrum disinfectant that it was one of the three disinfectants used in the Apollo space program's post-recovery operation of the spaceships that had landed on the moon.

MATERIALS AND METHODS

A. Sampling

The microbial sampling protocol employed in this study was the same as previously reported. Additional postembalming sampling was performed to comparatively evaluate the microbial effectiveness of the test chemicals. Preembalming body fluid and tissue aspirate samples were withdrawn from test cases (human remains) that had been dead for from 6 to 11 hours. These postmortem time intervals were selected as a result of previous temporal indications that the postmortem microbial populations were in a state of exponential growth.[13]

B. Embalming Procedures

1. Injections and drainage procedures always involved multipoint selections, such as the carotid artery/jugular vein and the femoral artery/femoral vein sites.
2. The arterial "test" injection solution was administered using a moderate rate of flow (10–12 minutes to inject each gallon) and sufficient pressure (2–10 pounds) to maintain that rate of injection.
3. After visible discolorations were removed, the intermittent and/or restricted type of drainage was used for the remainder of the operation.
4. Following arterial injection; the contents of the abdominal and thoracic cavities were chemically treated with 32 ounces of "test" cavity chemicals per cavity.

All test cases were professionally embalmed at the Wayne State University Department of Mortuary Science by a licensed member of the embalming teaching staff. Medical certifications indicated the primary cause of death to be other than an infectious disease. *All cases were evaluated and deemed completely suitable for normal funeral service viewing purposes* following completion of investigational handling.

C. Test Chemical Solutions

1. "Test" Arterial Solutions. Solution *"A"*—Prepared by diluting concentrated, commercially available, formaldehyde–glutaraldehyde products so that each gallon contained 2.0% formaldehyde and 2.0% glutaraldehyde, plus 4 ounces EDTA-base chemical water conditioner.

Solution "B"—Prepared by diluting concentrated, commercially available, formaldehyde–glutaraldehyde products so that each gallon contained 3.3% formaldehyde and 2.0% glutaraldehyde, plus 4 ounces EDTA-base chemical water conditioner.

Solution "C"—Prepared by diluting concentrated, commercially available, formaldehyde–glutaraldehyde products so that each gallon contained 2.8% formaldehyde and 2.37% glutaraldehyde, plus 4 ounces EDTA-base chemical water conditioner.

2. "Test" Cavity Solution. Concentrated, commercially available biologic preservative–disinfectant containing 10% formaldehyde, 2.0% glutaraldehyde, and 8.5% phenol in an alcohol base.

D. Microbial Identification and Enumeration

All samples were initially diluted 1:10 in phosphate-buffered saline (PBS) and 0.1 ml of each diluted sample was impinged onto a 0.45-μm Millipore (Millipore Corp., Bedford, MA) membrane filter (MF), washed once with 10 ml of PBS and then with 10 ml of Dey–Engley universal neutralizing medium (broth) for antimicrobial chemicals.[14] The Dey–Engley antimicrobial neutralizer contains chemicals selective for the neutralization of formaldehyde and glutaraldehyde. A 6-place manifold with sterile funnels and accessory items (Millipore) was utilized throughout the study to standardize sample handling and microbial quantitation. The MFs, with impinged, washed, and neutralized samples, were rolled onto primary isolation media (MacConkey and Blood Agar plates) and incubated at 35–37°C for 24 to 48 hours. Colonial isolates were subcultured and characterized by pertinent methods.[15] The gram-negative and the gram-positive aerobic and facultatively aerobic "indica-

tor" isolates were previously reported by Rose and Hockett.[13]

RESULTS

In test cases II, IV, and V, the quantitative postembalming reduction of microbial densities exceeded 95% within 20 to 24 hours (Table 1). The total volume of arterial injection solution used in these three test cases was 3.5 to 4.0 gallons. In test case 1 *only 2 gallons* of arterial injection solution were used and the microbial populations increased progressively throughout the postembalming sampling period of 22 hours. This indicated to the investigators that both the volume of solution and the concentration of active ingredients employed were insufficient. While tissue fixation in terms of normal in-state preparation and appearance was adequate, the microbial effects were unsatisfactory.

In case III, no microbial agents were recoverable from the unembalmed body. The investigators believe that the extensive antemortem administration of therapeutic antimicrobial agents was responsible for the negative baseline or control densities. It is interesting to note, however, that throughout the postembalming period of 25 hours there was no evidence of microbial colonization or recolonization from exogenous or other sources. The embalming chemicals effectively prevented the possible resumption of microbial growth and proliferation.

The volume of arterial injection solution and the concentrations of active arterial and cavity chemical ingredients used in cases II, IV, and V produced irreversible or cidal reductions of the control or preembalming microbial densities.

DISCUSSION

While internal anatomic sterilization may be neither chemically achievable nor environmentally necessary, the

TABLE 1. MICROBICIDAL EFFECTS OF "TEST" EMBALMING SOLUTIONS

Case No.	Body Weight (lbs)	Interval Between Death and Embalming	Injection Solution Type[a]	Injection Solution Volume (gal)	Microbial Densities[b] Preembalming	Microbial Densities[b] Postembalming	Percent Reduction
I	180	8	A	2.0	1,000	10,000–100,000	Densities inc.[c]
II	90	11	B	4.0	100,000–1,000,000	0–100	>95
III	105	8	C	4.0	0	0	No change[c]
IV	160	6	C	4.0	1,000–10,000	0–400	>95
V	150	10	C	3.5	100,000–1,000,000	0–50	>95

[a]See "Test" chemicals.
[b]Average, all sampling sites.
[c]See text (Results section).

postembalming production of a nonhazardous index of hygienic safety is a reasonable and essential public health expectation of modern embalming chemistry and techniques. The investigators feel that the microbial inactivation properties of embalming chemicals should assure an 80% or greater reduction in the postmortem microbial flora. Such a reduction would help to reduce the possible transmission of infectious doses of microbial agents within a variety of environments associated with the presence of embalmed human remains. These environments might well include areas or sites of earth interment, above-ground facilities such as mausoleums and storage or receiving vaults, refrigerated and nonrefrigerated storage facilities in medical and paramedical science programs, schools of funeral service education, and funeral homes. It is reasonable to expect that the postembalming microbial survivors or persisters might exit via one or more of the body orifices and contaminate environmental surfaces adjacent to the temporary or permanent location of the embalmed human remains.

The investigators concluded that the use of arterial and cavity chemicals containing an in-use concentration of 2.0% alkalinized glutaraldehyde in conjunction with formaldehyde and/or formaldehyde derivatives will effectively accomplish both the preservation and the disinfection functions of embalming.

ACKNOWLEDGMENT

Support for this study was provided by the Champion Company, Springfield, Ohio. The commercial products employed in the study were PLX, FAX, Di-San, and Searine compounded by the Champion Company.

REFERENCES

1. Walker JF. *Formaldehyde.* 3rd ed. American Chemical Society Monograph Series. New York: Reinhold 1964.

2. Lawrence CA, Block SS. *Disinfection, Sterilization and Preservation.* Philadelphia: Lea & Febiger; 1968.

3. Spaulding EH. Role of chemical disinfection in the prevention of nosocomial infections. In: *Proceedings of the International Conference on Nosocomial Infections.* Atlanta: Centers for Disease Control; August 1970.

4. Pervier NC. *Textbook of Chemistry for Embalmers.* rev ed. Minneapolis: University of Minnesota Bookstores; 1956:131.

5. Meade GM, Steenken W. Viability of tubercle bacilli in embalmed human lung tissue. *Am Rev Tuberculosis* 1949;59:429.

6. Weed LA, Baggerstoss AH. The isolation of pathogens from tissues of embalmed human bodies. *Am J Clin Pathol* 1951;21:1114.

7. Weed LA, Baggerstoss AH. The isolation of pathogens from embalmed tissues. *Proc Soc Mayo Clin* 1952;27:124.

8. Rubbo S, Gardner J, Webb R. Biocidal activities of glutaraldehyde and related compounds. *J Appl Bacteriol* 1967;30(1):78–87.

9. Pepper R, Lieberman E. Dialdehyde alcoholic sporicidal composition. U.S. Patent 3,016,328 to Ethicon, Inc., 1962.

10. Stonehill A, Krop S, Borick P. Buffered glutaraldehyde—A new chemical sterilizing solution. *Am J Hosp Pharm.* 1963;20:458–465.

11. O'Brien HA, Mitchell JD, Haberman S, Rowan DF, Winford TE, Pellet J. The use of activated glutaraldehyde as a cold sterilizing agent for urological instruments. *J Urol* 1966;95.

12. Haselhuhn DH, Brason FW, Borick PM. "In use" study of buffered glutaraldehyde for cold sterilization of anesthesia equipment. *Anesth Analg Curr Res* 1967;46.

13. Rose GW, Hockett RN. The microbiologic evaluation and enumeration of postmortem specimens from human remains. *Health Lab Sci* 1971;8:75–78.

14. Engley FB, Dey BP. A universal neutralizing medium for antimicrobial chemicals. In: *Proceedings of the 56th Mid-year Meeting, Chemical Specialities Manufacturers Association,* May 1970.

15. Blair JF, Lennette EH, Truant JP *Manual of Clinical Microbiology.* Bethesda, MD: American Society for Microbiology;1970.

The Antimicrobial Activity of Embalming Chemicals and Topical Disinfectants on the Microbial Flora of Human Remains*

Peter A. Burke and A.L. Sheffner
Department of Microbiology, Foster D. Snell, Inc.,
Florham Park, New Jersey

The antimicrobial activity of embalming chemicals and topical disinfectants was evaluated to determine the degree of disinfection achieved during the embalming of human remains. The administration of arterial and cavity

*Reprinted from *Health Lab Sci* 1976;13(2):267–270, with permission from the American Public Health Association.

embalming chemicals resulted in a 99% reduction of the postmortem microbial population after 2 hours of contact. This level of disinfection was maintained for the 24-hour test period. Topical disinfection of the body orifices was also observed. Therefore, it is probable that present embalming practices reduce the hazard from transmission of potentially infectious microbial agents within the immediate environment of embalmed human remains.

INTRODUCTION

For many years embalming chemicals have been utilized to preserve and disinfect biological tissues for anatomical studies, environmental storage, and hygienic safety. The majority of these embalming chemicals are formaldehyde-based products, whose disinfectant properties have been described by Walker,[1] Lawrence and Block,[2] and Spaulding.[3] It has been reported that pathogenic organisms, such as *K. pneumoniae, H. Influenzae, M. tuberculosis,* and *H. capsulatum,* are recoverable from embalmed human remains.[4-6] Thus, conceivably, infection could occur from contact with postembalming microbial fluids and swabs of areas around orifices from cadavers to determine if commercially available embalming chemicals produce a significant reduction in the microbial flora.

MATERIALS AND METHODS

Samples of biological fluids and swabs of the area around orifices were taken from eight cadavers to determine the antimicrobial activity of embalming fluids in vivo as a function of time. Four of the bodies were embalmed while the other four cadavers were not and served as controls. The primary cause of death of the subjects was diagnosed to be other than an infectious disease (i.e., coronary thrombosis, cerebrovascular accident, arteriosclerosis).

Embalming Procedure

The bodies were embalmed by a professional licensed mortician using the following procedure: The body was washed with an antiseptic soap containing 0.75% hexachlorophene and thoroughly rinsed. The cadaver was sprayed with a topical embalming disinfectant and the orifices swabbed with the same disinfectant. This disinfectant was a solution of 1.0% (w/v) formaldehyde and 0.5% (w/v) quaternary ammonium compounds in a base of isopropanol and ethylene dichloride.

Prior to dilution of the arterial embalming chemical, the tap water was treated with a water conditioning mixture formulated specifically for embalming use. This conditioner is a complexing agent that removes chemical constituents found in municipal water supplies which could interfere with the preservative and disinfecting properties of the arterial solutions. This conditioner is basically a mixture of trisodium ethylenediaminetetraacetate and polyvinylpyrrolidone in a base of various glycols.

The arterial embalming chemical consisted of 29.8% (w/v) formaldehyde, 3.8% (w/v) anionic detergents, 4.0% (w/v) borate and germicides, 9.6% (w/v) alcohol, and various inert ingredients in a water base. The arterial embalming chemical was then diluted 6 ounces to a half gallon of water. An equal amount of coinjection chemical for the purpose of stimulating drainage and inducing penetration was added to the solution. This chemical consisted of 8.9% (w/v) chelating agents, 0.1% (w/v) reducing agents, 0.7% (w/v) preservatives, 2.0% (w/v) plasticizers, 9.9% (w/v) humectants, and various inert ingredients in a water base.

The total amount of solution injected into the body was approximately 2 to $3\frac{1}{2}$ gallons, depending on the body size and weight. Two pints of cavity embalming chemical (24–28% [w/v] formaldehyde) were injected into each subject, one into the thoracic cavity and the other into the abdominal cavity. All products used in the study were commercially available embalming chemicals.

Sample Collection

Samples were drawn from superior and inferior anatomical sites, with sterile 18-gauge needles and 30-ml syringes. Needle puncture sites were topically disinfected with 95% ethanol. Swab samples were taken with sterile polyester swabs which just prior to swabbing were immersed in steril phosphate-buffered saline.* Biological fluids and swab cultures were taken from the following areas:

FLUID SAMPLES

- **Lung:** The needle was inserted 3 inches to the right of the midline, through the fifth intercostal space. Pulmonary fluids or aspirates were extracted from the middle lobe of the right lung.
- **Heart blood:** The needle was inserted 1 inch to the left of the midline, through the fifth intercostal space.
- **Descending colon:** A longitudinal incision 3 inches long was made midway between the tip to the 12th rib and the anterior iliac spine; the descending colon was identified and the fecal extracted from the lumen of the colon.
- **Urinary bladder:** The needle was inserted through the external urethral orifice and the urine extracted from the lumen of the bladder.

Dehydrated or coagulated sample sites were injected with sterile phosphate-buffered saline.

---

*Phosphate-buffered saline prepared by diluting 0.25 *M* phosphate buffer 1/1000 in physiological saline (0.9% NaCl).

SWABS OF ORIFICES

- **Oral cavity:** Samples were taken from the buccal furrow between the mucous membrane of the upper lip and the gingiva.
- **Nasal cavity:** Swabs were made from the vestibule of the left half of the nasal cavity.
- **Anus:** Swabs were taken from the terminal inch of the anal canal.

Immediately after taking samples, the swabs were placed in Stuart's transport medium.

Samples were taken prior to embalming and then 2, 4, 8, and 24 h after embalming. The bodies were covered with plastic sheeting while sampling procedure was not in process. All samples were packed in dry ice during transportation to the laboratories of Foster D. Snell, Inc., where they were immediately plated.

Quantitative Measurement of Microbiological Flora

Immediately following receipt in the laboratory, the biological fluids were serially diluted in thiotone peptone water blanks and subsequently plated on MacConkey and Heart Infusion Agar with 5% defibrinated sheep blood. Into both agar preparations, 0.5% Tween-80 and 0.1% lecithin were incorporated to neutralize residual microbial activity from the embalming fluids. The plates were incubated at 35-37°C for 48 h following which a colony count was performed.

Microbial Identification

Isolates were identified using standard morphological and biochemical tests with the general outline utilized for identification as defined in Bergey's Manual of

Determinative Bacteriology, eighth edition,[7] and Skerman's *Identification of the Genera of Bacteria*, second edition.[8]

RESULTS AND DISCUSSION

In vitro, germicidal activity of formaldehyde has been established and documented for many years.[2] However, the amount of microbiological data concerning the in vivo efficacy of embalming chemicals on human remains is scant. In the present study, formaldehyde-based embalming fluids were found to be highly active in reducing the microbial flora in human remains. The microbial population was reduced greater than 99% at every site 2 hours after embalming; with control bodies, as anticipated, a continuous microbial growth pattern was observed (Table 1). The antimicrobial action of formaldehyde-based embalming chemicals was apparently not limited or adversely affected by the proteinaceous material or other macromolecules present in the biological fluids and tissues.

Following topical disinfection of the areas around the orifices, no growth or limited growth could be detected after 24 h of exposure. Disinfection of the orifices occurred within 2 h of contact. Random positive results after disinfection, however, were seen because the bodies were not protected from the environment with the exception of a nonsterile plastic cloth.

Differential monitoring of the microbial population revealed that microorganisms translocate across anatomical barriers which during life prevent penetration and translocation. These body defenses are as follows: epithelial and mucous membrane coverings, reticuloendothelial system, blood drainer barrier.

TABLE 1. ANTIMICROBIAL ACTIVITY OF EMBALMING CHEMICALS AND TOPICAL DISINFECTANTS ON MICROFLORA OF HUMAN REMAINS

| Treatment | Anatomical Site | Pre-embalming | Treatment Period (hours) | | | | % Reduction After 24 Hours |
| | | | 2 | 4 | 8 | 24 | |
			Mean Microbial Populations[a]				
Embalmed	Heart	8.0×10^5	1.8×10^2	1.6×10^2	2.0×10^2	70	> 99%
Embalmed	Lung	2.5×10^1	< 10	< 10	< 10	< 10	> 99%
Embalmed	Colon	7.4×10^1	80	< 10	< 10	< 10	> 99%
Embalmed	Bladder	1.3×10^5	3.8×10^2	< 10	< 10	< 10	> 99%
Embalmed	Oral cavity	+ +[b]	0	0	0	0	—
Embalmed	Nasal cavity	+	0	0	+	0	—
Embalmed	Anus	+ + +	0	+	0	0	—
Unembalmed	Heart	2.8×10^5	7.2×10^5	7.8×10^5	7.5×10^5	9.0×10^5	—
Unembalmed	Lung	2.5×10^5	3.2×10^5	3.0×10^5	2.4×10^5	3.8×10^5	—
Unembalmed	Colon	1.5×10^6	1.6×10^6	1.7×10^6	1.5×10^6	2.2×10^6	—
Unembalmed	Bladder	2.9×10^6	2.3×10^6	2.3×10^6	2.4×10^6	2.5×10^6	—
Unembalmed	Oral cavity	+	+	+	+	+	—
Unembalmed	Nasal cavtity	+	+	+	+	+	—
Unembalmed	Anus	+ + +	+ + +	+ +	+ +	+ + +	—

[a]Organism ml (mean of 4 subjects per group).
[b]Scale of growth from swab cultures: 0 = none, + = slight, + + = moderate, + + + = heavy.

TABLE 2. ISOLATION AND DISTRIBUTION OF MICROFLORA ASSOCIATED WITH HUMAN REMAINS: ANATOMICAL SITES

Heart	Lung	Colon	Bladder
Proteus mirabilis	*Escherichia coli*	*Escherichia coli*	*Escherichia coli*
Pseudomonas sp.	*Pseudomonas aeruginosa*	*Micrococcus* sp.	*Klebsiella aerogenes*
Staphylococcus aureus	*Staphylococcus aureus*	*Proteus mirabilis*	*Proteus vulgaris*
Staphylococcus epidermidis	*Staphylococcus epidermidis*	*Proteus vulgaris*	*Proteus morganii*
Streptococcus	*Streptococcus* sp.	*Pseudomonas aeruginosa*	*Pseudomonas aeruginosa*
Bacillus sp.	*Alcaligenes faecalis*	*Staphylococcus aureus*	*Staphylococcus aureus*
Escherichia coli		*Staphylococcus epidermidis*	*Staphylococcus epidermidis*
		Streptococcus sp.	*Bacillus* sp.
		Bacillus sp.	
		Klebsiella aerogenes	

The organisms which were isolated from the human remains are listed in Table 2.

Comparison of the microbial flora prior to and after embalming produced no pattern or general trend. Specific microbial resistance to the antimicrobial action of formaldehyde-based embalming chemicals was not observed. No pathogenic bacteria were found following embalming.

In conclusion, it was found that the use of formaldehyde-based embalming chemicals is a satisfactory disinfectant when applied as a public health measure to reduce microbial hazards when human remains are handled.

ACKNOWLEDGMENTS

We thank J. B. Christensen of the George Washington School of Medicine, Department of Anatomy, Washington, DC, and R. Swaminathan, Foster D. Snell, Inc., for their professional assistance. This study was supported by the Embalming Chemical Manufacturers Association.

REFERENCES

1. Walker JF. *Formaldehyde.* American Chemical Society Monograph Series. 3rd ed. New York: Reinhold; 1964.
2. Lawrence CA, Block SS. *Disinfection, Sterilization, and Preservation.* Philadelphia: Lea & Febiger; 1968.
3. Spaulding EH. Role of chemical disinfection in the prevention of nosocomial infection. In: *Proceedings of the International Conference on Nosocomial Infections.* Atlanta: Centers for Disease Control; 1970.
4. Meade GM, Steenken W. Viability of tubercle bacilli in embalmed human lung tissue. *Am Rev Tuberculosis* 1949;59:429.
5. Weed, LA, Baggerstoss AH. The isolation of pathogens from tissues of embalmed human bodies. *Am J Clin Pathol* 1951;21:1114.
6. Weed LA, Baggerstoss AH. The isolation of pathogens from embalmed tissues. *Proc Soc Exp Biol Med* 1952;27:124.
7. Buchanan RE, Gibbons NE (Eds). *Bergey's Manual of Determinative Bacteriology.* 7th ed. 1957.
8. Skerman VK. *Identification of the Genera of Bacteria.* 2nd ed. 1967.

The Microbiologic Evaluation and Enumeration of Postmortem Specimens from Human Remains*

Gordon W. Rose, Ph.D.
Associate Director, Department of Mortuary Science, Wayne State University, Detroit, Michigan

Robert N. Hockett, M.S.
Research Associate, School of Dentistry, University of Michigan, Ann Arbor, Michigan

Several recognized and potential pathogens, both bacterial and mycotic, were recovered consistently from body fluids and/or aspirates withdrawn from human cases certified to have died from causes other than an infectious disease. Samples were taken from 5 anatomic sites of varying postmortem time intervals. Filter membrane culture techniques were used for primary isolation and enumeration. Some isolates seemed to imitate classical growth curve indications of exponential increase at the 6–8 hr postmortem interval. Densities reached a level of 3.0–3.5 million organisms per milliliter or gram of sam-

*Reprinted from *Health Lab Sci* 971;8(2), with permission from the American Public Health Association. Presented before the laboratory section at the Ninety-eighth Annual Meeting of the American Public Health Association, Houston, TX, Oct. 29, 1970.

ple at the 12–14 hr interval, the time period of maximal microbiologic translocation and proliferation. These studies indicate that unembalmed human remains are capable of contributing a multitude of infectious doses of microbial agents to a body handler, the body storage area, or to the environment adjacent to the body storage area.

INTRODUCTION

Research in postmortem microbiology is not new; Achard and Phulpin presented data on the recovery of microorganisms from human remains in 1895.[1] Sampling has generally followed the opening of body cavities.[2–4] One improvement in technique was the use of animal model systems[5] as an investigational tool. The amount of scientific data originating from this area of microbiologic investigation remains scant. The bibliography of the Embalming Chemical Manufacturers Association[6] is to be recommended for background.

The study utilized the application of the relatively new technique of membrane filtration (MF) to the qualitative and quantitative microbiological evaluation of body fluids and/or aspirates. Winn et al. reported the use of this technique in postmortem studies in 1966[7]. They described two advantages of the MF technique: (1) the MF method provides a three-dimensional approach to the cultivation of microorganisms; (2) it yields more accurate and reproducible quantitative results.

METHOD

Death certifications on all human remains sampled indicated the primary cause of death to be other than an infectious disease (e.g., coronary thrombosis, cerebrovascular accident, arteriosclerotic disease). Samples were secured from refrigerated cases over a postmortem period of 72 hr for temporal profile purposes. Samples were withdrawn from upper or superior to lower or inferior anatomic sites, with 18-gauge needles and 25-ml Luer syringes. Dehydration or coagulation of some samplings required aspirates of injected sterile phosphate-buffered saline (PBS). Topical disinfection of needle puncture sites was effected with an iodophore (Hi-Sine (R), Huntington Laboratories, Huntington, IN). The sampling needle was directed into the cisterna magna (cisterna cerebellomedullaris) at the base of the cerebellum via the foramen magnum for the withdrawal of cerebrospinal fluid. Heart blood samples were taken from the left ventricle by directing the needle to the upper border of the fifth rib just to the left of the sternum. Pulmonary fluids and/or aspirates were taken from the lungs for the third sampling. The needle was directed into the tranverse colon at the level of the umbilicus to sample the lumen contents. Finally, urinary bladder needle taps were made from a site marking the intersection of the median line and the pubic bone.

All samples were initially diluted 1 : 3 or 1 : 4 in PBS, and 0.1 ml of each diluted sample impinged on 0.45-μm MF, and then washed with 10.0 ml of PBS. The MFs with impinged organisms were rolled onto primary isolation agar plates of MacConkey, phenylethyl alcohol/blood, and chocolate blood. Aerobic incubation at 35–37°C for 24–48 hr and preliminary picking of isolates were routinely practiced. Isolates were characterized by pertinent methods.[8,9]

RESULTS AND DISCUSSION

Table 1 lists the bacterial isolates from the five anatomical areas sampled.

TABLE 1. BACTERIAL ISOLATES FROM FIVE ANATOMICAL SITES

Organism	Cerebrospinal Fluid	Lung	Heart Blood	Transverse Colon	Bladder Urine
Alcaligenes faecalis	x	x		x	x
Bacillus sp.			x	x	
Corynebacterium diphtheriae[a]	x	x		x	
Escherichia coli	x	x	x	x	
E. coli (A-D)					x
Klebsiella aerogenes	x	x	x	x	x
Micrococcus sp.	x	x	x	x	x
Proteus mirabillis			x	x	x
Proteus vulgaris				x	x
Providencia				x	
Pseudomonas aeruginosa	x	x	x	x	x
Shigella flexneri		x		x	
Staphylococcus aureus	x	x	x	x	x
Staphylococcus epidermidis	x	x	x	x	x
Streptococcus (Group D)	x	x	x	x	x
Streptococcus pneumoniae		x		x	x

[a]Not a typical isolate.

The selection of sampling sites was based on anatomic considerations of the normal microbial flora associated with specific anatomic areas during life. The epithelial and mucous membrane coverings and linings are normally during life intact anatomic barriers to bacterial penetration and translocation. The reticuloendothelial system is a second nonselective barrier which helps to deter translocation during life. The blood–brain barrier is probably the last line of anatomic defense against many potential microbial invaders. The cerebrospinal fluid, a filtrate of circulating blood, maintains its biologic integrity in a closed system of circulation.

All of the selected sampling sites were easily accessible and, with the exception of the colon, yielded essentially liquid specimens. The colon contents occasionally required a presampling injection of sterile PBS. Needle penetration of the selected sites involved minimal manipulation of the body areas and permitted the rapid procurement of specimens in a state best suited for MF processing.

Thorough washing of each impinged MF reduced or removed the possible effects of specific and nonspecific inhibitors that might have been associated with the specimens. Each MF was quickly transferred to the basic group of primary isolation agars. The direct rolling of the MFs onto the agar surfaces facilitated contact between the matrix- and surface-oriented microorganisms and growth substrates.

The MF allowed the impingement of a standardized volume (0.1 ml) of diluted specimen which gave total plate colony counts that were mathematically referable to densities per milliliter or per gram of original sample. Gridded MFs improved the accuracy of colony counting; plate counts in excess of 200 per plate were not recorded.

Processed MFs were sterilized with ethylene oxide and stored for possible future serotaxonomic or other studies.

Bacteria *normally* associated with the transverse colon during life, with the exception of clinically opportunistic conditions, do not translocate. They are, by description of the U.S. Public Health Service Ad Hoc Committee on the Safe Shipment and Handling of Etiological Agents,[10] "Agents of no . . . [to] ordinary potential hazard." This general statement assumes a knowledge of infectious disease and immunology. There might well be logical disagreement originating from those who have attempted the treatment of infections from enteric "commensals."

The colon was chosen as the translocation reference baseline for indicator organisms isolated from other sampling sites. The brain, lung, and heart samples frequently yielded recognized pathogens in addition to the indicator commensals and opportunists. Many of the same indicator organisms were isolated from all 5 sampling sites. This is indicative of the extent to which bacteria, both pathogenic and nonpathogenic, can be translocated within a period of 6–8 hr after death.

The quantitative results (Fig. 1) of the study indicate that a postmortem multiplication of the isolates begins approximately 4 hr after death and assumes a logarithmic-like increase between 6 and 8 hr after death. The bacterial cell densities reach a peak of approximately 3 to 3½ million organisms/ml or g of fluid or tissue within 24–30 hr after death.

Within a postmortem interval of 4–6 hr there is a body-wide redistribution of endogenous flora. Postmortem chemical changes in and manual manipulation of human remains may cause these organisms to exit from

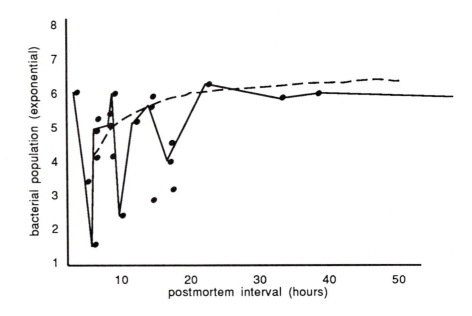

Figure 1. Bacterial population versus postmortem interval.

any of the body orifices and contribute contamination to adjacent environments. This places the body handlers and other personnel in or near the body storage area at higher risk.

ACKNOWLEDGMENT

Support for this study was received from the National Funeral Directors Association.

REFERENCES

1. Achard C, Phulpin E. Contribution a l'etude de l'envahissement des organes par les microbes pendant l' agonie et apres le mort. *Arch Med Expert Anat Pathol* 1895;7:25–47.
2. Burn CG. Experimental studies of postmortem bacterial invasion in animals. *J Infect Dis* 1934; 54:388–394.
3. Carpenter HM, Wilkins RM. Autopsy bacteriology: Review of 2,033 cases. *Arch Pathol* 1964;77: 73–81.
4. De Jongh D, Lottis JW, Green GS, Shinely JA, Minckler TM. Postmortem bacteriology. *Am J Clin Pathol* 1968;49:424–428.
5. Burn CG. Postmortem bacteriology. *J Infect Dis* 1934;54:395–403.
6. Hinson MR. Final report on literature search on the infectious nature of dead bodies for the Embalming Chemical Manufacturers Association. Mimeo, 1968.
7. Winn WR, White ML, Carter WT, Miller AB, Finegold SM. Rapid diagnosis of bacteremia with quantitative differential membrane filtration culture. *JAMA* 1966;197:539–548.
8. Cowan ST, Steel KJ. *Manual for the Identification of Medical Bacteria*. London: Cambridge University Press; 1966.
9. Harris AH, Coleman MB. *Diagnostic Procedures and Reagents*. Washington, DC: American Public Health Association; 1963.
10. Anonymous. *Classification of Etiologic Agents on the Basis of Hazard*. Atlanta: Centers for Disease Control (U.S. DHEW, USPHS);1970.

Recommendations for Prevention of HIV Transmission in Health-Care Settings*

INTRODUCTION

Human immunodeficiency virus (HIV), the virus that causes acquired immunodeficiency syndrome (AIDS), is

*Reprinted from *MMWR* 1987;38(25).

transmitted through sexual contact and exposure to infected blood or blood components and perinatally from mother to neonate. HIV has been isolated from blood, semen, vaginal secretions, saliva, tears, breast milk, cerebrospinal fluid, amniotic fluid, and urine and is likely to be isolated from other body fluids, secretions, and excretions. However, epidemiologic evidence has implicated only blood, semen, vaginal secretions, and possibly breast milk in transmission.

The increasing prevalence of HIV increases the risk that health-care workers will be exposed to blood from patients infected with HIV, especially when blood and body fluid precautions are not followed for all patients. Thus, this document emphasizes the need for health-care workers to consider **all** patients as potentially infected with HIV and/or other bloodborne pathogens and to adhere rigorously to infection-control precautions for minimizing the risk of exposure to blood and body fluids of all patients.

The recommendations contained in this document consolidate and update CDC recommendations published earlier for preventing HIV transmission in health-care settings; precautions for clinical and laboratory staffs[1] and precautions for health-care workers and allied professionals[2]; recommendations for preventing HIV transmission in the workplace[3] and during invasive procedures[4]; recommendations for preventing possible transmission of HIV from tears[5]; and recommendations for providing dialysis treatment for HIV-infected patients.[6] These recommendations also update portions of the "Guideline for Isolation Precautions in Hospitals"[7] and reemphasize some of the recommendations contained in "Infection Control Practices for Dentistry."[8] The recommendations contained in this document have been developed for use in health-care settings and emphasize the need to treat blood and other body fluids from **all** patients as potentially infective. These same prudent precautions also should be taken in other settings in which persons may be exposed to blood or other body fluids.

DEFINITION OF HEALTH-CARE WORKERS AND HEALTH-CARE WORKERS WITH AIDS

Health-care workers are defined as persons, including students and trainees, whose activities involve contact with patients or with blood or other body fluids from patients in a health-care setting.

As of July 10, 1987, a total of 1875 (5.8%) of 32,395 adults with AIDS, who had been reported to the CDC national surveillance system and for whom occupational information was available, reported being employed in a health-care or clinical laboratory setting. In comparison,

6.8 million persons—representing 5.6% of the U.S. labor force—were employed in health services. Of the health-care workers with AIDS, 95% have been reported to exhibit high-risk behavior; for the remaining 5%, the means of HIV acquisition was undetermined. Health-care workers with AIDS were significantly more likely than other workers to have an undetermined risk (5% versus 3% respectively). For both health-care workers and non–health-care workers with AIDS, the proportion with an undetermined risk has not increased since 1982.

AIDS patients initially reported as not belonging to recognized risk groups are investigated by state and local health departments to determine whether possible risk factors exist. Of all health-care workers with AIDS reported to CDC who were initially characterized as not having an identified risk and for whom follow-up information was available, 66% have been reclassified because risk factors were identified or because the patient was found not to meet the surveillance case definition for AIDS. Of the 87 health-care workers currently categorized as having no identifiable risk, information is incomplete on 16 (18%) because of death or refusal to be interviewed; 38 (44%) are still being investigated. The remaining 33 (38%) health-care workers were interviewed or had other follow-up information available. The occupations of these 33 were as follows: five physicians (15%), three of whom were surgeons; one dentist (3%); three nurses (9%); nine nursing assistants (27%); seven housekeeping or maintenance workers (21%); three clinical laboratory technicians (9%); one therapist (3%); and four others who did not have contact with patients (12%). Although 15 of these 33 health-care workers reported parenteral and/or other nonneedlestick exposure to blood or body fluids from patients in the 10 years preceding their diagnosis of AIDS, none of these exposures involved a patient with AIDS or known HIV infection.

RISK TO HEALTH-CARE WORKERS OF ACQUIRING HIV IN HEALTH-CARE SETTINGS

Health-care workers with documented percutaneous or mucous-membrane exposures to blood or body fluids of HIV-infected patients have been prospectively evaluated to determine the risk of infection after such exposures. As of June 30, 1987, 883 health-care workers have been tested for antibody to HIV in an ongoing surveillance project conducted by CDC.[9] Of these, 708 (80%) had percutaneous exposures to blood, and 175 (20%) had a mucous membrane or an open wound contaminated by blood or body fluid. Of 396 health-care workers, each of whom had only a convalescent-phase serum sample obtained and tested > 90 days postexposure, one—for whom heterosexual transmission could not be ruled out—was seropositive for HIV antibody. For 425 additional health-care workers, both acute- and convalescent-phase serum samples were obtained and tested; none of 74 health-care workers with nonpercutaneous exposures seroconverted, and 3 (0.9%) of 351 with percutaneous exposures seroconverted. None of these 3 health-care workers had other documented risk factors for infection.

Two other prospective studies to assess the risk of nosocomial acquisition of HIV infection for health-care workers are ongoing in the United States. As of April 30, 1987, 332 health-care workers with a total of 453 needlestick or mucous-membrane exposures to the blood or other body fluids of HIV-infected patients were tested for HIV antibody at the National Institutes of Health.[10] These exposed workers included 103 with needlestick injuries and 229 with mucous-membrane exposures; none had seroconverted. A similar study at the University of California of 129 health-care workers with documented needlestick injuries or mucous-membrane exposures to blood or other body fluids from patients with HIV infection has not identified any seroconversions.[11] Results of a prospective study in the United Kingdom identified no evidence of transmission among 150 health-care workers with parenteral or mucous-membrane exposures to blood or other body fluids, secretions, or excretions from patients with HIV infection.[12]

In addition to health-care workers enrolled in prospective studies, eight persons who provided care to infected patients and denied other risk factors have been reported to have acquired HIV infection. Three of these health-care workers had needlestick exposures to blood from infected patients.[13-15] Two were persons who provided nursing care to infected persons; although neither sustained a needlestick, both had extensive contact with blood or other body fluids, and neither observed recommended barrier precautions.[16,17] The other three were health-care workers with nonneedlestick exposures to blood from infected patients.[18] Although the exact route of transmission for these last three infections is not known, all three persons had direct contact of their skin with blood from infected patients, all had skin lesions that may have been contaminated by blood, and one also had a mucous-membrane exposure.

A total of 1231 dentists and hygiensts, many of whom practiced in areas with many AIDS cases, participated in a study to determine the prevalence of antibody to HIV; one dentist (0.1%) had HIV antibody. Although no exposure to a known HIV-infected person could be documented, epidemiologic investigation did not identify any other risk factor for infection. The infected dentist, who also had a history of sustaining needlestick injuries and trauma to his hands, did not routinely wear gloves when providing dental care.[19]

PRECAUTIONS TO PREVENT TRANSMISSION OF HIV (UNIVERSAL PRECAUTIONS)

Since medical history and examination cannot reliably identify all patients infected with HIV or other blood-borne pathogens, blood and body-fluid precautions should be consistently used for **all** patients. This approach, previously recommended by CDC,[3,4] and referred to as "universal blood and body-fluid precautions" or "universal precautions," should be used in the care of **all** patients, especially including those in emergency-care settings in which the risk of blood exposure is increased and the infection status of the patient is usually unknown.[20]

1. All health-care workers should routinely use appropriate barrier precautions to prevent skin and mucous-membrane exposure when contact with blood or other body fluids of any patient is anticipated. Gloves should be worn for touching blood and body fluids, mucous membranes, or nonintact skin of all patients, for handling items or surfaces soiled with blood or body fluids, and for performing venipuncture and other vascular access procedures. Gloves should be changed after contact with each patient. Masks and protective eyewear or face shields should be worn during procedures that are likely to generate droplets of blood or other body fluids to prevent exposure of mucous membranes of the mouth, nose, and eyes. Gowns or aprons should be worn during procedures that are likely to generate splashes of blood or other body fluids.

2. Hands and other skin surfaces should be washed immediately and thoroughly if contaminated with blood or other body fluids. Hands should be washed immediately after gloves are removed.

3. All health-care workers should take precautions to prevent injuries caused by needles, scalpels, and other sharp instruments or devices during procedures; when cleaning used instruments; during disposal of used needles; and when handling sharp instruments after procedures. To prevent needlestick injuries, needles should not be recapped, purposely bent or broken by hand, removed from disposable syringes, or otherwise manipulated by hand. After they are used, disposable syringes and needles, scalpel blades, and other sharp items should be placed in puncture-resistant containers for disposal; the puncture-resistant containers should be located as close as practical to the use area. Large-bore reusable needles should be placed in a puncture-resistant container for transport to the reprocessing area.

4. Although saliva has not been implicated in HIV transmission, to minimize the need for emergency mouth-to-mouth resuscitation, mouthpieces, resuscitation bags, or other ventilation devices should be available for use in areas in which the need for resuscitation is predictable.

5. Health-care workers who have exudative lesions or weeping dermatitis should refrain from all direct patient care and from handling patient-care equipment until the condition resolves.

6. Pregnant health-care workers are not known to be at greater risk of contracting HIV infection than health-care workers who are not pregnant; however, if a health-care worker develops HIV infection during pregnancy, the infant is at risk of infection resulting from perinatal transmission. Because of this risk, pregnant health-care workers should be especially familiar with and strictly adhere to precautions to minimize the risk of HIV transmission.

Implementation of universal blood and body-fluid precautions for **all** patients eliminates the need for use of the isolation category of "Blood and Body Fluid Precautions" previously recommended by CDC[7] for patients known or suspected to be infected with bloodborne pathogens. Isolation precautions (e.g., enteric, "AFB"[7]) should be used as necessary if associated conditions, such as infectious diarrhea or tuberculosis, are diagnosed or suspected.

PRECAUTIONS FOR INVASIVE PROCEDURES

In this document, an invasive procedure is defined as surgical entry into tissues, cavities, or organs or repair of major traumatic injuries in (1) an operating or delivery room, emergency department, or outpatient setting, including both physicians' and dentists' offices; (2) cardiac catheterization and angiographic procedures; (3) a vaginal or caesarean delivery or other invasive obstetric procedure during which bleeding may occur; or (4) the manipulation, cutting, or removal of any oral or perioral tissues, including tooth structure, during which bleeding occurs or the potential for bleeding exists. The universal blood and body-fluid precautions listed above, combined with the precautions listed below, should be the minimum precautions for **all** such invasive procedures.

1. All health-care workers who participate in invasive procedures must routinely use appropriate barrier precautions to prevent skin and mucous-membrane contact with blood and other body fluids of all patients. Gloves and surgical masks must be worn for all invasive procedures. Protective eyewear or face shields should be worn for procedures that commonly result in the gen-

eration of droplets, splashing of blood or other body fluids, or the generation of bone chips. Gowns or aprons made of materials that provide an effective barrier should be worn during invasive procedures that are likely to result in the splashing of blood or other body fluids. All health-care workers who perform or assist in vaginal or caesarean deliveries should wear gloves and gowns when handling the placenta or the infant until blood and amniotic fluid have been removed from the infant's skin and should wear gloves during the postdelivery care of the umbilical cord.

2. If a glove is torn or a needlestick or other injury occurs, the glove should be removed and a new glove used as promptly as patient safety permits; the needle or instrument involved in the incident should also be removed from the sterile field.

PRECAUTIONS FOR DENTISTRY*

Blood, saliva, and gingival fluid from **all** dental patients should be considered infective. Special emphasis should be placed on the following precautions for preventing transmission of bloodborne pathogens in dental practice in both institutional and noninstitutional settings.

1. In addition to wearing gloves for contact with oral mucous membranes of all patients, all dental workers should wear surgical masks and protective eyewear or chin-length plastic face shields during dental procedures in which splashing or spattering of blood, saliva, or gingival fluids is likely. Rubber dams, high-speed evacuation, and proper patient positioning, when appropriate, should be utilized to minimize generation of droplets and spatter.

2. Handpieces should be sterilized after use with each patient, since blood, saliva, or gingival fluid of patients may be aspirated into the handpiece or waterline. Handpieces that cannot be sterilized should at least be flushed, the outside surface cleaned and wiped with a suitable chemical germicide, and then rinsed. Handpieces should be flushed at the beginning of the day and after use with each patient. Manufacturers' recommendations should be followed for use and maintenance of waterlines and check valves and for flushing of handpieces. The same precautions should be used for ultrasonic scalers and air/water syringes.

---

*General infection-control precautions are more specifically addressed in previous recommendations for infection-control practices for dentistry.

3. Blood and saliva should be thoroughly and carefully cleaned from material that has been used in the mouth (e.g., impression materials, bite registration), especially before polishing and grinding intraoral devices. Contaminated materials, impressions, and intraoral devices should also be cleaned and disinfected before being handled in the dental laboratory and before they are placed in the patient's mouth. Because of the increasing variety of dental materials used intraorally, dental workers should consult with manufacturers as to the stability of specific materials when using disinfection procedures.

4. Dental equipment and surfaces that are difficult to disinfect (e.g., light handles or x-ray unit heads) and that may become contaminated should be wrapped with impervious-backed paper, aluminum foil, or clear plastic wrap. The coverings should be removed and discarded, and clean coverings should be put in place after use with each patient.

PRECAUTIONS FOR AUTOPSIES OR MORTICIANS' SERVICES

In addition to the universal blood and body-fluid precautions listed above, the following precautions should be used by persons performing postmortem procedures:

1. All persons performing or assisting in postmortem procedures should wear gloves, masks, protective eyewear, gowns, and waterproof aprons.

2. Instruments and surfaces contaminated during postmortem procedure should be decontaminated with an appropriate chemical germicide.

ENVIRONMENTAL CONSIDERATIONS FOR HIV TRANSMISSION, STERILIZATION, AND DISINFECTION

Standard sterilization and disinfection procedures for patient-care equipment currently recommended for use[25,26] in a variety of health-care settings—including hospitals, medical and dental clinics and offices, hemodialysis centers, emergency-care facilities, and long-term nursing-care facilities—are adequate to sterilize or disinfect instruments, devices, or other items contaminated with blood or other body fluids from persons infected with bloodborne pathogens including HIV.[21,23]

Instruments or devices that enter sterile tissue or the vascular system of any patient or through which blood flows should be sterilized before reuse. Devices or items that contact intact mucous membranes should be sterilized or receive high-level disinfection, a procedure that kills vegetative organisms and viruses but not necessarily large numbers of bacterial spores. Chemical germicides that are registered with the U.S. Environmental Protection Agency (EPA) as "sterilants" may be used either for sterilization or for high-level disinfection depending on contact time.

Contact lenses used in trial fittings should be disinfected after each fitting by using a hydrogen peroxide contact lens disinfecting system or, if compatible, with heat (78–80°C [172.4–176.0°F]) for 10 minutes.

Medical devices or instruments that require sterilization or disinfection should be thoroughly cleaned before being exposed to the germicide, and the manufacturer's instructions for the use of the germicide should be followed. Further, it is important that the manufacturer's specification for compatibility of the medical device with chemical germicides be closely followed. Information on specific label claims of commercial germicides can be obtained by writing to the Disinfectants Branch, Office of Pesticides, Environmental Protection Agency, 401 M Street, SW, Washington, DC 20460.

Studies have shown that HIV is inactivated rapidly after being exposed to commonly used chemical germicides at concentrations that are much lower than used in practice.[27–30] Embalming fluids are similar to the types of chemical germicides that have been tested and found to completely inactivate HIV. In addition to commercially available chemical germicides, a solution of sodium hypochlorite (household bleach) prepared daily is an inexpensive and effective germicide. Concentrations ranging from approximately 500 ppm (1 : 100 dilution of household bleach) sodium hypochlorite to 5000 ppm (1 : 10 dilution of household bleach) are effective depending on the amount of organic material (e.g., blood, mucus) present on the surface to be cleaned and disinfected. Commercially available chemical germicides may be more compatible with certain medical devices that might be corroded by repeated exposure to sodium hypochlorite, especially to the 1 : 10 dilution.

SURVIVAL OF HIV IN THE ENVIRONMENT

The most extensive study on the survival of HIV after drying involved greatly concentrated HIV samples, i.e., 10 million tissue-culture infectious doses per milliliter.[31] This concentration is at least 100,000 times greater than that typically found in the blood or serum of patients with HIV infection. HIV was detectable by tissue-culture techniques 1–3 days after drying, but the rate of inactivation was rapid. Studies performed at CDC have also shown that drying HIV causes a rapid (within several hours) 1–2 log (90–99%) reduction in HIV concentration. In tissue-culture fluid, cell-free HIV could be detected up to 15 days at room temperature, up to 11 days at 37°C (98.6°F), and up to 1 day if the HIV was cell-associated.

When considered in the context of environmental conditions in health-care facilities, these results do not require any changes in currently recommended sterilization, disinfection, or housekeeping strategies. When medical devices are contaminated with blood or other body fluids, existing recommendations include the cleaning of these instruments, followed by disinfection or sterilization, depending on the type of medical device. These protocols assume "worst-case" conditions of extreme virologic and microbiologic contamination, and whether viruses have been inactivated after drying plays no role in formulating these strategies. Consequently, no changes in published procedures for cleaning, disinfecting, or sterilizing need to be made.

HOUSEKEEPING

Environmental surfaces such as walls, floors, and other surfaces are not associated with transmission of infections to patients or health-care workers. Therefore, extraordinary attempts to disinfect or sterilize these environmental surfaces are not necessary. However, cleaning and removal of soil should be done routinely.

Cleaning schedules and methods vary according to the area of the hospital or institution, type of surface to be cleaned, and the amount and type of soil present. Horizontal surfaces (e.g., bedside tables and hard-surfaced flooring) in patient-care areas are usually cleaned on a regular basis, when soiling or spills occur, and when a patient is discharged. Cleaning of walls, blinds, and curtains is recommended only if they are visibly soiled. Disinfectant fogging is an unsatisfactory method of decontaminating air and surfaces and is not recommended.

Disinfectant–detergent formulations registered by EPA can be used for cleaning environmental surfaces, but the actual physical removal of microorganisms by scrubbing is probably at least as important as any antimicrobial effect of the cleaning agent used. Therefore, cost, safety, and acceptability by housekeepers can be the main criteria for selecting any such registered agent. The manufacturers' instructions for appropriate use should be followed.

CLEANING AND DECONTAMINATING SPILLS OF BLOOD OR OTHER BODY FLUIDS

Chemical germicides that are approved for use as "hospital disinfectants" and are tuberculocidal when used at recommended dilutions can be used to decontaminate spills of blood and other body fluids. Strategies for decontaminating spills of blood and other body fluids in a patient-care setting are different than for spills of cultures or other materials in clinical, public health, or research laboratories. In patient-care areas, visible material should first be removed and then the area should be decontaminated. With large spills of cultured or concentrated infectious agents in the laboratory, the contaminated area should be flooded with a liquid germicide before cleaning, then decontaminated with fresh germicidal chemical. In both settings, gloves should be worn during the cleaning and decontaminating procedures.

LAUNDRY

Although soiled linen has been identified as a source of large numbers of certain pathogenic microorganisms, the risk of actual disease transmission is negligible. Rather than rigid procedures and specifications, hygienic and commonsense storage and processing of clean and soiled linen are recommended.[26] Soiled linen should be handled as little as possible and with minimum agitation to prevent gross microbial contamination of the air and of persons handling the linen. All soiled linen should be bagged at the location where it was used; it should not be sorted or rinsed in patient-care areas. Linen soiled with blood or body fluids should be placed and transported in bags that prevent leakage. If hot water is used, linen should be washed with detergent in water at least 71°C (160°F) for 25 minutes. If low-temperature (<70°C [158°F]) laundry cycles are used, chemicals suitable for low-temperature washing at proper use-concentration should be used.

INFECTIVE WASTE

There is no epidemiologic evidence to suggest that most hospital waste is any more infective than residential waste. Moreover, there is no epidemiologic evidence that hospital waste has caused disease in the community as a result of improper disposal. Therefore, identifying wastes for which special precautions are indicated is largely a matter of judgment about the relative risk of disease transmission. The most practical approach to the management of infective waste is to identify those wastes with the potential for causing infection during handling and disposal and for which some special precautions appear prudent. Hospital wastes for which special precautions appear prudent include microbiology laboratory waste, pathology waste, and blood specimens or blood products. While any item that has had contact with blood, exudates, or secretions may be potentially infective, it is not usually considered practical or necessary to treat all such waste as infective.[23,26] Infective waste, in general, should either be incinerated or should be autoclaved before disposal in an sanitary landfill. Bulk blood, suctioned fluids, excretions, and secretions may be carefully poured down a drain connected to a sanitary sewer. Sanitary sewers may also be used to dispose of other infectious wastes capable of being ground and flushed into the sewer.

IMPLEMENTATION OF RECOMMENDED PRECAUTIONS

Employers of health-care workers should ensure that policies exist for:

1. Initial orientation and continuing education and training of all health-care workers—including students and trainees—on the epidemiology, modes of transmission, and prevention of HIV and other bloodborne infections and the need for routine use of universal blood and body-fluid precautions for **all** patients
2. Provision of equipment and supplies necessary to minimize the risk of infection with HIV and other bloodborne pathogens
3. Monitoring adherence to recommended protective measures. When monitoring reveals a failure to follow recommended precautions, counseling, education, and/or retraining should be provided, and, if necessary, appropriate disciplinary action shoud be considered. Professional associations and labor organizations, through continuing education efforts, should emphasize the need for health-care workers to follow recommended precautions.

REFERENCES

1. Centers for Disease Control. Acquired immunodeficiency syndrome (AIDS): Precautions for clinical and laboratory staffs. *MMWR* 1982;31:577–580.
2. Centers for Disease Control. Acquired immunodeficiency syndrome (AIDS): Precautions for health-care workers and allied professionals. *MMWR* 1983; 32:450–451.
3. Centers for Disease Control. Recommendations for preventing transmission of infection with human T-lymphotropic virus type III/lymphadenopathy-associated virus in the workplace. *MMWR* 1985;34:681–686, 691–695.
4. Centers for Disease Control. Recommendations for preventing transmission of infection with human T-lymphotropic virus type III/lymphadenopathy-associated virus during invasive procedures. *MMWR* 1986;35:221–223.
5. Centers for Disease Control. Recommendations for preventing possible transmission of human T-lymphotropic virus type III/lymphadenopathy-associated virus from tears. *MMWR* 1985;34: 533–534.

6. Centers for Disease Control. Recommendations for providing dialysis treatment to patients infected with human T-lymphotropic virus type III/lymphadenopathy-associated virus infection. *MMWR* 1986;35:376–378, 383.

7. Garner JS, Simmons BP. Guideline for isolation precautions in hospitals. *Infect Control* 1983; 4(suppl):245–325.

8. Centers for Disease Control. Recommended infection control practices for dentistry. *MMWR* 1986;35:237–242.

9. McCray E. The Cooperative Needlestick Surveillance Group. Occupational risk of the acquired immunodeficiency syndrome among health care workers. *N Engl J Med* 1986;314:1127–1132.

10. Henderson DK, Saah AJ, Zak BJ, et al. Risk of nosocomial infection with human T-cell lymphotropic virus type III/lymphadenopathy-associated virus in a large cohort of intensively exposed health care workers. *Ann Intern Med* 1986;104:644–647.

11. Gerberding JL, Bryant-LeBlanc CE, Nelson K, et al. Risk of transmitting the human immunodeficiency virus, cytomegalovirus, and hepatitis B virus to health care workers exposed to patients with AIDS and AIDS-related conditions. *J Infect Dis* 1987; 156:1–8.

12. McEvoy M, Porter K, Mortimer P, Simmons N, Shanson D. Prospective study of clinical, laboratory, and ancillary staff with accidental exposures to blood or other body fluids from patients infected with HIV. *Br Med J* 1987;294:1595–1597.

13. Anonymous. Needlestick transmission of HTLV-III from a patient infected in Africa. *Lancet* 1984;2: 1376–1377.

14. Oksenhendler E, Harzic M, Le Roux JM, Rabian C, Clauvel JP. HIV infection with seroconversion after a superficial needlestick injury to the finger. *N Engl J Med* 1986;315:582.

15. Neisson-Vernant C, Arfi S, Mathez D, Leibowitch J, Monplaisir N. Needlestick HIV seroconversion in a nurse. *Lancet* 1986;2:814.

16. Grint P, McEvoy M. Two associated cases of the acquired immune deficiency syndrome (AIDS). *PHLS Commun Dis Rep* 1985;42:4.

17. Centers for Disease Control. Apparent transmission of human T-lymphotropic-associated virus type III/lymphadenopathy-associated virus from a child to a mother providing health care. *MMWR* 1986;35:76–79.

18. Centers for Disease Control. Update: Human immunodeficiency virus infections in health-care workers exposed to blood of infected patients. *MMWR* 1987;36:285–289.

19. Kline RS, Phelan J, Friedland GH, et al. Low occupational risk for HIV infection for dental professionals (Abstract). In: *Abstracts from the III International Conference on AIDS, 1-5 June 1985, Washington, DC*, p. 155.

20. Baker JL, Kelen GD, Sivertson KT, Quinn TC. Unsuspected human immunodeficiency virus in critically ill emergency patients. *JAMA* 1987; 257:2609–2611.

21. Favero MS. Dialysis-associated diseases and their control. In: Bennett JV, Brachman PS (eds): *Hospital Infections*. Boston: Little, Brown; 1985;267–284.

22. Richardson JH, Barkley WE (eds). *Biosafety in Microbiological and Biomedical Laboratories*. Washington, DC: U.S. Department of Health and Human Services, Public Health Service; 1984: HHS Pub. No. (CDC) 84-8395.

23. Centers for Disease Control. Human T-lymphotropic virus type III/lymphadenopathy-associated virus: Agent summary statement. *MMWR* 1986; 35:540–542, 547–549.

24. Environmental Protection Agency. *EPA Guide for Infectious Waste Management*. Washington, DC: U.S. Environmental Protection Agency; May 1986: Pub. No. EPA/530-SW-86-014.

25. Favero MS. Sterilization, disinfection, and antisepsis in the hospital. In: *Manual of Clinical Microbiology*. 4th ed. Washington, DC: American Society for Microbiology; 1985;129–137.

26. Garner JS, Favero MS. *Guideline for Handwashing and Hospital Environmental Control*. Atlanta: Public Health Service, Centers for Disease Control: 1985:HHS Pub. No. 99-1117.

27. Spire B, Montagnier L, Barre-Sinoussi F, Chermann JC. Inactivation of lymphadenopathy associated virus by chemical disinfectants. *Lancet* 1984; 2:899–901.

28. Martin LS, McDougal JS, Loskoski SL. Disinfection and inactivation of the human T lymphotropic virus type III/lymphadenopathy-associated virus. *J Infect Dis* 1985;152:400–403.

29. McDougal JS, Martin LS, Cort SP, et al. Thermal inactivation of the acquired immunodeficiency syndrome virus-III/lymphadenopathy-associated virus, with special reference to antihemophilic factor. *J Clin Invest* 1985;76:875–877.

30. Spire B, Barre-Sinoussi F, Dormont D, Montagnier L, Chermann JC. Inactivation of lymphadenopathy-associated virus by heat, gamma rays, and ultraviolet light. *Lancet* 1985;1:188–189.

31. Resnik L, Veren K, Salahuddin SZ, Tondreau S, Markham PD. Stability and inactivation of HTLV-III/LAV under clinical and laboratory environments. *JAMA* 1986;255: 1887–1891.

32. Centers for Disease Control. Public Health Service (PHS) guidelines for counseling and antibody testing

to prevent HIV infection and AIDS. *MMWR* 1987;3:509–515.

33. Kane MA, Lettau LA. Transmission of HBV from dental personnel to patients. *J Am Dent Assoc* 1985; 110:634–636.

34. Lettau LA, Smith JD, Williams D, et al. Transmission of hepatitis B with resultant restriction of surgical practice. *JAMA* 1986;255:934–937.

35. Williams WW. Guideline for infection control in hospital personnel. *Infect Control* 1983;4(suppl): 326–349.

36. Centers for Disease Control. Prevention of acquired immune deficiency syndrome (AIDS): Report of interagency recommendations. *MMWR* 1983;32: 101–103.

37. Centers for Disease Control. Provisional Public Health Service inter-agency recommendations for screening donated blood and plasma for antibody to the virus causing acquired immunodeficiency syndrome. *MMWR* 1985;34:1–5.

CDC's Universal Precautions in the Context of Medical Waste Management*

Michael P. Kiley, Ph.D.
Office of Biosafety, Centers for Disease Control and Prevention, Atlanta, Georgia

BACKGROUND

This report is a synopsis of information previously published in the references listed at the back of this section as well as from an unpublished document entitled *The Center for Disease Control's Recommendations on Infective Waste* developed by the Office of Biosafety and the Hospital Infections Program at CDC.

INTRODUCTION

Prior to discussing "universal precautions" in the context of medical waste management, it is necessary to define what is meant by "universal precautions." Since medical history and examination cannot reliably identify all patients infected with HIV or other blood-borne pathogens, blood and body-fluid precautions should consistently be used for *all* patients. This is especially true

---

*From *MMWR*. September 27, 1989.

for emergency-care settings in which the risk of blood exposure is increased and the infection status of the patient is usually unknown. Universal precautions include the following recommendations intended to decrease the probability of infection of health-care workers:

1. All health-care workers should use appropriate barrier precautions to prevent skin or mucous membrane exposures. Barrier protection includes gloves, masks, gowns, aprons, and eye protection devices.
2. Hands and other skin surfaces should be washed immediately if contaminated with blood or other body fluids.
3. All health-care workers should take precautions to avoid injuries caused by needles, scalpels and other sharp instruments during all procedures using these devices. Needles should not be recapped, purposely bent, or manipulated by hand. All sharps should be disposed of in a puncture-resistant container that is capable of decontamination without further handling of the sharps.
4. Resuscitation bags or mouthpieces should be used for mouth-to-mouth resuscitation whenever possible.
5. Health-care workers with exudative lesions or weeping dermatitis should refrain from all direct patient care and from handling patient-care equipment until the condition resolves.

Universal precautions are meant to apply to blood, semen, and vaginal secretions as well as to cerebrospinal fluid, synovial fluid, pleural fluid, peritoneal fluid, pericardial fluid, and amniotic fluid. Universal precautions do not apply to feces, nasal secretions, sputum, sweat, tears, urine, and vomitus unless they contain visible blood. A more detailed description of these precautions can be found in the references.[1,2]

MEDICAL WASTE

As defined in the Medical Waste Tracking Act of 1988, medical waste means "any solid waste that is generated in the diagnosis, treatment or immunization of human beings or animals, in research pertaining thereto, or in the production or testing of biologicals." Although there may be other slightly different definitions of "medical waste" or "infective waste," each medical institution must develop a plan to deal with waste generated by such a facility.

Introduction

There is no epidemiologic or microbiologic evidence to suggest that most waste from hospitals, other health-care facilities, or clinical/research laboratories is any more infective than residential waste. Nor is there evidence that presently accepted waste disposal methods are contributing to human or environmental health hazards. Moreover, there is no documented epidemiologic evidence that current health-care related waste disposal practices have ever caused disease in the community. Therefore, identifying wastes for which special precautions are indicated is largely a matter of judgment about the estimated relative risk of disease transmission. This is necessary, since there are no reasonable tests to allow objective identification of infective waste. Aesthetic and emotional considerations or perceived health risks may override the actual risk of disease transmission.

The most practical approach to infective waste management is to identify those wastes that are judged to represent a sufficient potential risk of causing infection during handling and disposal and for which some special precautions appear prudent. Health-care related wastes for which special precautions appear prudent include microbiology laboratory waste, pathology waste, and blood specimens or blood products. Moreover, the risk of either injury or infection associated with the disposal of certain sharp items (e.g., needles and scalpel blades) contaminated with blood also needs to be considered. While any item that has had contact with blood, exudates, or secretions may be potentially infective, it is not normally considered practical or necessary to treat all such waste as infective.

Recommended Program

CDC recommends that a health-care facility establish an infective waste disposal plan. An integral part of an effective waste disposal plan is the designation of the person or persons responsible for establishing, monitoring, and periodically reviewing the plan. Such plans should consist of three basic elements for infective waste:

- Identification of potentially infective material
- Proper handling, transportation, and storage
- Appropriate processing and disposal

Identification of Potentially Infective Waste

CDC suggests that microbiology and pathology wastes, blood and blood products, and sharp items, especially needles, should be considered as potentially infective and handled and disposed of with special precautions. Other items may be designated for special handling based upon local and state ordinances. The most practical approach to infective waste management starts with identifying those wastes that are judged to represent sufficient potential risk of causing infection during handling and disposal and for which some special precautions would appear prudent. This identification process is very im-

portant because the separation of the waste stream that develops from it will have a perceived effect on the health and safety of the employees and a substantial effect on the cost of disposal. Items defined as infectious need to be identified at the source, segregated, and prepared for special handling. At the same time, it is important to eliminate non-infective waste from the special waste stream so as to keep disposal costs at a minimum. This step is sometimes difficult to implement because of the reticence of some staff to take the extra time to segregate waste material. Some infection control people have taken the position of designating most, if not all, waste from certain locations, for example, the operating room, for special handling so as to minimize distractions. On the other hand, we have heard of some hospitals designating *all* of their waste as infectious, a practice that comes under scrutiny soon after the first disposal bill arrives. A related circumstance was reported by a colleague who visited an infectious waste incinerator that was found to be malfunctioning because it was filled with computer printouts.

Handling, Transport, and Storage of Potentially Infective Waste

Persons involved in the handling, transportation, and storage of infective waste should be informed of the potential health and safety hazards and trained in appropriate handling and disposal methods. These employees should also be provided with appropriate personal protective equipment and trained in how to use it. If processing or disposal facilities are not available at the site of generation of infective waste, it may be safely transported in sealed impervious containers to another area or to another facility for appropriate treatment. To minimize the potential risk for accidental transmission of disease or injury, infective waste awaiting terminal processing should be stored in an area accessible only to personnel involved in the disposal process.

Processing and Disposal of Potentially Infective Waste

Waste that has been designated as infective should either be incinerated or should be decontaminated before disposal in a sanitary landfill. Acceptable decontamination methods include autoclaving, chemical disinfection, and exposure to gamma radiation. Disposable syringes with needles still attached, scalpel blades, broken glass, and other sharp items capable of causing injury should be placed intact into puncture-resistant containers located as close as practical to the site of origin. If the filled containers are to be autoclaved before disposal, they should be made of material that will maintain its impermeability after autoclaving in order to prevent subsequent injuries. Bulk blood, suctioned fluids, excretions, and secretions may be carefully poured down a drain connected to a sanitary sewer. Sanitary sewers may also be used for the disposal of other infectious wastes, provided they can be ground and flushed into the sewer.

Universal Precautions Applied to Infective Waste

The concept of universal precautions, that is, that blood and body-fluid precautions should be consistently used for *all* patients, does not alter the application of any of the preceding recommendations.[2] Universal Precautions are meant to supplement an infection control program, not replace it. As an example, isolation procedures would not be changed and only the waste material identified as being potentially infectious, for example, bulk blood and sharps, would be segregated for special handling. This would, of course, mean that not all of the waste from an isolation room would be designated as potentially infectious.

NON-TRADITIONAL HEALTH CARE PROVIDERS

CDC believes that our recommendations should apply to all health care facilities regardless of size. For example, strategies for the disposal of blood or sharps would apply both to large acute care hospitals as well as to small clinics. Obviously, there should be some judgment based on local and state ordinances.

SUMMARY

We are not aware of any significant public health problem posed by the disposal of infectious waste in the United States. In recent years there appears to have been improper disposal of some medical waste in areas where problems apparently peculiar to the eastern seaboard have received public attention. We believe that these problems can be addressed by state and local agencies. Procedures suggested by the EPA under the Medical Waste Tracking Act of 1988 should focus attention on the problem of proper disposal of medical waste. It may not be necessary to handle infectious waste with the same degree of management caution as hazardous chemical or radioactive waste. It may, however, be advisable for local communities to develop means of handling medical waste using the Medical Waste Tracking Act as a guideline.

We believe that the most frequent problem encountered in health-care facilities concerns the definition of infectious waste. When the definition is too broad, and virtually all waste is considered infective, waste management becomes oppressive and expensive and provides a misconception to the public that such waste is a significant health hazard.

REFERENCES

1. CDC. Recommendations for prevention of HIV transmission in health-care settings. *MMWR* 1987;36 (Suppl. No. 2S).
2. CDC. Update: Universal precautions for prevention of transmission of human immunodeficiency virus, hepatitis B virus, and other bloodborne pathogens in health-care settings. *MMWR* 1988;36:377,387–388.

Can Magnesium Sulfate Be Safely Used to Rid the Body of Fluid in the Lower Extremities?

Murray Shor
Instructor,
American Academy, McAllister Institute, New York, New York

Considering the wide distribution of news media, the public in general and basic medical science students in particular are surely aware that the major causes of death in both the preceding and current decade are neoplasms and cardiovascular diseases. This is of special interest to the embalmer because these different pathologies, vascular disorders and malignancies, may lead to edema. Considering that the combined deaths from these causes combined account for about 90% of the mortalities in this country, a large number of the bodies received by the embalmer have edema.

Generally, lymph, the fluid of the tissue spaces, is derived from the blood plasma by filtration. If more lymph enters the interstitial spaces than is carried off by the lymphatic vessels, edema results. Therefore, any abdominal neoplasm at the level of the second lumbar vertebra or higher could press against the thoracic duct, obstruct it, and cause lymphatic fluid to gather in the lower extremities. Because such tumors are involved in a large percentage of deaths, edema of the lower extremities is a common finding in bodies received by the mortician.

PRESSURE FROM HEART DISEASES

Many diseases of the heart have a similar effect on the fluid content of the lower extremities and the abdomen. If, for example, the right atrium remained filled after systole because of an inefficient right atrioventricular valve, blood attempting to enter the right atrium from the inferior vena cava during diastole would be prevented from doing so. A high intravenous pressure would result, preventing the reentry of fluid into the venous end of the capillary, and edema would ensue.

Complicating the problems of patients in the terminal stages of severe gastrointestinal or cardiac disease is the fact that they are unable to chew or swallow or retain protein foods such as meat. This reduces the protein content of the blood and, in turn, renders it hypotonic to the fluids of the surrounding tissues. Consequently, the outpouring of fluid from the capillary bed to the intercellular spaces is increased. The result is nutritional edema.

In addition to the disease just described, myriad circulatory disorders and infectious diseases can result in edema. So, without belaboring the point, I submit that edema is an embalming problem of some significance.

Now, let's get to the treatment.

Some embalmers treat edema of the lower extremities simply by elevating those parts. Others treat the condition by wrapping a spiral bandage from the ankle to the hip. These are tried and accepted methods. Were it not for still another, controversial technique, I would not feel compelled to write this article.

Most qualified operators agree that addition of magnesium sulfate to arterial fluid solution helps dehydrate the affected parts. Some, however, argue that the solution reaches the features and overdehydrates them. I believe this treatment can be applied with impunity.

We know that fluids pass through a membrane by osmosis and filtration. If pressure within the vascular system is kept high, it would favor the passage of fluids into the interstices by filtration. If fluids within the small blood vessels are hypotonic to extravascular fluids, again the condition would favor flow into the extravascular spaces.

USE OF SOLUTION AT LOW PRESSURE

Therefore, prudence dictates that we use a hypertonic solution at low pressure to encourage flow in the direction of the capillaries and eventually out of the body via venous drainage. According to Professor Pervier, a 6.77% solution exerts the same osmotic pressure as the human circulatory system. Because the extent of edema and the volume of fluids that can be tolerated vary in each case, it is impossible to recommend a specific concentration or volume. If, however, 6.77% solution exerts the same osmotic pressure as human circulatory tissue, 10% would be a good concentration at which to start.

To arrive at the volume of Epsom salt required to make a 10% solution, multiply the volume of solution required by the percentage desired. For use in a lower extremity, where 2 quarts of solution seems a reasonable quantity, multiply 64 ounces by 10%. The result is 6.4. Weigh out 6.4 ounces of Epsom salt and add it to enough arterial fluid solution to make 2 quarts. This gives you 2 quarts of 10% solution.

To overcome the possibility that the strong salt solution will reach the face and cause undue dehydration of the features, it is imperative that the embalmer raise and open both the femoral vein and the great saphenous vein. It must be remembered that the great saphenous vein enters the femoral vein about an inch and a half below the inguinal ligament. The embalmer usually raises the femoral vessels distal to this point, so that drainage from the lower extremity bypasses the femoral drainage point and reaches the face via the superficial return. In view of the fact that more return is accomplished by the superficial return than the deep return, failure to open the great saphenous vein would result in passage of the salt solution to the features by vascular channels too numerous to describe here.

Still another benefit derived by opening both the femoral and great saphenous vessels is the low intravenous pressure achieved by this procedure. With both major vessels of return wide open, it is obvious that pressure in the veins will not be high. If intracellular fluid pressure is high, due to accumulation of excess fluids, flow into the capillaries is favored, promoting drainage.

Removal of edematous fluids from the extremities is only one of the problems posed by the degenerative diseases of older members of the population. In the future, we shall discuss edema of other areas.

REFERENCE

Pervier NC. *Textbook of Chemistry for Embalmers*. Minneapolis: University of Minnesota; 1961.

Index

Note: Page numbers followed by f and t indicate Figures and Tables respectively. Page numbers in *italics* are glossary terms

Abdominal anatomical regions, *481*
Abdominal aorta
   arterial embalming, 174–175
   in infants, 288, 288f
Abdominal autopsy, 315, 317, 317f
Abdominal cavity
   aspiration, 263–264
   autopsied bodies, 306
   cavity embalming, 257–258
   closure of opening, 265–266, 266f
   in complete autopsy, 306
   contents, 259f, 259t, 259–260, 260f
   edema, 381
   organ removal from, 323–324, 324f
Abdominal feeding tubes, 209
Abdominal surgery, preembalming analysis
      and, 185
Abortion, 16
Abrasions, *481*
   dehydration of, 372
   discolorations, 355, 356–357, 358–359,
      359f
   preembalming treatment of, 212–213
   razor, (razor burn), 356–357, *491*
Abut, *481*
Accessory chemicals, 137–140, *481. See also*
      specific chemicals and fluids
Accidental death, 16
Accreditation, of mortuary schools, 452
Acetone (dimethyl ketone), 10
Acids, fatty, *486*
Acquired immunodeficiency syndrome. *See*
      AIDS
Action level, *481*
Active dyes, 123
Actual pressure, 223, *481*
Adair, Maude Adams, 471–472
Adhesives, 272, 276
Adipocere, *481*
Adolescents, 294
Adsorption, 233, *481*
Advanced decomposition, 344–345
Adventitia, 385
Aerobic, *481*
Aerosolization, *481*
Age considerations, 160, 183, 285. *See also*
      Children; Elderly; Infants
Agglutination, *481*
Agonal algor, 88, *481*
Agonal coagulation, 88, *481*
Agonal dehydration, 88, *481*
Agonal edema, 88, *481*
Agonal fever, 88, *481*

Agonal hypostasis, 88
Agonal period, of death, 88–89, *481*
Agonal translocation, 88–89, *481*
AIDS, *481. See also* Human
      immunodeficiency virus
   in health-care workers, 525–526
Air, from embalming apparatus, 407. *See*
      also Ventilation
Airborne pathogens, 39, *500. See also*
      Infection
Air brush kits, 475f, 476, 476f
Air conditioning, preparation room, 67
Air pressure machine, 71, 71f, 256
AL. *See* Action level
Alcohol, as preservative, 433, 434, 436
Alcoholism, 413
Aldehydes, 115
Alekton, 454
Aleutian Islanders, 430
Alexander, Dr. Joseph B., 436, 439,
      441–442
Alexander V, Pope, 432
Alexander the Great, 428
Algor, agonal, 88, *481*
Algor mortis, 90–91, 91f, *481*
Alkaline compounds, 117–118
Alternate drainage, 249, *481*
Aluminum salts, 421
American College of Embalming, 452
Amino acids, *481*
Anaerobic, *481*
Anal purge, 405
Analysis. *See* Embalming analysis
Anasarca, 375, *481*
Anatomical extent. *See* Anatomical guide
      and limits
Anatomical guide and limits, *481*
   axillary artery, 146, 147f
   brachial artery, 147, 148f
   carotid artery, 144, 145f
   femoral artery, 153, 153f
   popliteal fossa, 153
   radial artery, 149
   tibial arteries, 154
   ulnar artery, 149
Anatomical position, *481*
Anatomist period of embalming, 422,
      430–439
Anatomists, 430–431, 432–439
Anatomy. *See also* Anatomical guide and
      limits; Linear guide
   embalming techniques and, 422
   medieval instruction in, 430–431

Aneurysm, *481*
   aortic, 161, 388
Aneurysm hook, 74, *481*
Aneurysm needle, 73f, 73–74, *481–482*
Angstadt, Earle K., 474
Angular spring forceps, 248, *482*
Anomaly, *482*
Antecubital, *482*
Antemortem, *482*
Antemortem period, 87
   blood discoloration
      extravascular, 351f, 351–353, 352f
      intravascular, 349t, 349–351, 350f
   clots, 243
   dehydration in, 371
   subcutaneous emphysema, 261
Anterior, *482*
Anterior horizontal incision, 165, 166f
Anterior lateral incision, 165, 166f
Anterior superior iliac spine, *482*
Anterior tibial arteries. *See* Tibial arteries,
      anterior and posterior
Anterior triangle, of neck, 144
Anterior vertical incision, 165
Anthropology, physical, restorative art and,
      473
Antibiotic chemotherapy, 396
Anticlotting agents. *See* Anticoagulants
Anticoagulants, 112, 120–121, *482*
Antidehydrants. *See* Humectants
Antiinflammatories, 396
Antimetabolites, 393, 396–397
Antimicrobials
   embalming fluids and disinfectants as,
      517–522, 518t, 521t, 522t
   procedures/exposure intervals, 47t, 48
Aorta
   abdominal, 174–175, 288, 288f
   aneurysm of, 161, 388
   arterial solution distribution and,
      225–226, 226f
   ascending, 288–289, 289f
   preembalming analysis for repair, 184
   thoracic, 174–175
Apparatus. *See* Instrumentation and
      equipment
Apparent death, *482*
Arabs, 422, 428
Arch of the aorta, 164
   arterial solution distribution and, 226,
      226f
Armed services, deceased personnel care,
      34–36

Arms
  edematous, 380–381
  positioning of, 82, 198–199, 199f
Arsenic, 433, 436
  prohibited use of, 437, 455
Arterial coagula, 390, 390f
Arterial embalming, 22, 164, *486. See also*
      Arterial solution; Arterial solution
      injection
  abdominal aorta, 174–175
  axillary artery, 169–70, 170f
  brachial artery, 170
  carotid artery, 165–166, 166f, 167f
  cavity treatment in, 254
  dehydration, 372, 372t
  evaluation of body after, 187–188
  external iliac artery, 175, 175f
  facial artery, 168–169, 169f
  femoral artery, 171–172, 172f, 173f
  femoral vein, 172
  iliac artery, 175
  inferior vena cava, 175
  jugular vein, 165–166, 166f–168f
  popliteal artery, 172, 174, 174f
  processes in. *See* Arterial solution,
      distribution and diffusion of; Arterial
      solution injection; Drainage
  processes involved, 215
  radial artery, 170, 171f
  refrigerated bodies and, 340
  right atrium of heart, 175
  thoracic aorta, 174–175
  tibial arteries, 174, 174f
  ulnar artery, 170, 171f
Arterial fluid, *482. See also* Arterial
      solution; Embalming fluids
Arterial hemostat, 74, 74f
Arterial relationships
  axillary to axillary vein, 147
  brachial with basilic vein, 147
  carotid to internal jugular vein, 144
  femoral to femoral vein, 153
  popliteal artery and vein, 153–154
  radial to venae comitantes, 149
  ulnar to venae comitantes, 149
Arterial scissors, 74, 75f
Arterial solution, 109, 129, *482
  in autopsied bodies, 305
  chemical composition, 32, 43, 109, 217
  in children, 292–293
  classification, 129, 130t, 131, 132t
  delayed embalming, 334–335
  dilution of, 131, 132t
  distribution and diffusion of, 215–217,
      216f
    arterial fluid diffusion, 217, 229, 230f,
        231f
    center of distribution, 225–226, 226f
    combination resistance, 220
    diffusion methods, 229–232
    extravascular resistance, 217, 219–220,
        220f
    improving distribution, 228–229, 229f
    by injection, 217–218, 218f. *See also*
        Arterial solution injection
    intravascular resistance, 217, 218–219
    movement from outside capillaries to
        inside cells, 232f, 232–233
    paths of least resistance, 221–223, 222f
    primary dilution, 231
    resistance advantages, 221, 221f
    restricted cervical injection, 240
    routes, 215, 217

semipermeable membrane, 232
  signs of, 222, 226–228, 227f
  drainage of, 215–216, 216f
  dyes, 136, 226–227
  edema, 378–379, 380f
  firming speed and degree, 129
  fumeless, 136
  humectants, 136
  hypertonic solution, 231, 377, 377f
  injection of. *See* Arterial solution injection
  interstitial fluid, 216
  moisturizing qualities, 129
  osmosis, 379
  pH of, 131
  postembalming treatments, 270
  retention of, 191, 192f, 215–216, 216f
  short-circuiting, 237, 238f
  special purpose fluid, 334
  special-purpose fluid, 129
  strength, 162, 187, 292–293, 295,
      334–335
  temperature of, 131
  volume, 162, 292–293, 295, 335
Arterial solution injection, 217–218, 218f
  artery selection for, 235
    criteria, 236
  body preparation after. *See*
      Postembalming treatments
  body preparation prior to. *See* Body
      preparation
  clinical discussion, 225
  development, 433
  devices for, 67–69, 68f–73f, 71–73
  embalming analysis prior to. *See*
      Preembalming analysis
  historical methods, 422, 434, 436–440,
      438f, 442, 444, 453–454
  jaundice effects, treatment, 468
  nonpreservative, 431
  observations prior to, 228
  pressure and rate of flow, 32, 42,
      223–225, 224f
  restorative art and, 467
  selection criteria, 236
  sites for. *See also* Vessel selection, for
      arterial solution injection
    comparisons, 159, 159f
    primary, 157–158, 159–162
    secondary, 158, 162–163
  techniques, 235–242, 237f–238f, 240f,
      242f
  undertakers' instruction in, 446, 447
  volume used, 32, 42
Arterial tubes, 75, 77f, *482
Arterioles, 223, 237
Arteriosclerosis, 297, 298f, 387f, 387–388,
      388f, *482
Artery(ies). *See also individual arteries*
  branches of, 144, 146, 146f, 153, 154
  as injection site, 159, 159t. *See also* Vessel
      selection, for arterial solution
      injection
    primary, 157–158, 159–160
    secondary, 158, 162–163
  origins of, 144, 146, 147, 149, 153
Arthritic conditions, 296f, 296–297
Articulation, *482
Artificial cold, as preservative, 422
Ascending aorta in infants, 288–289, 289f
Ascites, 374, 381, *482
  extravascular resistance, 219–220
  preembalming treatment of, 214
Asepsis, 45, *482

Asheworth, Don, 469
Aspergillosis, 415
Asphyxia, *482
Aspirating instruments, 78, 79f, 80, 80f, 81f,
      255–257. *See also individually named
      instruments*
Aspiration, 22, 254, *482
  abdominal cavity, 263–264
  cranial, 264, 265f
  environmental issues, 456
  partial, arterial treatment and, 260–261,
      261f
  and reaspiration of cavities, 254, 266
  techniques, 262
  thoracic cavity, 263
Aspirators, 455–456, *489
Astor, Jacob, 466–467
Atheroma, *482
Atrium, right, *491
Auracius, Princess, 432
Authorization forms, 17, 18f, 19f
Autoclave, *482
Autolysis, 96, 100, 104, *482
  delayed embalming and, 342
Autopsied bodies, 303
  additional examinations, 313f, 313–314
  adult, chronology for embalming, 24–25
  cavity embalming, 262
  ethics, 15
  infants. *See* Infants, autopsied
  preparation of, 306–309, 308f
    cavity closure, 311–313, 312f
    final procedures, 313
    order for, 306–307
    supplemental hypodermic injection,
        309–310, 310f
    viscera, treatment of, 310
  restoration protocol for, 317–318
  secondary injection sites, 158
  suturing, 274
  treatment, 304–305
  vessel sites and selections, 158
Autopsy, *482
  abdominal, 315, 317, 317f
  complete, 305f, 305–306, 306f
  cranial, 314
  forensic, 303
  HIV transmission precautions, 528
  medicolegal, 303
  partial, 305, 306, 314–317, 315f–317f
  thoracic, 314–315, 315f, 316f
  treatment considerations. *See* Autopsy
      treatment
  types, 303–304
  when to perform, guidelines for, 304
Autopsy aspirator, 78, 79f, 256–257
Autopsy gels, 137–138, 312f, 313
  in postembalming treatments, 270–271
Autopsy treatment, 304–305
Axilla, surface anatomy, 145–146
Axillary artery
  anatomy of, 146–147, 147f
  in arterial embalming, 169–170, 170f
  incision for raising, 147
  injection and drainage techniques, 237,
      237f
  suturing of, 274
Axillary vein
  anatomy of, 147
  incision for raising, 147
  injection and drainage techniques, 237,
      237f
Aztecs, 429

Babylonians, 428
Bach, Johann Sebastian, 473
Backflow, preparation room, 41, 60–64, 61f–65f
Bacteremia, agonal translocation of microbes and, 88–89
Bacteria, saprophytic, 492
Bacterial infection
 embalming fluids, antimicrobial effects, 517–522, 518t, 521t, 522t
 postmortem presence and transmission, 499–501, 515, 516, 522–524, 523t, 524f
Bactericidal agent, 45, 482
Bacteriostatic agent, 45, 482
Baillie, Matthew, 435
Baker, Colonel L. C., 442
Baker, E. D., 441
Ball, Lafayette C., 468
Balsamic substance, 482
Bandages, 220
Bandage scissors, 75, 75f
Barnes, Carl Lewis, 450f, 451, 451f, 454, 466
Barnes, Dr., 444
Barnes, Thorton B., 454, 466
Barnes School, 466, 467
Barrow, Clyde, 469
Bartholin (1585-1629), 431
Baseball sutures, 274, 467
 autopsied bodies, 311, 313, 314
Base of the axillary space, 482
Basilic vein, 147
BCME (bischloromethyl ether), 482
Bedsores, 360–361
Beinhauer, F. C., 444
Berengarius, Jacobus, 431
Berkley, Sir William, 433
Bernard, Mrs. E. G., 452
Bernard School of Embalming, 452
Biohazard, 482
Biological death, 482
Bischloromethyl ether, 482
Bistoury knife, 74, 74f
Blanchard, Stephen, 433
Bleach, household, 487
Bleaching, of tissues, 227, 468
 as jaundice treatment, 354
Bleaching agent, 482
Bleaching solutions, 140, 468
Blind stitching, 467
Blisters, 359, 359f
Blood, 482
 removal
  agitation devices and, 456
  formalin and, 455
  historical methods, 431, 432, 433, 434
 spills, cleaning and decontamination of, 529–530
 vessels, injection. See Arterial solution injection
Bloodborne pathogen rule, 482–483
Bloodborne pathogens, 13–14, 39, 482
 effects of, 39
 infection risks, 44
 opportunistic, 39
 precautionary requirements, 30–33, 31f
Blood discoloration, 348
 ecchymosis, 352, 352f
 extravascular
  antemortem, 351f, 351–353, 352f
  postmortem, 351f, 351–353, 352f
 formaldehyde gray, 349t, 349–351, 350f

hematoma of the eye, 352, 352f
 hypodermic treatment, 352
 hypostasis, 349t, 349–351, 350f
 intravascular
  antemortem, 349t, 349–351, 350f
  clearing of, 227, 227f
  postmortem, 349t, 349–351, 350f
 livor mortis, 349t, 349–351, 350f
 postmortem stain, 349t, 349–351, 350f, 352–353
 surface embalming, 352
Blood drainage, 227
Blood pressure, 483
Blood vascular system, 483
Blood vessel
 distension during arterial solution distribution and diffusion, 227
 injection into. See Arterial solution injection
 selection for. See Vessel selection
Blood viscosity, 95
Blunt dissection, 483
Board of Health, 3, 39
Body cavity edema, 374
Body classification, 181–182
Body conditions, in preembalming analysis
 age, 183
 treatments, 189, 189t
 weight, 183
Body donation, 15. See also Organ donation
Body fluid spills, cleaning and decontamination of, 529–530
Body identification, 15
 Curry system, 472
 by facial reconstruction, 473
 physical anthropology and, 473
Body moisture, 369–371, 371f
Body pH, shift in, 96
Body preparation, 191
 after arterial injection. See Postembalming treatments
 before arterial injection. See Preembalming treatments
 arterial solution retention and, 191, 192f
 of autopsied bodies, 306–309, 308f
 cast removal, 211
 dehydration and, 371–373, 372t, 373f
 desiccation and, 371–372
 eye closure, 208–209, 210f
 feature setting. See Feature setting
 feeding tubes, 209
 hair care, 194
 intravenous tubes, 209, 211
 invasive procedures, treatment of, 209, 211
 legal requirements, 192
 mouth closure. See Mouth Closure
 and organ donation. See Organ donation
 orifices, packing of, 209
 packing the orifices, 209
 positioning of the body, 196f, 196–198, 197f, 198f
  hands and arms, 198–199, 199f
  head, 198
  problems, 199f, 199–200
  preliminary, 192–193, 193f
 for reembalming. See Reembalming
 setting the features. See Feature setting
 shaving the body, 194–196, 195f
 topical disinfection, 193–194
 treatments
  for abrasions, 212–213, 372
  for ascites, 214

following invasive procedures, 209, 211
 for fractures, 212, 212f
 for gas in cavities and tissues, 213–214, 214t
 for lacerations, 212
 for skin lesions, 211–212
 for skin-slip, 213, 213f
 for torn skin, 213, 213f
 for ulcerations, 211–212
 washing the body, 194
Body preservation, 421–424, 428–431. See also specific method
Body proteins, 17–19
Body rests, 82
Body trunk. See Trunk
Body typing, Slocum method, 181–182
Boil, 483
Bone marrow, treatment after vertebral body removal for, 325
Boniface, Pope, 431
Book of the Dead, 425
Borates, 117, 121
Boston College, 466
Bowsher, Ivan P., 471
Brachial artery
 anatomy, 147–148, 148f
 in arterial embalming, 170
 suturing of, 274
Brain purge, 405
Brain treatment
 Egyptian technique, 425
 historical accounts, 424, 432
 trocar methods, 454
Bridge suture, 274, 483
British Embalmer, 450
British Embalmers Society, 450
Broken bones, 212, 212f
Broken skin discolorations, 358–359, 359f
Brown, Dr. Charles D., 436, 439
Bruising, postmortem, 357
Buccal cavity, 483
Buckesto, Dr. J. P., 442–443
Buffers, 112, 117, 140, 483
Building permits, preparation room, 52
Bulb syringe, 68–69, 69f, 483
Bullet wound discolorations, 365f, 365–366
Bunnell, Chester, 441
Bunnell, George Holmes, 441
Bunnell, Milton, 441
Bunnell, William J., 439, 441, 443
Bureau of Vital Records, 3
Burgundy, Lady Johanna of, 432
Burial rites
 ancient Egyptian, 423, 423f
 Native American, 430
 Peruvian, 429
Burned bodies
 discolorations, 362–363, 363f
 edema, 382
Burr, Dr. Richard, 439, 443–444

Cadaver, 483
 preservation of, 421–424, 428–431
 for study and dissection, 430, 431, 435, 436
 theft of, 431, 435
Cadaveric lividity, 92f, 92–93, 94t, 483. See also Livor mortis
Cadaveric spasm, 483
Callaway, C. F., 470
Caloricity, postmortem, 96
Calvarium, 311–313, 312f, 483
 autopsied bodies, 311–313, 312f

Calvarium clamp, *483*
Campbell, Frank E., 464
Canalization, 387, *483*
Canary Islanders, 428–429
Cancer patients, infection as cause of death, 515
Candidiasis, 414–415
Canopic urns, 426, 426f
Capillaries, *483*
    arterial solution distribution and diffusion via, 218, 223, 232, 232f
Capillary embalming, 44, 215. *See also* Arterial embalming
Capillary expansion, agonal, 88
Capillary permeability, *484*
Capillary wash. *See* Preinjection fluid
Carbohydrate, *484*
    decomposition, 102
Carbolic acid, 116
Carbonates, 118
Carbon monoxide poisoning discoloration, 363–364, 364f
Carbuncle, *484*
Carcinogen, *484*
Cardiac disease, 299
Cardiac procedures, invasive, HIV transmission precautions, 527–528
Cardiovascular disease, edema effects, 534–535
Carmine dye, 123
Carotid artery, 143–144
    anatomy of, 144, 145f, 146f
    arch of the aorta and, 164
    in arterial embalming, 164–165, 166f, 167f
    and carotid sheath contents, 144, 147f
    in infants, 287
    injection and drainage techniques, 236, 238
    suturing of, 274
    in vessel selection, 287
Carotid sheath, 144, 147f
Carpenter, William S., 452
Cartonage, 427
Casket, The (journal), 446, 447, 447f, 463
Casket and Sunnyside (journal), 469, 471
Casketed remains, 282–283
Caskets, types and sizes, 197
Cast removal, 211
Catheter removal, 211
Catliff, Betty, 473
Cattell, Henry P., 439, 441–442, 442
Cause of death
    drug overdose, 314
    information on, 38f, 38–39
    in preembalming analysis, 183–184
    pulmonary embolism, 314
    unnatural, 361t, 361–367, 363f–365f, 367f
Cautery chemicals, 130, 138
Cavitation, *484*
Cavity contents, treatment of, 254, 254t
Cavity embalming, 22, 253–254, *484, 486.* *See also* Cavity treatment
    abdominal contents
        nine-region method, 259, 259f, 259t
        quadrant method, 259, 260f
        trocar guides, 259–260, 260f
    antemortem subcutaneous emphysema and, 261
    autopsies and, 291–292, 311–313, 312f
        partial, 262

chemical injection for, 32, 264–265, 422
closure of cavities, 311–313, 312f
    abdominal opening, 265–266, 266f
direct incision method, 263
filler, 467
historical methods, 422, 442–443, 453–454
in infants, 289, 291–292
reaspiration, 254, 266
reinjection, 266
Cavity fluid, 43, 109, 130, 136–137, *484*
    as jaundice treatment, 354
Cavity fluid injector, 80, 80f
Cavity treatment
    aspiration for
        abdominal cavity, 263–264, 265–266, 266t
        cranium, 264, 265f
        partial, prior or during arterial treatment, 260–261, 261f
        techniques, 262
        thoracic cavity, 263–264
    chronology of, 254t, 254–255, 255t
    instrumentation and equipment required, 255
        for aspiration, 256–257
        for vacuum creation, 255–256
    male genitalia, 264
    order of, 263
    organ donation and, 262
    organ removal and, 262
    purge in, 255, 255t
    refrigerated bodies, 340
    of skull. *See* Head
    surgical procedures and, 262
    time period for, 261–262
    of trunk. *See* Trunk
    visceral anatomy, 257–259
CDC/CDCP. *See* Centers for Disease Control and Prevention
Cecum guide, 260, 260f
Cedar, oil of, 424, 425
Ceilings, preparation room, 58–59, 59f
Cellular death, 87, *484*
Cellular edema, 374
Cemeteries
    grave robbing, 423, 423f, 427, 431, 435
    national system origins, 440
Center of drainage, 245, 245f, *484*
Center of fluid distribution, *484*
    arterial solution, 225–226, 226f
Centers for Disease Control and Prevention, *484*
    infective waste recommendations, 533, 534
    universal precautions, 532
        on HIV transmission, 527
Central America, 429
Centrifugal pump, 71f, 71–73, 72f, 73f
Cervical injection. *See* Restricted cervical injection
Chamberlain, C. B., 439, 444, 445, 446
Chaussier, Francois, 436
Cheeks, postembalming treatments, 271
Chelate, *484*
Chemical adduct system, 140
Chemical solutions, properties of, 131–133
Chemotherapy, *484*
    effect on embalming process, 393, 394–397, 395f, 399–400
    neutralizing effects of, 399, 399t
    one-bottle embalming and, 498
    preembalming analysis, 184, 185f, 185t

Cheselden, William, 434
Children, 140, 286, 292. *See also* Infants
    feature setting, 293–294, 294f
    fluid strengths and volume, 292–293
    injection pressure, 293
    positioning the body, 293, 293f
    preembalming analysis, 183
    rate of flow, 293
    vessel selection, 292
Chin rest, 205, *484*
Christians, 422
Chronology
    of cavity treatment. *See* Cavity treatment, chronology of
    for embalming. *See* Embalming, chronology for
Churchill, Winston, 421
Cincinnati College, 467, 469, 471
Cincinnati School of Embalming, 448f, 449, 466
Circle needles, 75, 76f
Circulatory changes, agonal, 88
Cisterna cerebellomedullaris, 38
Citrates, 120–121
Civil War embalming
    injury repair, 461
    practices, 439–440
    rules and regulations, 440, 444
    surgeons, 440–445
Clarke, C. Horace, 449
Clarke, Joseph Henry, 444, 448–449, 449f, 454, 461
Clarke School of Embalming, 448
Clauderus, Gabriel, 422, 433, 454
Cleaning, defined, 45
Clinical death, 87, *484*
Clostridium perfringens, 88–89, 140, *484.* *See also* Tissue gas
    embalming analysis, 181
Closure
    of abdominal opening, 265–266, 266f
    of cavities, 311–313, 312f
    of incisions. *See* Incisions
Clothing of deceased, 17, 20f, 193
Clotting, 161–162
Coagulating agents, *484*
Coagulation, *484*
    agonal, 88, *481*
    tissue, *493*
Cochineal dye, 123
Coffins, 197
    Egyptian, 427, 427f
    hermetically sealed, 461
    lead, 432
    patents, 444
Coinjection fluids, 130, 135–136, 295, *484*
Cold, as preservative
    artificial, 422
    dry, 421
Collection of Voyages, 430
Colleges. *See* Mortuary colleges
Collier, William G., 469–470
Collins, Floyd, 469
Colloidal dispersion, 233
Color change. *See* Discoloration
Coloring agents. *See* Dyes
Colostomy closures, 211, 277, 277f
Coma, *484*
Combination antibiotic chemotherapy, 396
Combination postembalming treatments, 272
Combination resistance, 220

Combined resistance, in arterial solution distribution and diffusion, 220
Common carotid artery. *See* Carotid artery
Communicable disease, *484*. *See also* Bloodborne pathogens
Community Right-to-Know Rule, 5
Company of Barbers, 434
Company of Barber-Surgeons, 434
Complete autopsy, 305f, 305–306, 306f
Compound, hardening, *487*
Comprehensive written hazard communication program, 9
Concurrent disinfection, 40, 45, *484*
    public health guidelines, 40–41, 41f
Concurrent drainage, 249, *484*
    arterial treatment for edema, 377
Condensation products as preservatives, 115
Condyle, *484*
Conference to Funeral Service Examining Boards, 452
Confidentiality, 15
Congealing, *484*
Congestive heart failure, 389
Conjunctiva, *484*
Consent for organ donation, 319–320
Contact lenses, sterilization, 529
Contact pressure, 220
Contagious disease, *484*. *See also* Bloodborne pathogens
Container labeling, 7
Contaminated material, definitions, *483*
Continuous drainage, 249
    arterial treatment for edema, 377
Continuous suture, 275–276, 276f
Copper, in embalming fluids, 455
Copper salts, as preservative, 421
Cornea, *484*
    removal, treatment after, 325
Corneal sclera button, *484*
Cornelius, W. P., 439, 445
Coroner, *484*
    autopsy by, 304
    and legal aspects of embalming, 16–17
    and organ donor consent, 320
Corpulence, *484*
Corticosteriods, 396
Cosmetic, opaque, *489*
Cosmetic fluid, 111, 129, *484*
Cosmetic treatment, 466, 467, 469, 473–474, 476
    classification, 129
    corrections, 282
    origins, 445, 464
    refrigerated bodies, 340
Counterstaining compound, *484*
Coupling compound system, 140
Coveralls, 272, 280, *484*
Craig, Golden, 452
Craig, Helene, 452
Crandall, Caroline Andrews, 463
Crandall, Joel E., 451, 462–467, 463f, 465f, 469, 474
Crandall, Norris, 463
Crane, C. H., 446
Cranial aspiration, 264, 265f
Cranial autopsy, 314
Cranial cavity, 306
Cranial embalming, *484*
Cremated remains, *484*
Crepitation, *485*
    postembalming treatments, 279
    preembalming treatments, 213

Creutzfeldt-Jakob disease, *485*
Cribriform plate, *485*
Criminals, remains of, 428, 430, 434, 439
Crosslinking reactions, 105f, 105–107, 106f, 107f
Crusades, handling of dead in, 431
Crystalloids, 232
Cudbear dye, 123
Curry, Gladys P., 472
Cytomycosis reticuloendothelial, 415–416
Cytotoxic drugs, 393, 396–397

Da Costa Brown, Dr. Charles, 439, 441–442
Darko, L. G., 452
Databases, 9–11
Davenport, L. Roy, 473
Da Vinci, Leonardo, 431
Death, *485*
    agonal period, 88–89
    antemortem period, 87
    apparent, *482*
    cause of. *See* Cause of death
    cellular, 87, *484*
    determination of, 85–86, 319
        organ donation and, 319
    early signs of, 86
    expert tests of, 86, *486*
    inexpert tests of, 86
    later signs of, 86
    legal, 87
    postmortem changes. *See* Postmortem changes
    somatic, 87, *492*
    tests of, 86–87, *492*
    types and stages of, 87–88
    unnatural, 361t, 361–367, 363f–365f, 367f
Death masks, 461, 464f, 469, 474
Death rattle, *485*
Death struggle, *485*
Debilitation from disease, postmortem treatment. *See* Restorative art
De Bils, Ludwig, 433
Decay, *485*. *See also* Decomposition
Deceptive acts or practices, 4
Decomposition, 342–344, *485*
    advanced, 344–345
    of ancient corpses, 423, 427
    autolysis, 104
    carbohydrates, 102
    catalysts of, 103f, 103–104
    crosslinking reactions, 105f, 105–107, 106f, 107f
    decay, 101–103
    dehydration, 342
    delayed embalming in bodies exhibiting, 341f, 341–345, 342f
    desquamation, 105
    discoloration, 104–105, 105f, 341, 349, 357
    disinfection by embalming, 105
    enzymes, 100–102
    gases from, 105, 213, 214t, 342, 408–409
    identification following, 472
    lipids, 102
    livor mortis, 341
    odors, 105, 342
    preservation by embalming, 105
    protein, 100–102, 101f, 102f
    ptomaines, 101
    purge, 105, 342, 342f

    putrefaction, 101–103
    signs of, 104–105, 105f
    skin-slip, 105, 342
    trunk discoloration, 341
    vascular discoloration, 341
Decontamination, of blood and body fluid spills, 529–530. *See also* Concurrent disinfection; Disinfection; Terminal disinfection
Decubitus ulcers, 360–361
Defamation, of other professionals, 15
Deformities, repair of, 426
Degenerative diseases, 187
De Graaf, Regnier, 431
Dehydrated body, preparation of, 371–373, 372t, 373f
Dehydrating high-index fluids, 139
Dehydration, 371, 371f, *485*. *See also* Moisture considerations
    agonal, 88, *481*
    in arterial embalming, 372, 372t
    delayed embalming and, 342
    discolorations, 355–356, 356f
    local problems, 372
    postembalming, 271, 372–373, 373f
    postmortem, 93–95, 95f, 371
    preparing body in cases of, 371–373, 372t, 373f
    of refrigerated bodies, 338–340
Delayed embalming, 333–334
    in decomposed bodies, 341f, 341–345, 342f
    injection protocol, 334–335
    of refrigerated bodies, 338–341, 339f
    in rigor mortis, 335–338, 336t, 337f
De Lessups, Ferdinand Marie, 437
Demisurgery, 462–469. *See also* Restorative art
Denatured protein, *485*
Density of chemical solutions, 131–133
Dental tie, 205, 206f, *485*
Dentistry, HIV transmission in
    precautions against, 527–528
    prevalence, 526
Deodorants. *See* Perfuming agents
Depilatories, use in restoration, 467
Dermasurgery, 467, 469. *See also* Restorative art
Dermatome, 328
Desiccation, 371–372, *485*
Desquamation. *See* Skin-slip
Dhonau, Charles O., 128, 449, 466–469, 471
Diabetes, 390–391, 391f
    in elderly, 300, 300f
Diabetic agents (oral), 398–399
Dialdehydes, 115–116
Dialysis, 231f, 232, *485*
Differential pressure, 223, *485*
Diffusion (fluid), 232, *485*
    of arterial solution. *See* Arterial solution, distribution and diffusion of
Digits, *485*
    arterial solution distribution and diffusion, 228
    treatment in mummies, 427
Dillinger, John, 469
Dilution
    of arterial solution, 131, 132t
    primary, 110, 131, 231, *491*
    secondary, 231, *492*
Dimethyl ketone (acetone), 10
Diodorus siculus, 424–425

Direct heart drainage, 246–247, 247f
Direct incision method, 263
Disasters
    human behavior during, 506
    response handbook for, 502–507
Disaster worker, disaster response protocol,
        502–505, 506–507
Discoloration, 347–349, 485. See also Blood
        discoloration
    classifications, 347–349
    conditions related to, 357–361
        in unnatural causes of death, 361–367
    from decomposition, 104–105, 105f, 357
    delayed embalming and, 341
    from embalming, treatment of, 355–357
    embalming considerations, 349, 355–357,
        356f
    extravascular blood, 351f, 351–353, 352f,
        486
    formaldehyde gray and, 198, 349t,
        349–351, 350f, 356
    intravascular blood, 349t, 349–351,
        350f
        clearing of, 227, 227f
    and jaundice treatment, 353f, 353–354,
        356
    livor mortis, 341, 349t, 349–351, 350f
    in nephritis, treatment of, 354–355
    postembalming treatments, 277–278
    on surface, treatment of, 355
    trunk areas, 341
    vascular, 341
    vessel selection and, 161–162
Disease, 485. See also individually named
        diseases
    cause of death and, 38f, 38–39
    preembalming analysis, 183–184
    transmission prevention procedures,
        529–530
    vessel selection and, 160–161
Disfigurement, treatment of. See Restorative
        art
Disinfectant, 45, 485
    antimicrobial effects, 517–522, 518t,
        521t, 522t
    checklist, 281
Disinfection, 13–14
    antimicrobial procedures/exposure
        intervals, 47t, 48
    concurrent. See Concurrent disinfection
    of drainage, 250
    by embalming, 105
    of equipment, 410. See also Terminal
        disinfection
    levels of, 45–46, 46t
    methods, 45, 46t
    microbicides activity levels, 46t
    primary, 45, 491
    procedures to prevent HIV transmission,
        528–529
    survey results, 44–45
    topical, 193–194
Dismemberment, 431
    of mummies, 427
Dissection
    ban on, 431
    blunt, 483
    of criminals' remains, 430, 434
    as educational tool, 422, 430–431, 439,
        469
Distal forearm, 148f, 148–149
Distal leg, 154, 154f
    in infants, 287

Distension
    autopsied bodies, 305
    facial tissue, 162
    gases causing, postembalming treatments
        for, 213–214, 214t, 278–279, 279f
    small surface vessels, 227
Distribution (fluid), 485
    of arterial solution. See Arterial solution,
        distribution and diffusion of
Doctors. See Physicians
Documentation
    of embalming, 17, 21f
    organ donors, 319
    postembalming treatments, 281–282
Dodge, A. Johnson, 463, 473
Doors, preparation room, 54, 58
Dorsal approach, spinal cord removal, 306,
        306f
Dorsalis pedis artery, 155
Double-base fluid, 116
Double intradermal sutures, 275, 275f
Drainage, 242, 485
    alternate, 249, 481
    arterial solution, 215–216, 216f
    in autopsy treatment, 305
    center of, 245, 245f, 484
    concurrent, 249, 484
    contents of, 242–244, 243f
    direct heart, 246–247, 247f
    disinfection, 250
    instrumentation for, 78, 79f, 247–248, 248f
    intermittent (restricted drainage), 249,
        250f, 488
    of interstitial fluid, 216
    purpose of, 244–245
    site for arterial treatment of edema, 377
    sites for, 245–246, 246f
    techniques for improving, 249–250
    veins for, 235
        selection criteria, 236
Drain tubes, 78, 79f, 247–248, 248f, 485
    jugular, 488
Drench shower, 485
Dressing forceps, 74, 74f
Drill, securing mandible and, 205
Droplet nucleus, 38
Drowning discolorations, 364–365
Drugs
    effect on embalming process, 393–400,
        400. See also individual drugs
    mummy remains as, trafficking in, 428
Dry abrasions, treatment of, 212
Dry gangrene, 485
Drying, of tissues
    arterial solution distribution and diffusion
        and, 227
    artificial, 422
        following restorative art, 467
        Gaunche method, 428–429
        Tranchina method, 436
    natural, 421, 423, 431
        following natron treatment, 426
        Native American practices, 429, 430
Dyes, 112, 123–124, 130, 485
    in arterial solution, 136, 226–227
    in autopsy treatment, 305
    fluorescent, 226–227, 456
Dyne, 122

Ecchymosis, 485
    blood discoloration, 352, 352f
    in elderly, 297–298

ECG (electrocardiogram), 485
Eckels, Howard S., 451, 462–463
Eckels Chemical Company, 469
Eckels College of Embalming, 450, 467
Eckels College of Mortuary Science, 472
Eckels molding masks, 464f
Ecuador, 429
Edema, 370, 383t, 485
    agonal, 88, 481
    anasarca and, 375
    arterial treatment of
        arterial solutions, 378–379, 380f
        arterial treatment for, 375–376
            methods, 376f, 376–378, 377f
    of body cavities, 374
    cellular, 374
    classification, 374
    corrective coinjection fluids, 130
    embalming analysis, 187
    intercellular, 374, 374f
    pitting type, 374, 490
    postmortem, 94
    problems created by, 374–375
    restricted cervical injection, 240
    skeletal, extravascular resistance, 220,
        220f
    solid, 374
    treatment of, 373–374
        abdominal cavity, 381
        arms, 380–381
        in burned bodies, 382
        hydrocele, 381–382
        hydrothorax, 381
        legs, 379–380, 534–535
        in renal failure, 382–384
        trunk, 381
EDTA (ethylenediaminetetraacetic acid), 121
Education, 27–29, 29f
    public health precautionary
        requirements, 33
EEG. See Electroencephalogram
Effigies, medieval, 461, 462f
Egypt, ancient burial rites, 421, 423, 423f,
        424–425, 426
Egyptian period of embalming, 422,
        423–430
EKG (electrocardiogram), 485
Elderly, 296
    arteriosclerosis, 297, 298f
    arthritic conditions, 296f, 296–297
    cardiac disease, 299
    diabetes mellitus, 300, 300f
    ecchymosis, 297–298
    gangrene, 300, 300f
    glycosuria, 300
    hyperglycemia, 300
    ketosis, 300
    malignancy, 298–299
    mouth closure problems, 297
    preembalming analysis, 183
    senile purpura, 297–298
Electric aspirator, 61, 61f, 485
    in cavity embalming, 256
Electric-heated spatula, 469, 470f
Electricity
    application to corpses, 454–455
    equipment innovations and, 455–456
Electric spatula, 485
Electrocardiogram, 485
Electrocution discolorations, 363
Electroencephalogram, 485
Elevation, of vessels, 163–164
Ellsworth, Colonel Elmer, 440, 441

Emaciation, preembalming analysis and, 183
Embalmers
    associations, 450, 499
    doctors as, 422
    Gaunche, 428–429
    historical figures, 432–438
    regulations governing, 456
    undertakers as. *See* Undertakers
    women as, 452
Embalmers and Funeral Directors, State
    Board of, 3
Embalmer's gray. *See* Formaldehyde gray
"Embalmer to the trade," 450
Embalming, 17–19, 21–22, 421, 422, *486*
    arterial. *See* Arterial embalming
    body proteins, 17–19
    cavity. *See* Cavity embalming
    chronology for, 434
        autopsied adult, 24–25
        unautopsied adult, 23–24
    cranial, *484*
    faulty theories, 37–38
    first U.S. book on, 437f, 438
    fluids. *See* Embalming fluids
    historical accounts, 424–425, 432–435,
        439–430
    history and origins, 421–457
    history of, 422, 423–424
        ethnic methods, non-Egyptian, 428–430
    hypodermic, *486*
    minimum standards, 42–43
    of multiple dead, 456
    mummification. *See* Mummies
    natural, 421
    order/sequence. *See* Embalming,
        chronology for
    periods. *See* Embalming periods
    preservation of body, 17–19, 21–22
    process, summarized, 17–19, 21–22
    professionalism in, 455
    purposes, 422–423, 427
        educational instruction, 422–423,
            430–431
        funereal. *See* Funerals
        public transport, 422, 431
        religious, 422, 429
    regulations, 456
    restoration of appearance, 19
    sites, residence *versus* funeral home, 446,
        455
    standards for. *See* Standards, for
        embalming practices
    surface, *486*
    training in. *See* Training
    treatment concerns, 453–455
    vascular (arterial), *486*
    vessel site and selection. *See* Vessel
        selection
    in wartime
        Civil War. *See* Civil War embalming
        Crusades, 431
        World War I, 467
    waterless, *493*
Embalming analysis, 179–181, *486*
    body conditions and treatments, 189, 189t
    classification of bodies, 181–182
    evaluation of body after arterial
        embalming, 187–188
    extrinsic factors, 179, 186
    general issues, 190
    injection of the body, 186–187
    intrinsic factors, 179, 183, 186, 186t
    postembalming, 269–270

preembalming, 182–186, 185f, 185t. *See
    also* Preembalming analysis
purpose of, 181
time periods, 179
treatments, 188t, 188–189
Embalming Chemical Manufacturers
    Association, 499
Embalming chemicals, 109–110. *See also
    specific fluids and chemicals*
    accessory, 137–140
    of anatomist period, 430–439
    ancient, 424–426, 428–430
    anticoagulants, 112, 120–121, *482*
    antimicrobial effects, 517–522, 518t,
        521t, 522t
    for arterial solution, 109
    for cavity fluids, 109
    dyes. *See* Dyes
    EPA regulations, 456
    germicides. *See* Germicides
    historical use, 432–456, 468
    modifying agents, 111–112, 117–120,
        489
    one-bottle embalming, 497–499
    preservatives. *See* Preservatives
    reodorants. *See* Perfuming agents
    research, 448, 456–457
    sales, 446–448
    surfactants, 112, 121–123, 122f, *492*
    use of, general precautions, 128–129,
        129f
    vehicles for, 123–124
Embalming delays. *See* Delayed embalming
Embalming fluids, 110, 127–128, 431,
    448f
    autopsied infants and, 290
    chemical components of, 111f, 111–113
    chemical principles of, 110–111
    classification of, 130t
    coinjection fluids, 130, 135–136
    dilution of, 131, 132t
    dyes added to, 130, 136
    fumeless, 137
    high-index fluids, 139
    humectants in, 136
    for infants and children, 140
    pH of, 131
    preinjection fluids, 130, 134–135
    as preservative, 129, 130, 291
    properties of, 131–133
    standards for, 110
    supplemental. *See* Supplemental fluids
    temperature of, 131
    tissue gas fluid, 130, 140
Embalming periods, 422
    anatomist, 430–439
    Egyptian, 423–430
    modern, 439–452
Embalming powder, 138
Embalming schools
    demisurgery/restorative art instruction,
        464, 467–469
    development, 422–423, 447–448,
        450–452
    industry sponsored, 451
Embalming surgeons, Civil War, 439–445
Embolus, 386t
Emergency response handbook, 502–507
Emphysema, subcutaneous. *See*
    Subcutaneous emphysema
Emulsified oils, 118
Endogenous invasion, 38
Engineering controls, *486*

England, embalming practice history, 433,
    434–435, 450
Enucleation. *See* Eye enucleation
Environment, *486*
    HIV and, 528–529
    and personal health considerations, 37–48
Environmental Protection Agency, 3, *486*
    Community Right-to-Know Rule, 5
    embalming regulations, 456
    germicide information, 529
    material safety data sheets, 5
Environmental regulations
    regulatory agencies, 456. *See also specific
        agency*
    water systems, aspirated materials and,
        456
Environmental surfaces, cleaning, 529
Enzymes, 100–102, 394, *486*
EPA. *See* Environmental Protection Agency
Epigastric cavity embalming, 259
Equipment. *See* Instrumentation and
    equipment
Esophageal varices, 403
Ethics, 14–16
Ethiopians, 428
Ethylenediaminetetraacetic acid, 121
Ethylene glycol, 118
Eustaschio, Bartolomeo, 431
Evisceration, ancient techniques, 422,
    424–425, 428–430
Excision, *486*
Expert tests of death, 86, *486*
Exposure
    occupational, *489*
        to formaldehyde, 455, 507–514, 510t
    permissible limit, *490*
    short-term limit, *492*
Exposure incident, *486*
Exsanguination discolorations, 367
External carotid artery. *See* Carotid artery
External compresses, 291
External iliac artery. *See* Iliac artery and vein
Extravascular, *486*
Extravascular blood discoloration, 351f,
    351–353, 352f, *486*
Extravascular resistance, in arterial solution
    distribution and diffusion, 217,
    219–220, 391
Extrinsic, *486*
Extrinsic factors
    in algor mortis, 90
    in embalming analysis, 179
    postmortem interval, 186
Eyecaps, 80, 81f, 208, *486*
Eye enucleation, 306, *486*
    in complete autopsy, 306
    discoloration, *486*
    restricted cervical injection, 240
    treatment after, 324–325, 326f
Eyelids, 271, 271f, 409–410
    overlap, *486*
Eye process, 454
Eyes
    ancient restoration and, 426
    closure, 208–209, 210f, 286
    ecchymosis. *See* Ecchymosis
    infants, 286
    tissue gas, 409–410
Eyewash station, *486*

Facial area
    destruction of features, 429

Facial area (*cont.*)
　discolorations
　　formaldehyde gray, 198
　　vessel selection, 161–162
　distension of tissue
　　restricted cervical injection, 240
　　vessel selection, 161–162
　facial artery, 168–169, 169f
　instant tissue fixation, 411
　restoration, 465, 467–468. *See also*
　　Cosmetic treatment; Modeling
　restricted cervical injection, 240
　tissue gas, 409, 410, 410f
　trauma to, 240, 410–411
　variation of features, 468
Falconry embalming method, 438
Family of deceased, 15
Fat, *486*
Fatty acids, *486*
Feature setting, 200
　in children, 293–294, 294f
　delayed embalming and, 344
　devices, 80, 81f
　eyecap, 208
　eye closure, 208–209, 210f
　lips, positioning of, 207f, 207–208, 208f
　modeling the mouth, 205, 207f
　mouth closure sequence, 200–201, 201f
　mucous membranes, 200
　nasal spine, 201
　postembalming treatments, 279–280, 280f
　during rigor mortis, 336
　securing mandible, 201–205, 202f–204f,
　　206f
Febrile, *486*
Federal Trade Commission, 3–4, 456
Feeding tubes, 209
Femoral artery
　anatomy, 152–153, 153f
　arterial embalming, 171–172, 172f, 173f
　in infants, 287
　injection and drainage techniques, 236,
　　237f, 238
　suturing of, 274
　vessel selection, 287
Femoral triangle, 150–152, 152f
Femoral vein
　arterial embalming, 172
　injection and drainage techniques, 236,
　　237f, 238
Fermentation, *486*
Fever, agonal, 88, *481*
Fever blisters, *486*
Filtration gravitation, 233, *487*
Fingers. *See* Digits
Firming, *486. See also* Tissue fixation
Firmness. *See also* Tissue fixation
　degree and speed of, 129
　restricted cervical injection and, 240
First call vehicles. *See* Vehicles
First degree burns, 363
Fixation
　of tissue. *See* Tissue fixation
　of tissues, *486*
Fixative, *486*
Flaccidity, primary and secondary, 99
Flap incision, 165, 166f
Flesh treatment, 429–430, 438f
Flies, 193–194, 283
Flooring, preparation room, 55–57
Fluid diffusion, *485*
　arterial solution. *See* Arterial solution,
　　distribution and diffusion of

Fluid distribution, center of, *484*
Fluorescent dye, 226, 456
Flush (flushing), *486*
Fly eggs, 193–194, 283
Foot, 154–155
Foot rests, 82
Forceps
　angular spring, *482*
　packing, *490*
Forearm, distal, 148f, 148–149
Forensic autopsy, 303
Forestus, Peter, 431–432
Formaldehyde, 10, *486. See also*
　　Formaldehyde gray
　advantages of, 109–110
　aldehydes, 115
　antimicrobial effects, 517–522, 518t,
　　521t, 522t
　chemical principles of, 110–111
　condensation products, 115
　disadvantages of, 109
　facial discolorations, 198
　formalin solution. *See* Formalin
　index, 114
　minimum standards for, 110
　occupational exposure, 455, 507–514,
　　510t
　paraformaldehyde, 114
　regulations governing, 456. *See also*
　　Formaldehyde Rule
　restricted cervical injection, 240
　trioxane, 115
　ventilation, 64–67
Formaldehyde gray, *486*
　blood discoloration, 349t, 349–351, 350f,
　　356
　body preparation, 198
Formaldehyde rule, 11–13, 457, *486*, 507,
　　509, 510
Formalin, 113–114, 455, 468, 507. *See also*
　　Formaldehyde
　occupational exposure to, 455
Fractures
　embalming induced, 428
　preembalming treatment of, 212, 212f,
　　426
Franchini, G., 436
Freezing, natural preservation via, 421
Frozen tissues, 341
FTC. *See* Federal Trade Commission
Fumeless arterial solution, 137
Fumeless cavity fluid, 137
Funeral coach, cleansing of, 31, 41
Funeral directors. *See* Undertakers
Funeral Directors Association. *See* National
　　Funeral Directors Association
Funeral Director's Encyclopedia, The,
　　465
Funeral homes, 28, 446, 455
Funeral Rule, 3–4
Funeral service, 422, 431, 439
　FTC rule governing, 3–4
　medieval, 461, 462f
Funeral service database, 9–11
Funeral Service Examining Boards, 452
Fungal infections, 414–417
Furuncle, *486*

Galen, Claudius, 430
Gallows, theft of bodies from, 431
Gangrene, *486*
　in elderly, 300, 300f

types of, definitions, *486–487*
vessel selection in, 161
Gannal, Adolphe Antoine, 437
Gannal, Felix, 437
Gannal, Jean Nicolas, 422, 436–437, 437f,
　　438, 454
Garfield, James A., 449
Gases, causing distension, 406–410, 407t.
　　See also specific gases
　decomposition and, 105, 408–409
　delayed embalming and, 342
　embalming protocol, 408–409
　extravascular resistance and, 219
　instrument disinfection and, 410
　preembalming treatment of, 213–214,
　　214t
　removal from tissues, 409–410, 410f
　types found in tissues, 406–408, 408f
　venting (Prunk correspondence), 442–443
Gas gangrene, 407–409, *487*
Gaunche method, 422, 428–429
Genitalia, male, 264
Germicides, 45, 111, 117, *487*
　boosters, 130
　HIV transmission prevention, 528–530
Gilding, of mummies, 426–427
Giliani, Alessandra, 431
Gluing, of features, 279–280, 280f
　lips, 205
Glutaraldehyde, 115–116, 517–519, 518t
　research on, 457
Glycerin, coagulation/jelling effect, 474
Glycerine, 118
Glycosuria, 300
Glyoxal, 115, 457
Gold, in ancient burial rites, 426–427, 429
Good luck charms, 428
Gooseneck, *487*
Grafts, in restorative art, 467
Grant, Ulysses S., 441, 448–449
Graves, theft from, 423, 423f, 427, 431,
　　435
Grave wax, *487*
Gravity bowl, 455
Gravity filtration, 233, *487*
Gravity injection, 67–68, 69, 69f
Gravity injector, 438, 438f, *487*
Green jaundice, 356
Greer, Colonel, 445
Greer, Prince, 439, 445
Griggs, J. Horace, 476
Groove director, 78, 79f, *487*
　drainage techniques, 248
Guild of Surgeons, 434
Gums, 118–119
Gunshot wound discolorations, 365f,
　　365–366

Hair
　destruction, 427
　preservation, 429
Hair care, 194
Half-curved needles, 75, 76f
Hand cream, 476
Handless injector, 451f
Hand pump, 69, 70f, 71, *487*
　in cavity embalming, 256
Hand rests, 82
Hands, positioning of, 198–199, 199f
　formalin effects, 455
Hanging, discoloration from, 362
Hannum, Ronald F., 452

Hardening compound, autopsied body preparation, 306
Hardening compounds, 138, *487*
 autopsied bodies and, 306
Hard water, *487*
Harlan, Richard, 438
Harper, Robert C., 469
Hauptmann, Bruno, 469
Hautekerken, Countess, 432
Hazard Communication Standard, 4–9, *487*. *See also* Material safety data sheet
Hazardous material, *487*
 chemicals, 11. *See also individual chemical names, i.e.* Formaldehyde
HBV (hepatitis B virus), *487*
HCHO. *See* Formaldehyde
Head
 in cavity embalming, 257, 424, 425, 432, 454
 facial features. *See* Facial area; Feature setting
 instructional use, 469
 positioning of, 198
 shrinking technique, 429
Headrests, 80, 81f, *487*
Health-care workers, 525
 with AIDS, 525–526
 HIV exposure and transmission, 525
  prevention guidelines, 526–530
Hearse, cleansing of, 31, 41
Heart
 anatomy of, 388–389
 diseased. *See* Heart disease
 drainage, 246–247, 247f
 removal for organ donation, 322–323
 right atrium of, 175
 surgery, preembalming analysis and, 184
Heart disease, 388–389
 congestive failure, 389
 edema effects, 534–535
 in elderly, 299
Heart guide, 259, 260f
Heat, as preservative, 421, 422
Heintzelman, Dr. R. B., 441
Hematemesis, *487*
Hematoma, *487*
 of the eye, 352, 352f
Heme, *487*
Hemoglobin, *487*
Hemolysis, *487*
Hemophilus influenzae, 517, 520
Hemostat, 74, 74f
Henry VIII, King of England, 434
Hensen, Ralph, 470
Hepatitis, *487*
 postmortem presence and transmission, 515, 516
Hepatitis B virus, *487*
Herbs, historical use, 428, 429, 432–433
Herodotus, 424, 426, 431
Herpes, *487*
Hidden sutures, 274, 274f
High-index fluids, 139, 334, *487*
High-level disinfection, 45, 46t
His, Wilhelm, 473
Histoplasma capsulatum, 517, 520
Histoplasmosis, 415–416
History of Egyptian Mummies, 429, 438
History of Embalming, 437, 437f, 438, 439
History of Virginia, excerpt, 429–430
HIV. *See* Human Immunodeficiency virus
Hohenschuh, William Peter, 451–452

Hohenschuh-Carpenter School of Embalming, 452
Hollow viscera
 in cavity treatment, 254, 254t
 expansion of, 219
Holmes, Dr. Thomas H., 422, 439–441, 445, 446
Holmes, Mr., 449
Holmes removal bag, 441, 441f
Homicide, 16
Hook, aneurysm, *481*
Hospital autopsy, 303–304
Hospital waste. *See* Infective waste; Medical waste
Household bleach, *487*
Housekeeping personnel, 526
Human immunodeficiency virus, *487*. *See also* AIDS
 in general population, transmission methods, 525
 in health-care settings, transmission prevention, 527–530
  risks, 525, 526
 survival, in the environment, 529
Human remains, *487*
 care of, 30
 embalming standards for, 42–43
 public health guidelines, 40
 removal/transfer of, 31–32
Humectants, 112, 118, 130, 136, *487*
Hunter, Dr. John, 435
Hunter, Dr. William, 434–435, 439
Hunter's canal, 435
Hutton, Frank A., 439, 442, 444, 461
Hydroaspirator, 61, 61f, 62, 63f, 78, 79f, *487*
 in cavity embalming, 255–256
Hydrocele, 381–382, *487*
Hydrocephalus, 374, 382, *487*
Hydrolysis, 100, *487*
Hydropericardium, 374, *487*
Hydrothorax, 374, 381, *488*
 extravascular resistance, 219–220
Hygroscopic, *488*
Hyperglycemia, 300
Hypertonic solution, 132–133, 373, 377, 377f, *488*
Hypochondriac cavity embalming, 259
Hypo-Derma Molding Cream, 475f
Hypodermic embalming, 22–23, *488*
 autopsied bodies, 309–310, 310f
 autopsied infants, 290–291
 blood discoloration, 352
 postembalming treatments, 271–272
Hypodermic injection, of tissue builders, 474, 475f, 476. *See also* Hypodermic embalming
Hypogastric cavity embalming, 259
Hypostasis, 91–92, 92f, *488*
 agonal, 88
 of blood and body fluids, 94–95, 95f
 blood discoloration, 349t, 349–351, 350f
Hypotonic solution, 132–133, 231, *488*
Hypovalve trocar, 80, 80f

Ice refrigeration method, 439
Ideal fluid strength and volume, 295
Ideal pressure, 295–296, 296f
 arterial injection, 224, 225
Ideal rate of flow, 295–296, 296f
 arterial injection, 224, 225

Identification, of body. *See* Body identification
Iliac artery and vein, 149–150, 152f
 arterial embalming, 175, 175f
 cavity embalming, 259
 drain tube for, 78, 79f
Imbibition, *488*
Immersion methods, 422
 ancient, 428
Immunizations, 41–42
Inactive dyes, 123
Incisions, *488*. *See also individually named incisions*
 for axillary artery and vein, 147, 169
 for brachial artery, 148
 for carotid artery and jugular vein, 165, 165f
 closure of. *See* Adhesives; Suturing
 for femoral artery and vein, 172
 in head shrinking process, 429
 Y type, 305f
Index, *488*
Indian College of Embalming, 450f, 451
Individual sutures, 274
Inexpert tests of death, 86
Infants, 140, 286, *488*
 abdominal aorta, 288, 288f
 ascending aorta, 288–289, 289f
 autopsied, 290–292
 carotid artery, 287
 cavity embalming, 289
 distal leg, 287
 eye closure, 286
 femoral artery, 287
 mouth closure, 286–287
 positioning, 287
 preembalming analysis, 183
 stillborn, 286
 vessel selection, 287–289, 288f, 289f
Infant trocar, 256
Infection
 bloodborne. *See* Bloodborne pathogens
 embalming fluids and, antimicrobial effects, 517–522, 518t, 521t, 522t
 fungal. *See* Mycotic infections
 HIV, transmission prevention in health-care settings, 525–530
 postmortem presence and transmission, 499–501, 514–516
  hepatitis, 515, 516
  toxoplasmosis, 515
  tuberculosis, 501, 515, 516
Infectious disease, *488*
Infectious hepatitis, postmortem presence and transmission, 515, 516
Infectious waste, *488*
Infective waste, 530, 533–534
 universal precautions, 534
Inferior, *488*
Inferior vena cava, 175
Inflammation, 220
Influenza pathogens, 517, 520
Inguinal ligament, *488*
Inguinal region
 anatomy of, 150
 cavity embalming, 259
Injection, *488*. *See also* Arterial solution injection
 of cavity chemicals, 264–265
 in degenerative diseases, 187
 edema and, 187
 embalming analysis and, 186–187
 and reinjection of cavities, 266

Injection (*cont.*)
in renal failure, 187
techniques, 235–242. *See also specific techniques*
of tissue builders, 474, 475f, 476
in wasting diseases, 187
Injection pressure, 72f, 72–73, 295–296, 296f, *488*
in autopsy treatment, 305
in children, 293
delayed embalming and, 335
filtration and, 230–231, 231f
and rate of flow, 223–225, 224f
Injection solutions. *See* Arterial solution; Embalming fluids
Injuries
embalming induced, 428
postmortem treatment of. *See* Restorative art
preembalming treatment of, 212, 212f, 426
Inorganic salts, 112, 119
Instantaneous rigor mortis, *488*
Instant tissue fixation, *488*
facial trauma, 411
injection and drainage techniques, 241, 242f
Instrumentation and equipment. *See also specific items*
for arterial solution injection, 67–69, 68f–73f, 71–73
raising artery and vein, 164
disinfection of, 280–281, 281f, 410
innovations, 455–456
patents, 441, 442, 444–446, 454
for preparation room, 67–82, 68f–82f
autopsied infants, 290
dermatome, 328
vessel site and selection, 164
in restorative art. *See* Restorative art
sterilization of, 517, 528–529
Intercellular, *488*
Intercellular edema, 374, 374f
Intercellular fluid, *488*
Intercostal space, *488*
Interlocking suture, 275
Intermediate-level disinfection, 46, 46t
Intermittent drainage, 32, 43, 249, 250f, *488*
Internal bleach, 130
Internal compresses, 291
Internal iliac artery. *See* Iliac artery and vein
Internal jugular vein. *See* Jugular vein
Interrupted injection, 377–378
Interruption, of vascular system, 161
Interstitial fluid, 216, *488*
Interstitial spaces, 230, 230f, 231
Intestines. *See* Viscera
Intima, 385
Intradermal sutures, 274, 274f
Intravascular, *488*
Intravascular blood discoloration, 93, 349t, 349–351, 350f
clearing of, 227, 227f
Intravascular disease processes, 385, 386t, 387t
embalming procedures, 219
Intravascular fluid, *488*
Intravascular resistance, in arterial solution distribution and diffusion, 217, 218–219, 385, 386t, 387t
Intravenous tubes, 209, 211
Intrinsic, *488*

Intrinsic factors
in algor mortis, 90
body conditions, 183
in embalming analysis, 179
postmortem interval, 186, 186t
Invasive procedures
HIV transmission precautions, 527–528
treatment and removal of devices, 209, 211, 276–277, 277f
Inversion suture, 275, 276f
autopsied bodies, 312f, 313
Inversion sutures, autopsied bodies, 312f, 313
Invisible stitching, 467
Iodophor, 40, 41
Iran (Persia), 428
Isotonic solution, *488*

James, Dr. Emory S., 453
Jaundice, 353f, 353–354, *488*
bleaching fluids, 140
buffer system fluids, 140
chemical adduct system, 140
coupling compound system, 140
green, 356
preembalming analysis, 183
treatment, 468, 469
Jaundice fluid, 139–140, 354, *488*
Jaw closure, 456
Jewelry, of deceased, 17, 20f, 193
Jews, 428
Jivaro Indians, 429
Johanna of Burgundy, Lady, 432
Johnson, Edward C., 469, 471, 474, 477
Jones, Hilton Ira, 457
Judicious counsel, 15
Jugular drain tube, *488*
Jugular vein
anatomy, 143–144
in arterial embalming, 165–166, 166f–168f
injection and drainage techniques, 236, 238

Karaya, 119
Ketosis, 300
Kidney, removal for organ donation, 320–322
Klebsiella pneumoniae, 517, 520
Kodiak archipelago, 430

Laboratory technicians, with AIDS, 526. *See also under* Health-care workers
Lacerations, *488*
preembalming treatment of, 212
Landig, R. Victor, 474
Larvicides, 194, *488*
Lateral, *488*
Laundry, disease transmission prevention, 530
Leakage
postembalming treatments, 282–283
from punctures, 228
Leg
distal, anatomic considerations. *See* Distal leg
edematous, 379–380, 534–535
Legal death, 87
Legal issues, 3
abortion, 16

accidental death, 16
body preparation, 192
coroner or medical examiner, 16–17
documentation, 17, 21f
embalmer ethics and, 14–16
embalming authorization, 3, 17, 18f, 19f, 20f
homicide, 16
multiple death disasters, 506
organ donation, 17, 22f, 319–320
personal property of deceased, 17, 20f
sudden death, 16–17
suicide, 16
Legionnaires' disease, *488*
Lepers, 428
Lesions, 277–278, *488*
pustular, *491*
Lewis, Dr. E. C., 439, 445
Lids. *See* Eyelids
Ligament, inguinal, *488*
Ligate, *488*
Ligation, of vessels, 163–164
Ligatures, 164
Lighting, preparation room, 57, 57f
Lime, as preservative, 422
Lincoln, Abraham, 442, 445–446
Lincoln, Willie, 442
Lindbergh, Charles A., 469
Linear guide, 143, *488*
axillary artery, 146
brachial artery, 147
carotid artery, 144
dorsalis pedis artery, 155
femoral artery, 152
popliteal fossa, 153
radial artery, 149
tibial arteries, 154
ulnar artery, 149
Lipid decomposition, 102
Lipolysis, *488*
Lips
arterial solution distribution and diffusion, 228
dehydration effects, 371f
in mouth closure sequence, 205
Liver, removal for organ donation, 322
Lividity, 92f, 92–93, 94t
cadaveric, *483*
Livor mortis, 92f, 92–93, 94t, *488*
blood discoloration, 349t, 349–351, 350f
delayed embalming and, 341
Local incision, and evisceration and immersion method, 422
Local ordinances, 52–53
Locking forceps, 74, 74f
Lock suture, 275
Long, Esmond R., 421
Long bone recovery and treatment, 325, 327f, 327–328
Loopuypt needles, 75, 76f
Louis XIX, King of France, 431
Low-level disinfection, 46, 46t
Luer-Lok arterial tubes, 75, 77f
Lumbar cavity embalming, 259
Lumen, *489*
intravascular resistance, 218–219
vascular considerations, 385
Lungs
purge, 389, 403
removal for organ donation, 322–323
Lyford, Dr. Benjamin F., 444–445
Lymphatic circulation, 242–243, 243f

Lymph nodes, swollen, 219
Lysin, *489*
Lysosomes, 100, *489*

Maggots, *489*
 body preparation and, 193–194
 postembalming treatments and, 283
Magnesium sulfate, leg edema reduction, 534–535
Magoluetus, Bishop, 432
Maintenance personnel, 526
Male genitalia, 264
Malignancy, 298–299
Mandible
 recovery of, 330
 securing for mouth closure, 201–205, 202f–204f, 206f
Mandibular suture, 204, 204f, *489*
Mannix, Honora D., 473
Mantoux skin test, 41
Manual aids, body preparation, 198, 199
Margolis, Dr. Otto S., 472
Marshall, Dr. Thomas, 438
Martiques, Monsier de, 432
Masking agents. *See* Perfuming agents
Masks
 oral-nasal, for personnel, 42
 preparation of, 461, 464f, 469, 474
Massage, *489*
Master Nuance Aire-Tynt Unit, 476f
Material Safety Data Sheet (MSDS), 4–9, *489*
Mayans, 429
Mayer, Robert G., 477
Mayer, J. Sheridan, 472–473
McEwen, Dr., 449
mCi. *See* Millicurie
Media, intravascular, 385
Medial, *489*
Medical autopsy, 303–304
Medical examiner, 16–17, *489*
 autopsy by, 304
 organ donation consent, 320
Medical schools, cadaver acquisition, 430, 431, 435, 436
Medical waste, 532
 infective nature of, 530. *See also* Infective waste
Medicine, embalmers and, 422
Medicolegal autopsy, 303
Meningitis, *489*
Mercury, 436
 prohibited use of, 437, 455
Merritt, Stephen, 449, 464
Methanol (methyl alcohol), 110–111, 116
Mexico, 429
Meyers, Dr. Eliab, 454
Microbes, *489*
 agonal translocation of, 88–89
Microbial flora
 embalming fluids and, 517–522, 518t, 521t, 522t
 postmortem presence and transmission of, 499–501, 514–516, 522–524, 523t, 524f
Microbicides, 46t
Midaxillary line, *489*
Military, care of deceased personnel in, 34–36
Millicurie (mCi), *489*
Modeling, 464, 468, 472, 474
 the mouth, 205, 207f

Modern period of embalming, 422, 439–457
Modifying agents, 111–112, 117–120, *489*. *See also specific agents*
Moist abrasions, treatment of, 212–213
Moist gangrene, 487
Moisture considerations, 369
 agonal changes, 88
 in anasarca, 375
 in arterial embalming, 372, 372t
 burned bodies, 382
 in dehydrated body preparation, 371–373, 372t, 373f
 dehydration and. *See* Dehydration
 in edema. *See* Edema
 embalming chemicals and, 129
 local problems, 372
 normal body moisture, 369–371, 371f
 postembalming dehydration, prevention treatments, 372–373, 373f
 in renal failure, 382–384
Mold (biological), 283
 preventive agents, *489*
Molding cream, 475f, 476
Molding masks, 464f
Mondino, 431
Moniliasis, 414–415
Mood-altering drugs, 398
Morgan, Dr. John, 438–439
Morgue site, temporary
 development and equipage, 503–504, 504f
 removal of remains, 505
Moribund, *489*
Morticians, 474. *See also* Undertakers
Morticians' Oath, 453
Mortuary colleges
 accreditation, 452
 curricula, 472
 development, 452–453
 faculty degree requirements, 473
 national association, 453
Mortuary cots, cleansing of, 31, 41
Mortuary putty, 312f, 313
 autopsied bodies, 312f, 313
Mortuary science, 27–28
Mortuary trays, cleansing of, 31, 41
Motion pictures, use in restoration, 467, 474
Mouth, 271
Mouth closure
 in elderly, 297
 in infants, 286–287
 instrumentation, 476
 lips, positioning of, 207f, 207–208, 208f
 modeling the mouth and, 205, 207f
 mucous membranes, 200
 nasal spine, 201
 securing mandible in, 201–205, 202f–204f, 206f
 sequence for, 200–201, 201f
Mouth formers, 80, 81f, *489*
MSDS (Material Safety Data Sheet), 4–9, *489*
Mucous membranes, 200
Multiple-agent chemotherapy, 393
Multiple dead, 502–507
 preservation of, 456
Multiple Death Disaster Response Handbook, 502–507
Multiple-site injection. *See* Multisite injection
Multipoint injection. *See* Multisite injection

Multisite injection, 157, *489*. *See also* Six-point injection
 and drainage, 32, 42, 239
Mummies, 421, 425–429, 427f, 462f
Murder victims, evidence preservation, 437
Musculature
 preembalming analysis, 202, 203f, *489*
 suturing, 202, 203f, *489*
Museums, human remains in, 434
Mutilations
 discolorations, 366–367, 367f
 postmortem treatment. *See* Restorative art
Mycobacterium tuberculosis, 517. *See also* Tuberculosis
Mycotic infections, 414–417

Nasal aspirator, 256
Nasal cavity, *489*
Nasal postembalming treatments, 271
Nasal process, 454
Nasal spine, 201
Nasal tube aspirator, 78, 80f, *489*
National Association of Colleges of Mortuary Science, 453
National Cemetery System, 440
National Funeral Directors Association, 448, 452, 474, 477
National Institute for Occupational Safety and Health, 8
National Selected Morticians, 474
Native American indians, 429–430
Natron (natrum), 424, 425–427
Neck
 cavity embalming, 257
 organ removal, in complete autopsy, 306
 surface features of, 143–144
 tissue gas, 409
Necrobiosis, 87, *489*
Necropsy, *489*. *See also* Autopsied bodies
Necrosis, 87, *489*
Needle, aneurysm, *481*
Needle embalming, 454
Needle injector, 80, 81f, *489*
 mouth closure and, 201–202, 202f
Neonates. *See* Infants
Nephritis, 354–355, *489*
Nerves, 159, 159t
Newborns. *See* Infants
New York School of Embalming, 467
New York State Embalmers Convention, 466
Nine-region method, of cavity embalming, 259f, 259t, 259–260, 260f
NIOSH (National Institute for Occupational Safety and Health), 8
Nitrogenous waste, *489*
Nocardia asteroides, 517
Noncosmetic fluid, 111, 129, *489*
Nondehydrating high-index fluids, 139
Nurses, with AIDS, 526. *See also under* Health-care workers
Nursing assistants, with AIDS, 526. *See also under* Health-care workers

Obese, *489*
Obesity, 413–414
 preembalming analysis and, 183
 vessel selection, 160
O'Brien (Irish giant), 435

Obstetric procedures, HIV transmission precautions, 527–528
Occupational exposure, 489
  to formaldehyde, 455, 507–514, 510t
Occupational Safety and Health Administration, 3, 456, 489
  bloodborne pathogen standard, 13–14
  disinfection, 13–14
  formaldehyde rule, 11–13, 457, 507, 509, 510
  hazard communication standard. See Hazard Communication Standard
  noncompliance penalties, 5
  preparation room, 52
  terminology definitions, 483
  universal precautions, 13–14
Odors, 105, 342
Odou, Mme. Linda, 452, 453
Odou Embalming Institute, 452, 453f
Offenbach, Peter, 432
Ohio, embalming room regulations, 52–53
Oils
  emulsified, 118
  historical use, 424, 425, 432, 434
O'Leary, Lydia, 472
One-bottle embalming, 497–499
One-point injection, 157, 236–237, 237f, 489
Opaque cosmetic, 489
Operative aids, 198, 199
Operative corrections, 489
Ophthalmoscope, 489
Opportunistic pathogens, 39–40
Optimum, 489
Oral Cavity, 489
Oral diabetic agents, 398–399
Oral-nasal masks, 42
Orbital area tissue gas, 409–410
Organ donation, 15, 17, 22f
  consent for, 319–320
    by coroner, 320
    by medical examiner, 320
  determination of death for, 319
  documentation, 319
  legal considerations, 319–320
  organ removal for. See Organ removal
  pronouncement of death for, 319
  uses for, 321f
Organ removal
  from abdominal cavity, 323–324, 324f
  bone marrow, 325
  in complete autopsy, 305–306
  cornea, 325
  eye enucleation, 324–325, 326f
  heart/lungs, 322–323
    treatment after, 323
  incisions used, closure protocol, 262
  kidney, 320–321, 321f
    removal method, 322
  liver, 322
  long bone recovery, 325, 327f, 327–328
  mandible recovery, 330
  pancreas, 323
  rib recovery, 330
  skin recovery, 328–330, 329f
  temporal bone recovery, 330f, 330–331
  tissue, 320, 321t
  vertebral body for bone marrow, 325
  viscera, 323
Orifices, packing of, 209
OSHA. See Occupational Safety and Health Administration
Osiris, 426

Osmosis, 133, 231, 231f, 379, 489
Oxalates, 121
Oxygen debt, 95–96

Pacemakers, 277
Packing forceps, 490
Packing materials
  for mummies, 426, 462f
  the orifices, 209
Paint sprayers, 476f, 476–477
Palpate, 490
Pancreas, removal for organ donation, 322–323
Paraformaldehyde, 114
Parallel incision, 490
Pare, Ambroise, 432–433
Parenteral, 490
Parker, Bonnie, 469
Partial autopsy, 305, 306, 314–317, 315f, 316f, 317f. See also Autopsied bodies
  cavity embalming in, 262
Parts per million (ppm), 490
Passive transport systems, 230–232, 490
Patents, embalming methods/equipment, 441–442, 444–446, 454
Path of least resistance, 221–223, 222f
  injection and drainage techniques, 237, 238f
Pathogens
  airborne, 39, 500
  bloodborne. See Bloodborne pathogens
  opportunistic, 39–40
Pathological discoloration, 348, 490
Patrick, General Rudolf, 445
Peat bogs, preservative qualities, 421
Pediculicide, 490
PEL (permissible exposure limit), 11–13, 490
Pelvic cavity, 258–259
  autopsied bodies, 306
  removal in complete autopsy, 306
Penetrating agents, 110
Pennsylvania, embalming room regulations, 52–53
Percutaneous, 490
Perfuming agents, 112, 124–125, 490
  in ancient embalming, 424, 425
Perfusion, 490
  of arterial solution, 215. See also Arterial solution, distribution and diffusion of
Period of the Anatomists. See Anatomist period
Peritonitis, 490
Permeability, capillary, 484
Permissible exposure limit, 11–13, 490
Permission to embalm, 3
Perphry, 425
Persia, 428
Personal health, environmental considerations and, 37–48
Personal hygiene, 281
Personal property, of deceased, 17, 20f, 193
Personal protective equipment, 33, 40, 42, 490
Peru, 429
Petechia, 490
Peter the Great, 433
Petroleum jelly, as tissue builder, 476
Pettigrew, Thomas Joseph, 429, 438
pH. See Potential of hydrogen (pH)
Pharmaceutical, 490
Phenol, 10–11, 116

Photographs. See under Restorative art
Phycomycosis, 415
Physical anthropology, 473
Physicians
  with AIDS, 526
  embalmers as, 422
Pitting edema, 490
Plants, historical use, 428, 429
Plaster
  as filler, 464
  as protective wrap, 427, 428
Plaster beds, 434, 435
Plaster masks, practice, 474
Plastic garments, 82, 82f, 280
Plastic surgery, 451, 470
Plastic work, 467
Plutarch, 425
Pneumonia, 490
Pneumonia pathogens, 517, 520
Poisoning discolorations, 366
  carbon monoxide, 363–364, 364f
Poisons, in embalming fluids, effects, 455
Polyhydric compounds. See Humectants
Popliteal artery
  anatomy of, 153–154
  arterial embalming, 172, 174, 174f
  suturing of, 274
Porti Boy, 456
Positioning devices, 490
Positioning the body, 196f, 196–198, 197f, 198f
  children, 293, 293f
  devices, 80, 81f, 82
  hands and arms, 198–199, 199f
  head, 198
  infants, 287
  lips, 207f, 207–208, 208f
  problems, 199f, 199–200
  during rigor mortis, 336
Postembalming dehydration, 372–373, 373f
Postembalming purge, 405–406
Postembalming treatments, 269–270
  areas needing arterial solution, 270
  disinfection and, 280–281, 281f
  distension, 278–279, 279f
  documentation and shipping preparation after, 281–282
  incision closure, 272, 273f–276f, 274–276. See also Adhesives; Suturing
  invasive devices, removal of, 276–277, 277f
  monitoring casketed remains after, 282–283
  personal hygiene and, 281
  plastic garments used, 280
  purge, 278, 283
  resetting and gluing features, 279–280, 280f
  supplemental embalming, 270–272, 271f
  ulcerations, lesions, and discolorations, 277–278
  washing and drying of body, 277, 278f
Posterior, 490
Posterior tibial arteries. See Tibial arteries, anterior and posterior
Posterior vertical incision, 165
Postmortem, 490. See also Autopsied bodies
Postmortem bruising, 357
Postmortem caloricity, 490
Postmortem changes, 89, 89f
  chemical, 90t, 95, 484
    autolysis, 96, 100, 104, 342

caloricity, 96
carbohydrate decomposition, 102
catalysts, 103f, 103–104
decomposition signs, 104–105, 105f
delayed embalming and, 342–344
embalming significance of, 102t
hydrolysis, 100
lipid decomposition, 102–103
oxygen debt, 95–96
pH shift, 98
protein decomposition, 100–102, 101f, 102f
rigor mortis, 98–100, 99f
stain, postmortem, 97–98
physical, 89–90, 90t
algor mortis, 90–91, 91f
blood viscosity, 95
dehydration, 93–95, 95f
embalming significance, 96t
hypostasis, 91–92, 92f
livor mortis, 92f, 92–93, 94t
principal types, 89f
Postmortem clots, 243
Postmortem coagula, 243
Postmortem dehydration, 371
Postmortem examination, 490
Postmortem extravascular blood
discoloration, 351f, 351–353, 352f
Postmortem interval between death and
embalming, 185–186, 186t
Postmortem intravascular blood
discoloration, 349t, 349–351, 350f
Postmortem needles, 75, 76f
Postmortem physical change, 490
Postmortem procedures, HIV transmission
precautions, 527–528
Postmortem stain, 96, 490
blood discoloration, 349t, 349–351, 350f,
352–353
delayed embalming and, 341
refrigerated bodies, 339–340
Potential of hydrogen (pH), 490
arterial solution, 131
shift in, 96
Potential pressure, 223, 490
Powders
as historical preservatives, 422, 432–433
as preservatives, 434–435
PPE. See Personal protective equipment
ppm (parts per million), 490
Prager, G. Joseph, 471
Precipitant, 490
Preembalming analysis, 182–183. See also
Body preparation
cause of death, 183–184
chemotherapy, 184, 185f, 185t
delayed embalming and, 342
disease process, 183–184
drug treatments, 184, 185f, 185t
intrinsic body conditions, 183
postmortem interval between death and
embalming, 185–186, 186t
surgical procedures, 184–185
Preembalming purge, 404t, 404–405
Preembalming treatments, 211–214, 212f,
213f, 214t. See also Body preparation
and postmortem dehydration, 371
preembalming purge and, 404t, 404–405
Preinjection fluid, 130, 134–135, 295, 490
delayed embalming, 343
as jaundice treatment, 354
Preparation rooms, 446, 490
equipment for, 67–73, 68f–73f

floor covering for, 56–57
flooring for, 55–56
health and safety standards, 51–52
health protection in, 16
infectious agents transmission in, 45t
instrumentation for, 73f–82f, 73–82
lighting, 57, 57f
locations for, 53, 54
physical design, 54–55, 55f
plastic garments use, 82, 82f
plumbing in, 60f–62f, 60–64, 64f, 65f
primary purpose, 51
regulations relating to, 52–53
size requirements, 54
sound insulation, 59–60
terminal disinfection in, 41
ventilation in, 64–67
public health guidelines, 40–41, 41f
walls, 59, 59f
windows, doors, and ceilings, 57–59
Preservation, 421–424, 428–431, 490. See
also specific method
Preservative demand, 490
Preservative powder, 490
Preservatives, 17–19, 21–22, 105, 111,
113–117. See also Arterial solution;
specific agents
for autopsied infants, 291
inactivation of, 395–396
Pressure
definitions of, 491
injection. See Injection pressure
Pressure filtration, 230–231, 231f, 491
Primary dilution, 110, 131, 231, 491
Primary disinfection, 45, 491
Primary flaccidity, 99
Primary injection fluid. See Preinjection fluid
Primary injection sites, 157–158
artery selection for, 159f, 159–162
Principles and Practice of Embalming, 452
The Principles of Restorative Art, 452
The Principles of Restorative Art As the
Embalmer Should Know Them,
470–471, 471f
Procurement, 491
Professional ethics. See Ethics
Professional performance standards. See
Standards
Professional responsibility, three-tiered
spectrum of, 37
Prognathism, 491
Prophylactic antibiotics, 42
Propylene glycol, 118
Protective equipment. See Personal
protective equipment
Proteins, 491
decomposition, 100–102, 101f, 102f
and embalming process, 17–19
Proteolysis, 491
Protocol. See Standards
Prunk, Dr. Daniel H., 439, 442–443, 443f
Ptomaine, 101, 491
Pubic symphysis, 491
Public health, embalming practices and
guidelines, 39–42, 41f, 45t
precautionary requirements and
standards, 30–33, 31f
Pulmonary embolism, 314
Pump, hand, 487
Puncture leakage, 228
Purges, 389, 403–404, 405, 491
during arterial injection, 161
in cavity embalming, 254–255, 255t

as decomposition sign, 105
delayed embalming and, 342, 342f
postembalming, 278, 283, 405–406
preembalming, 404, 404t, 404–405
refrigerated bodies, 340
restricted cervical injection and, 240
skin protection, 404
Pursestring suture, 491
Pus, 491
Pustular lesions, 360, 360f, 491
Putrefaction, 101–103, 491

Quadrant method, cavity embalming, 259
Quality care, 16
Quaternary ammonium compounds,
116–117

Radial artery
anatomy of, 149
arterial embalming, 170, 171f
suturing of, 274
Radiation fatalities, handling and
decontamination, 504–505
Radiation protection officer, 491
Radioactive isotopes, 397–398
Radionuclide, 491
Ramazzini, Bernardino, 439
Ramby, John, 434
Rate of flow, 32, 42, 295–296, 296f, 491
arterial treatment for edema, 377
centrifugal pump, 72
children, 293
delayed embalming, 335
injection pressure and, 223–225, 224f
Rates of flow, in autopsy treatment, 305
Razor burn (razor abrasion), 356–357,
491
Reaspiration, 254, 266, 491
Record keeping, 33
Red tagging, 39
Reducing agent, 491
Reembalming, 411–412
Refrigerated bodies, 338–341, 339f
discolorations, 361–362
Regulations, 440, 444, 456
for preparation rooms, 52–53
Reichle, Richard G., 477
Reinjection of cavities, 266
Release authorization, 17, 18f, 19f, 20f
Religion
body preservation, 422, 429
dissection prohibition, 431
Reminiscences of Early Embalming, 449f
Removal bag, Holmes, 441, 441f
Renal failure, 187, 382–384, 412–413
Renouard, Charles A., 448, 450, 466, 474
Renouard, Dr. Auguste, 446–448, 447,
447f, 454
Renouard Training School for Embalmers,
448
Reodorants. See Perfuming agents
Resinous substance, 491
in ancient embalming, 424, 426, 427, 428,
429
Resistance, in arterial solution distribution
and diffusion
advantages of, 221, 221f
combination type, 220
extravascular. See Extravascular resistance
intravascular. See Intravascular resistance
least, 221–223, 222f, 237, 238f

Restoration, 19, *491*
    autopsied bodies, 317–318
Restorative art, 451, 461
    advertising, emergence of, 467
    alternative terminology, 462, 466, 467
    arterial injection and, 467, 468
    case histories, 426, 450, 461, 466–469
    equipment/supplies, 464–476
    founder of, 462–467
    for identification purposes, 472, 473
    instruction/training in, 465f, 465–469,
        472–474
    for jaundice treatment, 468, 469
    photographs, use in, 464–469, 474
    techniques
        ancient, 426–427
        modern, 451, 461–477
Restorative fluid (humectant), *491*
Restricted cervical injection, 157, 334, *491*
    advantages of, 239–241, 240f
    carotid artery, 164
    jugular vein, 168
Restricted drainage. *See* Intermittent
        drainage
Resurrection, 422, 429
Retained fluid, 216
Reticuloendothelial cytomycosis, 415–416
Reynold, Joshua, 435
Rhodes, George M., 446
Rib recovery, 330
Richardson, Clyde E., 469
Richardson, Dr. B. W., 454
Right atrium, of heart, 175, *491*
"Right to know" laws, 52
Rigor mortis, 98–100, 99f, *491*
    body preparation, 197
    delayed embalming, 335–338, 336t, 337f
    extravascular resistance, 219
    instantaneous, *488*
Robbins (of Boston), 466, 467
Robinson, W. G., 449
Rochester School of Embalming, 448
Rodgers, Samuel, 439, 454
Rounding, of fingers, lips, and toes, 228
Rousevell, Mrs. G. A., 468
Royal College of Surgeons Museum, 434
Rubella vaccinations, 41
Ruysch, Frederick, 433

Saccharolysis, *491*
Safety issues, 31–32, 40–42, 44, 45t
St. Louis College of Mortuary Science, 452
Salts, in embalming process, 117, 421, 424,
        437–439
    inorganic, 112, 119
    natron (natrum), 424, 425–427
    use in reducing leg edema, 534–535
Sands, Frank T., 444
Sanitation, 16, *491*
Sanitation survey, 44–48
Sanitizer, 45
Saponification, *492*
Saprophytic bacteria, *492*
Sarcophagi, 423. *See also* Coffins
    Egyptian, 423, 428
Scaling skin discolorations, 358
Scalpel, 74, 75f, *492*
Scar tissue, 161
Schade, Charles T., 454
School of Embalming and Organic
        Chemistry, 448
Scissors, 74–75, 75f

SCM (sternocleidomastoid), 144
Scollay, G. W., 439, 444
Sealing agents, 139, *492*
Secondary dilution, 231, *492*
Secondary flaccidity, 99
Secondary injection sites, 158
    selection of, 162–163
Second degree burns, 363, 363f
Sectional injection. *See* Multisite injection
Seepage, of tissue builders, 474, 476
Segato, Girolamo, 438
Semilunar incision, 165, 166f
Semipermeable membrane, 232
Senile purpura, 297–298
Separated tissues, 282
Separator, 75, 76f
Sepsis, *492*
Septicemia, *492*
Sequence of embalming. *See* Embalming,
        chronology for
Sequestering agent, *492*
Serrated, *492*
Serrated edge hemostat, 74, 74f
Service vehicle, cleansing of, 41
Setting the features. *See* Feature setting
Sharps, *492*
Sharps container, *492*
Shaving, 194–196, 195f
Shaving cream, use in restorative art, 467
Shippen, Dr. William, 439
Shipping, preparation for, 281–282
Short-circuiting, of arterial solution, 237,
        238f
Short-term exposure limit, 11–13, *492*
Shoulder rests, 82
Simmons, Baxter, 452
Simmons, Lena, 452, 466, 467
Simmons School of Embalming, 452
Simple heat, as preservative, 422
Simple immersion, 422
Single-point injection, 157, 236–237, 237f,
        489
Sinks, preparation room, 63–64, 65f
Six-point injection, 157–158, 239. *See also*
        Multisite injection
Size requirement, preparation room, 54
Skeletal edema, 220, 220f
Skin
    discoloration of. *See* Discoloration
    elasticity loss, arterial solution distribution
        and diffusion and, 227
    grafting for restorative purposes, 467
    Native American treatment of, 429–430
    recovery and treatment, 328–330, 329f
Skin lesions
    discoloration, 357, 358f
    preembalming treatment of, 211–212,
        213, 213f
Skin-slip, *485*. *See also* Desquamation
    delayed embalming and, 342
    discolorations, 359–360
    preembalming treatment of, 213, 213f
    refrigerated bodies, 340–341
    as sign of decomposition, 105
Skull. *See* Head
Slip-type hub arterial tubes, 75, 77f
Slocum, Ray, 181–182, 471
Smith, G. Elliot, 428
Snow, Clyde, 473
Sodium hypochlorite, *492*
Soil, preservative qualities, 421
Solid edema, 374
Solid waste management, 31

Solutes, 232, *492*
Solution, *492*
    arterial, *482*
    hypertonic, *488*
    hypotonic, *488*
Solvents, 232, *492*
Somatic death, 87, *492*
Sorbitol glycols, 118
Sound insulation, preparation room, 59–60
Space, intercostal, *488*
Spasm, cadaveric, *483*
Spatula, electric-heated, 469, 470f
Speas, C. J., 465
Special-purpose fluid, high-index, 334
Specific gravity, chemical solutions, 131–133
Spices, historical use, 424–426, 428,
        432–433
Spinal cord, removal in complete autopsy,
        306, 306f
Spinal deformity, repair during restoration,
        426
Split injection, 157, 237–238, *492*
Spray applicators, 476f, 476–477
Spriggs, A. O., 474
Spring forceps, 75, 77f, *482*
Stain, postmortem. *See* Postmortem stain
Stain removers, 130
Stallard, Frank, 471
Standards, for embalming practices, 32,
        42–43
    armed services specifications, 34–35
    federal. *See* Environmental Protection
        Agency; Federal Trade Commission;
        Occupational Safety and Health
        Administration
    procedures, 43–44
    professional performance, 27–29, 29f
    public health guidelines, 30–31, 39–42,
        41f, 45t
State Board of Embalmers and Funeral
        Directors, 3
State codes, 52–53
State Department of Environmental
        Protection, 3
State Funeral Directors convention, 450
STEL (short-term exposure limit), 11–13,
        492
Sterilization, 45, *492*, 517, 528–529
Sterilizers, *492*
Sternocleidomastoid, 144
Stethoscope, *492*
Stillborn infants, 286, *492*
Stomach guide, 260, 260f
Stomach purge, 403
Stopcock, 75, 78f
Storage cabinet, preparation room, 54
Strap line incision, 165, 166f
Strub, Clarence G., 452–453, 470–471,
        471f
Subcutaneous, *492*
Subcutaneous emphysema, *492*
    cavity embalming, 261
    embalming protocol, 408
    gases, 406–407
    preembalming treatment of, 213, 214t
Subcutaneous sutures, 467
Sucquet, J. P., 422, 436, 439, 454
Sudden death, 16–17
Suicide, 16
Sullivan, Felix A., 448–450, 452, 454
Sunnyside, The (journal), 441, 446, 449,
        462, 465, 467
Superficial, *492*

Superior, *492*
Supplemental embalming, 270–272, 271f
Supplemental fluids, 43, 134–137, *492*
    classification of, 130t
Supraclavicular incision, 165, 166f
Surface compress, *492*
Surface discoloration, 348–349, *492*
    treatment of, 355
Surface disinfection, 281
Surface embalming, 22–23, *492*
    autopsied bodies, 307
    blood discoloration, 352
    postembalming treatments, 270–271
Surface evaporation, 93–94
Surface gels, 137–138
Surface vessels, distension of, 227
Surfactants, 112, 121–123, 122f, *492*
Surgeons, with AIDS, 526
Surgical procedures, 209, 262, 277
    HIV transmission precautions, 527–528
    preembalming analysis of, 184–185
Suture needles, 75, 76f, 272
Suture thread, 75, 272
Suturing
    common suture types, 274f, 274–276,
        275f, 276f. *See also individually
        named sutures*
    direction of, 272, 274
    materials for, 75, 76f, 272
    in postembalming treatments, 272
    techniques, 467
Swammerdam, Jan, 431, 433
Swelling, causes of, 338
Syria, 428
Syringes, 431, *483*
    use with tissue builders, 474, 475f, 476

Tables, preparation room, 67, 68f
    arrangement of, 54, 54f
Tabona, 428
Tannin, as preservative, 421, 437
Teachers' Institutes, 452–453, 453f
Technique of Restorative Art, 471–472
Temporal bone, recovery and treatment of,
    330f, 330–331
Temporary interrupted suture, 274, *483*
Temporary preservation, *492*
Tension breakers/reducers. *See* Surfactants
Terminal disinfection, 31, 32, 41, 45, *492*
    postembalming treatments, 280–281, 281f
    public health guidelines, 41f, 41–42
Tests of death, 86–87, *492*
Textbook of Facial Reconstruction, A, 472
Thanatology, *492*
Thenard, Louis Jacques, 436
Therapeutic discolorations, 348
Third-degree burns, 363, *492–493*
Thoracic autopsy, 314–315, 315f, 316f
Thoracic cavity, 174–175, 257
    aspiration, 263
    autopsied bodies, 306
    in complete autopsy, 306
Threaded hub arterial tubes, 75, 77f
Tibial arteries, anterior and posterior
    anatomy of, 154
    arterial embalming, 174, 174f
    suturing of, 274
Time-weighted average, 11–13, *493*
Tissue coagulation, *493*
Tissue donation. *See also* Organ donation
    consent for, 319–320
    uses for, 320, 321t

Tissue fixation, 464, 467
    arterial solution distribution and diffusion
        effects on, 227
    instant, 241, 242f
    product innovations, 474, 475f, 476
Tissue gas, 408, 408f, 408–409, *493. See
    also Clostridium perfringens*
    air from embalming apparatus, 407
    coinjection fluids, 130
    decomposition, 408
    fluid, 130, 140
    gas gangrene, 407–408
    preembalming treatment of, 213–214,
        214t
    subcutaneous emphysema, 406–407
    types, 406–408, 408f
Tissues
    arterial solution distribution and diffusion
        effects on, 227
    bleaching of. *See* Bleaching, of tissues
    distension, facial, 161–162
    donors. *See* Organ donation
    filler, 475f
Tobacco tar, *493*
Toes. *See* Digits
Toltecs, 429
Tombs. *See* Graves
Topical disinfection, 193–194, *493,*
    519–522, 521t, 522t
Torn skin, preembalming treatment of, 213,
    213f
Toxoplasma, 515
Tracheotomy tubes, 211
"Trade embalmer," 450
Tragacanth, 119
Training. *See also* Embalming schools;
        Mortuary Colleges
    in colonial America, 439
    early instructors, 434–439, 445, 448–452
    first U.S. textbook, 446
    in Hazard Communication Standard, 7–9
    in medieval period, 430–431
    modern era, 450–453, 452–453
    in restorative art, 465f, 465–469,
        472–474
Tranchina, G., 436
Tranquilizers, 398
Translocation, 38, *493*
    agonal, of microbes and bacteremia,
        88–89
Transplantation, *493*
Transport, of deceased
    disaster response protocol, 505–506
    preparation for, 422
        during Civil War, 440
        during Crusades, 431
        instruction in, 447
Transverse, *493*
Trauma, *493*
    postmortem treatment of. *See* Restorative
        art
Trioxane, 115
Triple-base fluid, 116
Trocar, 78, 80, 80f, *493*
    in cavity embalming, 254, 256
    development and initial use, 454
Trocar button, 80, 80f, 456, *493*
    applicator, 80, 81f
Trocar guide, 259–260, 260f, *493*
Trunk
    arteries of, 149, 150t, 151f
    autopsied infants, 291
    in cavity treatment, 442–443, 453–454

color changes on, 341
    edema of, 381
    tissue gas, 409
Tube aspirator, nasal, *489*
Tuberculosis, postmortem presence and
    transmission, 501, 515, 516
Tube/tubing, 256
    arterial, *482*
Tumors, 219
    edema effects, 534
    postmortem treatment of, 461, 467
Turpentine, 433, 434, 436
TWA (time-weighted average), 11–13, *493*
20-index fluid, 111
Typing, of bodies, 181–182

UAGA (Uniform Anatomical Gift Act),
    319–320
Ulcerations
    lesions, 360, 360f
    postembalming treatment of, 277–278
    preembalming treatment of, 211–212
Ulnar artery
    anatomy of, 149
    in arterial embalming, 170, 171f
    suturing of, 274
Umbilicus, 259
Undertakers. *See also* Embalmers
    HIV transmission precautions, 528
    professional organization, 444, 447–448,
        450, 452
    regulations, 456
    training, 446–448, 447f, 451. *See also*
        Embalming schools; Mortuary
        colleges
Undertaker's Manual, The, 447, 447f
Unembalmed remains, dangers of, 38
Uniform Anatomical Gift Act, 319–320
Uniform Determination of Death Act, 86
Uniform Organ Donor Card, 319
Unionalls, 82, 82f, 280, *493*
United States, development of embalming in,
    439–457
Universal precautions, 13–14, 30–31, *493,*
    527, 532, 534
Unnatural death, causes, 361t, 361–367,
    363f–365f, 367f
Urinary bladder trocar guide, 260
Urinary catheter, 211
Urns, canopic, 426, 426f
U.S. College of Embalming, 448

Vaccinations, 41–42
Vacuoles, 237
Vacuum, creation of, 255–256
Vacuum breaker, 41, 61–62, 62f, 63f, *493*
Valuables, of deceased, 17, 20f, 193
Valvular heart disease, 388–389
Van Butchell, Mrs. Martin, 434–435
Vascular considerations, 385
    in aortic aneurysm, 388
    arterial coagula and, 390, 390f
    in arteriosclerosis, 387f, 387–388, 388f
    in congestive heart failure, 389
    delayed embalming and, 341
    in diabetes, 390–391, 391f
    extravascular resistance and, 391
    intravascular disease processes and,
        386t–387t
    in valvular heart diseases, 388–389
    vasodilation and vasoconstriction, 390

Vascular discoloration, 341, 391f
Vascular embalming. *See* Arterial embalming
Vascular organ donation, 320–321, 321f
Vascular system interruption, 161
Vasoconstriction, 390
Vasodilation, 390
Vehicle (liquid), 112, 125, *493*
Vehicles (mortuary cots and trays), cleansing
    of, 31, 41
Veins, 159, 159t
    for drainage, 235, 236
Venae comitantes, and arterial relationship,
    149
Venous coagula, 390
Venous drainage, center of, *484*
Ventilation, 64
    air conditioning, 67
    within "at risk" environment, 31
    formaldehyde and, 64–67
    in preparation room, 40–41, 41f
Ventral approach, spinal cord removal, 306
Venules, 222, 223
Vertebral body removal, 325
Vessel distension, arterial solution
        distribution and diffusion and, 227
Vessel selection, for arterial solution
        injection site, 295
    abdominal aorta, 174–175, 288, 288f
    ascending aorta, 288–289, 289f
    in autopsied body, 158
        infants, 290
    axillary artery, 169–170, 170f
    brachial artery, 170
    carotid artery, 164–166, 166f–167f
    in children, 292
    comparisons, 159, 159t
    distal leg, 287
    elevation and ligation, 163–164
    facial artery, 168–169, 169f
    femoral artery and vein, 171–172, 172f
    iliac artery, 175, 175f
    incision technique, 176, 176f
    in infants, 287–289, 288f, 289f
    inferior vena cava, 175

instruments and ligatures, 164
jugular vein, 168, 168f
popliteal artery, 172, 174, 174f
primary site, 157–158, 159–162
radial artery, 170, 171f
right atrium of heart, 175–176
secondary site, 158, 162–163
thoracic aorta, 174–175
tibial arteries, 174, 174f
ulnar artery, 170–171, 171f
in unautopsied body, 158–159
Victim, of crime, evidence preservation, 437
Vigevano, 431
Viscera. *See also* Evisceration
    anatomy, 257–259
    autopsied bodies, 310
        infants, 291
    historical treatment, 424–426, 428–430,
        453–454
    organ removal, treatment after, 323
    weight, 220
Viscosity, *493. See also* Blood viscosity
Visual aids, for restoration, 474. *See also
    under* Restorative art

Walls, preparation room, 59, 59f
Warburton Act, 435
Wartime treatment of dead
    Civil War. *See* Civil War embalming
    during Crusades, 431
    World War I, 467
Washing the body, 194, 277, 278f
Waste
    infectious, *488*
    infective. *See* Infective waste
    medical. *See* Medical waste
    nitrogenous, *489*
Wasting diseases, 187
Water, hard, *487*
Water conditioner, 112, 119–120, 130, *493*
Water hardness, *493*
Waterless embalming, *493*
Waterlogged, *493*

Water supply, preparation room, 63
Wax, in restoration, 465, 467–469, 476
Weather line, 200
Weight of body
    obesity and, 413–414
    preembalming analysis of, 183
    vessel selection and, 160
Welch's bacillus. *See Clostridium
        perfringens;* Tissue gas
Werowance Indians, 430
Wet gangrene, *493*
Wetting agent, *493*
Whip suture, 275–276, 276f
Williams, E. A., 442
Windows, preparation room, 57–58
Wine, as preservative, 433, 436
Wire, securing mandible and, 205
Women, as embalmers, 452
Wood, Dr. Thomas, 439
Work practice controls, *493*
Work practices, 33
Works of Ambroise Pare, The, 432–433
World War I, treatment of war dead, 467
Worm suture, 275, 276f
    autopsied bodies, 312f, 313
Worm sutures, 312f, 313
Worsham, Albert H., 451, 467, 468, 474
Wrapping(s)
    historical accounts, 432
    mummy, 426, 427, 428

Xaxos, 429
X-ray examination, of mummified remains,
    428

Yarrow, H. C., 429
Y incision, 305f
Y tube, 75, 78f, 307, 309

Zinc chloride, 436
Zinc sulfate, 422